D1171650

Mucosal Biopsy
of the
Gastrointestinal
Tract

OTHER MONOGRAPHS IN THE SERIES
MAJOR PROBLEMS IN PATHOLOGY

Published

Azzopardi: *Problems in Breast Pathology*

Frable: *Thin-Needle Aspiration Biopsy*

Wigglesworth: *Perinatal Pathology*

Jaffe: *Surgical Pathology of Lymph Nodes and Related Organs*

Wittels: *Surgical Pathology of Bone Marrow*

Finegold: *Pathology of Neoplasia in Children and Adolescents*

Taylor: *Immunomicroscopy*

Fu & Reagan: *Pathology of the Uterine Cervix, Vagina and Vulva*

Wolf & Neiman: *Disorders of the Spleen*

Katzenstein & Askin: *Surgical Pathology of Non-neoplastic Lung Disease, 2nd ed.*

Livolsi: *Surgical Pathology of the Thyroid*

Striker, Olsen & Striker: *Interpretation of Renal Biopsy, 2nd ed.*

Forthcoming

Virmani, Atkinson & Fenoglio: *Pathology of the Heart*

Mackay, Lukeman & Ordonez: *Tumors of the Lung*

Nash & Said: *Pathology of Acquired Immune Deficiency*

Hendrickson & Kempson: *Surgical Pathology of the Uterine Corpus, 2nd ed.*

Frable: *Fine Needle Aspiration Biopsy, 2nd ed.*

Ordonez & Mackay: *Soft Tissue Tumors*

Crissman & Zarbo: *Surgical Pathology of the Upper Aerodigestive Tract Mucosa*

Variokojis & Vardiman: *Pathology of Myeloproliferative Disorders*

Ellis, Auclair & Gnepp: *Pathology of the Salivary Glands*

Jaffe: *Surgical Pathology of the Lymph Nodes, 2nd ed.*

Lloyd: *Surgical Pathology of the Pituitary Gland*

Lack: *Pathology of the Adrenal Medulla and Extra-adrenal Paraganglia*

Kornstein: *Pathology of the Anterior Mediastinum*

Tomazewski: *Surgical Pathology of the Urinary Bladder, Kidney, and Prostate*

Henson & Albores-Saavedra: *Pathology of Incipient Neoplasia, 2nd ed.*

Richard Whitehead, M.D., Ch.B., F.R.C. Path., F.R.C.P.A.

Professor of Pathology, Department of Pathology
Flinders University of South Australia
and Head of the Department of Histopathology
Flinders Medical Centre, South Australia

Mucosal Biopsy of the Gastrointestinal Tract

Volume 4 in the Series
MAJOR PROBLEMS IN PATHOLOGY

Fourth Edition

VIRGINIA A. LIVOLSI, M.D., *Consulting Editor*

Director, Surgical Pathology Section
Department of Pathology and Laboratory Medicine
University of Pennsylvania Medical Center
Philadelphia, Pennsylvania

1990

W. B. SAUNDERS COMPANY

Harcourt Brace Jovanovich, Inc.

PHILADELPHIA LONDON TORONTO MONTREAL SYDNEY TOKYO

W. B. SAUNDERS COMPANY

Harcourt Brace Jovanovich, Inc.

The Curtis Center
Independence Square West
Philadelphia, PA 19106

Library of Congress Cataloging-in-Publication Data

Whitehead, Richard.

Mucosal biopsy of the gastrointestinal tract /
Richard Whitehead.—4th ed.

   p. cm.—(Major problems in pathology; v. 3)

Includes bibliographical references.

ISBN 0–7216–3287-4

   1. Gastrointestinal system—Biopsy.   2. Gastric mucosa—
Biopsy.   3. Gastrointestinal system—Diseases—
Diagnosis.   I. Title.   II. Series. [DNLM: 1. Biopsy.
2. Gastric Mucosa—pathology.   3. Intestinal Mucosa—
pathology. W1 MA492X v. 3 / WI 141 W592m]

RC804.B5W47   1990   616.3′30758—dc20

DNLM/DLC   90–8170

Editor: Richard Zorab
Production Manager: Ken Neimeister
Manuscript Editor: Phyllis Skomorowsky
Illustration Coordinator: Peg Shaw
Indexer: Marie Coughlin

MUCOSAL BIOPSY OF THE GASTROINTESTINAL TRACT   ISBN 0–7216–3287–4
Fourth Edition

Copyright © 1990, 1985, 1979, 1973 by W. B. Saunders Company.

All rights reserved. No part of this publication may be reproduced or transmitted in any form or by any means, electronic or mechanical, including photocopy, recording, or any information storage and retrieval system, without permission in writing from the publisher.

Printed in the United States of America.

Last digit is the print number: 9   8   7   6   5   4   3   2   1

Editor's Foreword

Interpretation of mucosal biopsies from the gastrointestinal tract has been a major problem for pathologists since the diagnostic technique was introduced. When *Mucosal Biopsy of the Gastrointestinal Tract* was first published, biopsy access to the gastrointestinal tract was largely limited to regions within the reach of rigid endoscopic devices. The procedures involved represented more than a minor inconvenience to the patient. As a result, pathologists had relatively little occasion to see biopsies of the stomach, small bowel and proximal colon.

With the introduction of flexible endoscopy, direct visualization and biopsy of the entire gastrointestinal tract become routine. Today, mucosal biopsies make up a substantial part of the material seen by pathologists in their daily work. Because of the diversity of disease processes occurring in the oesophagus, stomach and small and large intestine, and the use of endoscopic biopsies to detect earlier and earlier stages of these diseases, pathologists are finding gastrointestinal mucosal biopsies a challenge out of proportion to their ever increasing numbers.

This authoritative monograph, written from the personal experience of Dr. Whitehead, is now in its fourth edition. It has been extensively updated since the preceding edition by inclusion of recently described diseases, clarification of previously recognized but poorly understood disease processes, and discussion of the application of new diagnostic methods. Thus, *Mucosal Biopsy of the Gastrointestinal Tract* remains the definitive reference for pathologists dealing with mucosal biopsies of the gastrointestinal tract.

JAMES L. BENNINGTON, M.D.
CONSULTING EDITOR

Preface

Since the last edition of this book, the use of endoscopic biopsy in the diagnosis of oesophageal and gastrointestinal disorders has burgeoned beyond expectations. The technique has in many instances replaced rather than been used as an adjunct to certain radiological procedures and is seen as the first line of investigation of a number of suspected disease processes. It is a most attractive diagnostic mode, and it is understandable that biopsy is likely to be more productive of interpretable tissue if it is taken under direct vision from lesions that are endoscopically abnormal. There has also been the steady realisation that even when endoscopic appearances are seemingly normal, biopsy tissues may reveal significant pathology that can dictate important patient management decisions. Moreover, as experience has grown in the interpretation of sighted endoscopic biopsies, the need for suction capsule biopsies has dwindled. In the oesophagus as elsewhere in the gastrointestinal tract, an increased range of endoscopic abnormalities has been categorised histologically, including inflammatory and premalignant lesions. The classification and delineation of subtypes of gastritis have undergone something of a revolution of late. Duodenal biopsies beyond the bulb have disclosed not only a new range of early proliferative lesions but have facilitated the investigation and categorisation of new malabsorptive conditions. Criteria for the diagnosis of colitis have been defined, and the recognition of new forms of inflammatory bowel disease has resulted. Finally, while not entirely new as independent entities, a plethora of cases of otherwise quite rare conditions has occurred in the setting of human immunodeficiency virus infection. Thus it is that new histological entities are being revealed in all regions of the bowel into which endoscopes are being passed.

As in previous editions, this book is aimed at guiding the practising histopathologist in the interpretation and reporting of these tiny fragments of the gut lining. Obviously many aspects of the pathology of the oesophagus and gastrointestinal tract will not be revealed in mucosal biopsies, and as a consequence this work does not pretend to supplant the larger texts that are concerned with the much wider aspects of pathology.

I am again indebted to my clinical colleagues at Flinders Medical Centre who have continued to support the process of interpretation of the biopsies from their patients by their constant readiness to enter into discussions. Once more my sincere thanks are due to Mr. Barry Gormley and his staff for their work in slide preparation and photography. Especially I thank Jenny Green, who has shown great patience and skills in handling these often tiny fragments of tissue. Mrs. Eugenie Efinger has been a dedicated worker in the preparation of the manuscript and bibliography and again deserves special mention. Figures 16–14 to 16–20 were made available by Dr. Robert Riddell and Figures 17–20 to 17–22 by Dr. Francisco Arnal and I am indebted to both for their kindness. Finally, W.B. Saunders Company has once more made every possible effort in facilitating production of this fourth edition.

Contents

General Comments on Procedure

The biopsy specimens produced by either suction or forceps procedures are inevitably small, but with technical expertise informative sections can usually be prepared. There is a case for handling multiple biopsies from the same patient and the same part of the digestive tract individually. This is especially true for the oesophagus, in which very small biopsies are the rule and orientation of them is difficult. It is also true for very small biopsies from other sites and especially those obtained by paediatric instruments. In the well-staffed laboratory, a case can easily be made for all intestinal biopsy tissues to be handled by the same scientific officer, and this is the author's practice. Rapid fixation is essential, and handling should be the minimum necessary to ensure that sections are cut at right angles to the mucosal surface. On the whole, suction biopsy specimens are easier to manage, because sections in the ideal plane are produced simply by cutting the disc-shaped piece of tissue at right angles to its long axis. When difficulty is experienced, for example with the small biopsies obtained by some of the fibreoptic instruments and especially if the specimen is irregular in shape, stereoscopic microscopy will often help in orientation, but in the hands of an experienced person this becomes increasingly unnecessary. The easy recognition of the mucosal surface comes with practice, and, this achieved, the biopsy can be flattened onto a piece of filter paper, luminal surface uppermost. Fixed flat in this way, the specimen is nearly always roughly laminar, and when sectioned at right angles to its long axis, the required result is produced. Forceps biopsies received already fixed are often rolled up into a ball reminiscent of a hedgehog having encountered an adversary. The mucosa is always outermost and the specimen cannot be flattened without producing a good deal of traumatic artefact. It is better to process these specimens as they are received, and although inevitably the first few sections will be tangential, deeper cuts nearly always produce sections at right angles to the mucosal surface.

Detailed stereo-microscopic examination of the biopsy specimens can give helpful preliminary information that later can be correlated with histology, particularly in small bowel diseases. However, there is no real indication for this in the majority of instances nowadays, because any mucosal abnormality would have been revealed to the endoscopist prior to biopsy by the comparable magnification of the instrument. In any case, it should never take the place of a proper histological examination, and delay in fixation, extra handling and the wiping away of adherent mucus in order to achieve a good stereoscopic view should be rigorously avoided because of the inevitable distortion, smearing and crushing artefacts that may result. Frequently, the net result is a loss of much more information than is gained by the stereoscopic study.

Pathologists will vary in their preference of fixatives, and some insist that the inclusion of mercury is an advantage. It probably matters little for ordinary haematoxylin and eosin (H & E) staining, but it is as well to remember that alcoholic and heavy metal fixatives containing mercury should be avoided if it is desirable to study enterochromaffin cells, and that Paneth cell granules are soluble in acetic acid and other acid fixatives. In this laboratory all biopsies are fixed in 10 per cent neutral buffered formal-saline and embedded in paraffin wax after passing through an automatic processing machine. Special fixation can always usefully be carried out on formalin-fixed material after the slides have been deparaffinised. The move some years ago towards glutaraldehyde fixation and resin embedding in order to facilitate thin sectioning has largely been reversed. With newer waxes, improved impregnation and vacuum embedding equipment, most good laboratories are able to cut sections of 2 microns for routine staining procedures; the advantage of this is the greater applicability of more staining methods to these thin paraffin sections.

In addition to H & E, any of the many specialised staining methods applicable to paraffin-embedded material may be employed. Individual pathologists often have their own preferences, and circumstances will sometimes dictate which particular method is used.

The improved quality of routine staining methods has in fact resulted in a decrease in the need to rely upon more sophisticated staining procedures. Consequently, the author routinely uses only H & E and, when indicated, a reticulin stain (James 1967) or Maxwell stain (Maxwell 1963); the diastase-periodic acid–Schiff method (Pearse 1968), which stains neutral mucins and some sialo-mucins magenta; the Alcian blue pH 2.5 periodic acid–Schiff method (Lev and Spicer 1964), which stains acid mucins blue and mixtures of acid and neutral mucins purple; and the high iron diamine Alcian blue pH 2.5 method of Spicer (1965), which stains neutral mucins magenta, acid sulphomucins brown and acid carboxylated sialomucins blue. These methods allow the recognition of the subtypes of intestinal metaplasia (see later).

Paneth cells can be characterised by using a phosphotungstic acid–haematoxylin or phloxine tartrazine stain, and, if early collagenisation of the subepithelial zone is suspected, a connective tissue stain such as a van Gieson is useful.

A PAS preparation is also used as a mucin stain in rectal biopsy examination because it doubles as a screen for the detection of amoebae. A better staining method in screening for amoebae in the author's view, however, is the Goldner modification of Masson's trichrome (Goldner 1938). Oesophageal biopsies can also be usefully routinely stained by the PAS method. It allows delineation of the glycogen-deficient basal layer and easy recognition of moniliasis and of glycogenic acanthosis. Perls' method used as a stain for haemosiderin may be indicated in the confirmation of ischaemic or other lesions. Many laboratories now also employ immunohistochemical procedures using specific, often monoclonal, antisera for the identification of plasma cell subtypes, neuronal tissues in Hirschsprung's disease, gastrin or other hormone-producing cells, viral or other antigens and in conjunction with lectins for the more detailed typing of mucins.

Electron microscopy is also being used more frequently, particularly in the delineation of disease processes, such as lipid malabsorption and viral and protozoal infections, and has helped to delineate new lesions, such as microvillous inclusion disease. In teaching hospital laboratories, a case can be made for taking biopsy tissue not only for electron microscopy but also for deep freezing so that this tissue is available for molecular biologically based investigations such as DNA hybridisation and gene rearrangement studies. Some frozen section immunohistochemical procedures can also be applied if indicated—in lymphoma diagnosis, for example.

REFERENCES

Goldner J. (1938) A modification of the Masson trichrome technique for routine laboratory purposes. American Journal of Pathology *14*:237–243.

James K. R. (1967) A simple silver method for the demonstration of reticulin fibres. Journal of Medical Laboratory Technology *24*:49–51.

Lev R. and Spicer S. S. (1964) Specific staining of sulphate groups with Alcian blue at low pH. Journal of Histochemistry and Cytochemistry *12*:309.

Pearse, A. G. E. (1968) Histochemistry: Theoretical and Applied. 3rd Edition. London: Churchill-Livingstone.

Spicer S. S. (1965) Diamine methods for differentiating mucosubstances histochemically. Journal of Histochemistry and Cytochemistry *13*:211–234.

I

Oesophageal Biopsy

1

NORMAL APPEARANCES IN OESOPHAGEAL BIOPSY SPECIMENS

Fibreoptic endoscopy and biopsy are fast becoming the usual diagnostic proce-dure in the investigation of oesophageal disorders. The tissue samples are small and superficial, only rarely including the muscularis mucosa. The normal epithe-lium is stratified and squamous (Fig. 1–1), and despite assertions to the contrary (Hendrix and Yardley 1976), is of nonkeratinising type, for although occasionally exhibiting a few keratohyalin granules, it lacks granular and keratin layers. It consists of a basal proliferative compartment which for all except the last 2 or 3 cm constitutes 10 to 15 per cent of the whole thickness of the mucosa. This layer contains both reserve cells that remain basal and cells that will eventually lose mitotic ability and become progressively superficial before desquamating at the surface. During this process, the cells acquire glycogen, which can be demonstrated in periodic acid–Schiff (PAS) preparations. The width of the zone of unstained basal cells, although not necessarily corresponding accurately with the population of cells still capable of division, is a useful indicator of it and of value in the diagnosis of reflux oesophagitis. Both melanoblasts and putative endocrine poly-peptide argyrophil cells can on occasion be demonstrated scattered among the cells of the basal layer. Tateishi et al (1974) found melanocytes in 4 and argyrophil cells in 14 of 50 oesophageal specimens obtained at autopsy. Intraepithelial lymphocytes and Langerhans cells similar to those present in the skin have also been described (Al Yassin and Toner 1976).

Extending into the epithelium from below are the subepithelial papillae of the lamina propria consisting of delicate vascular connective tissue. The number of papillae per unit length of epithelium has not been accurately determined, but in height they usually do not extend above half way to the surface. The lamina propria of the oesophageal epithelium is composed of loose connective tissue (Fig. 1–2) that contains scattered lymphocytes and plasma cells or small lymphoid aggregates that are mainly located around the ducts of the oesophageal glands and are obviously seen only in deep forceps biopsies of the type usually performed through rigid endoscopes. The ducts are lined by cuboidal cells as they leave the oesophageal glands but become of stratified squamous type after passing through the muscularis mucosa. The glands vary quite markedly in their number from patient to patient. They occupy the submucosa and are of mixed salivary type, being either purely mucinous, purely serous, or mucinous with serous crescents. At the lower end of the oesophagus, however, it is not rare to see in more

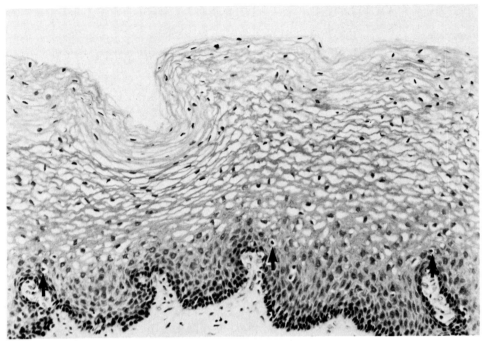

Figure 1–1. Normal oesophageal epithelium. Note the height of the papillae and the thickness of the basal layer; the clarity of cells in the upper layers is due to glucogen. Arrows indicate intraepithelial lymphocytes (H & E × 150).

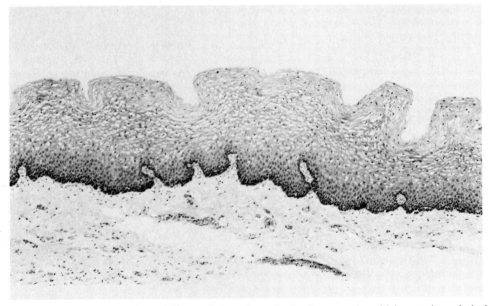

Figure 1–2. Low power view of Figure 1–1 to show the lamina propria, which contains relatively few lymphocytes (H & E × 75).

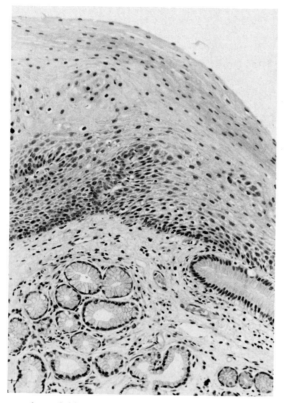

Figure 1–3. Lower oesophageal biopsy showing oesophageal cardiac-type glands in the lamina propria; glycogenic vacuolation of the squamous cells is not a feature (H & E × 150).

superficial biopsies a few simple mucinous glands in the lamina propria. These are similar to the gastric cardiac mucous glands (Fig. 1–3) and are referred to as oesophageal cardiac glands.

In premature infants, less commonly in term babies, and rarely in adults, scattered islands of ciliated epithelium may occur in patches throughout the oesophageal lining. This represents persistence of a developmental stage in the oesophageal mucosa and a simple variation from normal that is without significance (Raeburn 1951).

GASTRO-OESOPHAGEAL REFLUX AND OESOPHAGITIS, BARRETT'S OESOPHAGUS AND ECTOPIC GASTRIC MUCOSA

GASTRO-OESOPHAGEAL REFLUX AND OESOPHAGITIS

In geographic areas where the incidence of squamous carcinoma of the oesophagus is low, by far the most common diagnostic problem posed by oesophageal biopsy interpretation relates to the consequence of reflux of gastric contents. In the absence of ulceration or a Barrett's columnar lining there is debate as to what constitutes the histological grounds for the diagnosis of gastric reflux. It has long been held that a poor correlation exists between symptoms of reflux and inflammatory change of the oesophageal mucosa (Siegel and Hendrix 1963). Ismail-Beigi, Horton and Pope (1970), however, drew attention to basal cell hyperplasia and elongation of the papillae as an indication of reflux, whether or not inflammatory cells were present in the epithelium. Weinstein, Bogoch and Bowes (1975) subsequently showed that these changes are present in 57 per cent of asymptomatic volunteers in biopsies from the lower 2.5 cm of the oesophagus and in 19 per cent above this level. Using an automated image analyser, Adami, Eckardt and Paulini (1979) demonstrated an inter and intra observer error in excess of 20 per cent in the estimation of these parameters and concluded that assessment of basal cell thickness and papillary height as an index of gastro-oesophageal reflux was of limited value. This study was performed on autopsy material, but Seefeld et al (1977) had reached similar conclusions using biopsy tissues.

Central to this controversy is the fact that reflux is a normal phenomenon, and the likelihood is that the same degree of reflux will stimulate different levels of symptoms in different individuals. In addition, the effect of reflux depends upon its composition, its volume, its frequency, the effectiveness of the peristaltic clearance mechanism, the inherent resistance to damage due to the nature of the oesophageal epithelium, the neutralising effect of swallowed saliva and the protection afforded by the secretions of the oesophageal mucous glands. Given that the cause of oesophageal pain is not fully understood, it is hardly surprising that correlation of the histological consequences of reflux with symptoms is poor.

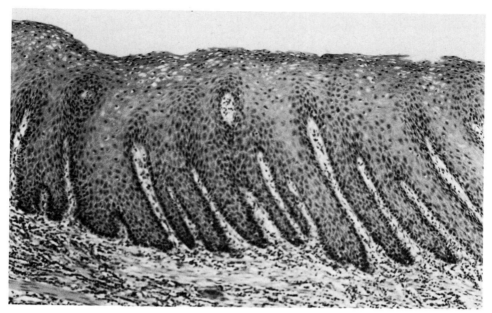

Figure 2–1. The epithelium shows elongation of the papillae, basal cell hyperplasia and loss of glycogenic vacuolation in all except the superficial layers (H & E × 100).

Indeed it is well recognized that patients with oesophagitis and stricture may have few or no reflux symptoms before dysphagia develops (Volpicelli, Yardley and Hendrix 1975).

The concern of the tissue pathologist, however, is the recognition of changes in oesophageal biopsies due to significant reflux of gastric contents (Figs. 2–1 to 2–4). Since reflux is a normal event, minor degrees of histological variations could be regarded as part of the normal spectrum of oesophageal histology, especially at

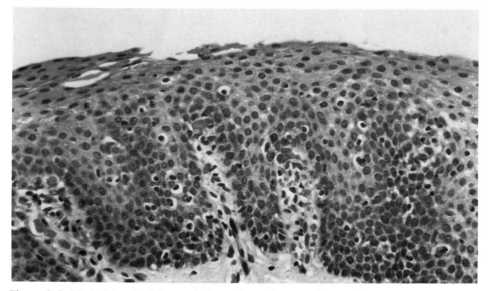

Figure 2–2. Marked basal cell hyperplasia maximum between the papillae and an obvious increase in intraepithelial lymphocytes (H & E × 175).

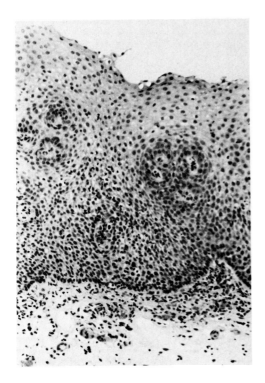

Figure 2–3. Features as in Figures 2–1 and 2–2 but the papillae are cross cut. The intraepithelial inflammatory cell infiltration contains polymorphonuclear leukocytes and there is obvious increased cellularity of the lamina propria (H & E × 150).

its very distal end. If we consider the pathophysiology of oesophageal damage due to reflux it is possible to predict the morphological changes that might ensue regardless of whether or not they are related to symptoms, and histological assessment of biopsies does provide a tangible piece of evidence of the evaluation of reflux disease (Funch-Jensen et al 1986). There is ample evidence of a damaging effect of acid, pepsin, and bile on the oesophageal mucosa in both humans

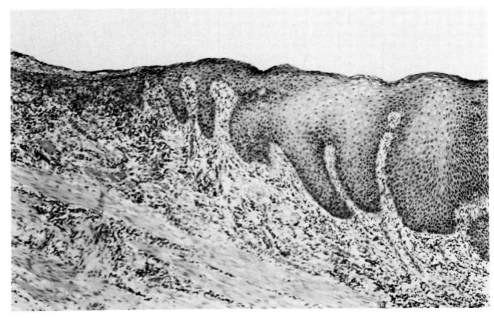

Figure 2–4. Reflux oesophagitis with impending erosion at left (H & E × 75).

(Hopwood et al 1981) and experimental animals (Carney et al 1981, Dodds et al 1981, Salo, Lehto and Kivilaakso 1983). This cell damage will result in a shortened cell life and increased surface exfoliation. In association with minor degrees of damage, the response of the oesophageal epithelium is to counteract the increased cell loss with increased cell production. Evidence for increased cell turnover in biopsies with proven reflux was provided by a morphometric analysis of various nuclear parameters in the different layers of the oesophageal epithelium (Jarvis, Dent and Whitehead 1985). The increased cell turnover results in a thickening of the basally situated proliferative component. This thickening tends to occur principally in the areas between subepithelial papillae. Damage to the basal cells due to diffusion of gastric contents across the oesophageal epithelium would be expected to be least marked in the cells furthest from the lumen, i.e., those lying between the subepithelial papillae. As already mentioned, this thickness, which is normally between 10 and 15 per cent of the whole mucosa, can be readily assessed in PAS stained sections. Another method is to arbitrarily define its upper extent as that level where the distance between nuclei equals the average nuclear diameter, but this only achieves the same purpose and is time consuming.

In association with basal cell hyperplasia, elongation of the subepithelial papillae occurs, and they tend to approach the surface. This is also a consequence of the mechanism of damage due to back diffusion. The lower cell turnover of damaged basal cells over the papillae and a uniform surface loss tends to bring the papillae nearer to the surface. Clearly when the damage is such that exfoliation exceeds the rate of cell renewal, erosions appear first over the papillae and then extend to the areas between. The tendency, with increased severity of damage, is for the epithelium as a whole to reduce in thickness. When ulceration occurs, a mixed inflammatory infiltration is seen in the related submucosa, and gradually a layer of granulation tissue is formed at its base.

Neutrophil polymorphonuclear leukocytes are a prominent component of the infiltrate and can also be seen in the neighbouring oesophageal epithelium. There has been a debate as to the importance of neutrophil or neutrophil polymorph infiltration of the non-ulcerated oesophageal epithelium as an indication of reflux damage, although in approximately 20 per cent of cases showing the epithelial changes of basal cell hyperplasia and elongation of papillae neutrophils are seen in the lamina propria below the epithelium. When neutrophil infiltration of the lamina propria is prominent, they are usually also seen in small numbers within the epithelium. This phenomenon is more obvious evidence of increasing damage and progressive thinning before ulceration occurs. Since lymphocytes occur in the lamina propria in normal circumstances, their presence is of no diagnostic significance, although their numbers do tend to increase along with polymorphs and plasma cells in severe oesophagitis with ulceration.

Winter et al (1982) and Brown, Goldman and Antonioli (1984) have drawn attention to the presence of intraepithelial eosinophils as a sensitive indicator of reflux in both children and adults. The infiltrate, it is claimed, may occur before other histological evidence develops.

The recognition of eosinophils is facilitated by examining Chromotrope 2R preparations in which they stand out brightly red against the weakly stained pale blue background of the epithelium (Figs. 2–5 and 2–6).

Certainly cases with a pronounced eosinophil infiltrate do occur in younger patients, but in cases seen by this observer, there has been no correlation with peripheral blood eosinophilia and no evidence that the phenomenon is related to eosinophilic gastroenteritis, although involvement of the oesophagus in this condition does apparently occur (see below). The claim that eosinophil infiltration

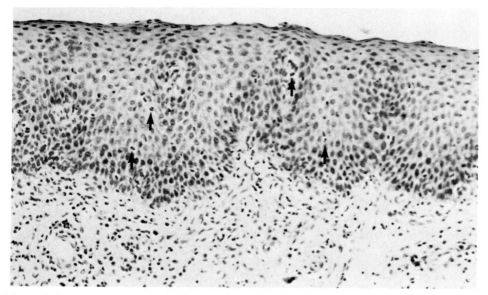

Figure 2–5. Oesophageal mucosa with a pronounced eosinophil polymorph infiltration. The nuclei are arrowed (H & E × 175).

is a good indication of reflux has been challenged in studies showing they have no diagnostic importance (Janisch et al 1984, Tummala et al 1987). Thus in the majority of cases that satisfy the histological criteria for reflux based upon basal cell hyperplasia, papillary elongation and the other features mentioned above, distinct eosinophil infiltration does not appear to be a feature and it is possible

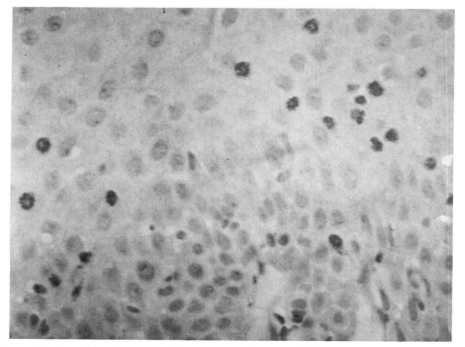

Figure 2–6. Oesophageal mucosa with a pronounced eosinophil leukocyte infiltration. The eosinophils stand out against the pale background; compare with Figure 2–5 (Chromotrope 2R × 400).

that cases characterised by eosinophils represent a subgroup in which a different aetiological mechanism operates. On rare occasions apparently it is a manifestation of eosinophilic gastroenteropathy and is associated with a peripheral eosinophilia and infiltrates in other parts of the bowel (Dobbins, Sheahan and Behar 1977, Lee 1985).

Intraepithelial cell nuclei other than those of the epithelium itself are certainly often observed in oesophageal biopsies. In ordinary haematoxylin and eosin stained slides these nuclei are small and variable in shape, seemingly being moulded between the epithelial cells themselves. Most of these are probably intraepithelial lymphocytes, but it is possible that some represent eosinophils or neutrophils that are degranulated. Certainly these irregular-shaped nuclear forms appear to be increased in number in oesophagitis. Geboes et al (1983) in a study using monoclonal antibodies have shown that in reflux oesophagitis Langerhans cells and cytotoxic T lymphocytes are present in increased numbers within the epithelium.

In summary, oesophageal biopsy appearances can indicate gastric reflux. A basal cell thickness in excess of 10 or 15 per cent and papillae extending into the upper half of the epithelium are the important features of minimal reflux and will be seen in very distal biopsies in approximately half of a normal asymptomatic population. This is to be expected, since some reflux is a normal phenomenon. Abnormal reflux will be associated with more severe alterations, thinning and eventual ulceration and secondary inflammatory changes. Although in a younger age group eosinophil infiltration may signify reflux, in most other patients this does not seem to be the case. It should be stated, however, that the morphological assessment of reflux oesophagitis by subjective histology and even by sophisticated image analysis still results in controversy, and some workers still express doubt as to its effectiveness (Collins et al 1989).

BARRETT'S OESOPHAGUS
(Columnar Lined Oesophagus)

Although there are still claims for a congenital origin for the columnar lined oesophagus (Haque and Merkel 1981, Stadelmann, Elster and Kuhn 1981), the consensus is that, when limited to the distal oesophagus or extending to involve most of its length, the condition is acquired and the end result of severe longstanding reflux. (See ectopic gastric mucosa following.)

The evidence for the acquisition of Barrett's mucosa following oesophagogastrectomy (Naef et al 1975, Hamilton and Yardley 1977), the healing of canine oesophageal lesions by columnar epithelium after destruction of the "anti-reflux" mechanism (Bremner, Lynch and Ellis 1970), the observation of orad migration of the squamo-columnar junction with time (Naef et al 1975) and the partial regression of Barrett's epithelium after anti-reflux operations (Brand et al 1980) all point to an acquired aetiology.

It would appear therefore that reflux of gastric or even intestinal contents following total gastrectomy (Meyer, Vollmar and Bar 1979) can lead to severe epithelial damage and erosion with a tendency to early healing by gastric type mucosa. It is most usual for the reflux to persist and possibly to increase in severity, and there is increasing evidence that Barrett's oesophagus is more common than is generally appreciated (Cooper and Barbezat 1987). The metaplastic change associated with recurrent ulceration and healing comes to occupy more and more of the oesophageal lining. The ulceration in Barrett's oesophagus is therefore found where expected, i.e., at the junction of squamous and columnar mucosa where attendant fibrosis may also produce a stricture. Barrett's oesophagus is occasionally familial (Prior and Whorwell 1986) and has been described in children following chemotherapy for leukaemia, apparently associated with reflux (Dahms et al 1987).

There has been some variance of opinion with respect to the type of mucosa that constitutes a Barrett's oesophagus; this results from the simple fact that the type of mucosa shows considerable variation in the same case and from case to case. At the lower gastric end it has been described as of fundic gastric type (Fig. 2–7) in that the mucosa contains both parietal and chief cells. The mucosa is, however, commonly gastritic and may be atrophic. In the author's experience this type of mucosa is never extensive and is usually located distally, although it may be seen at any level. When distal it is clearly responsible for difficulty in determining the precise gastro-oesophageal junction. It is not usual for this type of mucosa to be associated with intestinal metaplasia. A second type of columnar mucosa, which approximates gastric cardiac mucosa, is also seen (Fig. 2–8). A few parietal cells may occur among the cells forming the simple coiled mucinous glands (Fig. 2–9) that empty into the short crypts dipping down from the luminal epithelium of gastric superficial type. This type of mucosa can exhibit a variety of intermediate appearances as it progressively undergoes further metaplastic change.

These appearances are due to the acquisition of further cell types. First, there is the appearance of intestinal goblet cells (Figs. 2–10 and 2–11); second, there

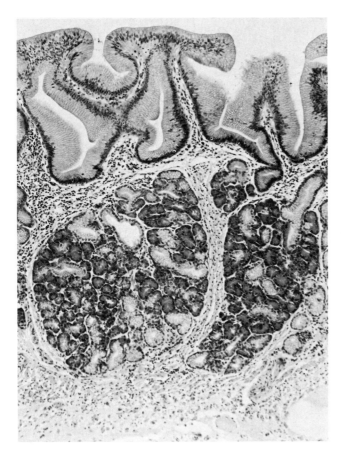

Figure 2–7. Barrett's oesophagus. Fundic (body) type mucosa. Note the mixed mucinous and body-type glands and the inflammation (H & E × 150).

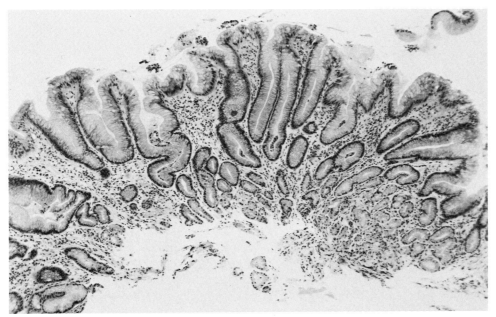

Figure 2–8. Barrett's oesophagus. Cardiac-type mucosa (H & E × 150).

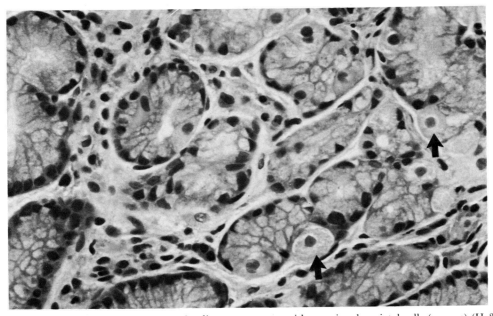

Figure 2–9. Barrett's oesophagus. Cardiac-type mucosa with occasional parietal cells (arrows) (H & E × 500).

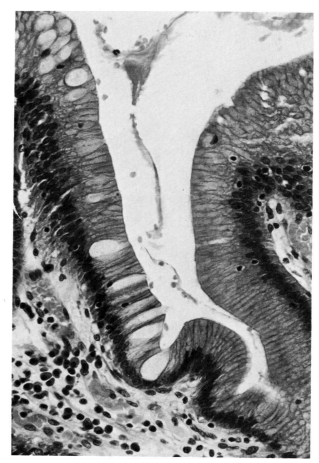

Figure 2–10. Barrett's oesophagus. A few goblet cells are beginning to appear, but most of the surface cells are gastric (H & E × 500).

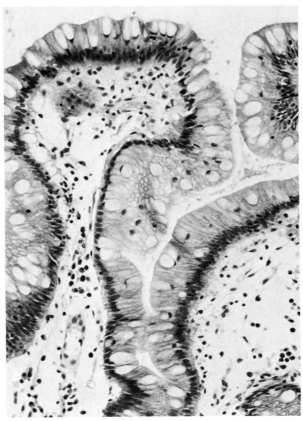

Figure 2–11. Barrett's oesophagus. Goblet cells are numerous and the remaining cells are difficult to identify (H & E × 250).

are cells with superficial cytoplasmic mucous droplets, but also with a luminal border equipped with microvilli (Fig. 2–12). These cells were described in electron microscope preparations by Trier (1970), who regarded them as unlike any other type of cell seen in the gastrointestinal tract. In fact, they are similar to gastric surface cells showing partial intestinalisation (Ming, Goldman and Freiman 1967) and to the intermediate stages of metaplastic gastric superficial cells in the duodenum (Patrick, Denham and Forrest 1974). Apparently, however, they do not possess the capacity to absorb lipid and do not have the fully developed histochemical characteristics of absorptive enterocytes. In the author's experience with Barrett's oesophagus in paraffin sections, some cells do have the appearance of enterocytes (Fig. 2–13) but the majority are best described as a half-way stage between an enterocyte and a gastric superficial epithelial cell.

These mucus-secreting cells in Barrett's oesophagus have been investigated by histochemical procedures (Jass 1981), and it is claimed that whereas the goblet cells secrete mainly acid sialomucins, the other mucus-secreting cells contain predominantly either neutral or acid sulphomucins. This form of intestinalisation is said to correspond to the incomplete metaplasia type IIA and IIB of Jass and Filipe (1981), but in reality the mucin pattern, based upon the use of the PAS Alcian blue and high iron diamine Alcian blue methods, is extremely variable in Barrett's oesophagus, showing a variety of combinations of mucins in both the goblet cells and the columnar mucinous cells. The real value of using these stains

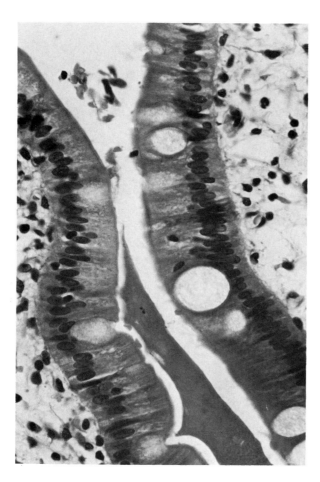

Figure 2–12. Barrett's oesophagus. Obvious goblet cells and intervening cells with both mucous droplets and a brush border (H & E × 500).

is easier recognition of the intermediate type of Barrett's epithelium. It has been shown by others, however, that there is a poor correlation between mucin type and cancer risk in Barrett's oesophagus and that its demonstration has no value in managing patients. Flow cytometry abnormalities of DNA content seemingly offer a better prospect in this regard (Reid et al 1987, Haggitt et al 1988). Other cells that also appear are enterochromaffin cells of intestinal type. In immunohistochemical studies these have been shown to contain 5-hydroxytryptamine, somatostatin, motilin, pancreatic polypeptide, glucose-dependent insulinotropic polypeptide, gastrin, glucagon, peptide tyrosine-tyrosine, secretin and neurotensin (Rindi et al 1987). Paneth cells, which are often easily recognized only in specially stained preparations, also occur. They are seen predominantly in areas where the mucosa most closely approximates to the small intestine (Fig. 2–14), even to the extent of exhibiting finger-like villous processes (Thompson, Zinsser and Enterline 1983). Pepsinogens A and C have also been demonstrated (Meuwissen et al 1988).

It is also worth noting that the junction of the squamous and columnar epithelium is often irregular. Sometimes squamous islands are left behind by the advancing edge of columnar epithelium. This may exhibit quite long tongue-shaped extensions upwards from the main columnar-lined area. Small squamous islands also tend to persist at the mouths of the ducts of the oesophageal glands (Fig. 2–15). In rare instances squamous epithelium can overlie Barrett's mucosa over quite extensive areas (Sampliner et al 1988).

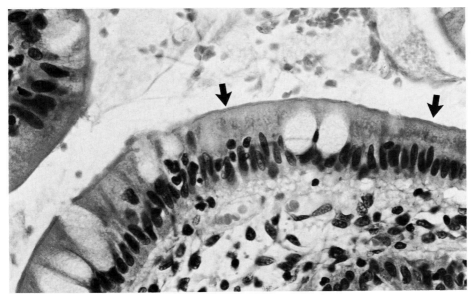

Figure 2–13. Barrett's oesophagus. Goblet cells and cells which cannot be differentiated from enterocytes (arrows) (H & E × 500).

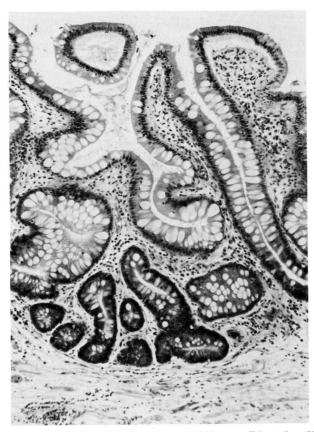

Figure 2–14. Barrett's oesophagus. Villous process mimicking small intestine (H & E × 250).

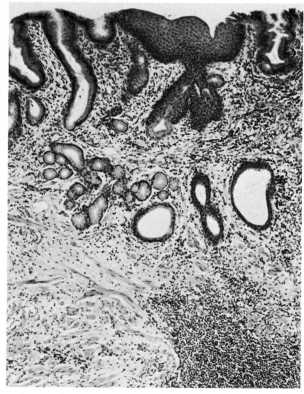

Figure 2–15. Barrett's oesophagus. Squamous island at the site of opening of the duct of an oesophageal gland (H & E × 200).

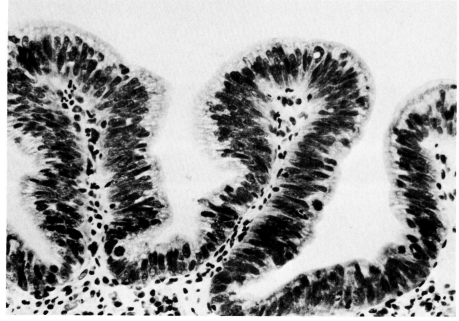

Figure 2–16. Barrett's oesophagus. Severe dysplasia. Note the mitotic figures (H & E × 500).

The metaplastic gastric epithelium in Barrett's oesophagus occasionally gives rise to hyperplastic polyps with appearances essentially similar to the same lesions arising in the stomach. As in the stomach, they probably represent a mucosal reaction to erosion or ulceration.

In longstanding cases of Barrett's oesophagus it is not unusual to see the additional features of dysplasia (Fig. 2–16). The range of dysplastic appearances is essentially similar to that which occurs in the stomach in atrophic gastritis with intestinal metaplasia, and all stages of severity up to carcinoma in situ can be recognized (Hamilton and Smith 1987, Reid et al 1988a). Levine et al (1989) have shown, however, that the recognition of these dysplastic changes can be greatly facilitated by the use of electron microscopy and flow cytometry. Neoplastic progression is characterised by abnormalities in the cytoplasmic organelles concerned with mucin production and by aneuploid or G_2/tetraploid nuclei. Elsewhere in the bowel the assessment of dysplasia is prone to significant observer variation (Reid et al 1988b). Sometimes the dysplastic epithelium occurs in the form of adenomatous polyps (McDonald, Brand and Thorning 1977, Thompson, Zinsser and Enterline 1983, Keeffe, Hisken and Schubert 1986). The invasive carcinoma that occurs in Barrett's oesophagus arises therefore from the partially or incompletely intestinalised epithelium and has as its counterpart in the stomach the intestinal type of carcinoma. Occasionally mucoepidermoid carcinoma is reported (Pascal and Clearfield 1987).

There is a further difficulty in the interpretation of biopsy specimens from patients with longstanding Barrett's oesophagus. In some cases fibrosis or fibromuscular proliferation entraps normal or dysplastic glands and can easily be mistaken for invasive adenocarcinoma (Rubio and Riddell 1988).

ECTOPIC GASTRIC MUCOSA

Heterotopia of ectopic gastric mucosa is known to occur in various sites in the gastrointestinal tract. Nevertheless its presence in the oesophagus has been the subject of some controversy. There are two reasons for this. First, some confusion has arisen between gastric ectopia proper and the presence of columnar epithelium, which is ciliated and has already been referred to (see Chapter 1). Second, the condition of gastric mucosal ectopia as a developmental defect has been discussed in the context of Barrett's mucosa but is an entirely separate entity.

Early autopsy studies (Rector and Connerley 1941) revealed microscopic evidence of ectopic gastric mucosa in 7.8 per cent of 1000 infant and child subjects, and in over half the abnormality was present in the upper one third of the oesophagus. With the increasing practice of endoscopy, evidence is now firm that heterotopic gastric mucosa, which is usually of body type, can be found in up to 4 per cent of cases, including in adults (Jabbari et al 1985). This mucosa is sometimes called "the inlet patch" and can show gastritis or ulceration; it may be associated with dysphagia or other symptoms and may lead to stricture (Raine 1983, Shah, DeRidder and Shah 1986, Truong, Stroehlein and McKechnie 1986, Wang, Spear and McGrew 1986, Schroeder, Myer and Schechter 1987, Steadman et al 1988).

3

NON-REFLUX OESOPHAGITIS AND ULCERATION

NON-SPECIFIC

This form of oesophagitis is part of the spectrum of oesophageal injury caused by the ingestion of strong acids or alkalis, physical agents, radiation, and drugs. The injury usually results in a localised oesophageal ulceration with or without subsequent fibrosis and stricture. Histologically it is normally non-specific, and biopsy specimens will reveal only the range of appearances seen in reflux oesophagitis with or without ulceration. In the early stages of acid/alkali injury, however, more tissue necrosis will be evident, and in ulcers secondary to radiotherapy deep biopsies will show the characteristic hyalinisation of vessels and bizarre fibroblasts. Epithelial nuclear abnormalities may also be found in more superficial biopsies, which, in the absence of a clinical history, can cause difficulties in interpretation because the changes may be similar to primary premalignant dysplasia. This is sometimes also a problem in oesophageal lesions that may complicate chemotherapy for malignancies in other parts of the body (Figs. 3–1, 3–2). Collins et al (1979), who reviewed drug-induced oesophageal ulceration, listed evidence for the implication of the following agents: emepronium bromide, Slow K, doxycycline, tetracycline, clindamycin, phenylbutazone, prednisone, fluouracil and carbachol. This list has been substantially lengthened to include non-steroidal anti-inflammatory drugs (NSAIDs); the most detailed list of drugs involved is given by Becouarn, Lamouliatte and Quinton (1983). There is evidence (Wilkins, Ridley and Pozniak 1984) for an association between the use of NSAIDs and benign oesophageal stricture. Oesophageal injury due to ingested chemicals or drugs tends to occur at sites of anatomical narrowing, e.g., at the level of the aortic arch or where there is pathological narrowing, e.g., due to an enlarged left atrium. It is more likely to occur if there is any disorder of oesophageal motility.

Necrotising lesions with secondary inflammatory changes have also been described in chronic graft versus host disease, particularly in the upper oesophagus (McDonald et al 1981). Ulceration of the oesophagus (Korula 1985) and the development of mucosal bridges, presumably due to healing of ulceration such as occurs in other ulcerative lesions of the bowel, have also been described (Gottfried and Goldberg 1985).

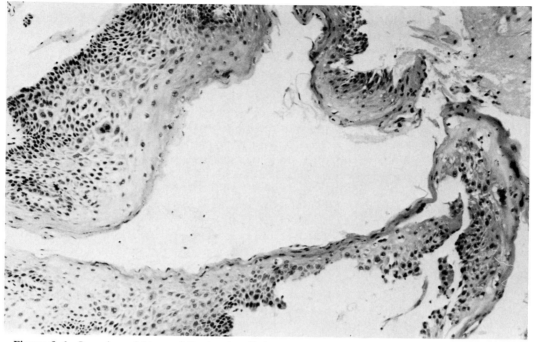

Figure 3–1. Oesophageal biopsy following irradiation of the mediastinum resulting in ulceration and dysphagia. Note irregular epithelial maturation and degenerative nuclear changes (H & E × 75).

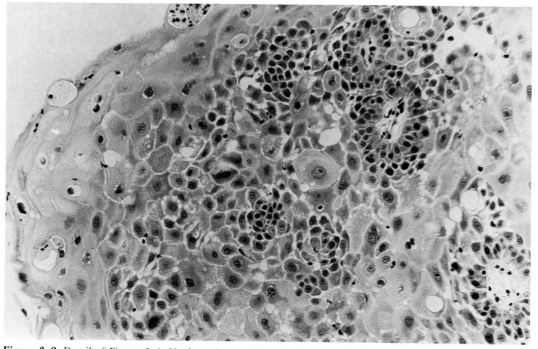

Figure 3–2. Detail of Figure 3–1. Nuclear abnormalities simulate neoplastic dysplasia (H & E × 500).

SPECIFIC

Specific forms of oesophagitis with or without ulceration and stricture are due to a variety of infective agents.

It is now well recognized that a wide range of gram-positive and gram-negative organisms can cause oesophagitis in the immunocompromised, and this can be diagnosed in biopsy specimens (Walsh, Belitsos and Hamilton 1986).

In tuberculosis the oesophagus is usually involved by extension of adjacent bony, lymph node or lung disease. Consequently oesophageal mucosal biopsies may or may not reveal diagnostic information (Dow 1981). Cases of primary tuberculous oesophagitis actually diagnosed by endoscopic biopsy on the basis of granulomata and the demonstration of acid-fast organisms are, however, on record (Seivewright, Feehally and Wicks 1984, Chase et al 1986, Catinella and Kittle 1988). In two of these cases the disease eroded an atherosclerotic aortic aneurysm and caused death. Sometimes primary oesophageal tuberculosis can present as a tumour (Laajam 1984). Syphilitic gummata of the oesophagus are extremely rare and their diagnosis on mucosal biopsy has not been described. Involvement by actinomycosis, blastomycosis, aspergillus and histoplasmosis is also uncommon, but distinctive histological appearances due to the presence of the respective agents have been described (Barrett 1950, Lee, Neumann and Welsh 1977, Hull 1979, Miller and Everett 1979, Knohe and Bernhardt 1980, McKenzie and Khakoo 1985). The same is true of candidal or monilial oesophagitis (Mathieson and Dutta 1983, Boylston et al 1987). Although candidal or monilial oeso-phagitis has commonly been an acute complication in patients with the acquired immunodeficiency syndrome (AIDS) (Porro, Parente and Cernuschi 1989) and in other immunodeficient hosts, in those with severe debilitating disease or diabetes, and in post-operative patients, especially after liver or renal transplantation (Alexander et al 1988), it is being recognized in a subacute or chronic form as a primary cause of oesophageal ulceration, tracheo-oesophageal fistula and stenosis (Kodsi et al 1976, Orringer and Sloan 1978, Agha 1984, Obrecht et al 1984). Occasionally it presents as an oesophageal polypoidal lesion (Ho, Cullen and Gray 1977). It is also described in neonates (Petru and Azimi 1984), in whom immaturity of the immune response may be implicated. The oval yeasts and hyphal forms can easily be recognized in biopsy tissue, especially if a PAS stain is examined (Fig. 3–3). Moniliasis also occurs as a secondary phenomenon in oesophageal ulcers due to other causes such as in Barrett's oesophagus (Scott and Jenkins 1982, Kalogeropoulos and Whitehead, 1988).

Viruses may also cause oesophageal ulceration. Cytomegalovirus infection is well recognized as a complication in immunosuppressed individuals and in those with AIDS (Freeman et al 1977, Allen et al 1981, Weller 1985) but occasionally causes erosive oesophagitis in healthy young adults (Villar, Massanari and Mitros 1984). The large intranuclear inclusions may be seen in fibroblasts and capillary endothelial cells in the ulcer base but usually not in the squamous epithelium. Herpes simplex Type 1 may also occur in the same type of patient or in one with severe debilitating disease (Agha, Lee and Nostrant 1986), but it is being described as a cause of dysphagia due to ulceration in previously healthy individuals (Depew et al 1977, DiPalma and Brady 1984, Desigan and Schneider 1985). Furthermore the great variability of both the clinical and endoscopic findings is being realised (Byard, Champion and Orizaga 1987). Apart from evidence of ulceration, the characteristic features in biopsies include multinucleate giant cells with their typical ground-glass nuclei. Cells in the ulcer margin less frequently contain intranuclear inclusions (Fig. 3–4). These are characteristically eosinophilic and are

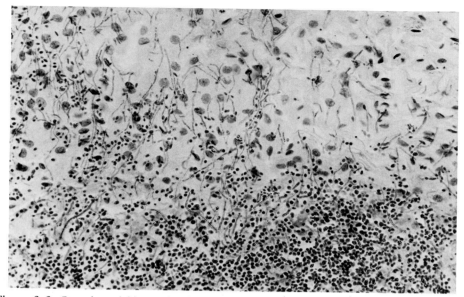

Figure 3–3. Oesophageal biopsy showing yeast and hyphal forms of *Candida* among squamous epithelial debris (PAS × 500).

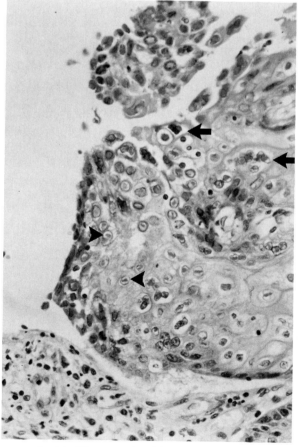

Figure 3–4. Herpes oesophagitis. Ulcer margin with multinucleate giant cells (arrows) and Cowdry type A inclusions (arrowheads) (H & E × 500).

surrounded by a clear zone with the nuclear chromatin condensed to a peripheral membranous ring (Cowdry Type-A cells). The endoscopic and light and electron microscopic appearances are described in detail by McKay and Day (1983), Burrig et al (1984), and Feiden et al (1984). Oesophagitis can also occur in patients who have concurrent cutaneous herpes zoster, and biopsy tissues show diffuse eosinophilic intranuclear inclusions (Gill et al 1984).

OTHER FORMS OF OESOPHAGITIS

Another cause of oesophageal ulceration is Behçet's syndrome. This has been reviewed by Kikuchi et al (1982). The pathology is not distinctive.

In systemic sclerosis the vascular changes and fibrosis affect the muscle layers and will not normally be seen in biopsy tissues. However, the functional alteration of the cardio-oesophageal junction allows excessive reflux, and reflux oesophagitis is common (Zamost et al 1987). This may progress to the acquisition of a Barrett's columnar lining (Cameron and Payne 1978). A similar range of pathological lesions is described as a less common complication of other collagen diseases, e.g., rheumatoid arthritis (Nishikai, Asaba and Homma 1977, Schneider et al 1984), systemic lupus erythematosus (Saladin et al 1966) and dermatomyositis (Greamer, Andersen and Code 1956). Similar basically reflux mucosal changes are seen in the neuromuscular disorder secondary to Chagas' disease and in visceral myopathy and neuropathy (Schuffler and Pope 1976, Cohen 1979, McDonald et al 1981).

That involvement of the oesophagus in Crohn's disease occurs is well recognised. Freson, Kottler and Wright (1984) describe a case with granulomas in an oesophageal biopsy, but in most instances the appearances are non-specific. This is true of most of the cases that continue to be reported in the literature, and the diagnosis is presumptive because of documented Crohn's disease in other parts of the gastrointestinal tract (Davidson and Sawyers 1983, Tishler and Helman 1984, Pepe et al 1985). Huchzermeyer et al (1976), however, who report five cases, make the point that an exact diagnosis requires histological examination of a resection specimen. LiVolsi and Jaretzki (1973) describe the occurrence of oesophageal Crohn's disease in the absence of gastrointestinal involvement proven at subsequent autopsy.

Sometimes endoscopists see oesophageal rings or webs, and the appearances of the mucosa vary between normal and severe reflux oesophagitis with ulceration (Eastridge, Pate and Mann 1984). The biopsy appearances are also similar and are reviewed by Janisch and Eckardt (1982), who reported two patients with multiple webs.

4

OESOPHAGEAL PLAQUES AND MISCELLANEOUS CONDITIONS

There are several histological entities that in the gross at endoscopy appear as discrete, surface, white or yellow plaques. Some are due to previously referred to fungal infections.

GLYCOGENIC ACANTHOSIS

This is the most common cause of oesophageal plaques (Bender et al 1973, Stern et al 1980). They are seen most commonly in the lower third of the oesophagus and are usually a few millimetres and rarely up to a centimetre in size, occurring predominantly on the crests of the longitudinal folds. Histologically, the epithelium is thickened due to an obvious increase in the glycogen-filled layer above the basal zone, which itself does not usually show hyperplasia, nor is there any nuclear atypia or keratinisation (Fig. 4–1). The condition probably has no malignant potential or clinical significance, but it has been suggested that it may be part of the spectrum of human papilloma virus (HPV) infection (Morris and Price 1986).

LIPID ISLANDS

Lipid islands similar to the so-called xanthelasma of the stomach and intestine are also occasionally reported and on biopsy show the same histological appearance of collections of typical foam cells (Remmele and Engelsing 1984).

OESOPHAGEAL LEUKOPLAKIA

Despite claims to the contrary (Rotterdam and Sommers 1981), it is the experience of most pathologists dealing with large numbers of biopsies that leukoplakia of the oesophagus comparable to the oral lesion is somewhat rare. The oral lesion is white because of keratinisation of a normally non-keratinised epithelium. The latter may be either hyperplastic or somewhat atrophic. The importance of oral leukoplakia, however, lies in the fact that it can exhibit a range

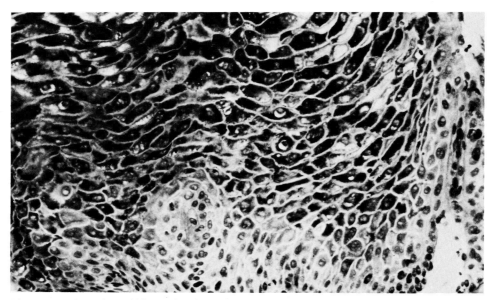

Figure 4–1. Oesophageal biopsy showing pronounced glycogen-rich zone above basal layer (PAS × 400).

of cellular atypia ranging up to carcinoma in situ and is regarded as premalignant, some 10 per cent of oral cases developing squamous carcinoma (King 1964). There are undoubted examples of oesophageal leukoplakia due to hyperkeratosis reported in the literature (Herschman et al 1978), but histological dysplasia has not been described. The malignant potential of this variety of oesophageal plaque therefore has yet to be determined. Hyperkeratotic white plaques may sometimes occur following acid/alkali burns and ulceration or in association with achalasia, scleroderma or severe reflux disease (Fig. 4–2).

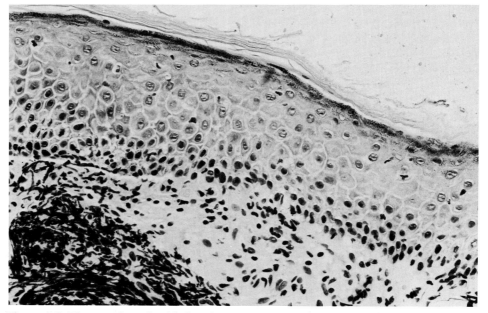

Figure 4–2. The oesophageal epithelium in prolonged achalasia has acquired a granular layer and is keratinised (H & E × 400).

OESOPHAGEAL PAPILLOMAS

In the past, single or multiple oesophageal papillomas were often reported as rarities, usually being diagnosed because they had produced symptoms due to their size (Walker 1978, Waterfall, Somers and Desa 1978, Colina, Solis and Munoz 1980). However, single or multiple small symptomless papillomas or polyps, sometimes described as low-domed plaques endoscopically, occur with an incidence of up to 0.45 per cent in upper gastrointestinal endoscopy examinations, and there are increasing numbers of reports of quite large series of cases (Javdan and Pitman 1984, Toet et al 1985, Fernandez-Rodriguez et al 1986, Sablich et al 1988). A single case of multiple oesophageal papillomas occurring in association with Goltz syndrome has also been recorded (Brinson et al 1987). Goltz syndrome is a congenital disease characterized by focal dermal hypoplasia, dysplasia of the skeleton, teeth and other structures of mesodermal and ectodermal origin, linear hyperpigmentation and sclerodactyly. Oesophageal papillomas are usually histo-logically benign (Figs. 4–3 and 4–4) and show the typical features of squamous papillomas in other sites, with irregular acanthosis and sometimes perinuclear cytoplasmic vacuolation of the superficial cells. Occasionally keratinisation may occur and the papillary stromal component may show an increase of lymphocytes and plasma cells. Although a relationship to human papillomavirus (HPV) was not demonstrated in early studies (Colina, Solis and Munoz 1980), there is more recent evidence based upon immunohistochemical methods that HPV infection may be implicated in a substantial number of cases (Winkler et al 1985). Further-more, it seems that at least some of these lesions may proceed through stages of increasing atypia and dysplasia to invasive squamous carcinoma (Hille et al 1986). Morris and Price (1986) have drawn a comparison with the role of HPV infection in squamous carcinomas in other epithelial surfaces such as the uterine cervix.

SEBACEOUS GLANDS IN THE OESOPHAGUS

Rarely have these lesions been diagnosed by endoscoy and biopsy (Salgado et al 1980, Bambirra et al 1983). They appear as yellow, raised plaques anywhere in the oesophagus and histologically are composed of mature sebaceous glands. They are presumably a developmental defect. Reconstructive surgery of the oesophagus that requires the use of skin flaps sometimes results in the condition known as hairy or hirsute oesophagus (Agha and Wimbish 1984, Llaneza, Menendez and Dunn 1987).

DYSPLASIA AND EARLY SQUAMOUS CARCINOMA OF THE OESOPHAGUS (Figs. 4–5 – 4–7)

In areas of low incidence, squamous carcinoma is usually diagnosed late in the course of the disease when the patient presents with dysphagia. In the past few years, workers in areas of high incidence have delineated the early stages of oesophageal squamous cancer (Crespi et al 1979, 1984, Dreyer 1980, Barge et al 1981, Munoz et al 1982, Mandard et al 1984). Wang (1981) described four endoscopic appearances in a group of 117 Chinese patients with early oesophageal cancer. The most common, occurring in 53 per cent, was a friable irregular erosion; 25.6 per cent presented as a raised polypoidal lesion with or without erosions; 12.8 per cent showed a hyperaemic roughening that bled easily; and 8.6 per cent showed one or more white plaques. In all cases the oesophagus exhibited

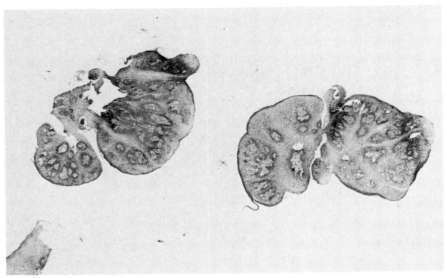

Figure 4–3. Oesophageal squamous epithelial papilloma removed endoscopically (H & E × 25).

a normal elasticity and peristaltic movement. It has become clear that squamous carcinoma of the oesophagus emerges in the main through a sequence of chronic oesophagitis, progressive dysplasia, carcinoma in situ and finally invasive carcinoma (Munoz et al 1982, Benasco et al 1985, Oettle et al 1986, Ohta et al 1986). There is also the evidence as outlined above that the situation is comparable to the same tumour arising in the uterine cervix and that, at least in a proportion of cases, HPV infection may play a role.

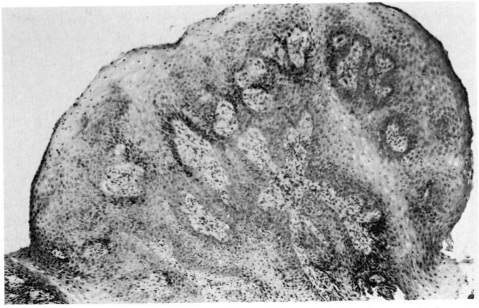

Figure 4–4. A higher power of one of the papillomas in Figure 4–3. Note the stromal inflammatory infiltrate and lack of epithelial atypia (H & E × 150).

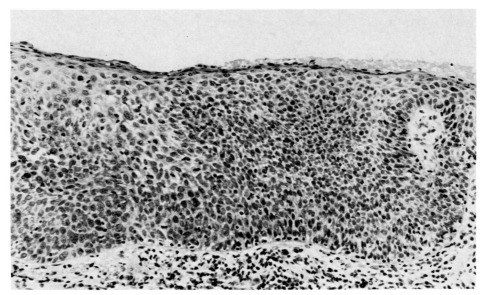

Figure 4–5. Dysplasia of the oesophageal epithelium, which is also thickened and shows inflammatory cell infiltration (H & E × 150).

Carcinoma in situ and early squamous carcinoma of the oesophagus have also been reported in low incidence areas (Seifert et al 1973), and it becomes increasingly likely that these curable lesions will be diagnosed more frequently outside China, South Africa, the Caspian littoral and parts of France and other areas where the incidence is high. It could well be that in these areas HPV plays a relatively more important role than do other factors.

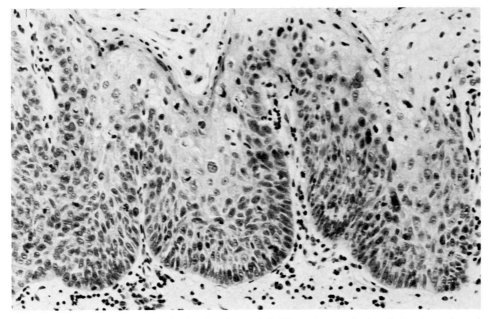

Figure 4–6. More severe dysplasia than in Figure 4–5. There is a marked variation in nuclear size, shape and polarity in the widened basal zone (H & E × 250).

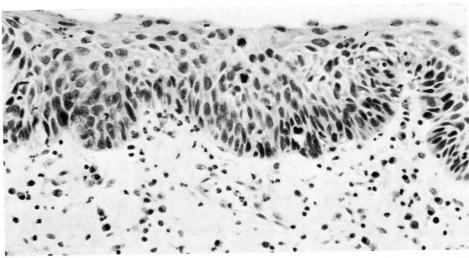

Figure 4–7. Severe dysplasia in a rather atrophic epithelium. Note the mitotic figures, one of them very near to the surface (H & E × 250).

The histological changes documented in high-risk populations include parabasal clear cell hyperplasia, which is PAS negative, as well as acanthosis and lymphocyte-plasma cell infiltrations. Sometimes the abnormal epithelium is thin and atrophic, but the important features are the dysplastic nuclear changes and kerato hyaline granules in the superficial cells. More severe dysplasia amounting to carcinoma in situ either in a thick or thin epithelium is also seen as a precursor of invasion. Similar dysplasia and carcinoma in situ are described in mucosa adjacent to invasive squamous carcinomas of the oesophagus (Mandard et al 1980). Those cases associated with HPV virus, in addition to dysplasia, exhibit typical koilocytosis with perinuclear halos and sometimes either pyknosis of the nuclei or a ground-glass appearance.

These precancerous changes appear to be identical in some cases to the postcricoid abnormalities that precede squamous carcinoma in patients with the Patterson-Kelly syndrome (Entwistle and Jacobs 1965). This entity occurs in women and consists of dysplasia, iron deficiency anaemia and gastric achlorhydria. It is rare except in northern Europe and is particularly common in Scandinavia. Because iron deficiency has a worldwide distribution, these changes are clearly not simply due to lack of iron, and it is of interest that post-cricoid carcinoma may also complicate pernicious anaemia (Jacobs 1962). In rare examples of biopsy material from patients with pernicious anaemia seen by this author, mild nuclear enlargement is observed in association with a chronic inflammatory infiltrate of the lamina propria (Fig. 4–8). Chronic oesophagitis, which may prove to be premalignant, could well be more common than previously believed. Cheli et al (1982) found chronic inflammation in biopsies of approximately 26 per cent of asymptomatic "Hungarian and Italian" subjects. The incidence was highest in the fifth and sixth decades of life.

RADIATION INDUCED OESOPHAGEAL CARCINOMA

With the increasingly successful use of radiation therapy for mediastinal malignancy and the resulting prolonged patient survival, reports of subsequent oeso-

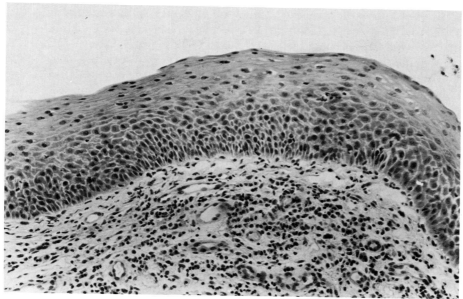

Figure 4–8. Oesophageal mucosa in pernicious anaemia. There is increased basal layer thickness and slight irregular nuclear enlargement most noticeable in the middle layer. A lymphoid infiltrate of the lamina propria is prominent (H & E × 250).

phageal radiation effect and subsequent malignancy have become increasingly common. (Morichau-Beauchant et al 1983, O'Connell, Seaman and Ghahremani 1984, Sherrill et al 1984, Ohta et al 1986). The evidence to date would indicate that this post-irradiation invasive carcinoma also develops via a progressively dysplastic phase, which has already been referred to.

DERMATOLOGICAL CONDITIONS

Although the oesophagus is affected by certain primarily dermatological entities, e.g., epidermolysis bullosa dystrophica, pemphigoid, pemphigus, bullous pemphigoid and toxic epidermal necrolysis, in the past reports of diagnosis based on oesophageal biopsy were few and only rarely was this made necessary when the oesophagus was affected in the absence of skin lesions (Wood, Patterson and Orlando 1982). However, reports of endoscopic biopsy diagnosis are becoming increasingly more common in cases of lichen planus (Lefer 1982), pemphigus vulgaris (Yamamoto et al 1983, Goldin and Lijovetzky 1985, Mobacken et al 1988), benign mucous membrane pemphigoid (Al-Kutoubi and Eliot 1984), Behçet's disease (Mori et al 1983, Anti et al 1986), Stevens-Johnson syndrome (Zweiban, Cohen and Chandrasoma 1986), lichen ruber (Van Maercke et al 1988) and bullous lesions associated with co-trimoxazole therapy (Heer et al 1985).

INTRAMURAL PSEUDODIVERTICULOSIS

This is a rare condition of unknown aetiology and is commonly diagnosed radiologically (Foxworthy 1985, Stephens et al 1986). Endoscopically the ostia may be visible, and biopsy may reveal the dilated excretory ducts of the oesophageal submucous glands, which are the basic pathological lesion in this condition (Hover et al 1982, Lax, Haroutiounian and Attia 1986). In a recent detailed autopsy study (Medeiros, Doos and Balogh 1988), chronic inflammatory changes around submucous glands and early pseudodiverticula formation were common findings, which suggests that chronic inflammation plays an aetiological role in this condition.

REFERENCES—SECTION ONE:
OESOPHAGEAL BIOPSY

Adami B., Eckardt V.F. and Paulini K. (1979) Sampling error and observer variation in the interpretation of esophageal biopsies. Digestion 19:404–410.

Agha F.P. (1984) Candidiasis-induced esophageal strictures. Gastrointestinal Radiology 9:283–286.

Agha F.P., Lee H.H. and Nostrant T.T. (1986) Herpetic esophagitis: a diagnostic challenge in immunocompromised patients. American Journal of Gastroenterology 81:246–253.

Agha F.P. and Wimbish K.J. (1984) Hirsute esophagus: clinical and roentgen features. Gastrointestinal Radiology 9:297–300.

Alexander J.A., Brouillette D.E., Chien M-C., Yoo Y-K., Tarter R.E., Gavaler J.S. and Van Thiel D.H. (1988) Infectious esophagitis following liver and renal transplantation. Digestive Diseases and Sciences 33:1121–1126.

Al-Kutoubi M.A. and Eliot C. (1984) Oesophageal involvement in benign mucous membrane pemphigoid. Clinical Radiology 35:131–135.

Allen J.I., Silvis S.E., Sumner H.W. and McClain C.J. (1981) Cytomegalic inclusion disease diagnosed endoscopically. Digestive Diseases and Sciences 26:133–135.

Al Yassin T.M. and Toner P.G. (1976) Langerhans cells in the human oesophagus. Journal of Anatomy 122:435–445.

Anti M., Marra G., Rapaccini G.L., Barone C., Manna R., Bochicchio G.B. and Fedeli G. (1986) Esophageal involvement in Behcet's syndrome. Journal of Clinical Gastroenterology 8:514–519.

Bambirra E.A., de Souza Andrade J., de Souza L.A.H., Savi A., Lima G.F. and de Oliveira C.A. (1983) Sebaceous glands in the esophagus. Gastrointestinal Endoscopy 29:251–252.

Barge J., Molas G., Maillard J.N., Fekete F., Bogomoletz W.V. and Potet F. (1981) Superficial oesophageal carcinoma: an oesophageal counterpart of early gastric cancer. Histopathology 5:499–510.

Barrett N.R. (1950) Chronic peptic ulcer of the oesophagus and "oesophagitis." British Journal of Surgery, 38:175–182.

Becouarn Y., Lamouliatte H. and Quinton A. (1983) Drug induced acute esophageal lesions. Gastroenterologie Clinique et Biologique 7:868–876.

Benasco C., Combalia N., Pou J.M. and Miquel J.M. (1985) Superficial esophageal carcinoma: a report of 12 cases. Gastrointestinal Endoscopy 31:64–67.

Bender M.D., Allison J., Cuartas F. and Montgomery C. (1973) Glycogenic acanthosis of the esophagus: a form of benign epithelial hyperplasia. Gastroenterology 65:373–380.

Boylston A.W., Cook H.T., Francis N.D. and Goldin R.D. (1987) Biopsy pathology of acquired immune deficiency syndrome (AIDS). Journal of Clinical Pathology 40:1–8.

Brand D.L., Ylvisaker J.T., Gelfand M. and Pope C.E. (1980) Regression of columnar esophageal (Barrett's) epithelium after anti-reflux surgery. The New England Journal of Medicine 302:844–848.

Bremner C.G., Lynch V.P. and Ellis F.H. Jr. (1970) Barrett's esophagus: congenital or acquired? An experimental study of esophageal mucosal regeneration in the dog. Surgery 68:209–216.

Brinson R.R., Schuman B.M., Mills L.R., Thigpen S. and Freedman S. (1987) Multiple squamous papillomas of the esophagus associated with Goltz syndrome. American Journal of Gastroenterology 82:1177–1179.

Brown L.F., Goldman H. and Antonioli D.A. (1984) Intraepithelial eosinophils in endoscopic biopsies of adults with reflux esophagitis. American Journal of Surgical Pathology 8:899–905.

Burrig K-F., Borchard F., Feiden W. and Pfitzer P. (1984) Herpes oesophagitis II. Electron microscopical findings. Virchows Archiv 404:177–185.

Byard R.W., Champion M.C. and Orizaga M. (1987) Variability in the clinical presentation and endoscopic findings of herpetic esophagitis. Endoscopy 19:153–155.

Cameron A.J. and Payne W.S. (1978) Barrett's esophagus occurring as a complication of scleroderma. Mayo Clinic Proceedings 53:612–615.

Carney C.N., Orlando R.C., Powell D.W. and Dotson M.M. (1981) Morphologic alterations in early acid-induced epithelial injury of the rabbit esophagus. Laboratory Investigation 45:198–208.

Catinella F.P. and Kittle C.F. (1988) Tuberculous esophagitis with aortic aneurysm fistula. Annals of Thoracic Surgery 45:87–88.

Chase R.A., Haber M.H., Pottage J.C., Schaffner J.A., Miller C. and Levin S. (1986) Tuberculous esophagitis with erosion into aortic aneurysm. Archives of Pathology and Laboratory Medicine *110*:965–966.

Cheli R., Simon L., Elster K. and Bocchini R. (1982) Oesophagitis in Italian and Hungarian asymptomatic subjects. Endoscopy *14*:1–3.

Cohen S. (1979) Motor disorders of the esophagus. The New England Journal of Medicine *301*:184–192.

Colina F., Solis J.A. and Munoz M.T. (1980) Squamous papilloma of the esophagus. American Journal of Gastroenterology *74*:410–414.

Collins F.J., Matthews H.R., Baker S.E. and Strakova J.M. (1979) Drug-induced oesophageal injury. British Medical Journal *1*:1673–1676.

Collins J.S.A., Watt P.C.H., Hamilton P.W., Collins B.J., Sloan J.M., Elliott H. and Love A.H.G. (1989) Assessment of oesophagitis by histology and morphometry. Histopathology *14*:381–389.

Cooper B.T. and Barbezat G.O. (1987) Barrett's oesophagus: a clinical study of 52 patients. Quarterly Journal of Medicine *62*:97–108.

Crespi M., Grassi A., Munoz N., Guo-Quing W. and Guanrei Y. (1984) Endoscopic features of suspected precancerous lesions in high-risk areas for esophageal cancer. Endoscopy *16*:85–91.

Crespi M., Munoz N., Grassi A., Aramesh B., Amiri G., Mojtabai A. and Casale V. (1979) Oesophageal lesions in northern Iran; a premalignant condition? Lancet *2*:217–221.

Dahms B.B., Greco M.A., Strandjord S.E. and Rothstein F.C. (1987) Barrett's esophagus in three children after antileukemia chemotherapy. Cancer *60*:2896–2900.

Davidson J.T. and Sawyers J.L. (1983) Crohn's disease of the esophagus. The American Surgeon *49*:168–172.

Depew W.T., Prentice R.S.A., Beck I.T., Blakeman J.M. and Da Costa L.R. (1977) Herpes simplex ulcerative esophagitis in a healthy subject. American Journal of Gastroenterology *68*:381–385.

Desigan G. and Schneider R.P. (1985) Herpes simplex esophagitis in healthy adults. Southern Medical Journal *78*:1135–1137.

DiPalma J.A. and Brady C.E. (1984) Herpex simplex esophagitis in a nonimmunosuppressed host with gastroesophageal reflux. Gastrointestinal Endoscopy *30*:24–25.

Dobbins J.W., Sheahan D.G. and Behar J. (1977) Eosinophilic gastroenteritis with oesophageal involvement. Gastroenterology *72*:1312–1316.

Dodds W.J., Hogan W.J., Helm J.F. and Dent J. (1981) Pathogenesis of reflux esophagitis. Gastroenterology *81*:376–394.

Dow C.J. (1981) Oesophageal tuberculosis: four cases. Gut *22*:234–236.

Dreyer L. (1980) The incidence of dysplasia and associated epithelial lesions in the oesophageal mucosa of South African blacks. South African Medical Journal *58*:406–408.

Eastridge C.E., Pate J.W. and Mann J.A. (1984) Lower esophageal ring: experience in treatment of 88 patients. Annals of Thoracic Surgery *37*:103–107.

Entwistle C.C. and Jacobs A. (1965) Histological findings in the Paterson-Kelly syndrome. Journal of Clinical Pathology *18*:408–413.

Feiden W., Borchard F., Burrig K-F. and Pfitzer P. (1984) Herpes oesophagitis I. Light microscopical and immunohistochemical investigations. Virchows Archiv *404*:167–176.

Fernandez-Rodriguez C.M., Badia-Figuerola N., del Arbol L.R., Fernandez-Seara J., Dominguez F. and Aviles-Ruiz J.F. (1986) Squamous papilloma of the esophagus: report of 6 cases with long-term follow-up in 4 patients. American Journal of Gastroenterology *81*:1059–1062.

Foxworthy V. (1985) Diffuse intramural pseudodiverticulosis of the oesophagus. British Journal of Clinical Practice *39*:449–450.

Freeman H.J., Shnitzka T.K., Piercey J.R.A. and Weinstein W.M. (1977) Cytomegalovirus infection of the gastrointestinal tract in a patient with late onset immunodeficiency syndrome. Gastroenterology *73*:1397.

Freson M., Kottler R.E. and Wright J.P. (1984) Crohn's disease of the oesophagus. S.A. Medical Journal *66*:417–418.

Funch-Jensen P., Kock K., Christensen L.A., Fallingborg J., Kjaergaard J.J., Andersen S.P. and Teglbjaerg P.S. (1986) Microscopic appearance of the esophageal mucosa in a consecutive series of patients submitted to upper endoscopy. Scandinavian Journal of Gastroenterology *21*:65–69.

Geboes K., De Wolf-Peeters C., Rutgeerts P., Janssens J., Vantrappen G. and Desmet V. (1983) Lymphocytes and Langerhans cells in the human oesophageal epithelium. Virchows Archiv (A) *401*:45–55.

Gill R.A., Gebhard R.L., Dozeman R.L. and Sumner H.W. (1984) Shingles esophagitis: endoscopic diagnosis in two patients. Gastrointestinal Endoscopy *30*:26–27.

Goldin E. and Lijovetzky G. (1985) Esophageal involvement by pemphigus vulgaris. American Journal of Gastroenterology *80*:828–830.

Gottfried E.B. and Goldberg H.J. (1985) Mucosal bridge of the distal esophagus after esophageal variceal sclerotherapy. Gastrointestinal Endoscopy *31*:267–269.

Greamer B., Andersen H.A. and Code C.F. (1956) Esophageal motility in patients with scleroderma and related diseases. Gastroenterologia *86*:763–775.

Haggitt R.C., Reid B.J., Rabinovitch P.S. and Rubin C.E. (1988) Barrett's esophagus. American Journal of Pathology *131*:53–61.

Hamilton S.R. and Smith R.R.L. (1987) The relationship between columnar epithelial dysplasia and invasive adenocarcinoma arising in Barrett's esophagus. American Journal of Clinical Pathology *87*:301–312.

Hamilton S.R. and Yardley J.H. (1977) Regeneration of cardiac type mucosa and acquisition of Barrett mucosa after esophagogastrostomy. Gastroenterology 72:669–675.

Haque A.K. and Merkel M. (1981) Total columnar-lined esophagus. Archives of Pathology and Laboratory Medicine 105:546–548.

Heer M., Altorfer J., Burger H-R. and Walti M. (1985) Bullous esophageal lesions due to co-trimoxazole: an immune-mediated process? Gastroenterology 88:1954–1957.

Hendrix T.R. and Yardley J.H. (1976) Consequences of gastro-oesophageal reflux. Clinics in Gastroenterology 5:155–174.

Herschman B.R., Uppaputhangkule V., Maas L. and Gelzayd E. (1978) Esophageal leukoplakia: a rare entity. Journal of the American Medical Association 239:2021.

Hille J.J., Margolius K.A., Markowitz S. and Isaacson C. (1986) Human papillomavirus infection related to oesophageal carcinoma in black South Africans. South African Medical Journal 69:417–420.

Ho C-S., Cullen J.B. and Gray R.R. (1977) An unusual manifestation of esophageal moniliasis. Radiology 123:287–288.

Hopwood D., Bateson M.C., Milne G. and Bouchier I.A.D. (1981) Effects of bile acids and hydrogen ion on the fine structure of oesophageal epithelium. Gut 22:306–311.

Hover A.R., Brady C.E., Williams J.R., Stewart D.L. and Christian C. (1982) Multiple retention cysts of the lower esophagus. Journal of Clinical Gastroenterology 4:209–212.

Huchzermeyer H., Paul F., Seifert E., Froehlich H. and Rasmussen Ch. W. (1976) Endoscopic results in five patients with Crohn's disease of the oesophagus. Endoscopy 8:75–81.

Hull P.R. (1979) Systemic histoplasmosis with oesophageal obstruction due to histoplasma granulomas. South African Medical Journal 55:639–640.

Ismail-Beigi F., Horton P.F. and Pope C.E. (1970) Histological consequences of gastrooesophageal reflux in man. Gastroenterology 58:163–174.

Jabbari M., Goresky C.A., Lough J., Yaffe C., Daly D. and Cote C. (1985) The inlet patch: heterotopic gastric mucosa in the upper esophagus. Gastroenterology 89:352–356.

Jacobs A. (1962) Post-cricoid carcinoma in patients with pernicious anaemia. British Medical Journal 3:91–92

Janisch H.D. and Eckardt V.F. (1982) Histological abnormalities in patients with multiple esophageal webs. Digestive Diseases and Sciences 27:503–506.

Janisch H.D., Pfannkuch F., von Kleist D., Degenhardt U., Bauer E. and Hampel K.E. (1984) Histologic abnormalities in routine biopsies of patients with esophagitis and different gastric acid secretion. Applied Pathology 2:272–276.

Jarvis L.R., Dent J. and Whitehead R. (1985) Morphometric assessment of reflux oesophagitis in fibreoptic biopsy specimens. Journal of Clinical Pathology 38:44–48.

Jass J.R. (1981) Mucin histochemistry of the columnar epithelium of the oesophagus: a retrospective study. Journal of Clinical Pathology 34:866–870.

Jass J.R. and Filipe M.I. (1981) The mucin profiles of normal gastric mucosa, intestinal metaplasia and its variants and gastric carcinoma. Histochemical Journal 13:931–939.

Javdan P. and Pitman E.R. (1984) Squamous papilloma of esophagus. Digestive Diseases and Sciences 29:317–320.

Kalogeropoulos N.K. and Whitehead R. (1988) Campylobacter-like organisms and candida in peptic ulcers and similar lesions of the upper gastrointestinal tract: a study of 247 cases. Journal of Clinical Pathology 41:1093–1098.

Keeffe E.B., Hisken E.C. and Schubert F. (1986) Adenomatous polyp arising in Barrett's esophagus. Journal of Clinical Gastroenterology 8:271–274.

Kikuchi K., Suga T., Senoue I., Nomiyama T., Miwa M. and Miwa T. (1982) Esophageal ulceration in a patient with Behcet's syndrome. Tokai Journal of Experimental and Clinical Medicine 7:135–143.

King D.H. (1964) Intraoral leukoplakia? Cancer 17:131–136.

Knohe M. and Bernhardt H. (1980) Endoscopic aspects of mycosis in the upper digestive tract. Endoscopy 12:295–298

Kodsi B.E., Wickremesinghe P.C., Kozinn P.J., Iswara K. and Goldberg P.K. (1976) Candida esophagitis. Gastroenterology 71:715–719.

Korula J. (1985) Pseudotumor of the esophagus: an unusual complication of esophageal variceal sclerotherapy. American Journal of Gastroenterology 80:954–956.

Laajam M.A. (1984) Primary tuberculosis of the esophagus: pseudotumoral presentation. American Journal of Gastroenterology 79:839–841.

Lax J.D., Haroutiounian G. and Attia A. (1986) An unusual case of dysphagia: esophageal intramural pseudodiverticulosis. American Journal of Gastroenterology 81:1002–1004.

Lee J-H., Neumann D.A. and Welsh J.D. (1977) Disseminated histoplasmosis presenting with esophageal symptomatology. The American Journal of Digestive Diseases 22:831–834.

Lee R.G. (1985) Marked eosinophilia in esophageal mucosal biopsies. American Journal of Surgical Pathology 9:475–479.

Lefer L.G. (1982) Lichen planus of the esophagus. The American Journal of Dermatopathology 4:267–269.

Levine D.S., Reid B.J., Haggitt R.C., Rubin C.E. and Rabinovitch P.S. (1989) Correlation of ultrastructural aberrations with dysplasia and flow cytometric abnormalities in Barrett's epithelium. Gastroenterology 96:355–367.

LiVolsi V.A. and Jaretzki A. (1973) Granulomatous oesophagitis: a case of Crohn's disease limited to the oesophagus. Gastroenterology 64:313–319.

Llaneza P.P., Menendez A.M. and Dunn G.D. (1987) Hairy esophagus contributing to dysphagia. Gastrointestinal Endoscopy 33:331–332.

McDonald G.B., Brand D.L. and Thorning D.R. (1977) Multiple adenomatous neoplasms arising in columnar-lined (Barrett's) eosophagus. Gastroenterology 72:1317–1321.

McDonald G.B., Sullivan K.M., Schuffler M.D., Shulman H.M. and Thomas E.D. (1981) Esophageal abnormalities in chronic graft-vs-host disease in humans. Gastroenterology 80:914–921

McKay J.S. and Day D.W. (1983) Herpes simplex oesophagitis. Histopathology 7:409–420.

McKenzie R. and Khakoo R. (1985) Blastomycosis of the esophagus presenting with gastrointestinal bleeding. Gastroenterology 88:1271–1273.

Mandard A.M., Marnay J., Gignoux M., Segol P., Blanc L., Ollivier J.M., Borel B. and Mandard J.C. (1984) Cancer of the esophagus and associated lesions. Human Pathology 15:660–669.

Mandard A.M., Tourneux J., Gignoux M., Blanc L., Segol P. and Mandard J.C. (1980) In situ carcinoma of the esophagus: macroscopic study with particular reference to the Lugol test. Endoscopy 12:51–57.

Mathieson R. and Dutta S.K. (1983) Candida esophagitis. Digestive Diseases and Sciences 28:365–370.

Medeiros L.J., Doos W.G. and Balogh K. (1988) Esophageal intramural pseudodiverticulosis. Human Pathology 19:928–931.

Meuwissen S.G.M., Bosma A., van Donk E., Waalewijn R., Pals G., Pronk J.C., Eriksson A.W., Mullink H. and Meijer C.J.L.M. (1988) Immunohistochemical localization of pepsinogen A and C containing cells in Barrett's oesophagus. Virchows Archiv 413:11–16.

Meyer W., Vollmar F. and Baer W. (1979) Barrett-esophagus following total gastrectomy. Endoscopy 2:121–126.

Miller D.P. and Everett E.D. (1979) Gastrointestinal histoplasmosis. Journal of Clinical Gastroenterology 1:233–236

Ming S.C., Goldman H. and Freiman D.G. (1967) Intestinal metaplasia and histogenesis of carcinoma of the human stomach. Cancer 20:1418–1429.

Mobacken H., Al Karawi M., Mohamed A. and Coode P. (1988) Oesophageal pemphigus vulgaris. Dermatologica 176:266–269.

Mori S., Yoshihira A., Kawamura H., Takeuchi A., Hashimoto T. and Inaba G. (1983) Esophageal involvement in Behcet's disease. American Journal of Gastroenterology 78:548–553.

Morichau-Beauchant M., Touchard G., Battandier D., Maire P., Fontanel J-P., Daban A., Babin P. and Matuchansky C. (1983) Chronic radiation esophagitis after treatment of carcinoma of the oropharynx: a poorly recognized entity. Gastroenterologie Clinique et Biologique 7:843–850.

Morris H. and Price S. (1986) Langerhans' cells, papillomaviruses and oesophageal carcinoma. South African Medical Journal 69:413–417.

Munoz N., Crespi M., Grassi A., Qing W.G., Qiong S. and Cai L.Z. (1982) Precursor lesions of oesophageal cancer in high-risk populations in Iran and China. Lancet 1:876–879.

Naef A.P., Savary M., Ozzello L. and Pearson F.G. (1975) Columnar-lined lower esophagus: an acquired lesion with malignant predisposition. Journal of Thoracic Cardiovascular Surgery 70:826–835.

Nishikai M., Asaba G. and Homma M. (1977) Rheumatoid esophageal disease. American Journal of Gastroenterology 67:29–33.

Obrecht W.F., Richter J.E., Olympio G.A. and Gelfand D.W. (1984) Tracheoesophageal fistula: a serious complication of infectious esophagitis. Gastroenterology 87:1174–1179.

O'Connell E.W., Seaman W.B. and Ghahremani G.G. (1984) Radiation-induced esophageal carcinoma. Gastrointestinal Radiology 9:287–291.

Oettle G.J., Paterson A.C., Leiman G. and Segal I. (1986) Esophagitis in a population at risk for esophageal carcinoma. Cancer 57:2222–2229.

Ohta H., Nakazawa S., Segawa K., and Yoshino J. (1986) Distribution of epithelial dysplasia in the cancerous esophagus. Scandinavian Journal of Gastroenterology 21:392–398.

Orringer M.B. and Sloan H. (1978) Monilial esophagitis: an increasingly frequent cause of esophageal stenosis? Annals of Thoracic Surgery 26:364–374.

Pascal R. R. and Clearfield H. R. (1987) Mucoepidermoid (adenosquamous) carcinoma arising in Barrett's esophagus. Digestive Diseases and Sciences 32:428–432.

Patrick W.J.A., Denham D. and Forrest A.P.M. (1974) Mucous change in the human duodenum: a light and electron microscopic study and correlation with disease and gastric acid secretion. Gut 15:767–776.

Pepe G., Pepe F., Cali V., Sanfilippo G. and Pecorella G. (1985) Crohn's disease of the esophagus. A case report. The Italian Journal of Surgical Sciences 15:369–371.

Petru A. and Azimi P.H. (1984) Esophagitis associated with candida infection in a neonate. Clinical Pediatrics 23:179–181.

Porro G.B., Parente F. and Cernuschi M. (1989) The diagnosis of esophageal candidiasis in patients with acquired immune deficiency syndrome: is endoscopy always necessary? American Journal of Gastroenterology 84:143–146.

Prior A. and Whorwell P.J. (1986) Familial Barrett's oesophagus? Hepato-gastroenterology 33:86–87.

Raeburn C. (1951) Columnar ciliated epithelium in the adult oesophagus. Journal of Pathology and Bacteriology 63:157–159.

Raine C.H. (1983) Ectopic gastric mucosa in the upper esophagus as a cause of dysphagia. Annals of Otology, Rhinology and Laryngology 92:65–66.

Rector L.E. and Connerley M.I. (1941) Aberrant mucosa in the esophagus in infants and children. Archives of Pathology and Laboratory Medicine 31:285–294.

Reid B.J., Haggitt R.C., Rubin C.E. and Rabinovitch P.S. (1987) Barrett's esophagus. Gastroenterology 93:1–11.

Reid B.J., Weinstein W.M., Lewin K.L., Haggitt R.C., Van Deventer G., Den Besten L. and Rubin C.E. (1988a) Endoscopic biopsy can detect high-grade dysplasia or early adenocarcinoma in Barrett's esophagus without grossly recognizable neoplastic lesions. Gastroenterology 94:81–90.

Reid B.J., Haggitt R.C., Rubin C.E., Roth G., Surawicz C.M., Van Belle G., Lewin K., Weinstein W.M.. Antonioli D.A., Goldman H., MacDonald W. and Owen D. (1988b) Observer variation in the diagnosis of dysplasia in Barrett's esophagus. Human Pathology 19:166–178.

Remmele W. and Engelsing B. (1984) Lipid island of the esophagus. Endoscopy 16:240–241.

Rindi G., Bishop A.E., Daly M.J., Isaacs P., Lee F.I. and Polak J.M. (1987) A mixed pattern of endocrine cells in metaplastic Barrett's oesophagus. Histochemistry 87:377–383.

Rotterdam H. and Sommers S.C. (1981) In: Biopsy Diagnosis of the Digestive Tract. New York: Raven Press, 1981 p. 13.

Rubio C.A. and Riddell R. (1988) Musculo-fibrous anomaly in Barrett's mucosa with dysplasia. American Journal of Surgical Pathology 12:885–889.

Sablich R., Benedetti G., Bignucolo S. and Serraino D. (1988) Squamous cell papilloma of the esophagus. Endoscopy 20:5–7.

Saladin T.A., French A.B., Zarafonetis C.J.D. and Pollard H.M.(1966) Esophageal motor abnormalities in scleroderma and related diseases. American Journal of Digestive Diseases 11:522–535.

Salgado J.A., Filho J. de S. A., Lima G.F. Jr., Savi A., Fonseca L.M.A. and de Oliveira C.A. (1980) Sebaceous glands in the esophagus. Gastrointestinal Endoscopy 26:150.

Salo J.A., Lehto V-P. and Kivilaakso E. (1983) Morphological alterations in experimental esophagitis. Light microscopic and scanning and transmission electron microscopic study. Digestive Diseases and Sciences 28:440–448.

Sampliner R.E., Steinbronn K., Garewal H.S. and Riddell R.H. (1988) Squamous mucosa overlying columnar epithelium in Barrett's esophagus in the absence of anti-reflux surgery. American Journal of Gastroenterology 83:510–512.

Schneider H.A., Yonker R.A., Longley S., Katz P., Mathias J. and Panush R.S. (1984) Scleroderma esophagus: a nonspecific entity. Annals of Internal Medicine 100:848–850.

Schroeder W.W., Myer C.M. and Schechter G.L. (1987) Ectopic gastric mucosa in the cervical esophagus. Laryngoscope 97:131–135.

Schuffler M.D. and Pope C.E. II (1976) Esophageal motor dysfunction in idiopathic intestinal pseudo-obstruction. Gastroenterology 70:677–682.

Scott B.B. and Jenkins D. (1982) Gastro-oesophageal candidiasis. Gut 23:137–139.

Seefeld U., Krejs G.J., Siebenmann R.E. and Blum A.L. (1977) Esophageal histology in gastrooesophageal reflux. American Journal of Digestive Diseases 22:956–964.

Seifert E., Borst H.H., Ostertag H., Stender H. St., Braschke M., Misaki F. and Atay Z. (1973) Carcinoma in situ of the esophagus (early esophageal cancer). Endoscopy 5:147–153.

Seivewright N., Feehally J. and Wicks A.C.B. (1984) Primary tuberculosis of the esophagus. American Journal of Gastroenterology 79:842–843.

Shah K.K., DeRidder P.H. and Shah K.K. (1986) Ectopic gastric mucosa in proximal esophagus. Journal of Clinical Gastroenterology 8:509–513.

Sherrill D.J., Grishkin B.A., Galal F.S., Zajtchuk R. and Graeber G.M. (1984) Radiation associated malignancies of the esophagus. Cancer 54:726–728.

Siegel C.I. and Hendrix T.R. (1963) Oesophageal motor abnormalities induced by acid perfusion in patients with heartburn. Journal of Clinical Investigation 42:686–695.

Stadelmann O., Elster K. and Kuhn H.A. (1981) Columnar-lined oesophagus (Barrett's syndrome): congenital or acquired? Endoscopy 13:140–147.

Steadman C., Kerlin P., Teague C. and Stephenson P. (1988) High esophageal stricture: a complication of "inlet patch" mucosa. Gastroenterology 94:521–524.

Stephens W.P., Mossman A., Ratcliffe J.F., Gould D.A. and Oleesky S. (1986) Intramural pseudodi-verticulosis: an unusual cause of benign oesophageal stricture. Postgraduate Medical Journal 62:201–204.

Stern Z., Sharon P., Ligumsky M., Levij I.S. and Rachmilewitz D. (1980) Glycogenic acanthosis of the esophagus. American Journal of Gastroenterology 74:261–263.

Tateishi R., Taniguchi H., Wada A., Horai T. and Taniguchi K. (1974) Argyrophil cells and melanocytes in esophageal mucosa. Archives of Pathology 98:87–89.

Thompson J.J., Zinsser K.R. and Enterline H.T. (1983) Barrett's metaplasia and adenocarcinoma of the esophagus and gastroesophageal junction. Human Pathology 14:42–61.

Tishler J.M.A. and Helman C.A. (1984) Crohn's disease of the esophagus. Journal of Canadian Association of Radiologists 35:28–30.

Toet A.E., Dekker W., Op den Orth J.O. and Blok P. (1985) Squamous cell papilloma of the esophagus: report of 4 cases. Gastrointestinal Endoscopy 31:77–79.

Trier J.S. (1970) Morphology of the epithelium of the distal esophagus in patients with midesophageal peptic strictures. Gastroenterology 58:444–461.

Truong L.D., Stroehlein J.R. and McKechnie J.C. (1986) Gastric heterotopia of the proximal esophagus: a report of 4 cases detected by endoscopy and review of the literature. American Journal of Gastroenterology *81*:1162–1166.

Tummala V., Barwick K.W., Sontag S.J., Vlahcevic R.Z. and McCallum R.W. (1987) The significance of intraepithelial eosinophils in the histologic diagnosis of gastroesophageal reflux. American Journal of Clinical Pathology *87*:43–48.

Van Maercke Ph., Gunther M., Groth W., Gheorghiu Th. and Habermann U. (1988) Lichen ruber mucosae with esophageal involvement. Endoscopy *20*:158–160.

Villar L.A., Massanari R.M. and Mitros F.A. (1984) Cytomegalovirus infection with acute erosive esophagitis. The American Journal of Medicine *76*:924–928.

Volpicelli N.A., Yardley J.H. and Hendrix T.R. (1975) A histopathologic demonstration of the association between gastritis and reflux esophagitis. Gastroenterology *68*:1007.

Walker J.H. (1978) Giant papilloma of the thoracic esophagus. American Journal of Roentgenology *131*:519–520.

Walsh T.J., Belitsos N.J. and Hamilton S.R. (1986) Bacterial esophagitis in immunocompromised patients. Archives of Internal Medicine *146*:1345–1348.

Wang G-Q. (1981) Endoscopic diagnosis of early oesophageal carcinoma. Journal of the Royal Society of Medicine *74*:502–503.

Wang M.M.J., Spear M. and McGrew W. (1986) Heterotopic gastric mucosa of the esophagus. Southern Medical Journal *79*:633–635.

Waterfall W.E., Somers S. and Desa D.J. (1978) Benign oesophageal papillomatosis. Journal of Clinical Pathology *31*:111–115.

Weinstein W.M., Bogoch E.R. and Bowes K.L. (1975) The normal human esophageal mucosa: a histological reappraisal. Gastroenterology *68*:40–44.

Weller I.V.D. (1985) AIDS and the gut. Scandinavian Journal of Gastroenterology *20*(suppl. 114):77–89.

Wilkins W.E., Ridley M.G. and Pozniak A.L. (1984) Benign stricture of the oesophagus: role of non-steroidal anti-inflammatory drugs. Gut *25*:478–480.

Winkler B., Capo V., Reumann W., Ma A., la Porta R., Reilly S., Green P.M.R., Richart R.M. and Crum C.P. (1985) Human papillomavirus infection of the esophagus. Cancer *55*:149–155.

Winter H.S., Madara J.L., Stafford R.J., Grand R.J., Quinlan J-E. and Goldman H. (1982) Intraepithelial eosinophils: a new diagnostic criterion for reflux esophagitis. Gastroenterology *83*:818–823.

Wood D.R., Patterson J.B. and Orlando R.C. (1982) Pemphigus vulgaris of the esophagus. Annals of Internal Medicine *96*:189–191.

Yamamoto H., Kozawa Y., Otake S. and Shimokawa R. (1983) Pemphigus vulgaris involving the mouth and esophagus. International Journal of Oral Surgery *12*:194–200.

Zamost B.J., Hirschberg J., Ippoliti A.F., Furst D.E., Clements P.J. and Weinstein W.M. (1987) Esophagitis in scleroderma. Prevalence and risk factors. Gastroenterology *92*:421–428.

Zweiban B., Cohen H. and Chandrasoma P. (1986) Gastrointestinal involvement complicating Stevens-Johnson syndrome. Gastroenterology *91*:469–474.

Gastric Biopsy

NORMAL APPEARANCES IN GASTRIC BIOPSY SPECIMENS

The pyloric glands occupy a roughly triangular area in the lower third of the stomach. On the greater curve they occupy the immediate pyloric region, but on the lesser curve the upper limit, although commonly held to be in the region of the incisura angularis, is quite variable and rarely extends to the oesophagus. The cardiac glands are found distal to the cardio-oesophageal junction for a distance of about 1 cm, and the remaining mucosa is of body type. The junction between the three areas may be abrupt but is often occupied by a narrow transitional zone. At the pylorus-body junction in the lesser curve region the width of the transitional zone is variable, and rarely the whole lesser curve shows a transitional appearance.

Transitional zones also occur where the cardiac mucosa abuts the oesophagus and where the antral mucosa abuts the duodenum. At the former site the transition is usually abrupt, although in the gross it takes the form of the irregular or serrated so-called Z line. The transition zone between gastric and duodenal mucosae also tends to be serrated and up to 3 mm wide, but beyond this for another 3 mm a mucosa with mixed histological features may also be seen. In this, adjacent villi may be covered by antral type superficial epithelium or small bowel type epithelium in a varying mix (Lawson 1988).

BODY MUCOSA (Fig. 5–1)

Throughout the stomach the superficial epithelium is composed of a single layer of cells with a basal nucleus below a typical cup-shaped column of clear or faintly granular mucin. Occasionally one sees an intraepithelial lymphocyte that has insinuated itself between adjacent epithelial cells. The surface epithelium dips to form shallow gastric pits, into which open approximately four gastric glands. These are simple straight tubules, tightly packed together, roughly the same length, which occupy three quarters of the thickness of the mucosa. Most cells lining the upper part of the glands are parietal cells. These are eosinophilic and triangular with a central nucleus. Their longest side is applied to the basement membrane, and sometimes intracellular canaliculi are visible. At the junction of the glands with the pits, scattered among the parietal cells and sometimes deeper,

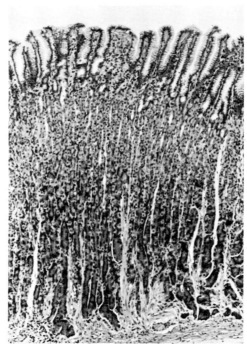

Figure 5–1. Normal body mucosa. Note regular superficial epithelium, short gastric pits, predominance of parietal cells in upper half and chief cells in lower half of tubules (H & E × 75).

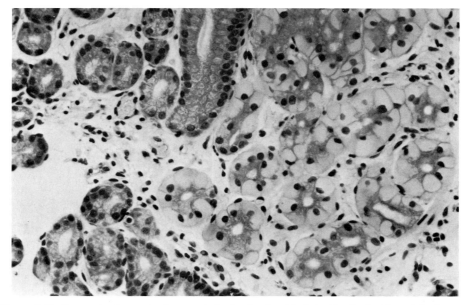

Figure 5–2. Oncocytic change in the gastric body gland epithelial cells. An incidental finding more common in old age (H & E × 350).

there are the mucin-secreting neck cells which, like the superficial epithelium, contain PAS-positive and diastase-resistant mucin. The lower half of the glands contains the chief cells, which mingle with the parietal cells in the region of the middle third. Chief cells have a basal nucleus and a cytoplasm filled with basophilic pepsinogen granules. The degree of basophilia of the granules varies from biopsy to biopsy. Sometimes in old age, gastric body gland cells show a focal cytoplasmic eosinophilic appearance similar to that which occurs in other glandular tissues and is usually referred to as oncocytic change (Fig. 5–2).

Occasionally, towards the base there is an argentaffin (enterochromaffin) cell. Rarely are the basal parts of the tubules cystic (Fig. 5–3), but the flattened cells always retain their special staining characteristics. An extreme form of this change that produces elevations of the mucosa is referred to later. However, this is in contrast to the cystic change that occurs in Menetrier's disease, in which the cysts are invariably larger and associated with abnormalities of the muscularis mucosa (see later).

The lamina propria is most obvious between the gastric pits where it contains a small number of plasma cells, lymphocytes, eosinophils and histiocytes, together with a fine capillary plexus and non-myelinated nerves. Owen (1986) has claimed that in normal gastric mucosa lymphatic capillaries are present in the superficial lamina propria and extend downwards between the gland tubules to form a plexus just superficial to the muscularis mucosae, which then drains into large lymphatics in the submucosa. However, in a combined light microscopic, electron microscopic and immunohistochemical study Listrom and Fenoglio-Preiser (1987) have shown that in normal mucosa the upper two thirds and the lamina propria are normally devoid of lymphatics. In such circumstances the ability of intramucosal gastric carcinoma to metastasize (Bogomoletz 1984) becomes difficult to understand. However, in mucosa that exhibits atrophic gastritis and is thin, lymphatic channels do in fact reach the surface. Because gastric cancer often arises in a background of atrophic gastritis the access of malignant cells to lymphatics is thus understandable.

There are no objective guidelines as to what constitutes a normal number of cells in the lamina propria. This, of course, is only a reflection of the difficulty,

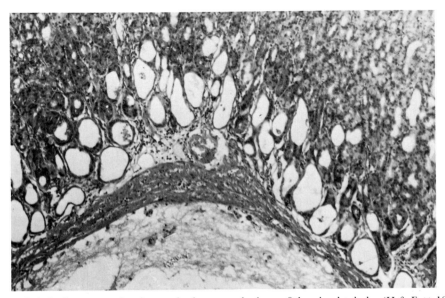

Figure 5–3. Body mucosa showing cystic change at the base of the gland tubules (H & E × 188).

firstly, in defining a normal population and secondly, in acquiring biopsy specimens from such a group. Illustration of this is seen in the study of Myren and Serck-Hanssen (1975), who found what they subjectively considered to be an increase in inflammatory infiltration in the interfoveolar lamina propria of four antral, three lesser curve and two greater curve biopsies from ten healthy medical student volunteers. At intervals along the mucosa the muscularis mucosa sends infrequent groups of smooth muscle fibres upwards between the glands. In reticulin preparations (Fig. 5–4) the basement membrane of the surface epithelium, pits and glands appears as a single layer of fibres, between which a delicate mesh of strands represents the supporting connective tissues between and in relation to the capillaries. The sharp division between the reticulin pattern of the lamina propria and the denser network around the fibres and vessels of the muscularis mucosa is broken only by occasional tent-shaped skeins of fibres that surround the upward muscularis prolongations.

PYLORIC MUCOSA (Fig. 5–5)

Here the gastric pits are deeper and sometimes branched, and the glands are shorter and less tightly packed than in the body, ending at different levels and occupying one half or less of the mucosal thickness. They are simple or branched coiled tubules, composed of mucin-secreting cells and occasional parietal cells (Fig. 5–6), especially near transitional zones. The incidence and distribution of parietal

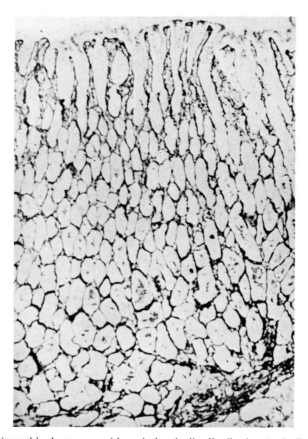

Figure 5–4. Normal body mucosa with typical reticulin distribution (reticulin stain × 102).

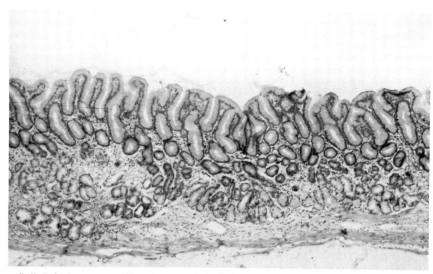

Figure 5–5. Pyloric mucosa. The pits are relatively long and some branch; they occupy one half the thickness of the mucosa. The glands are of simple mucin-producing type (H & E × 75).

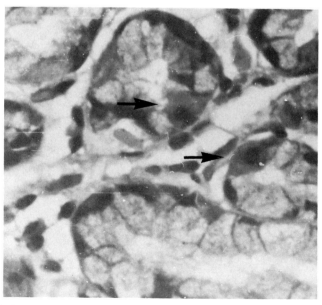

Figure 5–6. Pyloric mucosa. Occasional parietal cells in otherwise typical mucin-producing pyloric glands (arrows) (H & E × 400).

cells in antral mucosa were studied in an autopsy series by Tominaga (1975). Parietal cells were found in 98.3 per cent of patients ranging in age from newborn to elderly, and were considered to be a normal constituent of antral mucosa and not due to either metaplasia or dystopia. Very infrequently an isolated zone of chief cells may also be seen (Fig. 5–7).

Argentaffin cells are more frequent in this area of the gastric mucosa. They have a nucleus near the lumen of the gland and a strongly eosinophilic cytoplasm due to granules just too small to be resolved by the light microscope (Fig. 5–8). The interdigitation of fibres from the muscularis mucosa is more marked and there is more intertubular reticulin, so that the pattern is quite distinctive (Fig. 5–9).

CARDIAC MUCOSA (Fig. 5–10)

Cardiac mucosa is essentially similar to the pyloric mucosa except that the glands are even less tightly packed together. As a rule, parietal cells and argentaffin cells are absent. A characteristic feature is the presence of one or more dilated or cystic glands with a thin epithelial wall.

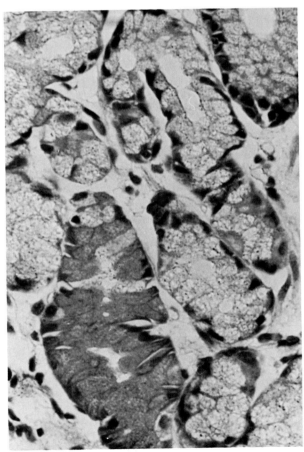

Figure 5–7. Pyloric mucosa. In addition to scattered parietal cells in other tubules, one tubule is filled predominantly with chief cells (H & E × 375).

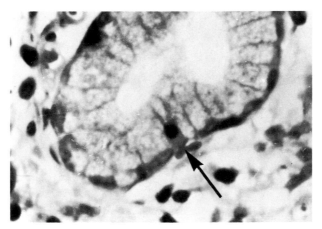

Figure 5–8. Pyloric gland, argentaffin cell (arrow). Note that nucleus is nearer to the lumen of the tubule than to the basement membrane (H & E × 500).

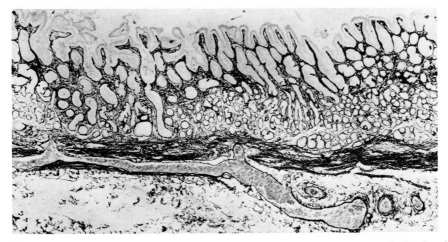

Figure 5–9. Pyloric mucosa. Distinctive reticulin pattern with more intertubular reticulin than in the body mucosa (reticulin stain × 42).

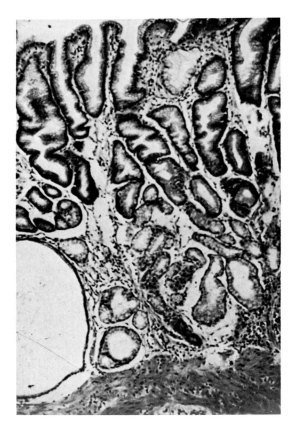

Figure 5–10. Cardiac mucosa. Like the pyloric mucosa the pits occupy one half of its thickness. The cystic gland is typical (H & E × 85).

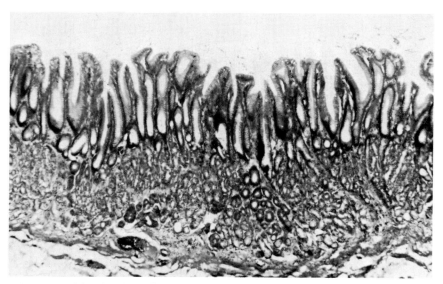

Figure 5–11. Transitional mucosa, from region of junction of body with pyloric area (H & E × 75).

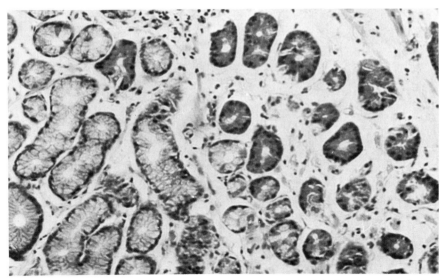

Figure 5–12. Detail of Figure 5–11 showing both pyloric (left) and body (right) glands (H & E × 150).

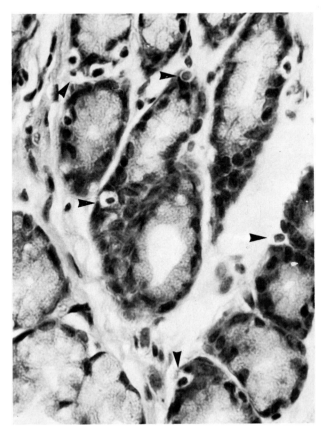

Figure 5–13. Pyloric mucosa. Note the numerous clear cells (arrowheads) (H & E × 300).

TRANSITIONAL MUCOSA (Figs. 5–11 and 5–12)

Transitional mucosa is composed of both body and pyloric or cardiac type glands. Like pyloric and cardiac mucosa the pits occupy about one half of the mucosal thickness.

Electron microscopic, histochemical and immunological studies have shown that in addition to argentaffin cells several other endocrine polypeptide cells are present in the gastric mucosa (Dawson 1970, Pearse et al 1970), but the characterisation of this complex system of cell types is still the subject of investigation.

In ordinary haematoxylin and eosin preparations many of the non-argentaffin endocrine cells appear as clear cells or halo cells (Fig. 5–13). The gastrin-producing cell of the antrum belongs to this group and constitutes some 50 per cent of the endocrine cells in this site.

Approximately 30 per cent of clear cells produce serotonin and 15 per cent produce somatostatin. In body mucosa the major portion of endocrine cells belong to the so-called enterochromaffin-like (ECL) group and secrete histamine, bombesin and vasoactive intestinal peptide. Others secrete serotonin and in some, identified by a variety of histochemical techniques, the secretions produced remain to be identified. Thus the list of hormones secreted by these cells in the gastric mucosa, as elsewhere in the gut, is growing rapidly. A comprehensive account of the gut hormone system is to be found in a multiauthor publication edited by Bloom and Polak (1981) and more recently has also been described by Falkmer and Wilander (1989). What is also being increasingly appreciated is that, with intestinalisation of the gastric mucosa due to metaplasia, new endocrine cell types also appear (Mingazzini et al 1984). Another cell type occasionally described in the gastric mucosa is the fibrillovesicular cell, or tuft cell, but it is only identified in electron microscopic studies (Wattel and Geuze 1978, Blom 1984).

GASTRITIS

6

It has been usual to subdivide gastritis into acute and chronic forms. However, accurate information is meagre concerning the mucosal histology of the putative "acute gastritis," referring to the symptom complex associated with alcohol and food overindulgence, drug ingestion and viral infections. It is only since the use of fibreoptic biopsy instruments that the spectrum of these changes has been better delineated. As a result many of the lesions produced by ingestion of certain drugs would be more accurately described as acute haemorrhagic erosions rather than acute gastritis.

The capacity of the gastric mucosa to withstand the deleterious effects of its own secretions is probably the result of several interacting phenomena that effectively constitute a mucosal barrier (Rees and Turnberg 1982, Rees 1987). All has yet to be revealed, but some of the mechanisms involved are its capacity for regeneration, factors that control its blood flow, its ability to maintain a luminal mucus layer and to secrete bicarbonate, the protective effect of prostaglandins and epidermal growth factors. Presumably any one or a combination of several circumstances that tend to interfere with this complex barrier may precipitate mucosal self-injury, which is manifested by superficial necrosis and haemorrhage. Cell death may be followed by an inflammatory reaction, so that, by a common pathway, an acute gastric inflammation is a predictable course of events following tissue damage initiated by several different means. In experimental animals there is ample evidence for the induction of mucosal injury by alcohol, aspirin and other non-steroidal anti-inflammatory drugs (NSAIDs), bile, pancreatic juice and a variety of stresses that induce a decreased mucosal blood flow.

It has also become evident of late that all chronic gastritis is not the same. Although there are histological similarities, there are clear pathophysiological differences between the chronic inflammation that accompanies a chronic erosion and the lesion of pernicious anaemia. Both are aetiologically different from the chronic gastritis associated with increasing age, and all are different in some ways from that which is associated with peptic ulcer. Latterly we have also seen claims for separate entities such as various forms of chronic erosive gastritis, lymphocytic gastritis, and the gastritis associated with campylobacter infestation. Thus the diverse disease processes that fall under the general heading of gastritis are becoming better delineated, and there is no doubt that further advances in our understanding of the inflammatory states of the gastric mucosa have yet to be made.

ACUTE (GASTRITIS) MUCOSAL INJURY

Clearly the gastric mucosa will be injured by a variety of chemicals and strong acids and alkalis. One case even reports extensive damage due to a saline emetic (Calam, Krasner and Haqqani 1982). In circumstances when these agents are inadvertently ingested, a variety of histological lesions results, ranging from hyperaemia and surface erosion to more massive mucosal necrosis and sloughing with or without secondary haemorrhage. The occasion rarely arises when these changes are seen in biopsy specimens, and our information is based upon findings in surgical and autopsy material. In milder forms of injury the initial lesion will stimulate an acute inflammatory reaction so that if resolution occurs at some stage an acute gastritis will, in fact, be seen. Furthermore, acute injuries may be superimposed on a mucosa showing chronic inflammatory changes.

Acute mucosal damage is induced by external x-ray therapy for peptic ulceration. Two weeks after treatment there is a patchy but severe coagulative necrosis with subsequent secondary inflammatory infiltration (Goldgraber et al 1954) and a tendency to revert to normal after about four months. After intragastric irradiation, however, permanent and histologically characteristic tissue damage occurs with ulceration, fibrosis and obliterative vascular hyalinisation (Fruin, Littman and Littman 1963, Berthrong and Fajardo 1981).

The majority of instances of acute mucosal injury in the form of haemorrhages or haemorrhagic erosions are due to the ingestion of aspirin or other NSAIDs (Pemberton and Strand 1979, Laine and Weinstein 1988a). In a group of healthy volunteers, Hoftiezer, O'Laughlin and Ivey (1982) have shown that this is true of aspirin even if buffered and when used in recommended daily doses. Aspirin and related drugs probably act by damaging the mucosal barrier; this is reviewed by Silen (1985), who highlighted that this barrier is a complex physiological mechanism involving mucosal blood flow and events involving local acid and alkaline metabolites. Salicylates accelerate epithelial cell turnover (Croft 1963), cause back diffusion of acid (Davenport 1967), and in common with many NSAIDs inhibit prostaglandin synthesis. Prostaglandins and epidermal growth factor are known to be cytoprotective for the gastric mucosa in a variety of experimental situations (Konturek et al 1981, Lacy and Ito 1982, Rainsford and Willis 1982). The overall result is to produce haemorrhagic erosions (Lanza 1984). These are not infrequently the cause of acute intragastric bleeding and are commonly visualised endoscopically though rarely biopsied (Figs. 6–1, 6–2). Sometimes aspirin-induced erosion and haemorrhage is diffuse, and urgent radical surgery is indicated. In the excised specimen histological examination reveals loss of the superficial epithelium and upper gastric pits with a diffuse haemorrhage into the upper layers of the mucosa (Fig. 6–3). This so-called acute haemorrhagic gastritis is sometimes the result of stress when ulceration in the form of either multiple erosions or as a diffuse lesion occurs mainly in the body of the stomach. It may be seen after major surgery or trauma (Flowers, Kyle and Hoerr 1970), sepsis, burns or head injury and is probably related to a reduced mucosal blood flow (Skillman and Silen 1972, Miller 1987) and tissue acidosis (Silen 1987).

Apart from diffuse lesions that necessitate surgery, evidence suggests that most acute mucosal erosions will heal completely, leaving a normal mucosa, but may be biopsied when the lesion is only partially resolved (Fig. 6–4). Chronic use of aspirin and NSAIDs, however, has been implicated in chronic peptic ulceration, although this is still controversial (Duggan et al 1986, Graham and Smith 1986). It seems possible that, in some patients at least, chronic use is associated with a

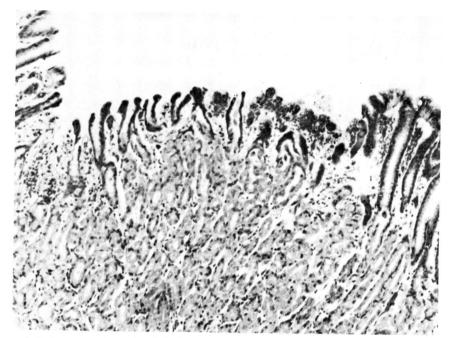

Figure 6–1. Acute gastric erosion in body mucosa following aspirin. The region of mucosa normally composed of pits is absent centrally and there is haemorrhage into the upper lamina propria (Trichrome × 80).

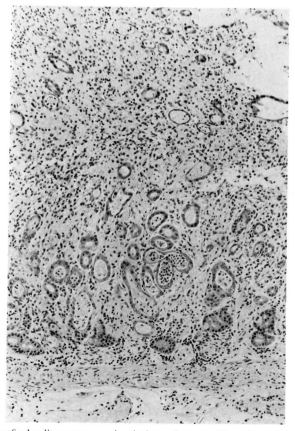

Figure 6–2. Biopsy of a healing acute erosion in its early stage. Note the mainly acute inflammatory reaction (H & E × 150).

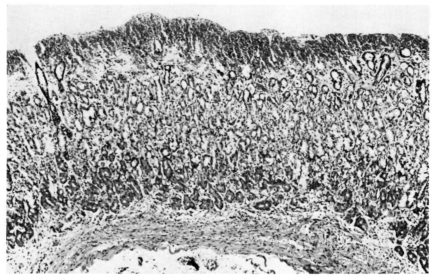

Figure 6–3. Body mucosa showing acute haemorrhagic gastritis. The superficial epithelium and gastric pits are eroded and a diffuse haemorrhagic zone occupies the surface layer (H & E × 70).

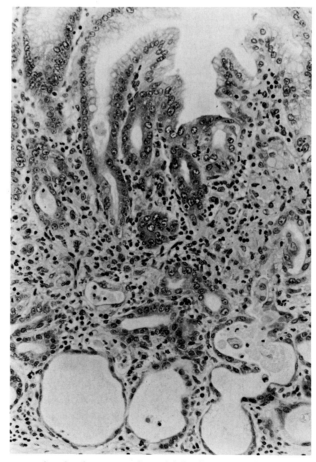

Figure 6–4. Acute erosion in the stage of partial healing. Note histiocytes in the often dilated atrophic tubules and a mild, mainly chronic inflammatory infiltrate of the lamina propria. The repair of the superficial epithelium is relatively more advanced (H & E × 300).

mucosal adaptation response and does not necessarily lead to chronic ulceration. Metzger et al (1976) described the gastric mucosa in biopsies from patients with rheumatoid arthritis during continuous or interrupted ingestion of aspirin. Although there was focal mucosal injury with haemorrhage and erosion, there was no significant increase in gastritis in the mucosa away from the focal lesions. MacDonald (1973) and Hamilton and Yardley (1980) have also shown that in gastric resections for gastric ulcer in patients who used aspirin regularly, about 50 per cent show a normal mucosa around the ulcer. This has practical applications in reporting biopsy tissues taken from gastric ulcer margins. The lack of a significant gastritis and an absence of pyloric or intestinal metaplasia raises the likelihood that an ulcer is drug induced, and this clearly has important implications in terms of management and prognosis.

It has long been held that alcohol ingestion is a cause of acute mucosal damage. While changes due to alcohol can be induced in experimental animals, the doses used are not always comparable to the amounts consumed by humans. Palmer (1954) reported without illustration an acute superficial gastritis in all of 34 men biopsied within six hours of a bout of acute alcohol intoxication. In 9 of 11 re-biopsied three weeks later the mucosa was said to have returned to normal. Gottfried, Korsten and Leiber (1978) observed the gastric mucosa in seven male alcoholic volunteers after the ingestion of the equivalent of 6–7 ounces of an 86 proof beverage. The changes described at three hours after ingestion consisted of an extravasation of red cells into the upper lamina propria in four of seven subjects. The superficial epithelium remained ostensibly normal, however, and appears so in their illustration. Similar changes were reported by Laine and Weinstein (1988b) in a group of actively drinking alcoholics, but it is interesting that the degree of haemorrhage observed was only statistically more severe in the alcoholics than in a non-alcoholic control group. Certainly these changes are not regarded by this author as specific for alcohol damage, since similar haemorrhages are seen in gastric biopsies in non-alcoholic patients who otherwise have a normal mucosa; the changes could easily be a traumatic biopsy artefact. It is possible that alcohol affects the gastric mucosa in such a way that a biopsy procedure is more likely to result in subepithelial haemorrhage.

Virtually nothing is known of the morphological changes that may be induced by the many oral drugs associated with gastric upsets, or the vast variety of exotic foodstuffs and condiments consumed. Certainly the ingestion of pickles can produce epithelial degeneration (Fig. 6–5A, B), and it is tempting to postulate that repeated minor damage of this type determined by dietary habits is responsible for the high incidence of chronic gastritis that occurs in countries such as Finland and Japan. Indeed, Fontham et al (1986) and Burr et al (1987) have produced evidence that there is a high incidence of gastritis in populations consuming diets rich in salty foods and deficient in fresh fruit and vegetables.

ACUTE GASTRIC INFECTIONS

In humans, unlike in some animals, the stomach does not harbour a permanent microbial flora. Bacteria entering with food are quickly killed by the action of free hydrochloric acid, but some, such as lactobacilli, being more resistant than usual, may persist for short periods. The achlorhydric stomach therefore, as expected, is usually heavily colonised. Gastric acidity is thus important in protecting the small bowel from potential pathogens. It is thus not surprising that in a normal stomach bacterial infection is unusual.

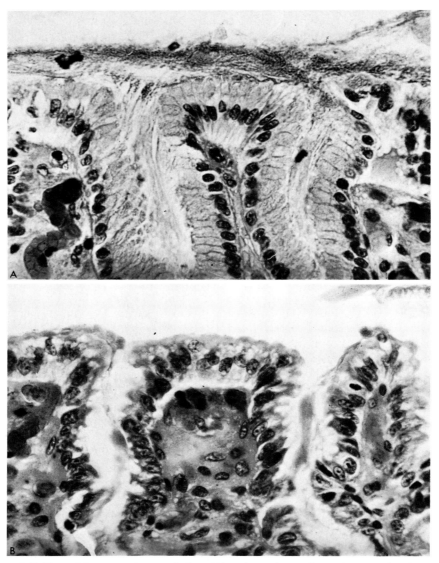

Figure 6–5. Normal human volunteer before **(A)** and one hour after **(B)** consuming 8 ounces of pickled gherkins. There are appreciable changes of possible damage to the surface epithelium (H & E × 420).

Pastore et al (1976) have described reversible gastric mucosal alterations due to infestation with *Vibrio cholerae*. These included degenerative changes of the superficial epithelium, oedema, vascular congestion and mononuclear cell infiltration of the lamina propria. The changes that Palmer (1951) described in acute staphylococcal food poisoning were principally those of epithelial necrosis and intraluminal sloughing in the region of the gastric pits. However, a critical appraisal of the illustrations published shows only a series of traumatic artefacts. Rarely is the gastric mucosa invaded by the haemolytic streptococcus (Gonzalez-Crussi and Hackett 1966, Nevin et al 1969). It is usually the consequence of a severe generalised infection elsewhere presenting as an acute abdominal crisis, and a diagnosis based on biopsy is unlikely. This is largely because the disease is an acute purulent necrotising lesion due to a diffuse spread of organisms throughout the mucosal, submucosal and muscular layers of the bowel. The mucosa sloughs and the stomach wall is grossly thickened, hyperaemic or infarcted and shows extensive vascular thrombosis. It is possible that the condition of emphysematous gastritis is a related lesion due to the involvement of gas-forming organisms.

With the exception of herpes simplex virus and cytomegalovirus infection in immunosuppressed patients (Malfertheiner 1988, Gazzard 1988), the putative gastritis that occurs as part of systemic viral illness has not been studied by biopsy. In cytomegalovirus infection, however, typical inclusions are often seen in the epithelial cells in the base of superficial erosions or neighbouring mucosa (Fig. 6–6). An uncommon presentation in cytomegalovirus gastritis is an appearance at endoscopy of multiple hyperaemic non-ulcerated nodules (Shuster et al 1989).

Candida can also invade the gastric mucosa in the immunocompromised patient and is fairly common in acquired immunodeficiency syndrome (AIDS) patients (Gazzard 1988), but it is more common as an invader of the base of chronic peptic ulcers. This has recently been studied in detail by Kalogeropoulos and Whitehead (1988), who found the organism in 26 per cent of gastric ulcers, 20 per cent of duodenal ulcers and 24 per cent of the ulcers associated with Barrett's oesophagus.

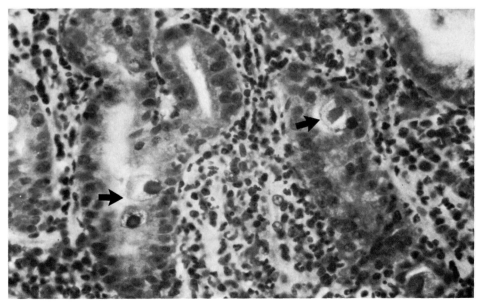

Figure 6–6. Biopsy of the edge of a gastric ulcer. There are a marked gastritis and typical cytomegalovirus inclusions in the epithelial cells (arrows) (H & E × 500).

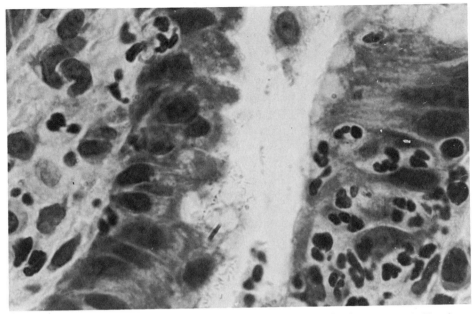

Figure 6–7. Gastric pits showing epithelial degenerative changes, polymorph infiltration and *Campylobacter* organisms applied to the mucous layer, and in the lumen (H & E × 1000).

Ramsey et al (1979) described an epidemic of transient gastritis characterised by abdominal pain, nausea and vomiting that ocurred among a group of volunteers being used for gastric secretory studies. Acute inflammatory changes mainly in the superficial parts of the gastric mucosa were coincident with decreased acid secretion, although the parietal cells were largely uninvolved in the inflammatory process. The agent responsible for the epidemic was not discovered at that time, but in retrospect has been ascribed to *Campylobacter pyloris* (Gledhill et al 1985). Indeed there are other isolated reports supporting the claim that *Campylobacter** can cause acute gastritis (Frommer et al 1988). This organism and its relationship to gastritis, duodenitis and peptic ulcer are now the subject of a vast literature. Despite this, opinion is still divided as to the significance of *Campylobacter pyloris* and as to whether it is directly responsible for the inflammation related to peptic ulceration. There are those who believe that it is a cause of acute gastritis because it may be seen in association with polymorph infiltration of the gastric epithelium (Fig. 6–7); that it is associated with the type B gastritis seen in prepyloric and duodenal ulcers; that it affects the metaplastic gastric epithelium in the duodenum, which is often present in association with duodenal ulcers; and that it is always associated with a neutrophil polymorph inflammatory cell infiltration of the epithelium in whose mucinous layer it resides (Bartlett 1988, Barthel et al 1988, Price 1988, Rauws et al 1988, Graham 1989). Some even advocate the use of therapy aimed at eradicating the organism when it is demonstrated in biopsy specimens of patients investigated for upper gastrointestinal symptoms (Marshall 1988). Of interest in this respect is the report by Berstad et al (1988) that antacids reduce *Campylobacter pylori* colonisation without affecting the gastritis in patients with non-ulcer dyspepsia and erosive prepyloric changes. There are other indi-

_____

*This organism has recently been reclassified as a *Helicobacter* (*Lancet*, 1989).

cations why its pathogenetic role in gastritis and peptic ulcer disease must be doubted. The organism is uncommon in association with gastric metaplasia of the duodenum in some circumstances, e.g., chronic renal failure (Shousha, Keen and Parkins 1989). It is not associated with some 30 per cent of gastric ulcers and not always associated with a neutrophil polymorph tissue reaction (Fig. 6–8), and the latter may be extreme in its absence (Fig. 6–9). It is seen in association with the gastritis and duodenitis found in asymptomatic volunteers (Fitzgibbons et al 1988) and in 25 per cent of humans with a normal gastric body mucosa. It is found fairly commonly in association with the gastric metaplastic epithelium in Barrett's oesophagus, yet has no consistent relationship to either inflammation or peptic ulceration (Kalogeropoulos and Whitehead 1988, Talley et al 1988). Indeed the role of gastric reflux in the pathogenesis of Barrett's oesophagus and ulceration seems to be confirmed in view of the report that it is known to regress under the influence of Omeprezole therapy (Deviere et al 1989). Furthermore it has long been recognised that spiral or curved organisms in histological material in gastric or duodenal biopsies are not all *Campylobacter pyloris* species (McNulty et al 1989). In many ways the presence of *Campylobacter pyloris* in the stomach and duodenum in association with peptic ulceration can be compared with the presence of other commensal organisms such as *Candida albicans*, and it is suggested that attempts to identify and treat *Campylobacter pyloris* infections are still very much in the realm of research activity (Marcheggiano et al 1987, Sethi et al 1987, Graham and Michaletz 1988, Kalogeropoulos and Whitehead 1988, Nedenskov-Sorensen et al 1988, Price 1988, Queiroz et al 1988).

As already mentioned, candidiasis may also affect the stomach. It is described as part of a systemic candidiasis complicating prolonged antibiotic, steroid or cytotoxic therapy (Eras, Goldstein and Sherlock 1972) and is seen fairly frequently in AIDS patients (Gazzard 1988). It is most usual, however, as a secondary local infection in a chronic peptic or malignant ulcer (Katzenstein and Maksem 1979, Scott and Jenkins 1982, Kalogeropoulos and Whitehead 1988). In these circum-

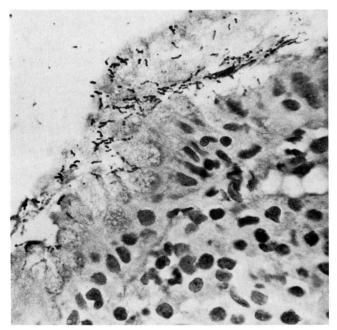

Figure 6–8. Gastric surface epithelium with numerous *Campylobacter*, but a conspicuous absence of neutrophil polymorph leukocytes. (Dieterle's silver × 750).

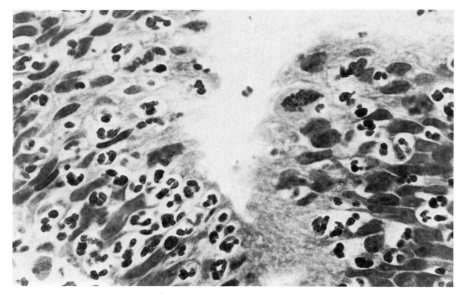

Figure 6–9. Gastric pit with marked epithelial polymorph infiltration but no *Campylobacter* (H & E × 1000).

stances it is regarded as a commensal organism, but it is natural to wonder whether its presence in a peptic ulcer has an influence on the chronicity of the lesion and its response to anti-ulcer therapy.

CHRONIC GASTRITIS

In pathological terms, chronic gastritis refers to an inflammatory lesion of the stomach that affects more or less of the mucosa, that may or may not be associated with peptic ulcer or pernicious anaemia and that increases in frequency with age. Histologically it is characterised by mucosal inflammation with or without destruction and architectural modification of the epithelial components. It emerged as an entity following the work concerned with the lesion of pernicious anaemia (Faber 1935, Magnus and Ungley 1938). Further studies were made by examination of laparatomy biopsies (Schindler 1947) and excised stomach specimens (Magnus 1946, 1952). It was, however, the advent of the flexible tube biopsy instruments (Wood et al 1949, Tomenius 1950) that marked the beginning of a new era of interest and investigation into mucosal lesions of the stomach.

A mass of literature soon appeared concerning the association of chronic gastritis with the anaemias, peptic ulceration, cancer and autoimmune phenomena. A good deal of discrepancy arose, due in part to the lack of good control studies in normal populations, but mainly due to the inherent shortcomings of the biopsy instruments. The instruments could provide biopsy specimens from only a limited area of the stomach, never from high in the fundus and hardly ever from the antrum. The site of the biopsy specimen, usually taken from the greater curve on the anterior wall, was never accurately known. It was with justification that MacDonald and Rubin (1967) wrote, "The definition and classification of chronic gastritis remains unsatisfactory."

With fibreoptic gastroscopes equipped with biopsy facilities, specimens can now be obtained from all parts of the gastric mucosa, which can also be clearly visualised and photographed at the same gastroscopic examination. The biopsy specimens are small but usually include the muscularis mucosa.

Multiple biopsy specimens from different anatomical sites, accurate evaluation of the samples and the facility of sequential studies have resulted in considerable advances in our knowledge about chronic gastritis, particularly in the recognition of subtypes.

Evaluation of Chronic Gastritis in Biopsies

In order to categorize chronic gastritis it has become increasingly plain that not only is the histological character of the mucosa important but equally so is the geographical distribution of the changes within the stomach, the presence of antibodies to gastric cell components, and, to a lesser extent, the macroscopic appearances at endoscopy. The subtypes of chronic gastritis that are now recognised have certain histological features in common. Thus in each biopsy the different components of the mucosa should be assessed separately and variations from normal carefully noted. The different combinations of features taken in conjunction with the other factors mentioned above will then allow the gastritis to be typed.

The *superficial epithelium* may show features suggesting degenerative or regenerative processes. The cells may appear flattened or cuboidal with hyperchromatic nuclei, partial or complete loss of the mucin column and increased basophilia of the diminished cytoplasm (Fig. 6–10). The cells may form a layer several cells thick, their limiting membranes becoming blurred and indistinct so that bud-like syncytial masses are formed (Fig. 6–11), and may seem to be in the process of exfoliation. On occasion mitotic figures occur in the superficial epithelium (Fig. 6–12). Normally they are rare and are seen only in the regenerative zone of the mucosa at the base of the gastric pits, and thus it seems that very immature cells still capable of cell division are reaching the surface. When degenerative changes are most marked, the epithelium may show invasion by polymorphonuclear leukocytes; this constitutes a striking picture (Fig. 6–13) suggestive of an active inflammatory destruction of the epithelium, and may be associated with epithelial erosions. Sometimes intraepithelial lymphocytes are the predominant feature, and when these are numerous, in the absence of a polymorph component, they frequently appear with a surrounding clear space or vacuole. The surface epithelium under these circumstances may show little change and appear relatively normal. This may also occur in the absence of intraepithelial lymphocytes, especially when the inflammatory infiltrate of the lamina propria is also minimal despite marked glandular atrophy. The superficial epithelium may also be the site of small intestinal metaplasia (see later).

These epithelial changes may also be seen in the gastric *pits*. Polymorph invasion of the crypt epithelium, with collections of polymorphs in the dilated lumen (see Fig. 6–12), mimics the appearance of a crypt abscess in ulcerative colitis. The increased activity of the regenerative zone is reflected not only in an increased basophilia and mitotic activity but also by a tortuosity and elongation of the pits. This may be a striking feature under some circumstances, and they may also be separated by inflammatory oedema of the lamina propria and congestion of capillary vessels. The pits may thus appear reduced in number. But a reduction in number and distortion of the normal pattern is usually the result of degenerative atrophy and incomplete restoration due to previous episodes of inflammation. An

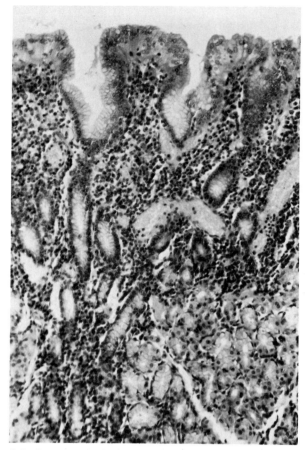

Figure 6–10. Gastric body mucosa in chronic gastritis showing degenerative changes of the superficial epithelium (H & E × 188).

intraepithelial lymphocyte population similar to that in the superficial epithelium may also be a striking feature (see Fig. 6–13).

The *gland tubules* may remain normal despite severe changes in the superficial epithelium and gastric pits. Frequently, however, a shrinkage or complete disappearance of groups of tubules occurs. The number that disappear varies, and no normal tubules may remain. Sometimes an acute inflammatory destruction is observed similar to that seen in the superficial epithelium and gastric pits (Fig. 6–14).

Pseudopyloric *metaplasia* (Figs. 6–15, 6–16) is recognised only in body glands, whereas intestinal metaplasia affects all types of glands, the superficial epithelium and pits. The earliest stage of pseudopyloric metaplasia consists of an increase in mucous neck cells, which later replace the remaining specialised cells in the rest of the tubule, so that the appearance mimics normal pyloric glands. This may reflect deficient differentiation whereby in the normal course of events mucous neck cells descend into the gastric glands and become chief and parietal cells. When there is intestinal metaplasia (Figs. 6–17, 6–18), epithelial cells of small intestinal type, including absorptive cells in various stages of maturation, goblet cells and Paneth cells, can be recognised. Argentaffin cells are also present in increased numbers. Sometimes structures covered by intestinal epithelium project from the surface, thus simulating intestinal villi closely, and rarely the transformation mimics a small intestinal mucosa with villi and a gland layer (Fig. 6–19).

Text continued on page 66

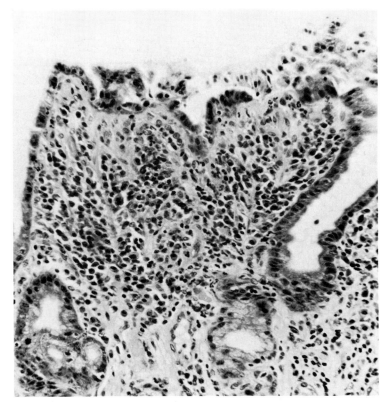

Figure 6–11. Gastric superficial epithelium showing regenerative syncytial masses of hyperchromatic cells, some of which appear to be in the process of exfoliation (H & E × 450).

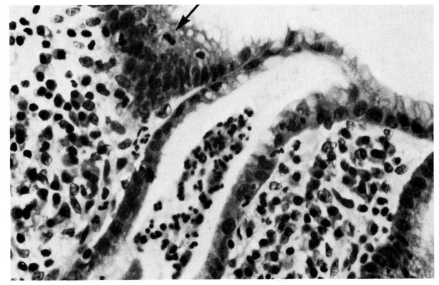

Figure 6–12. A gastric pit containing pus cells. Note the mitotic figure in the superficial epithelium (arrow) (H & E × 450).

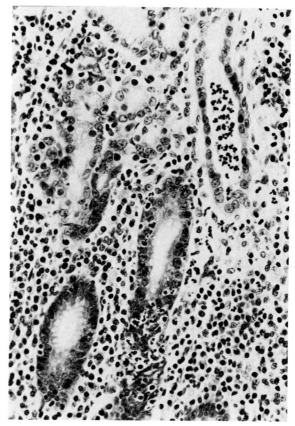

Figure 6–13. Gastric superficial epithelium and pits showing degenerative and regenerative features with an active inflammatory infiltration and distortion. Note intraepithelial polymorphs and lymphocytes seemingly in a vacuole (H & E × 425).

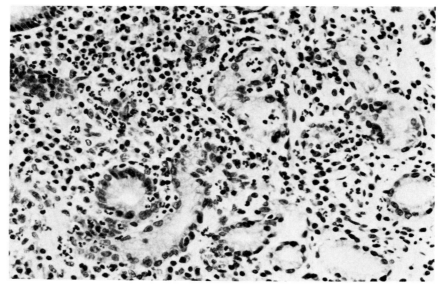

Figure 6–14. Gastric body gland tubules showing inflammatory destruction. Note the generalised cellular infiltrate and a prominence of polymorphs in the lamina propria (H & E × 200).

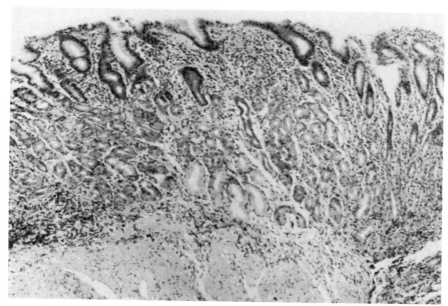

Figure 6–15. Body mucosa showing diffuse inflammatory infiltration and, centrally, loss of gland tubules with the earliest stage of pseudopyloric metaplasia in others (H & E × 70).

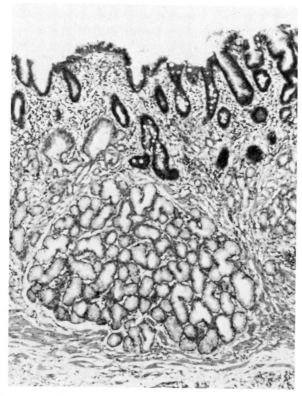

Figure 6–16. Body mucosa showing marked pseudopyloric metaplasia of glands. Note intestinal metaplasia of pits and superficial epithelium (H & E × 70).

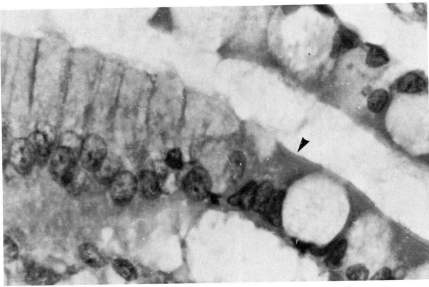

Figure 6–17. Metaplastic intestinal absorptive cells and goblet cells (right and above); note the brush border (arrowhead). Typical gastric superficial epithelium (left) (H & E × 420).

However, the transformation of gastric cells to intestinal cells will obviously result in intermediate forms. When it is complete, i.e., with enterocytes, intestinal goblet cells and Paneth cells, it has all the characteristics of small intestine, both ultrastructurally and histochemically (Lev 1966, Goldman and Ming 1968). An intermediate or incomplete form is also recognised (Iida, Murata and Nagata 1978), which has the combination of goblet cells and columnar cells with features resembling gastric foveolar cells. This type of intestinal metaplasia has been subdivided further on the basis of the histochemistry of the mucus they contain. In type IIA, neutral mucins are said to predominate, whereas in type B they are sulphomucins. Using immunohistological methods, Nardelli et al (1983) have

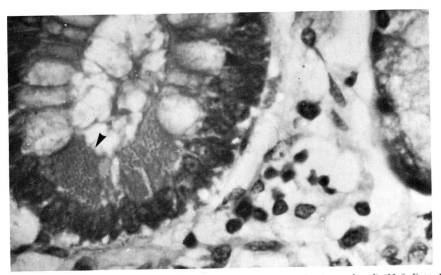

Figure 6–18. Metaplastic Paneth cells with typical refractile granules (arrowhead) (H & E × 420).

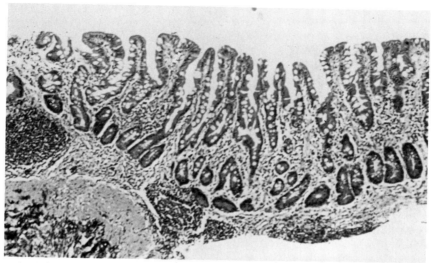

Figure 6–19. Gastric body mucosa showing a virtually complete small intestinalisation with villous processes and a gland layer. Note there is still a prominent inflammatory infiltrate of the lamina propria (H & E × 45).

shown that incomplete intestinal metaplasia has antigens common to foetal duodenum. Complete and incomplete intestinal metaplasia types A and B are now referred to as types 1, 2 and 3, respectively. This subject is referred to in greater detail later in relation to gastric carcinoma, but one should also note the association of intestinal metaplasia with other cell types normally not present in the gastric mucosa.

In Japanese subjects with peptic ulcer, epithelial dysplasia or early cancer seen in association with areas of intestinal metaplasia, it is not unusual to find cystically dilated glands containing ciliated cells (Rubio and Kato 1986). Sometimes such cells also contain argyrophilic basal granules, and ultrastructural studies show that the cilia have a shaft, neck and basal body comparable to those seen in respiratory epithelium (Torikata et al 1986, Torikata, Mukai and Kawakita 1989). Similar cells are apparently less common in Europeans (Rubio and Serck-Hanssen 1986). Another cytological phenomenon sometimes related to ciliated cells is the presence of cytoplasmic vacuolisation. The vacuoles may be mucin positive and may also contain neuroendocrine granules, but they may also be mucin negative and devoid of cilia and the vacuole may appear infranuclear in position. A further type is the vacuole that seemingly surrounds intraepithelial lymphocytes (Rubio and Kato 1987, 1988). In association with type IIB or type 3 intestinal metaplasia, Newbold, MacDonald and Allum (1988) have also described probable precursor cells that occur in the surface epithelium between gastric pits. They occur as groups of up to 25 cells, exhibit no mitotic activity, are mucin negative and have no brush border.

The *lamina propria* may show an inflammatory infiltrate that includes plasma cells, lymphocytes and eosinophil and neutrophil polymorphs. Neutrophil polymorphs or a mixture of lymphocytes and plasma cells may predominate. The infiltrate may be restricted to a part or the whole of the area between the gastric pits and, in addition, may involve part or the whole of the deeper parts when it is usually associated with glandular atrophy. A polymorph-rich infiltrate is commonly associated with vascular dilatation and a sero-fibrinous oedema with destructive inflammation of the related epithelium. When chronic inflammatory

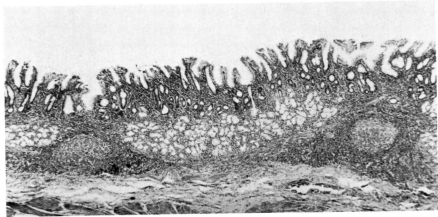

Figure 6–20. Gastric body mucosa showing pseudopyloric metaplasia and lymphoid hyperplasia (H & E × 14).

cells predominate, plasma cells are seen in the upper layers and lymphocytes in the lower layers, where follicular aggregates with or without germinal centres may form (Fig. 6–20). This has been referred to in the past as follicular gastritis. In mucosa with only minimal epithelial degenerative changes or widespread atrophy and metaplasia, the inflammatory infiltrate is often very scanty and always of plasma cell and lymphocyte preponderance type. Foci of fatty infiltration may appear in the lamina propria (Fig. 6–21) and in any lymphoid follicles present, which will also appear atrophic, being without germinal centres. Sometimes the lamina propria shows only oedema, vascular hyperaemia and, particularly in the antrum, a tendency for new strands of smooth muscle to grow up into the upper layers.

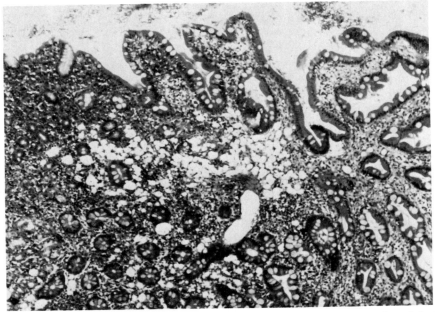

Figure 6–21. Gastric body mucosa showing intestinal metaplasia and fatty infiltration of the lamina propria (H & E × 150).

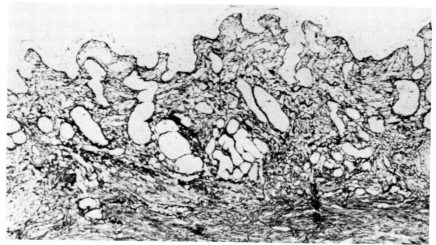

Figure 6–22. Gastric body mucosa in atrophic gastritis. There are subepithelial and intertubular condensation and deposition of new reticulin. Compare with Figure 5–4 (reticulin stain × 75).

The reticulin fibres may appear more widely spaced than normal when there is inflammatory oedema. A more frequent change is seen in association with atrophy. Under the superficial epithelium and in the inter-pit and inter-gland areas a felt-like mesh results when the reticulin fibres collapse together, as the tubules disappear and new fibres are formed as part of the inflammatory reaction. In severe atrophy the junction between the muscularis mucosa and lamina propria is less well defined than normal and the whole of the normal reticulin pattern is obscured (Figs. 6–22, 6–23).

Sometimes in biopsy interpretation there are difficulties in recognising mucosal type if severe gastritis is present and there is atrophy or metaplasia. When only metaplastic pseudopyloric or intestinal tubules remain, the mucosa cannot be classified, but if residual body glands remain and their recognition is facilitated in

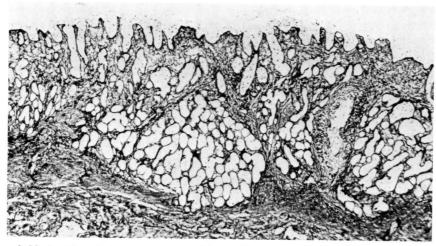

Figure 6–23. Gastric pyloric mucosa in atrophic gastritis. Features similar to those in Figure 6–22. Compare with Figure 5–9 (reticulin stain × 75).

Maxwell preparations, the mucosa must be of body or junctional type. If all the tubules that remain are of "pyloric" type, the mucosa could have originated in any part of the stomach, because gastritis in pyloric or cardiac mucosa will be similar to gastritis with complete pseudopyloric metaplasia in body or junctional mucosa. When fibreoptic instruments are used, the site of the biopsy specimen is fairly accurately located, except in stomachs altered by previous operations. Thus in usual practice difficulty arises only in biopsy specimens from the lesser curve area, where even in the normal stomach the demarcation of one region from its neighbour is often poorly defined. A helpful point in the differentiation of normal pyloric glands from pseudopyloric glands is that, whereas the former may contain occasional parietal cells, the latter do not.

If the inflammatory and reactive changes already outlined affect only the superficial epithelium, gastric pit region and related lamina propria, it is convention to refer to this as superficial gastritis. Atrophic gastritis, on the other hand, occurs if the changes affect the gland layer, and the difficult line of demarcation is between superficial gastritis and early atrophic gastritis, the later and more severe grades of atrophic gastritis being obvious. Deep extension of the inflammatory infiltrate around the tubules may be helpful in the recognition of atrophic gastritis, but the only satisfactory criterion is recognition of atrophy of the tubules. In this respect the preparations stained for reticulin are most valuable, since loss of tubules, even in small numbers, is reflected by the changes in reticulin pattern already outlined.

Atrophic gastritis could be quantitated by accurately measuring the number of glands that remain, but a convenient subdivision is into mild, moderate and severe. If only one or two groups of tubules have disappeared, the mucosa is classified as showing mild atrophy. It is this severity of involvement that is sometimes referred to as "focal atrophic gastritis." If all normal tubules are lost or only one or two groups remain, the diagnosis is severe gastritis, and all appearances between these two extremes are classed as moderate. It is important for this scheme that only normal glands be considered and those showing metaplasia be discounted.

In severe atrophic gastritis with widespread metaplasia, a negligible inflammatory cell infiltrate, atrophic lymphoid aggregates and fatty infiltration of the lamina propria, the appearances are often classified as "gastric mucosal atrophy" (Figs. 6–24, 6–25). A further feature in severe atrophic gastritis is an increase in the number of endocrine cells (Rubin 1969, Bordi, Ravazzola and De Vita 1983). In addition to cell types normally present in the stomach, new forms are acquired. Cells positive for somatostatin, motilin, glicentin and cholecystokinin have been demonstrated by immunofluorescence (Bordi and Ravazzola 1979). In some instances endocrine cells are so numerous that they can be recognised in ordinary H & E stained sections (Figs. 6–26, 6–27) and confirmed in a Gremelius preparation. It is now well recognized that pernicious anaemia or achylia are conditions most closely associated with carcinoids (Wilander 1981), and cases are recorded (Black and Haffner 1968, Goldman, French and Burbige 1981, Hodges, Isaacson and Wright 1981) of multiple gastric carcinoid tumours and endocrine cell hyperplasia that is grossly nodular (Sjoblom et al 1989).

Some biopsy specimens exhibit an invasion of polymorphs into, and degenerative changes of the epithelial elements of, the gastric mucosa. Crypt abscess formation may be present, and if these features reflect an acute inflammatory epithelial destruction, as seems likely, then clearly its presence should be recorded. It is surprising that this phenomenon received scant mention in the previous literature until reported by Whitehead, Truelove and Gear (1972). If epithelial degenerative changes are associated with an infiltrate of chronic type, this could be regarded

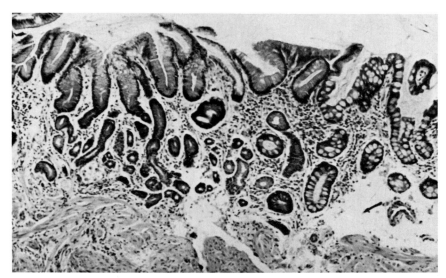

Figure 6–24. Gastric body mucosa showing "gastric atrophy." There is partial intestinal metaplasia but no evidence of epithelial degeneration. The density of the cellular infiltrate is comparable to that in the normal mucosa considering that there is severe tubular atrophy and a secondary condensation of the lamina propria (H & E × 75).

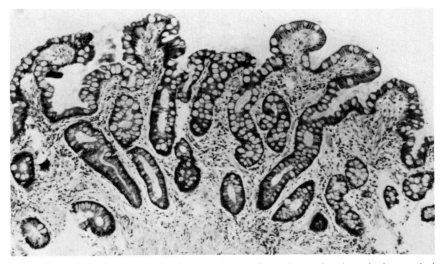

Figure 6–25. Gastric body mucosa showing gastric atrophy and complete intestinal metaplasia (H & E × 75).

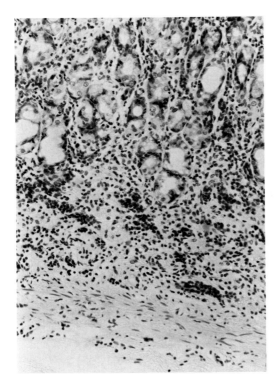

Figure 6–26. Severe atrophic gastritis with islands of endocrine cell hyperplasia both in association with the basal glands and in the neighbouring lamina propria (H & E × 500).

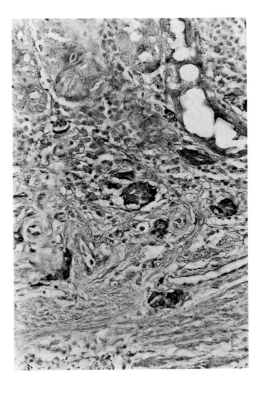

Figure 6–27. Comparable field to Figure 6–26 stained specifically for endocrine cells (Grimelius × 600).

as chronic activity, and in both types the activity could be graded simply on the basis of whether it was diffuse throughout the mucosa or patchy in distribution. In some cases the mucosa shows little or no epithelial degenerative change and either a very slight or imperceptible chronic inflammatory infiltrate, in spite of the fact that there may be evidence of distortion and atrophy of the normal mucosal architecture. These appearances are clearly suggestive of a quiescent or burnt-out stage of a previous inflammatory process. This quiescent phase is seen par excellence in mucosae with severe atrophy and metaplasia, i.e., those showing so-called gastric atrophy.

Intestinal metaplasia nearly always occurs in a mucosa that is the site of atrophic gastritis. Sometimes it is present in the superficial epithelium and pits in superficial gastritis, and very occasionally isolated islands are seen in biopsy specimens consisting of otherwise normal mucosa (Fig. 6–28). For practical purposes the presence of epithelium with intestinal morphology should always be regarded as abnormal. Pseudopyloric metaplasia also invariably occurs only in atrophic gastritis, but occasional gland tubules of simple mucus-secreting type are rarely seen among specialised gland tubules in otherwise normal body mucosa. Some evidence based upon surgically induced trauma of body mucosa, which initially causes a reversion to the more simple pyloric structure followed by recovery, indicates that at least in some circumstances this type of metaplasia may be reversible (Harvey 1907). Similar findings have been recorded in the repair of aspirin-induced erosions (Yeomans 1976). Both types of metaplasia should be recorded separately because they may have different significance, and the degree to which they are present can be conveniently graded. Reference has already been made to the possibility of subdividing intestinal metaplasia according to the mucins that predominate. Although there are claims as to the greater malignant potential of the incomplete type of metaplasia (Filipe 1983, Silva and Filipe 1986), which resembles colon rather than small intestine, there is a clear need for further elucidation of this; it may be that the metaplasia is a paraneoplastic rather than a preneoplastic phenomenon (Bedossa, Lemaigre and Martin 1987, Ramesar, Sanders and Hopwood 1987, Rubio et al 1987).

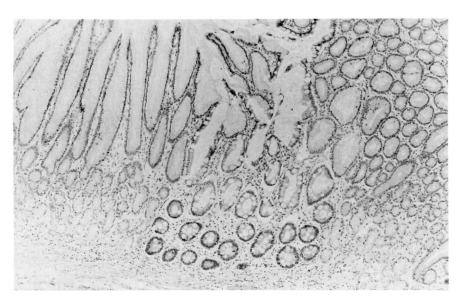

Figure 6–28. Normal pyloric mucosa with isolated island of intestinal metaplasia (H & E × 75).

Thus, in evaluating chronic gastritis according to the above principles, the following features should be considered.

Mucosal Type

Aided by knowledge of the site from which the biopsy specimen was obtained, it is usually possible to type the mucosa as of pyloric, body, cardiac or junctional zone origin. Junctional mucosa occurs not only at the sites of change between the main mucosal areas in the stomach, namely antral, body and cardiac, but also between the pylorus and duodenum and between the cardiac region and the oesophagus.

Site of Gastritic Process

It is of considerable value to register the predominant site of the inflammatory process in gastritis. A superficial inflammation is arguably an earlier or less severe form of tissue damage than a deeper form which is invariably associated with glandular destruction and atrophy.

Type of Inflammation

The inflammatory infiltrate seen characterising gastritis may be mainly acute, mainly chronic or mixed acute and chronic. This most certainly is a reflection of the "activity" of the pathogenetic process related to the factors causing the gastritis. It is also possible that differences in aetiology may be concerned in determining whether the inflammation also seems to centre upon the epithelium as well as the lamina propria or even in preference to it.

Metaplasia

Pseudopyloric and intestinal metaplasia are important histological features because they represent a reaction by the mucosa to a significantly severe pathological process tending to destroy the native cellular elements. There is some evidence that intestinal metaplasia represents a more severe expression of severity of mucosal injury. It is largely a non-reversible change and has an association with an increased malignant potential, the precise nature of which needs elucidation.

Lamina Propria Changes

Apart from inflammatory cell infiltration, important lamina propria changes include collapse of the reticulin framework and approximation of the surface and crypt epithelium to the deeper-lying lymphoid plexus, which is important in the metastatic process involved in early gastric cancer. In addition, the oedema, neomuscularisation and vascular ectasia appear to be a reaction to some forms of tissue injury, notably bile reflux.

The different combinations of these features in conjunction with other known circumstances, such as the presence of autoantibodies, family history and the geographic distribution of the lesions in the stomach, will usually allow allocation of the gastritis to one or another category that may have pathogenetic and clinical significance in terms not only of possible therapy but also of likely complications, such as anaemia, peptic ulcer disease, or malignancy. Thus it has become possible to recognise several subtypes of chronic gastritis.

7

SUBTYPES OF CHRONIC GASTRITIS

SUBTYPES, AETIOLOGY AND SIGNIFICANCE

Type A Gastritis

Strickland and Mackay (1973) designated this as type A gastritis, but it is also known as autoimmune gastritis. It is classically seen in patients with latent or overt pernicious anaemia in whom it is commonly claimed that the lesion diffusely affects all the gastric mucosa except for the antrum. It is now known, however, that the antrum is not always normal. A constant feature is hyperplasia of the middle third of the mucosa, which is due to an increase in gastrin-producing cells. These appear as clear cells in ordinary haematoxylin and eosin preparations. This feature, together with mucosal polyps of regenerative or hyperplastic type that are sometimes transitory, is well recognised (Lewin et al 1976, Elsborg et al 1977). In addition, Kekki et al (1983) have shown that the antral mucosa may also show gastritis of variable degree which tends to revert to normal in the later stages, especially if the initial gastritis was superficial.

In the remainder of the stomach the body and fundal areas show a severe atrophic gastritis that in the later stages, when the lamina propria inflammatory cell component tends to disappear, is better described as gastric mucosal atrophy. There is a progressive loss of the specialised body glands, which are replaced by pseudopyloric or intestinal metaplastic elements. In addition there is an epithelial endocrine cell proliferation and a predisposition to carcinoid tumours (Borch et al 1986, Bordi et al 1986, Mueller, Kirchner and Mueller-Hermelink 1987, Itsuno et al 1989) which is probably driven by the hypergastrinaemia. A biopsy showing all these features is not diagnostic, however, for similar changes are seen in other forms of chronic atrophic gastritis. Apart from minor changes, from megaloblastosis back to normal, the lesion is not reversed by vitamin B_{12} therapy, although it has been claimed that vitamin B_{12} absorption and histology may improve following cortisone administration (Jeffries 1965). This was not confirmed, however, in a similar study by Strickland et al (1973).

In latent pernicious anaemia, achlorhydria, low intrinsic factor secretion and atrophic gastritis are present, but although serum vitamin B_{12} may be low there are no manifestations of vitamin B_{12} deficiency. A proportion go on to develop pernicious anaemia, but the factors that determine this progression are not fully understood. Pernicious anaemia may rarely occur in juveniles and it appears to have several causes. There may be inadequate synthesis of intrinsic factor, a block to its secretion or the secretion of abnormal intrinsic factor (Levine and Allen 1985). Acid secretion and gastric mucosal histology are normal. In Imerslund's syndrome (Imerslund 1960) the same features are associated with the production of normal intrinsic factor, but it is not effective in promoting vitamin B_{12} absorption and there is a coexistent proteinuria.

The literature concerning immunological studies in chronic gastritis is enormous and often contradictory (Glass 1977). Limited sampling of the gastritic mucosa and the technical difficulties inherent in the immunological methods used have probably contributed to this. Antibodies against a microsomal fraction of parietal cells can be demonstrated both by fluorescence and by complement fixation methods. Two antibodies active against intrinsic factor have been demonstrated. One blocks the interaction of vitamin B_{12} with intrinsic factor, and the other combines with the vitamin B_{12} intrinsic factor complex.

Parietal cell antibodies are rarely found if the body mucosa is normal, and the incidence rises with increasing severity of the histological lesion. What determines whether parietal cell antibodies are produced in any case of chronic gastritis seems to depend upon the type of patient in which the gastritis occurs rather than on the gastritis itself; e.g., these antibodies are commonly associated with gastritis in patients with pernicious anaemia, iron deficiency anaemia, diabetes and the thyroid autoimmune disorders (Wright et al 1966).

Antibodies to intrinsic factor are less common than parietal cell antibodies and are associated with the more severe grades of gastritis. They are usually found in patients with pernicious anaemia or latent pernicious anaemia. When present in other conditions, e.g., thyroid diseases, they appear in the serum and not in the gastric juice. It seems that it is the gastric juice antibodies that are important in interfering with vitamin B_{12} absorption. There is no relationship between serial serum intrinsic factor antibody titres and the liability to develop the disease (Irvine, Cullen and Mawhinney, 1974).

The antibodies probably do not initiate the gastritis, although a lesion in monkeys equivalent to gastritis has been produced by Freund adjuvant and gastric mucosal injections (Andrada and Rose 1969). Cell-mediated immunity against intrinsic factor has also been shown (Chanarin and James 1974). Cytotoxicity of the antibodies has not been demonstrated, but this may only reflect the present difficulties in growing gastric mucosal constituents in tissue culture. Cell-mediated immunity against other mucosal antigens has, however, been demonstrated by Uibo and Salupere (1981) in patients who have no parietal cell antibodies. Clearly the question of the role of immune phenomena in the production of gastritis is still to be resolved, but the role of cytotoxic antibodies seems to be gaining acceptance (De Aizpurua et al 1983, Kaye, Whorwell and Wright 1983). It is possible that gastritis may well be initiated by environmental factors and subsequently perpetuated by autoimmune phenomena, especially in a prone and genetically determined group. It is pertinent in this respect that there is a considerable immunological overlap between pernicious anaemia, thyroid autoimmune disease and diabetes, and that patients with severe atrophic gastritis following gastrectomy operations rarely develop antibodies.

Type B Gastritis

This type of gastritis is seen in association with a negative parietal cell antibody test, a moderate or slight reduction in acid secretion and only rarely an impairment of vitamin B_{12} absorption. The gastritis is always distal in the stomach, involving the pyloric region and extending proximally to a variable extent along the lesser curve. Designated type B by Strickland and Mackay (1973), this type of mucosal inflammation is very prone to ulcerate (Ritchie and Delaney 1968). Since that time, it has attracted considerable attention because of its close association with hyperchlorhydria, duodenitis and prepyloric or duodenal peptic ulcers (Correa 1980, Kekki and Villako 1981, Varis 1981). Correa (1988) has stressed the density of the lymphoid infiltrate in this type of gastritis in which there are often concomitant reactive germinal follicles expanding the lamina propria. Wyatt and Dixon (1988), on the other hand, have proposed that type B gastritis is closely related to colonization with *Campylobacter pyloris* and that the inflammation so induced impairs mucosal defence mechanisms, predisposing both gastric mucosa and gastric metaplasia of duodenal mucosa to peptic ulceration.

The relationship between gastritis and peptic ulcer is nevertheless far from clear. From the very earliest of observations (Cruveilhier 1862) it became evident that ulcer and gastritis were invariably present in the same stomach.

The gastritis has a type B distribution in prepyloric and duodenal ulcers, but in ulcers higher in the stomach it extends proximally to involve a larger area although in a patchy fashion (Gear, Truelove and Whitehead 1971). This is referred to again in consideration of the entity that has been called type AB gastritis. All chronic peptic ulcers are situated in a pyloric type of mucosa, and thus occur either just distal to the junction of body with pyloric mucosa or in the pyloric mucosa beyond (Oi, Oshida and Sugimura 1959). Consequently, when the ulcer occurs high in the stomach, the antrum appears to be enlarged. This could clearly be the result of atrophic gastritis and pseudopyloric metaplasia involving the more proximal as well as the distal part of the stomach in a way that suggests that there is backwards extension of the process, but it could also be interpreted to mean that those individuals who possess an abnormally large antrum are prone to ulcer. There is some evidence that the former is the case and that high gastric ulcers are always associated with gastritis in the area of the stomach distal to the ulcer (Tatsuta and Okuda 1975). However, the possibility of mixed forms of gastritis opens this subject up for further research and debate.

Type AB Gastritis

The AB gastritis of Kekki and Villako (1981) and Varis (1981) corresponds to the multifocal atrophic gastritis of Correa (1980, 1988). It tends to occur with a geographic distribution in populations with a high risk of gastric cancer and also appears to be associated with gastric peptic ulcers that are situated high in the stomach. It is initially a patchy proximal atrophic gastritis affecting the antrum and lesser curve and develops as a more widespread lesion associated with increasing intestinal metaplasia involving the higher lesser curve region and both anterior and posterior walls of the body. The foci increase in size with duration and tend to coalesce, thus affecting most of the gastric mucosa, but the high fundus is usually spared. The associated gastric ulcer may heal as the disease progresses, which is possibly related to the tendency to develop hypochlorhydria. However, coexistent intrinsic factor and parietal cell antibodies are unusual and vitamin B_{12} deficiency does not occur. The progressive nature of this disease has been monitored in biopsy studies (Gear, Truelove and Whitehead 1971, Aukee and Krohn 1972, Kekki, Hakkiluoto and Siurala 1976, Pulimood, Knudsen and Coghill 1976, Ormiston, Gear and Codling 1982) and shown to be uninfluenced by ulcer treatment using histamine H2-receptor-antagonists (Pounder et al 1976).

Although there may well be a genetic susceptibility to acquire this type of gastritis in that it appears to run in families (Bonney et al 1986), the high incidence in populations consuming diets high in salt and deficient in fresh vegetables and fruit makes it highly likely that environmental influences are also important (Fontham et al 1986, Bevoc et al 1987). In low incidence areas, however, genetic influences seem to be of prime importance and may account for the familial occurrence of gastric carcinoma.

Bile Reflux Gastritis

The considerable literature relating to this entity is controversial for a number of reasons. There is good experimental evidence for a damaging effect of bile and pancreatic juice on the gastric mucosa (Davenport 1968, Cheng, Ritchie and Delaney 1969, Brooks, Wenger and Hersh 1975, Eastwood 1975, Mann 1976, Orchard et al 1977), and thus it is gaining acceptance that alkaline or enterogastric reflux may be of clinical importance in humans (Ritchie 1984, 1986). However, although reflux is said to be rare in normal people (Cocking and Grech 1973), it is claimed to be commonplace in patients attending gastroenterology clinics who do not have a gastric ulcer or a history of previous gastric operations (Niemela et al 1987), and when present at endoscopy has no clinical relevance and is not associated with histological injury (Nasrallah et al 1987). In patients who have had gastric operations for peptic ulcer, either duodenal or gastric, it is the accepted view that enterogastric bile alkaline reflux is usual (Hoare et al 1977), and concern has been expressed over a relationship between this and the subsequent development of gastritis, gastric mucosal dysplasia and carcinoma (Aukee and Krohn 1972, Watt, Sloan and Kennedy 1983, Watt et al 1983, Langhans, Bues and Bunte 1984, Houghton et al 1986), although the results of other workers would indicate that the case has been overstated (Ovaska et al 1986). The matter is further complicated by the report that in patients with gastric ulcer treated by certain types of operations, i.e., that of highly selective vagotomy, there may be a decrease in the degree of bile reflux, but that this has no effect on the gastritis present (Dewar, Dixon and Johnston 1984).

Clearly many of these previous studies have problems in defining what constitutes "bile reflux," in the parameters they have chosen for assessing gastric mucosal damage and because in patients with peptic ulcers there is, in any case, an associated chronic gastritis that may or may not be related to bile reflux. It has long been known that the gastritis associated with peptic ulcer persists and progresses in severity even when the ulcer has healed (Gear, Truelove and Whitehead 1971, Pulimood, Knudsen and Coghill 1976) and this may be independent of reflux. Of the different morphological aspects of chronic gastritis it seems theoretically possible that one or more parameters is aetiologically more closely related to reflux than the others. Thus Mosimann et al (1981) drew attention to elongation and tortuosity of the gastric pits as a specific association of bile in the stomach. Some further confirmation of this was supplied by Mosimann et al (1984) when this lesion was seen to regress in postoperative duodenal ulcer patients if bile diversion was achieved by a Roux-en-Y gastrojejunostomy procedure. A study by Dixon et al (1986) led to the claim that reflux-associated features in gastric biopsies are foveolar hyperplasia, oedema and smooth muscle fibres in the lamina propria, vasodilatation and congestion of superficial mucosal capillaries, and a paucity of acute and chronic inflammatory cells. It is not clear from this study, however, what was the extent of changes in the stomach that would normally be regarded as chronic gastritis or chronic atrophic gastritis, which is so typically present in at least part of the stomach in association with peptic ulcer. Bechi et al (1987) have addressed this issue, however, and shown that while foveolar hyperplasia is reflux related, chronic atrophic gastritis is not. These histological features can certainly occur in the stomach when obvious bile reflux is seen endoscopically (Figs. 7–1 to 7–4). However, they must be seen in proper perspective. Any or all of them, although claimed to be specific for reflux, can in fact be seen in other states of the gastric mucosa, such as the edge of erosions or ulcers, in Menetrier's disease, gastritis cystica profunda, hyperplastic polyps and the Canada-Cronkhite lesion, and they are simply part of the spectrum of the mucosa's response to injury. The claim that subnuclear vacuolisation of foveolar cells of fundic or body mucosa is a histological marker for protracted duodenogastric reflux (Rubio and Slezak 1988) will require confirmation, particularly since the vacuoles are usually empty and are negative with mucin and mucopolysaccharide stains.

Chronic Erosive Gastritis

In the late seventies endoscopists began to refer to certain gastric mucosal appearances as aphthous ulceration (Morgan et al 1976), chronic erosive verrucous gastritis (Green et al 1977) and varioliform gastritis (Lambert et al 1978). These had no relationship to acute haemorrhagic erosions, also known as acute erosive gastritis. One of the continuing problems associated with the definition of these disease states is the use of erosion by endoscopists for lesions which histologically have an intact surface epithelium (Karvonen et al 1983, Nesland and Berstad 1985, Nesland, Berstad and Serck-Hanssen 1986, Berstad and Nesland 1987). This was addressed in a multicentre European study in which both endoscopic

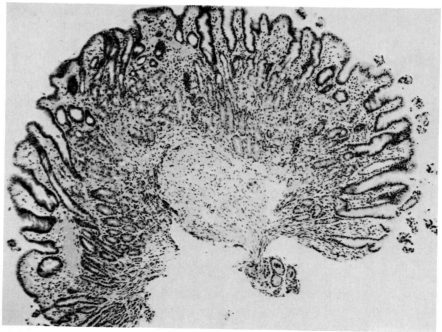

Figure 7–1. Antral mucosa in the presence of severe endoscopic bile reflux showing elongation and tortuosity of gastric pits (H & E × 50).

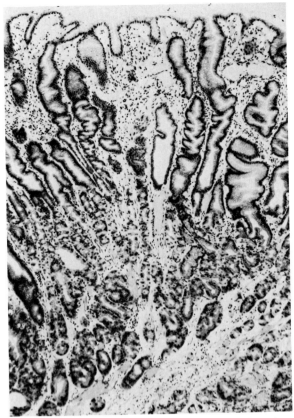

Figure 7–2. Body mucosa in the same stomach as Figure 7–1. There is marked tortuosity and elongation of pits in addition to increased vascularity and muscularisation of the lamina propria. Note the relative absence of inflammation (H & E × 200).

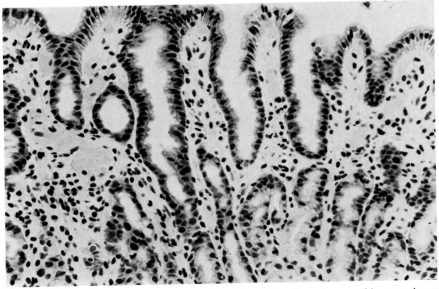

Figure 7–3. Detail of upper lamina propria in bile reflux. Note the oedema and increased vascularity and relatively scant inflammation (H & E × 350).

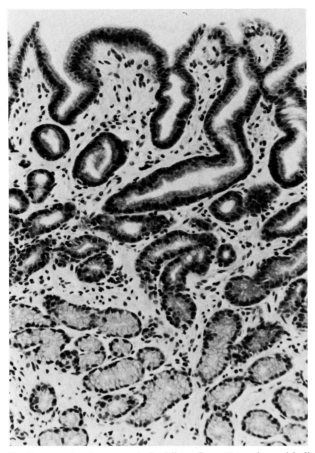

Figure 7–4. Detail of upper lamina propria in bile reflux. Note the epithelial changes and the muscularisation of the lamina propria (H & E × 350).

and histological features were correlated (Gad 1986). It was shown that as little as 42 per cent of lesions diagnosed endoscopically as erosions had histological evidence of surface loss of epithelium. Thus most of the lesions diagnosed as erosions macroscopically were revealed to be foci of acute inflammation with or without surface exudate, islands of intestinal metaplasia, areas of subepithelial capillary hyperaemia and a variety of other lesions. A further problem relates to the fact that as a basic principle it seems likely that an inflamed gastric mucosa will be prone to erosion of its surface epithelium, and so chronic erosive gastritis may be a stage in the evolution of different forms of gastritis. Indeed there is evidence that some forms of chronic erosions occur in patients with type B antral gastritis and that there is thus an association with prepyloric and duodenal ulceration (Karvonen et al 1987). Evidence also emerged gradually that a separate form of chronic erosive gastritis also existed and that this was unrelated to type B gastritis or peptic ulceration. It corresponded to the varioliform gastritis of earlier authors (Lambert et al 1978) and was characterized by raised nodular lesions with an ulcerated or an intact surface epithelium that tended to occur in rows in the body of the stomach situated on the rugae and only sometimes extended into the antrum (Elta et al 1983, Franzin et al 1984). Unfortunately some reports included inadequate histological examination of the lesions (Gallagher, Lennon and Crowe 1987).

As a follow-up study to previous work, Haot et al (1988) reviewed their cases characterized previously at endoscopy as erosive, varioliform or aphthoid gastritis.

When large folds predominated in the gastric body and were accompanied by nodules and erosions, then the histological appearance of the neighbouring mucosa was said to show a characteristic picture, namely, "lymphocytic gastritis." In this form of gastritis, lymphocytes appeared in the surface and foveolar epithelium and were surrounded by a typical clear halo; gastric pits were elongated and tortuous but otherwise normal; lymphocytes and plasma cells although present in the lamina propria were usually few and there was no correlation with the density of the intraepithelial lymphocyte population. In the vicinity of the erosions the picture was obscured by the presence of more acute inflammation and the accumulation of polymorphs within the crypts. In the remaining cases of chronic erosive gastritis, the histological findings in the surrounding mucosa were said to be "non-specific" and would usually be described as chronic atrophic gastritis. Seemingly, therefore, Haot would claim that lymphocytic gastritis has a typical endoscopic appearance with nodules, erosions and large folds predominating in the body, which contrasts with a non-specific, presumably type B gastritis affecting the antrum and associated with flat erosions. This has been reaffirmed (Haot et al 1989) after a review of the original cases of diffuse varioliform gastritis originally published by Lambert et al (1978). However, the entity of "lymphocytic gastritis" requires much more precise characterisation. Intraepithelial lymphocytes are seen in other forms of chronic gastritis (Fig. 7–5), and some objective determination of what numbers constitute a diagnosis are needed. On the basis of experience with the significance of intraepithelial lymphocytic infiltrates in conditions of the small and large intestine, much more investigative work is indicated. Dixon et al (1988), however, also recognize "lymphocytic gastritis" as a distinct entity and believe that it is possibly the result of an abnormal response to antigens produced by *Campylobacter pylori* and that the condition is comparable to coeliac disease. It is well to recall, however, that the small bowel appearances in coeliac disease are not entirely specific either. Nevertheless, Kawai et al (1970) postulated an immunological pathogenesis in the aetiology of chronic erosive gastritis, and Roesch and Warnatz (1974) demonstrated a decrease in IgM and an increase in IgG cells in the nodular lesions. Lambert et al (1977), however, have described an increase in IgE cells, but all these phenomena may be secondary. In follow-up studies spanning six years, Freise et al (1979) found that the lesions remained static in 50 per cent of cases and in the remainder either disappeared or showed a decrease in size. Farthing et al (1981) have reported healing in patients receiving prednisolone therapy and Elta et al (1983) following antacid treatment. Clarke, Lee and Nicholson (1977), no doubt also describing chronic erosive gastritis, drew attention to it as a cause of protein-losing enteropathy.

Thus what is the current status of knowledge concerning this condition? As pathologists we know that despite the limited number of ways that tissues can react to noxious stimuli, different diseases can be recognized by the combinations in which these reactions appear grouped together. Such examples are plentiful in the recognition of the different forms of colitis, for example, and it is being increasingly recognised that we should be striving in a similar way with the somewhat unsatisfactory position that prevails in the context of "chronic erosive gastritis." There appear to be two problems which are central to the debate. Firstly, there is the specificity or otherwise of the erosive aspect of the condition, and, secondly, there is the specificity or otherwise of the gastritis. In the stomach or duodenum pathologists accept the definition of erosion as a focus of loss of part of or the whole full thickness of the mucosa, but not including the muscularis mucosa. It implies the probability of healing without scarring and is a convenient way of differentiating erosion from the more advanced lesion of peptic ulcer. In

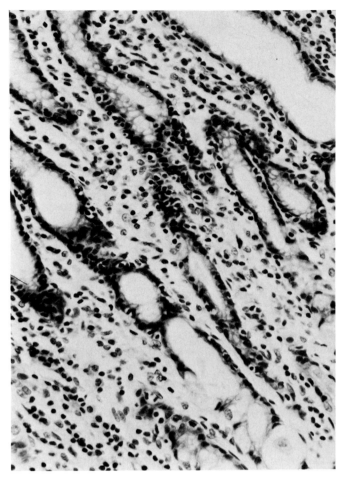

Figure 7–5. Chronic gastritis with no significant polymorph infiltration but a prominent intraepithelial lymphocyte population (H & E × 350).

reality this is somewhat artificial, since presumably every ulcer starts life as an erosion no matter how brief a life this may be. However, this does not deny the possibility that erosions may have different causes and a different natural life span related to the cause. In addition, it is likely that this cause will be reflected in the histological appearance of the mucosa immediately related to the site of the erosion. Application of this reasoning thus gives grounds for the view that there are at least two distinct forms of chronic erosive gastritis. One would appear to be related to type B gastritis and is associated with peptic ulceration, probably as a precursor lesion being more frequently antral. The other may well be related to so-called lymphocytic gastritis, have no association with peptic ulceration, more commonly involve the body and is associated with multiplicity, enlarged rugal folds and a characteristic macroscopic and radiological appearance. This would be in keeping with the author's experience and with all the previous studies in this condition. At the same time it explains some of the apparent discrepancies.

Histologically, therefore, the first type of erosion simply shows superficial necrosis surrounded by mucosa with features of chronic gastritis such as is seen in that with a type B distribution. This may have acute or chronic inflammatory elements and a varying degree of metaplastic features. Chronic erosions of the second type also show a central epithelial deficit with a necrotic base but are bordered by hyperplastic, elongated, tortuous and branched crypts composed of relatively undifferentiated cells. In this type of erosion the inflammatory changes in the surrounding mucosa appear to vary in severity. In the lamina propria it can be minimal or marked, but as outlined above it may be characterized by an intraepithelial lymphocyte population which is abnormally conspicuous. The muscularis mucosa is always intact but may show hyperplasia. Cystic dilatation of deeper glands may occur and they may also exhibit pseudopyloric metaplasia when the lesion involves the body mucosa. It is a combination of foveolar and pseudopyloric glandular hyperplasia, which adds bulk to the lesion. It is the overall structure of this lesion that accounts for its gross polypoidal character, and the central erosion gives it a classical volcano-like form easily identified both radiologically and endoscopically. Thus Japanese researchers have classified the lesion as a form of gastric polyp. It is a lesion that clearly requires further study. (For illustrations and further discussion see Chapter 8.)

AETIOLOGY AND SIGNIFICANCE OF THE SUBTYPES OF CHRONIC GASTRITIS

Aetiology

Although there is no direct evidence that repeated gastric mucosal injury or recurrent acute gastritis leads to chronic gastritis, this is commonly assumed. Much of the work in this area predated the recognition of the various types of chronic gastritis already discussed. Nevertheless, many of the observations are worthy of consideration because, even in retrospect, they can be related to the forms of chronic gastritis that are recognized in modern times. Chronic gastritis of the body mucosa has been linked with chronic alcoholism, although the reported incidence varies between 10 and 70 per cent (Joske, Finckh and Wood 1955, Williams 1956, Debray et al 1957, Parl et al 1979). Indirect evidence for a link comes from Dinoso et al (1972), who demonstrated an improvement in histological appearance in 12 alcoholics following abstinence of up to nine months' duration. The gastritis was described as either superficial or atrophic, but since these lesions are commonplace in subjects with type AB gastritis who are not alcoholics and increase in incidence with age (Kekki et al 1977), the significance of this observation loses some of its impact. Indeed, there is other evidence that would tend to refute an association. Brown et al (1981), for example, have reported that in patients with alcoholic cirrhosis the incidence of chronic gastritis is no higher than in control series. In the past, blind biopsy studies have also shown that the drinking of hot liquids is associated with an increased incidence of chronic gastritis of the body of the stomach (Edwards and Edwards 1956), and this would suggest repeated trauma as a causative factor. Correa (1982) makes a claim for dietary trauma from highly salted food and hard grains in the food of those living in high incidence areas of AB type chronic gastritis. This finds support in the fact that the incidence of body gastritis increases in frequency with age (Andrews et al 1967). Cigarette smoking also seems to be important in some way (Edwards and Coghill 1966), and it is perhaps significant that both age and cigarette smoking are also related to atherosclerosis. Chronic peptic ulceration, which is always associated with either type B or type AB chronic gastritis, is much more common in patients with severe atherosclerosis, especially if there is aortic calcification and particularly if atheromatous aneurysms are present (Elkeles 1964, Jones, Kirk and Bloor 1970). The effect of smoking on vessels and on the stomach may be quite separate effects. Jarvis and Whitehead (1980), for example, have shown that administration of nicotine to rats in their drinking water results in a decrease in the mucus-producing component of the gastric mucosa. Theoretically this would tend to decrease its ability to withstand the effect of any other ingested agents with a propensity for gastric mucosal injury.

The association between type B and AB gastritis and chronic peptic ulcer provides presumptive evidence for an association between gastritis and chronic renal failure, hyperparathyroidism, cardiovascular disease other than hypertension, cirrhosis of the liver and chronic respiratory disease in all of which peptic ulcer incidence is elevated (Langman and Cooke 1976).

Edwards and Coghill (1966) also showed an increased incidence of presumptive AB chronic gastritis in the lower social classes and in those subjects who have blue eyes, which suggests a possible genetic predisposition. Further evidence for this comes from the family studies of Varis (1981) and Kekki and Villako (1981) in Finnish and Estonian populations. In a blind biopsy follow-up study, Siurala and Salmi (1971) have shown that superficial gastritis develops with time into atrophic gastritis. However, this seems not to be so in all types of gastritis. Siurala, Sipponen and Kekki (1985), for example, have shown that although body gastritis of type A progresses rapidly, changes in the antrum tend to resolve. In type B associated with prepyloric or duodenal ulcer it persists and gets worse in the antrum but does not seem to progress to affect the body unless antrectomy is performed. In high gastric ulcers the body gastritis associated with it tends to progress rapidly, whereas that in the antrum does not. Thus it is becoming increasingly clear that not only are there different forms of simple gastritis but that the aetiology is complex. Combinations of environmental and genetic factors coupled with pathophysiological disturbances causing autoimmune phenomena, hypersecretion or reflux of duodenal contents all seem to interplay in the production of a chronic mucosal damage. At least in some forms this chronic damage seems to be punctuated by acute episodes characterized by more obvious epithelial injury and polymorphonuclear leukocyte infiltration. There is some biopsy evidence (McIntyre, Irani and Piris 1981) that this mechanism operates in the gastritis associated with prolonged NSAID therapy, but at least in the early stages, inflammation, acute or chronic, does not usually appear as part of the mucosal damage associated with these agents (personal observation). However, that prolonged use does cause gastric ulceration, which is most often prepyloric, seems proven (Roth and Bennett 1987), but the position is complicated by the fact that NSAIDs may be used by a large number of patients who already have a chronic gastritis related to other factors. The case for their ulceragenicity seems proven in the face of the evidence and the fact that prevention of NSAID-associated peptic ulceration can be achieved therapeutically by a synthetic prostaglandin E analogue (Graham, Agrawal and Roth 1988).

It therefore seems likely not only that superficial gastritis can progress to atrophic gastritis but that so-called gastric atrophy is an end stage of atrophic gastritis. This would appear to hold true of gastritis occurring both with and without peptic ulceration. It is well to remember, however, that early studies (Roesch, Demling and Elster 1975) showed that although progression is usual, regression from atrophic gastritis to normal may occur in gastritis that would now probably be called type AB if it is not associated with ulcers. The implication is considerable, i.e., the possible reversibility of a highly cancer-prone situation. Clearly more evidence related to this is desirable.

The controversy related to the role of *Campylobacter pylori* in the aetiology of acute gastric inflammation, chronic gastritis and peptic ulceration has already been referred to. Belief in such for an association stems in large measure from the claim by Marshall et al (1985) that they fulfilled Koch's postulates for the organism in that an acute transient gastritis followed ingestion of a laboratory culture by a human volunteer. The experience was repeated by another group (Morris and Nicholson 1987) with apparently similar results, but in both studies the organism only flourished in the stomach if drug-induced hypochlorhydria was artificially produced prior to challenge with the organism. Moreover, as we have seen, there is a considerable body of evidence that is counter to a simple aetiological role for this organism in causing either acute or chronic gastritis. It is obviously a ubiquitous bacterium and in the right circumstances can flourish in the stomach, but further investigation is required as to its precise role, if any, other than as a commensal in both acute and chronic gastritis in its many forms.

Significance

The ability to secrete acid, pepsinogen and intrinsic factor is reduced as the body mucosa atrophies (Glass et al 1960), but normally the ability to produce some intrinsic factor persists longer than the ability to secrete appreciable acid. This is interesting because in humans both are produced by the parietal cell (Hoedemaeker et al 1964). It may simply be a reflection of the volumes of the two products secreted normally and their relative biological activity.

As atrophic gastritis progresses the pattern of mucoprotein secretion alters, and albumin and globulin in high concentrations may be found in the gastric juice (Glass and Ishimori 1961, Glass 1965). Diffuse atrophic gastritis with a persistent loss of albumin from the gastric mucosa has been postulated as a cause of otherwise obscure hypoalbuminaemia that occurs in elderly patients (Coghill 1969).

Despite these disturbances of function the evidence that chronic gastritis of the body mucosa is associated with dyspepsia is far from convincing (Joske, Finckh and Wood 1955, Shiner and Doniach 1957, Coghill 1960, Hojgaard, Matzen and Christoffersen 1987, Talley and Phillips 1988). There can be no doubt that chronic gastritis of the body mucosa can be present in patients who have no symptoms referable to the stomach, whereas many who complain of persistent dyspepsia have neither peptic ulcer nor body gastritis. In a study of dyspepsia patients in whom gross gastric, duodenal, pancreatic and hepatic pathology was excluded as far as possible, Cheli, Perasso and Giacosa (1983) showed that the incidence of antral and body gastritis was the same as in a control group. They concluded that gastritis was not a cause of dyspepsia "sine materia."

It has been repeatedly shown that the incidence of body gastritis in patients with iron deficiency anaemia is between 30 and 60 per cent (Badenoch, Evans and Richards 1957, Coghill and Williams 1958) and gastritis of the body mucosa is more common in those who have no other known cause for iron deficiency. The view that iron deficiency causes gastritis is unfounded; follow-up studies (Ikkala and Siurala 1964, Ikkala, Salmi and Siurala 1970) show that gastritis persists after the anaemia has been treated, and that recurrent anaemia is seen more frequently in those patients in whom the gastritis progresses in severity. This would indicate that the gastritis might be the cause of the anaemia. In postgastrectomy patients, for example, there is a significant blood loss from the atrophic gastric mucosa of the gastric remnant (Holt, Gear and Warner 1970). In addition, patients with atrophic gastritis also show an increase in free iron loss (Sutton et al 1970) that undoubtedly is related to the markedly raised rate of cell turnover that occurs in this condition.

The levels of serum gastrin in relation to chronic gastritis have been studied intensively in peptic ulcer patients (Byrnes et al 1970, Korman, Soveney and Hansky 1971, 1972). The most usual findings are raised levels in gastric ulcer and in patients with Zollinger-Ellison syndrome, with low levels in duodenal ulcer. There is usually, however, a greater response in patients with duodenal ulcer than in normals or in patients with gastric ulcer after giving protein foods, but the highest stimulated levels are seen in patients with Zollinger-Ellison syndrome. It has also been shown that patients with pernicious anaemia have high levels (McGuigan and Trudeau 1970). Another study has directly related gastrin levels specifically to antral gastritis. Fasting serum levels are decreased in patients with atrophic gastritis only if the antrum is relatively unaffected (Strickland et al 1971).

Morson (1955) has shown that atrophic gastritis with intestinal metaplasia is seen in over 90 per cent of cases of cancer of the stomach. After 25 years the incidence of cancer in patients who have had a gastrectomy or gastroenterostomy for either duodenal or gastric ulcer is six times the expected rate (Stalsberg and Taksdal 1971), and gastritis in these patients is the rule (Schrumpf et al 1977). Deaths from gastric cancer occur between three and four times the expected frequency in patients with pernicious anaemia (Mosbech and Videbaek 1950, Blackburn et al 1968). In a follow-up study of atrophic gastritis of AB type unassociated with pernicious anaemia, Siurala and Seppala (1960) showed that approximately 10 per cent develop cancer, and since this form of gastritis occurs numerically so much more often, it constitutes a much larger risk and a more important precancerous condition than pernicious anaemia. Indeed, in a population-based study Schafer et al (1985) could find no strong indication for endoscopic surveillance of asymptomatic patients with pernicious anaemia with a view to detecting treatable carcinoma.

There is good evidence that carcinoma arising in chronic gastritis does so through progressive dysplasia involving the areas of intestinalisation (Morson et al 1980). Furthermore, the tumour arising in such circumstances is of the so-called intestinal type (Lauren 1965), and studies suggest that the intestinal mucosa from which it arises is of colonic (type 3) rather than small intestinal type. This has been based upon the histochemical characterisation of epithelial mucins (Jass and Filipe 1979, 1981, Filipe et al 1985, Silva and Filipe 1986). It is this type of carcinoma that forms the excess of tumours in those countries with a high incidence of gastric cancer, and it would be in keeping with the relative incidence of carcinoma arising in the small and large intestine, respectively. However, Ramesar, Sanders and Hopwood (1987) have found that typing intestinal metaplasia in biopsies is of little value in identifying patients at risk of gastric adenocarcinoma. Furthermore, type 3, or large intestinal type metaplasia, is uncommon in the gastric remnant harbouring a carcinoma (Bedossa, Lemaigre and Martin 1987a). Indeed, Rubio et al (1987) believe that incomplete or type 3 intestinal metaplasia may be a paraneoplastic rather than a preneoplastic phenomenon. It would certainly seem that dysplasia and preneoplastic changes can be seen in non-intestinalised epithelium (Ghandur-Mnaymneh et al 1988), and it is postulated that this phenomenon is important in the genesis of the diffuse type of gastric carcinoma. At the same time dysplasia can also be seen in association with intestinalised epithelium in stomachs that are also the site of intestinal type carcinomas (Saraga, Gardiol and Costa 1987). There would thus appear to be a strong association between chronic gastritis of type A, type B and type AB and the development of carcinoma of the stomach. The nature of this association is still in doubt. However, electron microscopic (Tarpila, Telkka and Siurala 1969), immunological (De Boer, Forsyth and Nairn 1969) and histochemical (Stemmermann 1967, Sasano et al 1969) studies have shown that almost all gastric cancers have a proportion of cells with characteristics of intestinal epithelium. Cells with intestinal characteristics are also found in normal gastric mucosa towards the bottom of the gastric pits, and this is known to be the area associated with proliferation and cell renewal. In gastritis there is a tendency for the intestinal type of cell to be produced, and in atrophic gastritis with a markedly increased cell turnover, cancer might well be expected to supervene in a proportion of cases. These circumstances may explain why cancer and intestinal metaplasia are so commonly associated. What is less easily understood is why, although gastric carcinoma and pernicious anaemia occur most frequently in association with blood group A, there is no increased incidence of blood group A in those patients with atrophic gastritis who have obvious intestinal metaplasia in their gastric mucosa (Glober et al 1972).

The association of widespread atrophic gastritis and intestinal metaplasia with the development of cancer has important clinical connotations. Skinner, Heenan and Whitehead (1975) have shown that the gastritis and intestinal metaplasia associated with peptic ulcer of the body of the stomach have a similar distribution and severity to that seen with gastric cancer, but it is more localised with pyloric ulcer. In cases of recurrent stomal or pyloric ulcer after gastrojejunostomy for duodenal ulcer, however, the gastrectomy specimen shows a distribution and severity of gastritis that is also like that seen in cancer. This similarity points to a higher cancer risk in the stomach with body ulcer and after gastrojejunostomy. Lundegardh et al (1988) have recently shown that stomach cancer is indeed more common in patients operated on for gastric ulcer than those operated on for duodenal ulcer. For duodenal ulcer the Polyagastrectomy operation as opposed to varieties of vagotomy and antrectomy or drainage appears to be associated with a higher cancer risk (Lygidakis 1986). Nevertheless, it is plain that the choice of surgical treatment of peptic ulcer that ensures cure must be influenced by the relative postoperative tendencies to accelerate the premalignant condition of chronic gastritis of both types B and AB and possibly that due to or accentuated by bile reflux (Kliems et al 1979, Assad and Eastwood 1980, Kekki et al 1980, Saukkonen et al 1980, Graem et al 1981, Dougherty, Foster and Eisenberg 1982). Whether the risk of cancer is wholly related to the surgical intervention for ulcer disease or whether the disease process itself is responsible and the surgery is incidental (Hermanek and Riemann 1982) has been debated. It seems much more likely that the addition of a further dimension of disturbance of gastric function increases the rate of progress of the basic disease process, i.e., the chronic gastritis. Thus if some form of gastric operation is found necessary for the treatment of peptic ulcers, the chances of subsequent development of cancer is so high that a case can be made for interval gastroscopy and multiple biopsy, since early asymptomatic cancer can be present in such stomachs (Schrumpf et al 1977). At this stage the cancer is more amenable to complete cure; and this has been highlighted by Pointner et al (1988) in their report of early gastric cancer in the gastric remnant.

There is no available information on a relationship between chronic erosive gastritis and susceptibility to gastric cancer.

GASTRIC EPITHELIAL DYSPLASIA AND EARLY GASTRIC CANCER, EPITHELIAL POLYPS, POLYPOSIS AND MUCOSAL HYPERPLASIA, LYMPHOID HYPERPLASIA AND LYMPHOMA

GASTRIC DYSPLASIA AND EARLY GASTRIC CANCER

In parallel with experience in other organs and epithelial surfaces, the identification of early cancer of the stomach has resulted in the delineation of even earlier stages of the disease, namely, malignant dysplasia (Schade 1974, Oehlert et al 1975, 1979, Borchard, Mittelstaedt and Kieker 1979, Cuello et al 1979, Meister et al 1979, Morson et al 1980, Farini et al 1981, Ming et al 1984). Dysplasia is commonly, but not always associated with areas of intestinal metaplasia of incomplete type, and it occurs in flat as well as polypoidal lesions (Jass 1983). It is perhaps significant that this type of metaplasia is similar to that which occurs in Barrett's oesophagus, another site of the dysplasia-cancer sequence. However, dysplastic features occur independently of intestinalisation, and there are claims (Ghandur-Mnaymneh et al 1988) that this type of metaplasia is related more closely to the development of the diffuse as opposed to the intestinal type of carcinoma. However, we have already seen that the distinction between intestinal and diffuse is somewhat artificial in terms of the pathobiology of gastric cancer, although it has some value in providing insight into possible aetiology and its precursor or associated lesions. It is thus not surprising that descriptions of dysplasia have involved the use of different terminology to describe a subjective impression of increasing architectural and cytological atypia, i.e., dysplasia which at its end point qualifies for carcinoma in situ. The difficulties that such exercises created in the past have resulted in categories such as "borderline" and "probably carcinoma" (Nagayo 1972) and the suggestion that "carcinoma in situ" as a term should be abandoned. Morson et al (1980), for example, suggested that any lesion still confined by epithelial basement membrane should be designated as severe dysplasia, and when invasion of lamina propria is demonstrated, the lesion should be called intramucosal carcinoma. This, however, is clearly not satisfactory for small endoscopic biopsy interpretation and reporting. It is not possible to make such a diagnosis unless the gastrectomy specimen is available, for the malignant tissue may not be entirely intramucosal. Consequently it is now advocated that the problem of differentiating between true dysplasia and regenerative dysplasia be recognized and that atypical features, such as nuclear enlargement, hyperchromasia, loss of differentiation, a high mitotic rate, glands sharing a common "party wall," abnormal patterns of cell orientation and mucin secretion, produce a range of true dysplastic appearances that culminate in an appearance that is histologically similar to some carcinomas, but is still confined by a basement membrane, i.e., carcinoma in situ (Figs. 8–1 to 8–6). For the time being these abnormalities are best conveyed to the clinician in terms of mild, moderate or severe dysplasia, for the use of the term carcinoma in situ may result in overexuberant treatment that at our present state of knowledge is not justified. In an 11 year histological follow-up study, Saraga, Gardiol and Costa (1987) showed that in 85 patients in whom dysplasia was diagnosed, 17 out of 18 diagnosed as severe dysplasia developed a carcinoma, whereas 1 from 41 with moderate dysplasia and 0 from 23 with mild dysplasia did so.

Hyperplasia and regeneration of ulcerated gastric mucosa may mimic dysplastic changes, but there is usually, though not always, a prominent inflammatory infiltration with polymorph invasion between the epithelial cells, which consequently may also show degenerative appearances in some areas (Fig. 8–7, 8–8). With experience, differentiation between true dysplasia and regenerative dysplasia is usually easy, but from the practical standpoint, if there is doubt it is advisable to repeat the endoscopy and to obtain further biopsy specimens. A useful pointer in regenerative atypia is for the cells to show a tendency to mature towards the

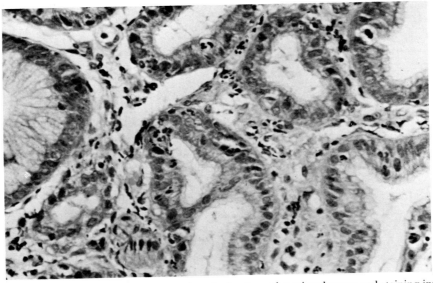

Figure 8–1. Mildly dysplastic appearances largely due to nuclear size changes and staining intensity. There is also an inflammatory component (H & E × 150).

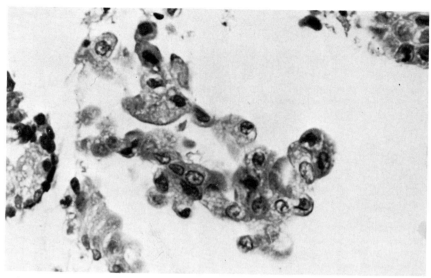

Figure 8–2. Detached epithelium that appears abnormal because of nuclear abnormalities and an abnormal disposition of cells (H & E × 300).

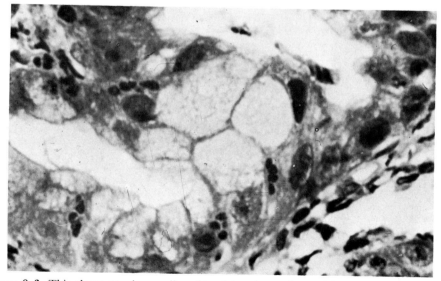

Figure 8–3. This shows an abnormality of nuclei and cytoplasm with "party-walling" giving an appearance of in situ signet ring cells (H & E × 600).

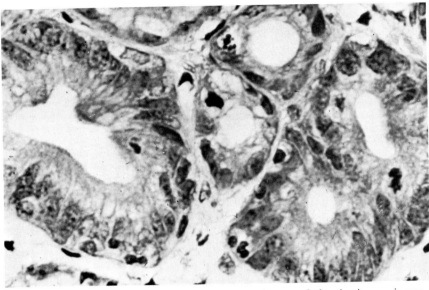

Figure 8–4. This shows sufficiently abnormal features to be regarded as in situ carcinoma (H & E × 300).

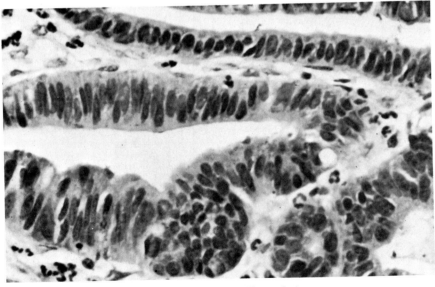

Figure 8–5. Same as Figure 8–4.

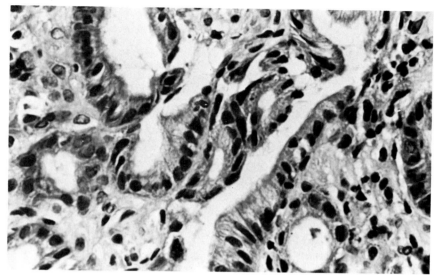

Figure 8–6. Same as Figure 8–4.

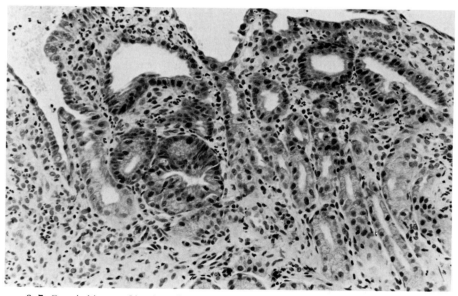

Figure 8–7. Gastric biopsy of benign ulcer edge. There are mild epithelial cell abnormalities due to regeneration. Note scarring of lamina propria (H & E × 300).

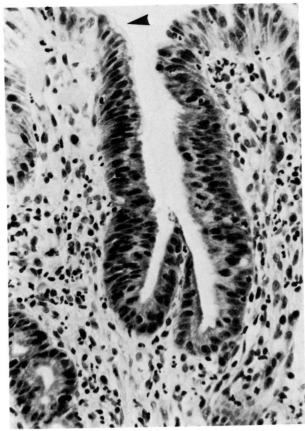

Figure 8–8. Gastric biopsy of benign ulcer edge. The abnormalities are more severe than in Figure 8–7, and there is more palisating of nuclei although the cells mature towards the surface (arrowhead) (H & E × 300).

surface, but even this may not be seen in earlier regenerative change and hence the need sometimes to rebiopsy. There will inevitably be an unclassifiable group, but this should be progressively smaller as experience increases. It is the persistence of abnormal features in sequential biopsies that justifiably supports a diagnosis of true dysplasia. There is some evidence that in situ dysplasia may even be recognisable cytologically (Seppala, Lehtola and Siurala 1976). Efforts to diagnose these possibly earlier stages of carcinoma also include the use of dyes. Just before endoscopy the dyes are introduced into the stomach for the purpose of directing the biopsy to areas of intestinal metaplasia, dysplasia or small foci of cancer. Methylene blue (Suzuki et al 1973), toluidine blue (Giler, Kadish and Urca 1976), indigo carmine (Ida et al 1975) and the combined Congo-red–methylene blue (Tatsuta et al 1982) are just some of the dye methods currently in use. Dysplasia apparently may exist for many years before becoming invasive carcinoma (Loux and Zamcheck 1969). Obviously the precise delineation of dysplasia or precancer constitutes a clear challenge that if met, would mean a great stride forward in the area of cancer prevention. There is real evidence that morphometric methods similar to those already applied in the cytological diagnosis of malignancy (Boon et al 1981) may also be developed for use in biopsy tissues. Already the subjective classification of dysplasia and its shortcomings have been the stimulus to use a computerised measuring system in the analysis of its various features (Jarvis and Whitehead 1985), and there is now increasing evidence that such methods may have a real place in the assessment of these early stages of gastric malignancy

(Tosi et al 1987). In the meantime pathologists need to begin to recognize true dysplasia so that patients can be sequentially endoscoped and rebiopsied. Much more of the natural history of carcinoma of the stomach will then surely unfold.

The diagnosis of the earlier stages of carcinoma of the stomach is now commonplace. These show certain distinctive macroscopic appearances which have been classified by the Japanese Gastroenterological Endoscopical Society according to whether or not the lesion is raised above the surface and whether or not there is ulceration. Raised carcinomas account for only one quarter of the cases and tend to occur more often either in the distal or the proximal stomach (Mori et al 1987, Ohta et al 1987) rather than the body. The principal application of the classification appears to be in the accurate communication of endoscopy appearances between endoscopists. However, it has a greater value if it serves to draw the attention of the would-be endoscopist to a different macroscopic form of stomach cancer that is curable. Although first described in Japan, early gastric cancer has since been recognized worldwide (Evans et al 1978, Elster et al 1979, Ostertag and Georgii 1979, Seifert et al 1979, Green et al 1981, Goldstein et al 1983, Bogomoletz 1984a, Grigioni et al 1984, O'Brien et al 1985, White et al 1985, Lehnert et al 1989). It is generally regarded not as a lesion fundamentally different from advanced gastric cancer but only at an early stage of development. Early and late gastric cancer have been shown, for example, to have similar DNA distribution patterns (Macartney, Camplejohn and Powell 1986, Czerniak, Herz and Koss 1987). Its recognition and study have made it clear that the evolution of the advanced stage of the disease occurs during a long period of up to 15 years or more (Fujita 1978). It has even been argued on the basis of follow-up endoscopic studies in high-risk patients that delaying surgery for early gastric cancer can be justified (Bodner, Pointner and Glaser 1988). Certainly cases are on record of early gastric cancer remaining unchanged for seven years (Eckardt et al 1984). Early gastric cancer is thus a useful term, for its diagnosis has meaning in a much better prognosis for the patient following appropriate therapy.

Early cancer is defined as a tumour that does not extend beyond the mucosa or submucosa even though there may be lymph node metastases. Clearly, early gastric cancer can (1) be in situ, i.e., confined by the epithelial basement membrane; (2) be intramucosal, i.e., confined by the muscularis mucosa, but invading the lamina propria; or (3) invade the muscularis mucosa and submucosa. Histological examination reveals the same tumour types as in the usual carcinoma of stomach, and it is likely that early gastric cancer is indeed the early stage of development of ordinary gastric cancer. Fukuda et al (1988) even describe a rare small cell early gastric carcinoma which like its advanced counterpart also exhibited argyrophilia and evidence of squamous differentiation.

One macroscopic variety deserves special mention in that it mimics peptic ulceration (Gear et al 1969, Mountford et al 1980) and intramucosal cancer has been observed to ulcerate and heal repeatedly (Sakita et al 1971). It cannot be stressed too forcibly that all stomach ulcers should be examined histologically. Biopsies should be taken from the base as well as the edge (Hatfield et al 1975), and six from each site appears to be the smallest number that ensures the maximum "pick-up" rate, those from the base giving only a slightly smaller yield than those from the edge (Lin et al 1989). It has even been shown that early carcinoma may only be revealed after repeated endoscopy and biopsy of apparently benign ulcers (Farinati et al 1987).

When biopsy examination is combined with brush cytology, the success rate is highest (Witzel et al 1976, Halter et al 1977, Chambers and Clark 1986), i.e., 95 to 100 per cent.

To the pathologist the diagnosis of early cancer does not differ from that of established cancer. The difficulties are the same, i.e., the problem of arriving at a definite diagnosis on relatively minute tissue samples. The histological diagnosis of carcinoma may be obvious where there is invasion beyond the muscularis mucosa (Fig. 8–9). However, the biopsy specimens frequently do not contain tissue deep to the muscularis mucosa and some other guidelines are then necessary. A common situation is the presence of abnormal but gland-forming epithelium in which the component cells are so bizarre that the diagnosis of carcinoma can be made with confidence. The question then arises as to whether or not this epithelium is still confined by the epithelial basement membrane, i.e., is it an in situ growth or is it invasive? The only guide to invasiveness when the biopsy is small and does not include deeper structures is the nature of the tissue that surrounds the abnormal glandular epithelium. Invasive carcinoma invariably excites around itself a more or less dense desmoplastic stromal reaction (Fig. 8–10). If abnormal glandular epithelium is surrounded by normal lamina propria, therefore, it should be regarded as in situ carcinoma (Fig. 8–11). Biopsies from benign gastric ulcers can mimic this appearance when the healing process traps glandular elements. Generally the glands are not atypical, and the fibrous tissue is not usually as homogeneous or dense but possesses more of the characteristics of granulation tissue (Fig. 8–12). Invasive carcinoma can also be diagnosed with confidence when individual or small abnormal groups of malignant cells can be identified in the lamina propria (Fig. 8–13). This may occur on occasion without an obvious stromal reaction, especially with signet ring cell carcinoma. Slides stained by a method for mucin are particularly useful in the diagnosis of this type of carcinoma. Sometimes only a few malignant cells are present that may be inconspicuous in ordinary H & E preparations but become obvious with a mucin stain (Fig. 8–14). Microscopically, therefore, early gastric cancer may have an adenocarcinomatous or tubo-papillary pattern or it may be anaplastic. The latter is usually of classical signet ring cell type or mucocellular, but mixtures of the two are also seen. The appearances do not differ from late gastric carcinoma (Elster

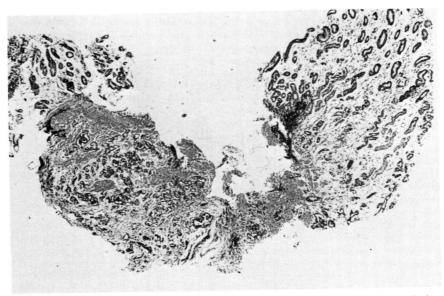

Figure 8–9. Carcinomatous tissue mingling with and deep to elements of the muscularis mucosa (left). Compare with uninvolved but traumatised mucosa (right) (H & E × 60).

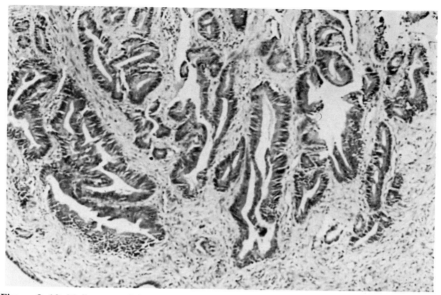

Figure 8–10. Malignant acini surrounded by dense fibrous tumour stroma (H & E × 90).

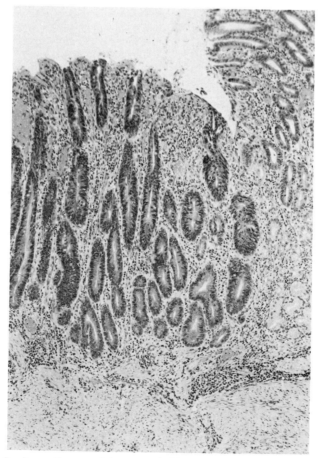

Figure 8–11. In situ malignant acini surrounded by normal lamina propria (H & E × 90).

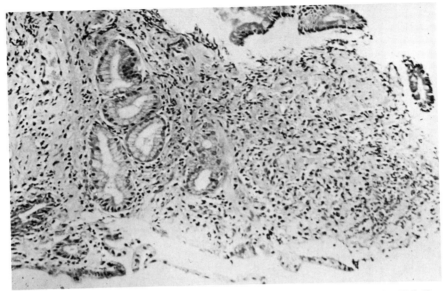

Figure 8–12. Normal acini surrounded by granulation tissue in benign ulcer margin (H & E × 150).

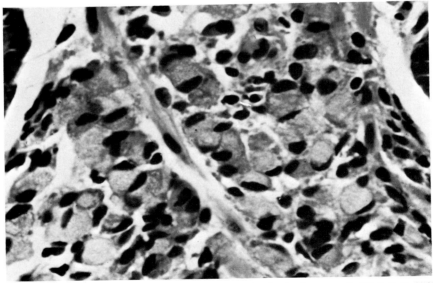

Figure 8–13. Individual signet ring carcinoma cells in the lamina propria (H & E × 350).

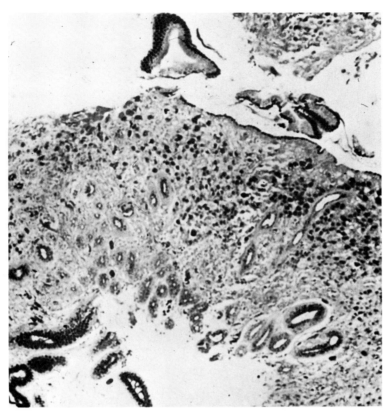

Figure 8–14. Individual malignant cells (dark dots) stained by the periodic acid-Schiff method (PAS × 40).

et al 1979). It is of some interest that it is the tumours of adenocarcinomatous pattern that are more likely to metastasize and, in contrast to advanced carcinoma of this type, have a worse prognosis than the diffuse form.

There seems to be no good reason that superficial spreading carcinoma (Figs. 8–15, 8–16) should be regarded as a separate entity. Unless it can be shown that it always remains intramucosal despite involving large areas of stomach, it is sensible to regard it as another macroscopic form of early cancer, since histologically it is usually anaplastic or signet ring type.

Since Balfour (1922) first described carcinoma in patients treated for ulcer by partial gastrectomy the subject has attracted a considerable literature (Farrands et al 1983, Totten, Burns and Kay 1983, Offerhaus et al 1984a,b, Pickford et al 1984, Clark, Fresini and Gledhill 1985, Lundegardh et al 1988, Pointner et al 1988). Although there are opinions to the contrary, most authors advocate follow-up endoscopy and biopsy of patients who have had previous gastric surgery. There is controversy, however, about when this surveillance should begin and how often it should be carried out. Certainly 20 to 25 years after the operation the chance of finding cancer is very real. In view of the probable time span associated with the development of advanced carcinoma in a non-operated stomach, a case for commencing surveillance soon after surgery could be made, although it may not be justifiable on grounds of cost effectiveness.

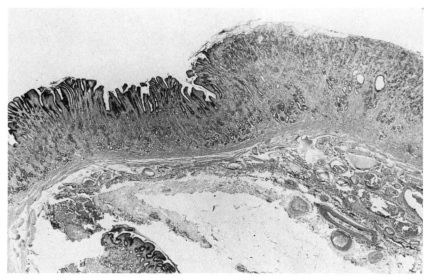

Figure 8–15. Excised stomach specimen, normal pyloric mucosa on the left and intramucosal carcinoma on the right (H & E × 315).

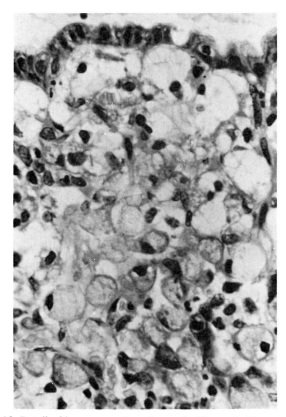

Figure 8–16. Detail of intramucosal carcinoma in Figure 8–15 (H & E × 375).

MUCOSAL HYPERPLASIAS AND POLYPS

Fibreoptic gastroscopy has revealed that gastric polyps are not as rare as was once held. In particular it is now commonplace for polyps of 1 cm or less in size to be removed at the endoscopic examination. Because of the diverse pathological nature of polypoidal lesions, polypectomy by snare may be neither possible nor the best form of treatment. Each case should be considered on its merits, but there would seem to be a place for biopsy of a majority of large polypoidal lesions, so that something of their nature can be ascertained before deciding appropriate therapy. However, polypoidal lesions caused by pathology of the deeper gastric tissues may not be revealed in the relatively superficial fibreoptic biopsy unless the lesion is ulcerated.

Although the term polyp embraces all manner of lesions of the mucosa, submucosa or muscularis that cause a protrusion into the gastric lumen, from the clinical standpoint it is most commonly used in reference to lesions composed of the mucosal elements. The particular importance of epithelial polyps lies in their relationship to carcinoma, for more than half of all polyps are asymptomatic. Symptoms are usually the result of erosion and bleeding, or are secondary to the polyp's bulk, or its obstruction of cardia or pylorus. There are several classifications of gastric polyps and polyposis syndromes (Nakamura 1970, Elster 1976, Ming 1977, Nakamura and Nakano 1985), and although it is possible to match one subtype in one classification with a similar one in another, the lack of uniformity of nomenclature and omissions of certain polyp types are unsatisfactory. Further-more, not all classifications address themselves to the problem of the definition of "polyposis" and its relationship, if any, to the stomach with more than one polyp, on the one hand, and a diffuse, polypoidal, hyperplastic mucosal lesion, on the other. Biopsy and the facility for excision of epithelial polyps demand a clear and comprehensive classification. It is important to recognise that epithelial polyps presumably arise by either an abnormal stimulation of cell growth in excess of that required for normal mucosal integrity, i.e., hyperplasia, or by a more complete loss of control over mucosal kinetics, i.e., neoplasia. Thus, broadly speaking, while a hyperplastic group and a neoplastic group of polyps might be recognised, there is every reason to believe that a hyperplastic process may at any time revert to normal or alternatively become truly neoplastic. By this reasoning it is possible to predict that hyperplastic polypoidal reactions will have histological similarities, not only if focal in form, but if they involve more or less the whole of the gastric mucosa, thus constituting a diffuse mucosal hyperplasia or a polyposis. Further-more the occasional development of neoplasia in a long-standing hyperplastic condition is also, as in other organs, a predictable event. The turnover of gastric surface epithelial mucus cells is rapid with a cell cycle time of two to three days and replacement in four to six days. Parietal and chief cells are replaced much more slowly, probably in excess of three months (Lipkin 1981). It seems that all these cell types are derived from a common precursor in the region of the base of the gastric pit, only this population being capable of cell division in normal mucosa. The controlling mechanisms for gastric cell turnover are largely unknown. Clearly there must be local ones that promote orderly healing of focal lesions, but there are others, e.g., the hormone gastrin, that exerts a generalised trophic action. Disorder of these mechanisms, which may be the result of exogenous or endogenous factors, could clearly result in local as well as generalised mucosal hyperplasia, and both focal and more widespread dysplastic or neoplastic lesions. In a consideration of gastric polyps, therefore, these facts need to be taken into account. If in prospective observations a lesion proves to be reversible, it would be logical to argue that it was hyperplastic rather than neoplastic in nature, even though the original stimulus was not known.

The basic pathological process in all forms of hyperplasia is essentially the same and differs only in extent of severity of variation or combination of the individual histological features in each instance. Similar changes are seen in the margins of a healing gastric ulcer, and the mechanism of polyp formation seems to be an exaggeration of the normal response of proliferation in the process of healing. However, an erosion or ulcer is not always present and the stimulus for hyperplasia is often obscure.

There is a proliferation of the foveolar cells and a tendency towards so-called pseudopyloric metaplasia of glands if body mucosa is involved. The foveolae or pits elongate and become tortuous and individual cells appear hypertrophied and sometimes have a metaplastic appearance with an eosinophilic cytoplasm. The simple mucinous glands have a tendency to form cysts. The lamina propria usually contains a mixture of lymphocytes, plasma cells and a few eosinophils and, especially if there is associated surface erosion, a population of polymorphs. Sometimes any increase in cellularity is minimal, but usually the intervening lamina propria is oedematous in places and, near the surface particularly, shows a profusion of thin-walled, dilated vascular spaces.

Another variable feature is a proliferation of muscular elements which spring from the muscularis mucosa and extend for varying distances into the lamina, sometimes almost reaching the surface. Sometimes intestinal metaplasia is present, but rarely is this extensive and is probably accounted for by the development of the polypoidal process on a background mucosa involved by chronic gastritis. Uncommonly, and usually in association with ulceration or other specific clinical situations, the cyst formation of the simple mucinous glands and the muscular hyperplasia is an extremely prominent feature. The resulting appearances have prompted the use of somewhat elaborate terminology. This is indeed true for all of the hyperplastic polypoidal states of the gastric mucosa, for whereas the basic tissue reactions are similar, clinical and other features seen in association with the various combinations of these reactions vary widely. Hence several types of hyperplastic lesions can be recognised.

Hyperplastic Polyps (Fig. 8–17)

Hyperplastic polyps comprise up to 90 per cent of gastric polyps in different reported series (Ming 1977, Nakamura and Nakano 1985). They rarely exceed 2 cm in largest diameter and are then commonly pedunculated. More usually they are much smaller and sessile with a smooth surface. Although they are usually single and most common in the antrum, multiple polyps can be seen in the same stomach and may involve all mucosal areas. Extensive multiple polyposis is uncommon. The background mucosa on which they occur may be essentially normal or it can show chronic gastritis.

Histologically the polyp consists of hyperplastic foveolae lined by tall epithelial cells with copious cytoplasm, but basal nuclei (Fig. 8–18). This epithelium extends onto the surface, which is generally non-ulcerated. The foveolae usually have complex branched outlines or are cystically dilated. The lamina propria contains a variable number of inflammatory cells, and, especially in polyps that are not ulcerated, they may be scant. Heavy infiltration is unusual and it may have a neutrophil component. The lamina is also frequently oedematous and exhibits a profusion of thin-walled vessels; another usual but variable feature in terms of its

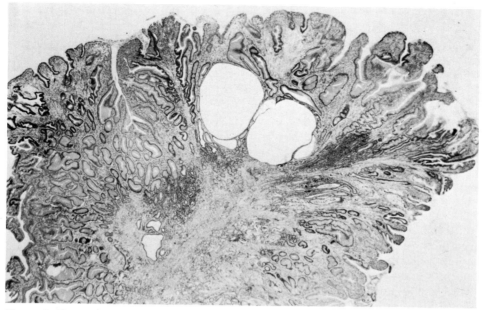

Figure 8–17. A sessile hyperplastic polyp removed endoscopically. Note the epithelial cysts and tortuous branched foveolae (H & E × 25).

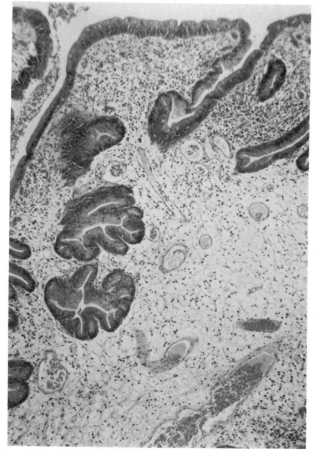

Figure 8–18. Hyperplastic branched foveolae composed of mucous-secreting cells with copious cytoplasm. Note the vascularity of the oedematous lamina propria and the inflammatory infiltrate (H & E × 300).

extent is proliferation of strands of smooth muscle that run between the glandular elements (Fig. 8–19). The deeper parts of the polyp frequently show a few pyloric type glands even when the polyp is located in the body region, and residual chief and parietal cells are unusual (Fig. 8–20). Intestinal metaplasia is never a prominent feature but occurs as small foci in approximately 15 per cent of polyps (Fig. 8–21). There is usually no evidence of significant dysplasia of the epithelial elements, although when surface ulceration is seen the neighbouring epithelium often reverts to a lower more basophilic proliferative type. A rather characteristic feature of hyperplastic polyps, especially of the sessile type, is the gradual transition of the appearances at the junction of the polyp and neighbouring mucosa (Fig. 8–22). As asserted by Ming (1977), there seems to be little point in recognizing a subgroup of so-called foveolar hyperplastic polyps (Elster 1974), for this lesion is nothing more than an early hyperplastic polyp (Fig. 8–23).

There is good evidence (Kamiya et al 1981) that the hyperplastic polyp is not a significant precancerous lesion, although it may coexist in the same stomach with carcinoma. In a prolonged follow-up study of between five and twelve years, they even showed the disappearance of a few lesions. However, the same authors also describe the development of increasing atypia and eventual carcinoma in two out of over 2,000 lesions. Polyps with mixed hyperplastic and adenomatous features are also encountered. (This subject is considered under Adenomatous Polyps.)

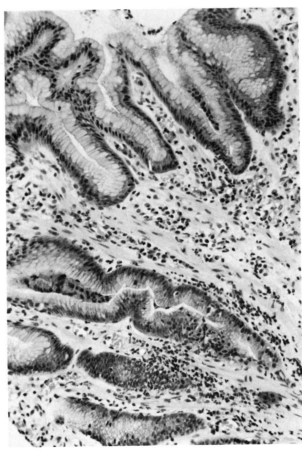

Figure 8–19. Muscle hyperplasia is sometimes seen almost extending to the surface (H & E × 300).

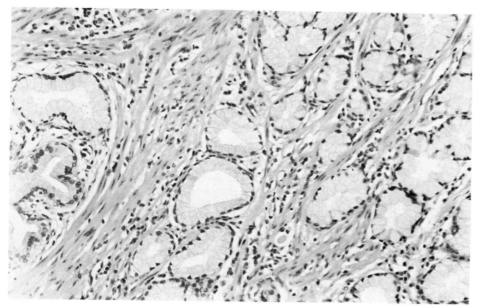

Figure 8–20. The deeper glands in this hyperplastic polyp are of pyloric type and there is obvious muscle hyperplasia (H & E × 300).

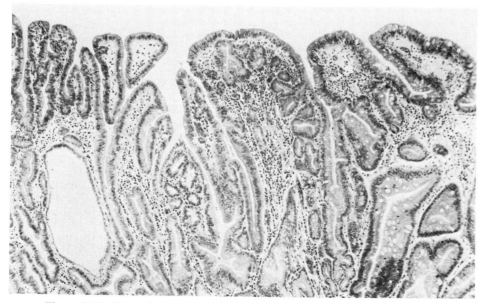

Figure 8–21. Hyperplastic polyp with intestinal metaplasia (right) (H & E × 300).

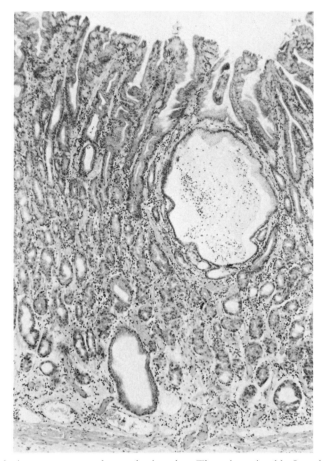

Figure 8–22. Pyloric mucosa near a hyperplastic polyp. There is noticeable foveolar tortuousity due to hyperplasia and occasional glandular cysts (H & E × 125).

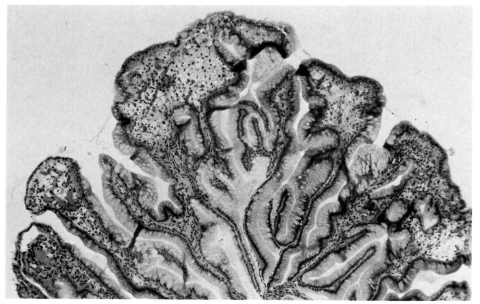

Figure 8–23. So-called foveolar hyperplastic polyp, which is only an early hyperplastic polyp without all the features seen in large lesions (H & E × 175).

Chronic Erosion

Chronic erosion has already been considered under Forms of Gastritis. The raised polypoidal lesions associated with erosion are rarely larger than 2 to 3 mm in diameter. Histologically the lesion consists of a central erosion with a necrotic base containing inflammatory debris that is bordered by hyperplastic, elongated, tortuous and branched crypts composed of relatively undifferentiated cells (Fig. 8–24A, B). Inflammatory changes in the lamina propria vary in severity from mild to marked and may be determined in part by the background mucosa upon which the lesion occurs, although it can be pronounced when the neighbouring mucosa is normal. It may be predominantly acute or chronic but is most frequently mixed; sometimes intraepithelial lymphocytes may be conspicuous. The erosion is always superficial and the muscularis intact. It is not usual for this lesion to involve a marked muscularis hyperplasia, but an element of cystic dilatation of both the crypts and underlying glands may be seen. The lesion occurs in the body mucosa where the deeper glands show a tendency to dedifferentiation and assume a pseudopyloric simple mucinous form which may undergo a hyperplasia, adding to the bulk of the lesion. Many of these features persist even when the erosion has healed (Figs. 8–25, 8–26). This is the type of lesion that Nakamura and Nakano (1985) classify as a type II polyp, and it has no known malignant potential. In view of the putative association with lymphocytic gastritis and claims outlined early of a relationship to *Campylobacter* infection, this polypoidal chronic erosion is clearly one which requires further study.

Gastritis Cystica Polyposa (et profunda)

This is a lesion characterised by all the histological features described in hyperplastic polyps. In addition, however, there is a marked proliferation of muscular elements and entrapment of numerous epithelial cysts. Sometimes, but not always, the cysts appear below the split and hypertrophied muscular mucosa, hence the use of "profunda" in the terminology (Figs. 8–27, 8–28). These lesions have been described at gastroenterology stomas, at peptic ulcer edges and in association with carcinoma (Ignatius, Armstrong and Eversole 1970, Mori, Shinya and Wolff 1971, Littler and Gleibermann 1972, Honore, Lewis and Ohara 1979, Stemmermann and Hayashi 1979, Franzin and Novelli 1981, Jablokow, Aranha and Reyes 1982, Fonde and Rodning 1986, Ozenc, Ruacan and Aran 1988). Because of the frequent association with chronic gastritis the lesions are also fairly frequently associated with areas of intestinal metaplasia. The condition has commanded attention because of its florid gross appearance. A typical lesion at a gastroenterostomy stoma is often several centimetres in diameter and consists of a local massive exaggeration of the normal mucosal rugal pattern. Presumably these lesions are due to a prolonged stimulated hyperplastic response to mucosal injury or erosion. Certainly erosions are not uncommonly present in the region of gastroenterostomy stomas and the regurgitation of bile and pancreatic juice, which is a regular event in this postoperative state, could well account for a prolonged mucosal injury. Indeed, in exaggerated form, most of the histological features seen in this condition are similar to those present in bile-reflux gastritis. In view of the increased incidence of cancer in the postoperative stomach it is not surprising that dysplastic changes have been described in this condition (Franzin et al 1985), which may also account for its coexistence with frank adenocarcinoma (Bogomoletz et al 1985).

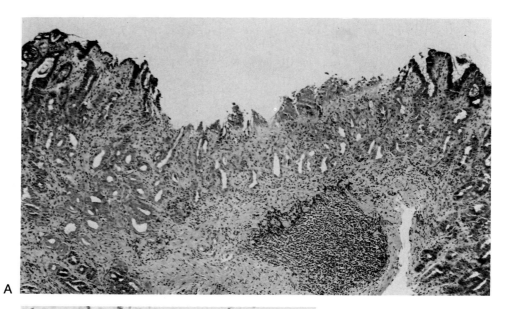

A

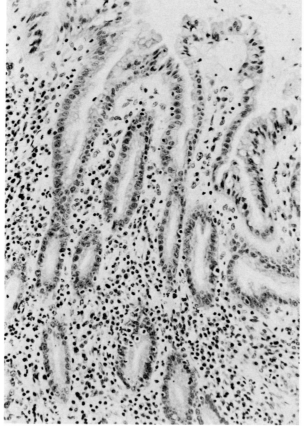

B

Figure 8–24. Chronic erosions. **A**, Early lesion with regenerative tortuousity of the marginal crypts and associated inflammatory changes (H & E × 100). **B**, Detail of the margin of a chronic erosion. Note the hyperplastic appearance and the inflammation characterised by numerous intra-epithelial lymphocytes (H & E × 300).

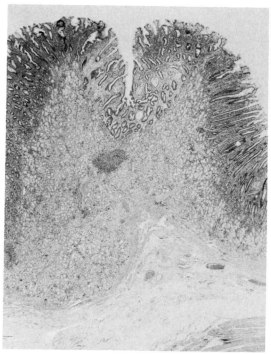

Figure 8–25. Healed chronic erosion with persistent tortuous and irregularly branched crypts and hyperplastic pyloric-type glands. Note the occasional cystic crypts and the mainly superficial inflammation (H & E × 75).

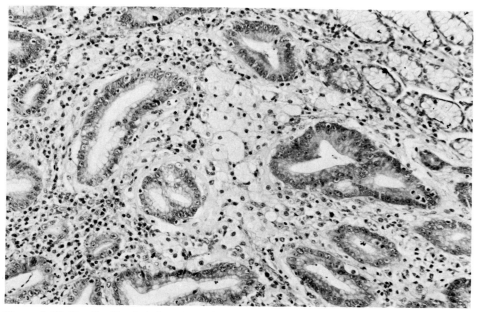

Figure 8–26. Detail of healed chronic erosion to show xanthelasmatous foamy macrophages in the lamina propria (H & E × 300).

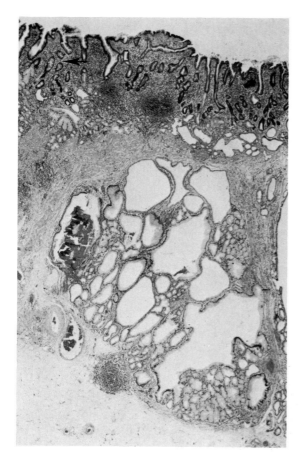

Figure 8–27. Gastritis cystica profunda. Note the inflammatory infiltration, intestinal metaplasia (arrow) and the deep cysts (H & E × 25).

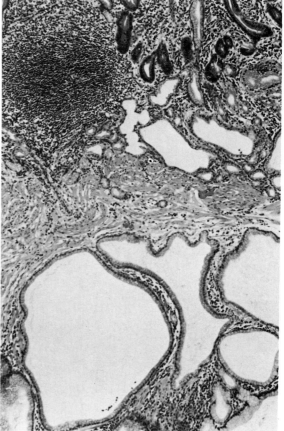

Figure 8–28. Detail of Figure 8–27. Cystic simple mucinous glands lie below the splayed and hyperplastic muscularis mucosa running across the centre (H & E × 175).

Other Forms of Mucosal Hyperplasia

The unusual prominence of normal gastric rugae was called état mammelonné by early French pathologists (Magnus 1952). An abnormal rugal hyperplasia, however, occurs in some patients with duodenal ulcer and the Zollinger-Ellison syndrome (Krag 1966, Zollinger and Moore 1968). Mucosal biopsies afford the means of estimating parietal cell mass by quantitative methods in these circumstances. Schmidt-Wilcke, Haake and Riecken (1974), for example, have shown a close relationship between parietal cell density and maximal acid output in duodenal ulcer patients.

Epithelial hyperplasia involving the gastric pits, glands or both (Fig. 8–29) has been described in association with carcinoma of the stomach and with peptic ulcer, both gastric and duodenal (Monroe, Boughton and Sommers 1964, Stamm and Saremaslani 1989). Usually, but not always, it occurs close to the primary lesion, and similar changes occur in the mucosa adjacent to colonic carcinoma (Saffos and Rhatigan 1977). It is important that this entity is recognised as being different from the lesion that results from gastritis with pseudopyloric metaplasia of body glands, which is seen in the distal stomach in relation to peptic ulcer. It is universally accepted that carcinoma of the stomach and peptic ulcer are associated with a degree of type AB or type B chronic gastritis involving the pyloric antrum, and to a variable degree more proximal parts of the stomach. The gastritis is

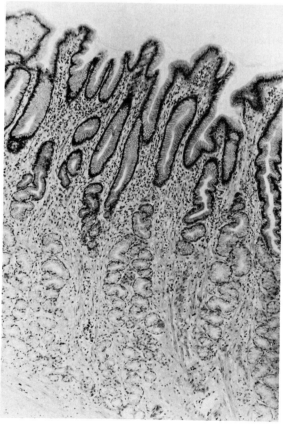

Figure 8–29. Antral type mucosa near a prepyloric peptic ulcer. There is pit, neck and glandular hyperplasia. Compare with Figure 5–5 (H & E × 100).

commonly severe, especially in conjunction with high gastric ulcer and carcinoma, and is frequently associated with both pseudopyloric and intestinal metaplasia. Distortion of the gastric pits by inflammatory oedema, and inflammatory infiltration with lymphoid aggregates when there is also pseudopyloric metaplasia of body glands, is easily interpreted as a hyperplastic state of the pyloric mucosa. It is for this reason that some authors, misinterpretating these changes, make the claim that high gastric ulcers occur in stomachs with an unusually large antrum. It has already been pointed out, however, that pyloric mucosa can often be differentiated from pseudopyloric metaplasia by the presence of parietal cells in the former.

Menetrier's Disease

Menetrier's disease (Menetrier 1888) is frequently referred to incorrectly as hypertrophic gastritis. In hypertrophy of a tissue or an organ there is an increase in size but not in number of its constituent parts, the latter being hyperplasia. Both may exist concomitantly, but in the case of Menetrier's disease the lesion is a hyperplasia and not hypertrophy.

The thickened mucosa (Fig. 8–30) is thrown into folds into which a spur of muscularis mucosa often projects. The pits are elongated, as are the glands, which nevertheless may retain a normal cellular component. There are areas, however, where simple mucin-secreting epithelium similar to gastric surface epithelium extends into the basal parts of the glands, which frequently show cystic change. This mucin-secreting epithelium may be flattened but will usually show histochemical evidence of a transition from gastric to intestinal type (Whitehead, unpublished observation). Sometimes frank intestinal metaplasia is seen (Fig. 8–31), but this seems to occur more commonly in areas where there is also inflammatory infiltration.

Smooth-muscle bundles can be traced from the muscularis mucosa between the

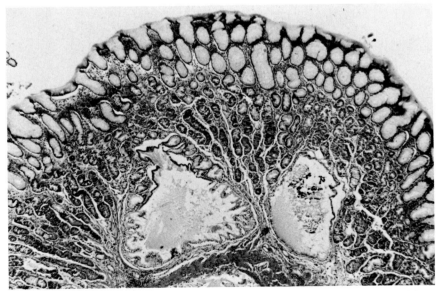

Figure 8–30. Gastric body mucosa in Menetrier's disease. There is overall thickening of the mucosa, and simple surface-type mucin-secreting epithelium extends into and lines deep cystic spaces (H & E × 56).

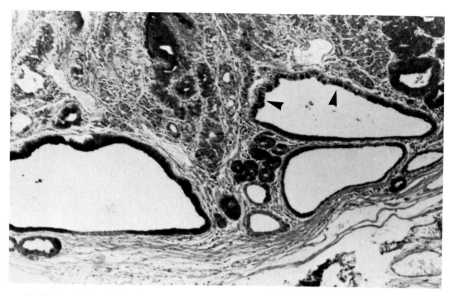

Figure 8–31. Cystic basal glands in Menetrier's disease tending to split the muscularis mucosa. Note the small-intestinal type of goblet cells (arrowheads) as compared to the gastric type of mucin-secreting epithelium lining other cysts (PAS × 150).

glands and often right up to the surface (Fig. 8–32). There is hyperplasia, splitting and irregularity of the muscularis mucosa, which is exaggerated where cystic glandular changes are most marked, and cystic glands may appear in the sub-mucosa.

In some cases of Menetrier's disease there is an overall depletion of specialised oxyntic and peptic cells, and it is not unusual for low acid secretion to accompany the disease. Parietal and peptic cells may be very obvious, however, and some cases are associated also with a normal (Gabreau et al 1982) or a high acid output (Brooks, Isenberg and Goldstein 1970, Overholt and Jeffries 1970, Kristensen and Nilsson 1985). Lam et al (1983) describe two brothers with pachydermoperiostosis, Menetrier's and peptic ulcer, and in large series of cases peptic ulcer disease appears to be not all that uncommon (Searcy and Malagelada 1984). Although other familial cases are on record (Larsen, Tarp and Kristensen 1987), heredity seems to be of minor significance in pathogenesis. Celik, Ettinger and Satchidanand (1984) describe a case associated with massive bleeding from a coexistent arteriovenous malformation, which in all probability is a fortuitous relationship.

The degree and distribution of an inflammatory infiltration or true gastritis vary in different cases, and some at least are related to rupture of cystic lesions (Fig. 8–33). The mucus released seems to evoke an inflammatory reaction characterised by an occasional giant cell.

There is now ample evidence that Menetrier's disease is sometimes reversible (Berry, Ben-Dov and Freund 1980, Walker 1981). Occasionally this has followed treatment with cimetidine (Vendelboe and Jespersen 1981, Gabreau et al 1982). An interesting case of Menetrier's lesion ascribed to increased local synthesis of prostaglandin E_2 has been described (Boyd et al 1988) in which the lesion regressed after successful treatment of a carcinoid syndrome.

Transient Menetrier's disease seems to occur particularly in childhood (Schar-

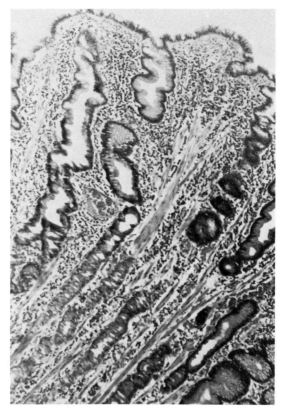

Figure 8–32. Gastric mucosa in Menetrier's disease showing smooth-muscle bundles extending almost to the surface epithelium (H & E × 255).

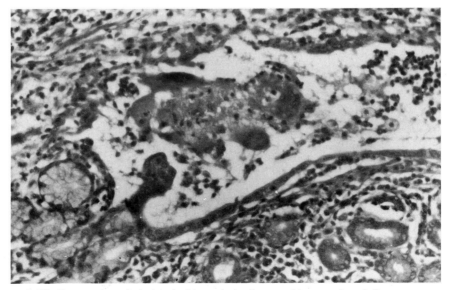

Figure 8–33. Ruptured cystic lesion in Menetrier's disease with secondary inflammatory reaction and mucin granuloma (H & E × 375).

schmidt 1977, Bloom 1981, Kraut et al 1981, Stillman et al 1981). In childhood it also appears that the mucosa can revert to normal (Baker et al 1986), whereas in adults resolution may result in residual atrophic gastritis (Berenson, Sannella and Freston 1976).

It is interesting that certain cases with typical histological features of Menetrier's disease are associated with multiple endocrine adenomata (Kenny, Dockerty and Waugh 1954) and sometimes with a Zollinger-Ellison syndrome, a pancreatic islet cell tumour, marked gastric hypersecretion and peptic ulceration (Whitehead, unpublished observation). Menetrier's disease has also been described in association with vitiligo. Berkowitz, Passaro and Isenberg (1977) and Ming (1977) identified three types of hyperplasia of the gastric mucosa, one primarily involving mucus cells of foveolar origin, one involving chief and parietal cells only, and a third affecting all cell types. However, cases reported in the literature make it plain the gastric mucosal hyperplasia that characteristically spares the antrum presents a spectrum of clinical and histological features. The more severe and prolonged disturbances of mucosal dynamics, whatever the precipitating stimulus, will be associated with the most severe histological disturbances, whereas relatively milder and shorter-lived stimuli will give rise to milder and potentially reversible lesions. This does not mean that one needs to advocate abolition of terms such as Menetrier's or Zollinger-Ellison syndrome, since they also have other clinical implications. This principle is also illustrated by consideration of the entity Cronkhite-Canada syndrome.

Cronkhite-Canada Syndrome

Diffuse gastrointestinal mucosal thickening and irregularity often referred to as polyposis, together with abnormal skin pigmentation, dystrophy of the nails, baldness and various biochemical abnormalities secondary to the gastrointestinal loss of protein and tissue fluid, was first described by Cronkhite and Canada in 1955. The disease often has a prolonged course and only a minority of patients are observed to recover spontaneously (Aanestad et al 1987).

The intestinal mucosal lesion is not a true neoplastic polyposis, and in the stomach it shares many features with Menetrier's disease. Not only in the stomach but also in the rest of the intestine (see Fig. 18–35) the lesions appear to be the result of a functional disorder of the mucin glands. Early lesions in the stomach show a progressive loss of specialised body glands by a process of mucin cell transformation. These become increasingly numerous, enlarged and often bizarre in morphology, and because of excessive and perhaps abnormal secretion the glands become cystic. Consequently there is deformity and thickening of the mucosa (Fig. 8–34). Some cysts are invaded by inflammatory cells, and others rupture into the lamina propria, causing a further secondary inflammatory response that has a conspicuous histiocytic element (Fig. 8–35). It is this excessive secretion, cystic dilatation of glands, their rupture and increased bulk of the lamina propria (Fig. 8–36) that accounts for the grossly polypoidal appearance of the mucosa. It is also because of these features that Johnson et al (1972) regarded the lesions as a diffuse gastroenterocolitis with inflammatory pseudopolyposis.

There is evidence that the non-polypoidal mucosa is also abnormal with a tendency for specialised cell type to be replaced by mucus cells (Freeman et al 1985). It is postulated, based upon an electron microscopic study, that the primary process or defect affects the regenerative zones of the mucosa involved (Jenkins, Stephenson and Scott 1985).

The Cronkhite-Canada syndrome has been reported in association with multiple

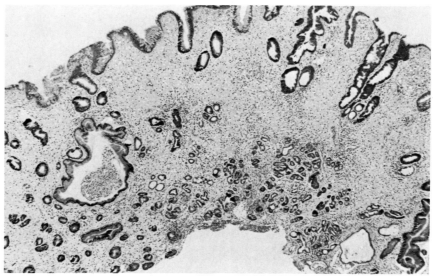

Figure 8–34. Gastric biopsy in Cronkhite-Canada syndrome. The mucosa is thickened and some glands are cystic. Note the apparent excess of lamina propria (H & E × 14).

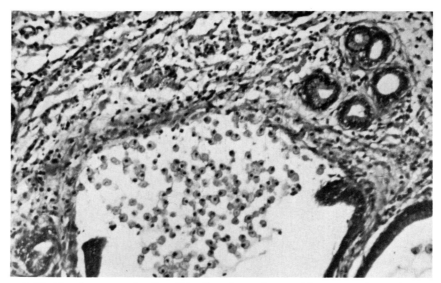

Figure 8–35. Gastric mucosa in Cronkhite-Canada syndrome. The ruptured cyst has produced secondary inflammation and a marked histiocytic reaction (H & E × 105).

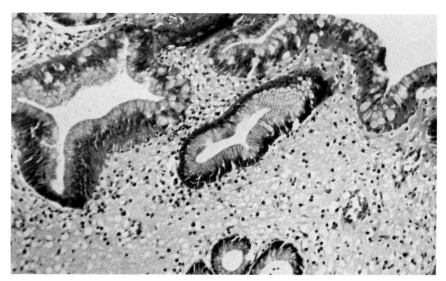

Figure 8–36. Gastric mucosa in Cronkhite-Canada syndrome. The lamina propria is bulky and distinctly oedematous. Note the enlargement and irregularity of form of the mucinous epithelium (H & E × 105).

myeloma (Rubin et al 1980) and cytomegalovirus infection (Lipper and Kahn 1977), but both are probably fortuitous. Nonomura et al (1980) describe a case associated with sigmoid carcinoma and in a review of the literature noted a 15 per cent incidence of complicating carcinoma in this rare condition. In cases described by Katayama, Kimura and Konn (1985) and Malhotra and Sheffield (1988), not only was colon carcinoma present but there were also adenomatous changes in the epithelium of the polypoidal lesions. Colonic tumours are thus not that rare, but in their review of 55 cases in the literature Daniel et al (1982) found only one complicated by gastric cancer. In contrast, an association between Menetrier's and gastric carcinoma appears real (Scharschmidt 1977). This does not mean that Menetrier's and Cronkhite-Canada are entirely unrelated. They certainly share histological similarities in the gastric mucosa, and like cases of Menetrier's disease, the features of Cronkhite-Canada syndrome are known to be completely reversible (Russell, Bhathal and St. John 1983, Peart et al 1984). The interrelationships of all the hyperplastic lesions of the stomach, although often distinct clinicopathological entities, can be illustrated by the reports of Krentz and Gohrband (1976) who followed 45 patients with gastric erosions for five years and witnessed the evolution in 26 of hyperplastic folds. Similarly, as Roesch (1978) reports, chronic erosions are not infrequently seen at the apices of the giant hyperplastic folds in Menetrier's disease. It seems that hyperplastic lesions of the stomach are in some instances a reaction to mucosal damage or ulceration, in others due to the trophic action of gastrin, but in the majority the stimulus to hyperplasia is as yet not determined.

Hamartomatous and Heterotopic Polyps

Primarily epithelial polyps may also be due to errors of development, i.e., they are hamartomas or heterotopias. In Peutz-Jeghers syndrome gastric involvement occurs in approximately one quarter of cases. The lesions, as elsewhere, are composed of a somewhat disorganised arrangement of the glandular elements normally present in that part, e.g., antral, body or cardiac together with muscle bundles extending from the muscularis mucosa (Figs. 8–37, 8–38). In Peutz-Jeghers disease as a whole there is now a well-recognized increased incidence of cancer not only of the intestine and stomach but also in a variety of other organs (Utsunomiya et al 1974, Halbert 1982). The exact relationship between gastric polyps and the evolution of carcinoma of the stomach still requires elucidation.

In colonic juvenile polyposis gastric involvement may also occur. Like juvenile polyps elsewhere, the sparse, often cystic, glandular elements are set in abundant lamina propria devoid of muscle. They are commonly infiltrated by inflammatory cells and have a rounded appearance and a smooth surface. Malignant potential has not been recorded. In the case of familial juvenile polyposis of the stomach described by Watanabe, Nagashima and Motoi (1979), who also review the previous literature, there is a remarkable similarity of the illustrated pathology to the lesions of the Cronkhite-Canada syndrome.

Another form of gastric polyposis that occurs in the region of the gastric body mucosa is also included in the hamartomatous group (Parks, Bussey and Lockhart-Mummery 1970, Tatsuta et al 1982). It occurs in patients with familial polyposis coli, or Gardners syndrome, but much more frequently is unassociated (Elster 1976, Lee and Burt 1986, Bedossa, Lemaigre and Martin 1987b, Justrabo et al 1987). The lesions are usually just a few millimetres in diameter and are rarely as large as 1 cm. They are caused by a cystic dilatation of the gastric body glands, and, although flattened, the lining cells usually retain the features of parietal and chief cells although occasional cysts are lined by mucous neck cells (Figs. 8–39, 8–40). The gastric pit zone and surface epithelium are largely normal, although stretched over the underlying cystic glands, and there is not usually a significant inflammatory change in the lamina propria unless a coincidental and probably

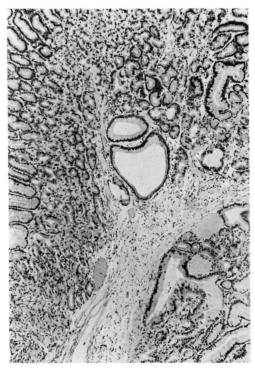

Figure 8–37. Peutz-Jegher gastric polyp with branching muscular core and cystic deep mucous glands (H & E × 125).

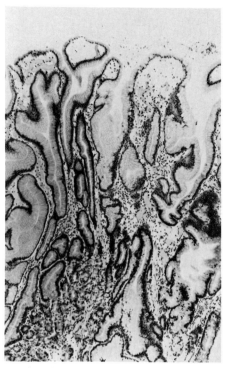

Figure 8–38. Peutz-Jegher gastric polyp in its upper part with irregular branching abnormal crypts and strands of interfoveolar muscle tissue (H & E × 250).

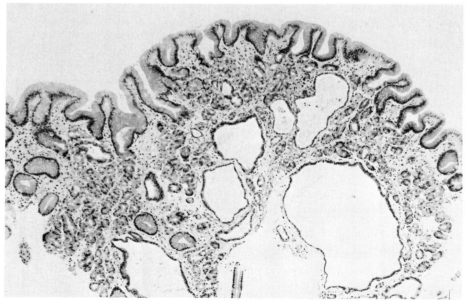

Figure 8–39. Cystic body gland polyp (H & E × 125).

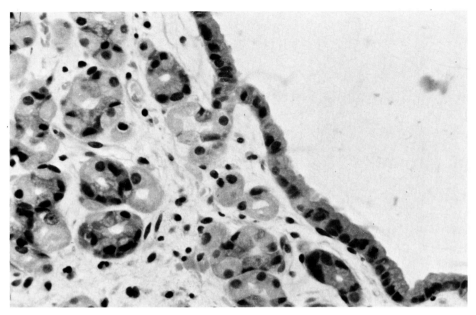

Figure 8–40. Detail of Figure 8–39 showing the characteristic lining of chief and parietal cells (H & E × 400).

unrelated gastritis is present. It is probably incorrect to regard these lesions as hamartomatous since the basic structure of the gastric mucosa is normal, the only abnormality being gland dilatation. Iida et al (1980) have described three patients in whom multiple polyps of this type spontaneously resolved; they are thus more likely to be the result of disordered function and secretion of the gastric glands. Watanabe et al (1978) in common with other Japanese pathologists have called these lesions fundic gland polyps. Cystic glandular fundic polypsis, a similar terminology, is favoured by Voigt et al (1983), but since the lesion can occur in all areas of the gastric mucosa that is of body type, the use of the term fundic, which is only part of the body mucosa, is incorrect. Elster (1976) prefers the descriptive term "cysts of the gastric glands" and Chakravorty and Schatzki (1975) call the lesion "gastric cystic polyposis." A more accurate descriptive terminology would, however, be "cystic body gland polyp" or "cystic body gland polyposis" if multiple.

Carfagna et al (1987) have reported a fundic polypoidal hamartoma in a patient with widespread gastritis. It consisted of cystic glands set in a framework of smooth muscle tissue. The glands were both body and antral in type and included endocrine cells. Heterotopic pancreatic tissue or Brunner's glands may also present as a polypoidal lesion usually in the region of the antrum.

Adenomatous Polyps

These lesions arising in intestinalised gastritic mucosa exhibit a range of macroscopic appearances identical to adenomatous polyps of the colon. It would seem that smaller sessile lesions are common in Japan (Nakamura 1970, Nakamura and Nakano 1985), whereas in most other countries polyps tend to be rather more pedunculated, larger and sometimes villous. Adenomatous polyps are the commonest of the two types of lesion seen in the stomach in familial adenomatosis patients, the other, as already mentioned, being cystic fundic gland polyps (Iida et al 1988). Because of the usual distribution of simple chronic gastritis, adenomatous polyps in non-adenomatosis patients are most frequent in the antrum but may arise in any site. In essence they constitute a focus of dysplastic epithelium whose growth characteristics determine that an accumulation of cells occurs at the site, thus raising them above the surrounding mucosa. Clearly the individual cytological features will be the same irrespective of whether the dysplastic focus is flat or polypoidal and the arguments relating to the use of the term carcinoma in situ are the same. Like colonic polyps, tubular and villous patterns may predominate, although most are mixed. There is no doubt as to the malignant potential of adenomatous polyps, and, indeed, all the arguments relating to the adenoma-cancer sequence in the colon apply to the stomach. Up to approximately one half of adenomatous polyps will also show invasive carcinoma, and this is more likely to be seen the larger the lesion. In addition to the cystic body gland polyps seen in patients with familial polyposis coli, adenomatous polyps of the gastric antrum also occur (Sugihara et al 1982, Jarvinen, Nyberg, Peltokallio 1983). It is also being recognised more commonly that adenomatous change may be superimposed on a hyperplastic polyp (Figs. 8–41, 8–42). Indeed, Nakamura and Nakano (1985) regard this type of lesion (type III) as being fundamentally different from the wholly adenomatous polyp (type IV), which has a greater malignant potential (Muratani et al 1989). Thus, although hyperplastic polyps are, as already stated,

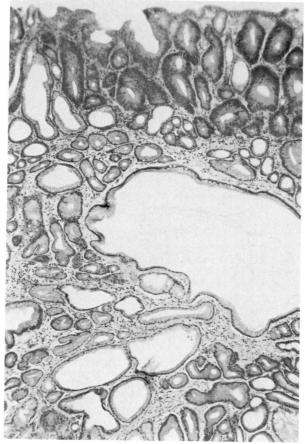

Figure 8–41. Gastric polyp with both hyperplastic and adenomatous features (H & E × 125).

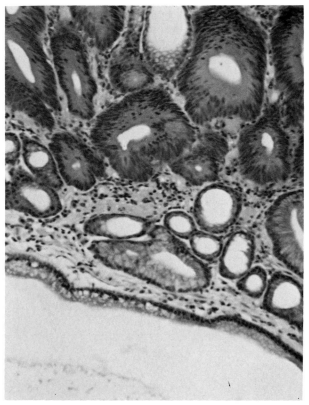

Figure 8–42. Detail of the polyp in Figure 8–41. The adenomatous features are mainly of tubular pattern and the dysplasia moderate in degree (H & E × 300).

predominantly without a significant cancer risk, they may on occasion, as illustrated, progress to exhibit adenomatous features, when as in an adenomatous polyp de novo, a further loss of cell growth control mechanisms may result in increased malignant potential and invasion. This no doubt accounts for the examples of malignancy occurring in hyperplastic polyps (Nakamura 1970, Ming 1977, Hattori 1985, Daibo, Itabashi and Hirota 1987), but the incidence of this change is less than 5 per cent.

Adenomatous and carcinomatous lesions consisting predominantly of neoplastic Paneth cells also are described sometimes in association with pernicious anaemia (Lev and DeNucci 1989, Rubio 1989).

LYMPHOID HYPERPLASIA AND MALIGNANT LYMPHOMA

The diagnosis of lesions that raise suspicions of being malignant because of their endoscopic appearance is a particularly difficult task when they are of lymphoid origin. Lymphoid infiltrates may be reactive as part of the picture of chronic gastritis or as a tissue response to ulceration (Hyjek and Kelenyi 1982) or they may be malignant. The difficulty for the pathologist in differentiating between benign and malignant infiltrates is accentuated by the fact that both may coexist in one and the same lesion. Furthermore, lymphoid tissue is absent from gastric mucosa at birth (Takaki 1986) and appears during life in association with the various inflammatory states of the mucosa and ulceration. Thus one would expect to find a reactive element in any malignant lymphoid process that supervened. If the malignancy derives from preexisting reactive elements, a further difficulty is predictable, namely, the criteria for deciding when the malignant process has definitively established itself. With the burgeoning of immunochemistry in histopathology, much new light is being cast on this problem area.

Claims in the past (Katz et al 1973) that gastroscopic appearances are of greater importance than biopsy histology or brush cytology for the diagnosis of some forms of gastric lymphoma can no longer be sustained. Since the introduction of the use of the Kiel classification and cell characterisation by the use of monoclonal antibodies, great strides forward have been accomplished (Van den Heule, Van Kerkem and Heimann 1979, Spinelli, Lo Gullo and Pizzetti 1980, Saraga, Hurlimann and Ozzello 1981, Brousse et al 1983, Isaacson and Wright 1984, Isaacson, Spencer and Finn 1986, Myhre and Isaacson 1987). Nevertheless, claims are still made for the existence of a tumour-like lesion occurring in association with past or present peptic ulcer, which is called gastric pseudolymphoma (Tokunaga, Watanabe and Morimatsu 1987, Graffner and Hesselvik 1987). The balance of opinion is, however, changing, and with the newer methods of investigation it appears that most if not all so-called pseudolymphomas are in fact low grade lymphomas (Myhre and Isaacson 1987). Light chain restriction has been convincingly demonstrated in lesions that would otherwise be diagnosed as pseudolymphoma (Isaacson, Spencer and Finn 1986, Burke et al 1987).

Most gastric lymphomas are B cell in type, of follicle centre cell origin and contain centrocyte-like cells or have plasma cell differentiation in a minority (Myhre and Isaacson 1987). Plasmacytomas have, of course, been recognised on simple morphological grounds for some time (Nakanishi et al 1982), some even containing crystalline cytoplasmic inclusions (Ferrer-Roca 1982), and lately cases have been adequately characterised using advanced immunoperoxidase and immunogold techniques (Ooi, Nakanishi and Hashiba 1987). Some have been associated with serum alpha heavy chain (Guardia et al 1980), and gastric immunoblastic lymphomas are described in patients with a preexisting angioimmunoblastic lymphadenopathy (Bauer et al 1982). Thus early claims that so-called pseudolymphoma was a premalignant lesion (Wolf and Spjut 1981, Brooks and Enterline 1983) seem now to be partly substantiated, although there are those who might argue that so-called pseudolymphoma is already a low grade lymphoma (Isaacson, Spencer and Finn 1986).

Isaacson and Spencer (1987) have argued that primary gastric B cell lymphoma, which often remains localised for long periods, involving regional lymph nodes in a minority of cases, and responding well to therapy and even surgical removal, is a tumour arising in centrocytic-like cells that are immunologically distinct from centrocytes proper. The malignancy arises thus in interfollicular areas but may invade the reactive follicles secondarily. These authors draw comparison with B cell lymphomas of similar type arising in the lymphoid tissue associated with other mucosal surfaces that are also known for their good prognosis, e.g., in the lung, salivary glands and thyroid. Mohri (1987), however, apparently believes that primary gastric lymphomas may arise not only in interfollicular cells but in follicular centre cells also. This is clearly a field for further study, but from the viewpoint of diagnosis in biopsy tissues several points can be made. The density of the infiltrate and the relative preservation of the native mucosal architecture despite some glandular atrophy in the absence of ulceration can sometimes be helpful in allaying a suspicion of lymphoma (Fig. 8–43). In lymphoma the phenomenon of epithelial tropism of the malignant cells and the formation of so-called lymphoepithelial lesions (Isaacson and Wright 1983, 1984) tends to lead to epithelial and glandular destruction (Figs. 8–44, 8–45A, B, C). These lymphoep-

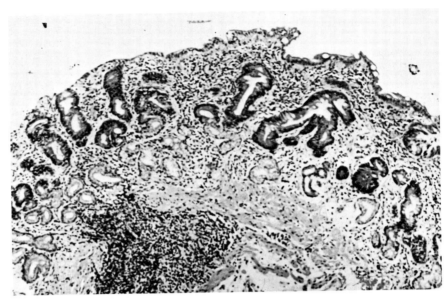

Figure 8–43. Chronic atrophic gastritis: cellular infiltrate although deep, is not particularly dense, and although there is glandular atrophy and intestinal metaplasia, an overall preservation of mucosal architecture is present, although somewhat collapsed (H & E × 100).

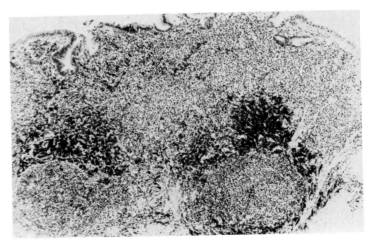

Figure 8–44. Malignant lymphoma. Note obliteration of glandular elements and density of infiltrate although the surface epithelium is intact. Two abnormal follicles are present and there is biopsy artefact above these (H & E × 100).

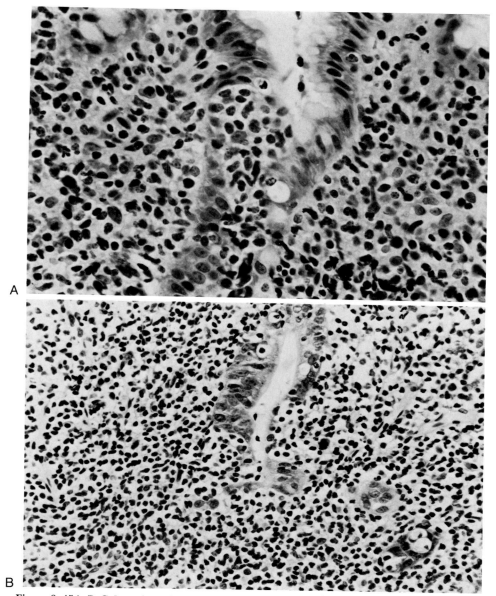

Figure 8–45A, B, C. Lympho-epithelial lesions in biopsies of a malignant lymphoma. Note progressive destruction of the epithelial element by the infiltrating islands of malignant cells (H & E × 500).

Illustration continued on following page

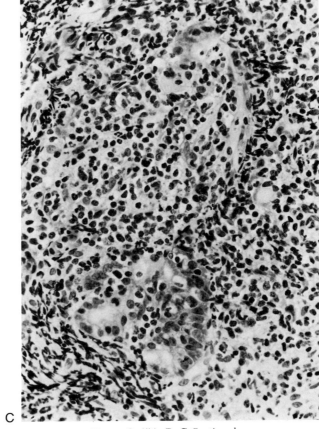

C

Figure 8–45A, B, C *Continued*

ithelial lesions tend to occur only in better differentiated tumours, and when cells resemble centroblasts or immunoblasts they are absent. The cells can usually be differentiated from non-malignant intraepithelial lymphocytes, which tend to occur as single cells surrounded by a clear halo whereas tumour cells occur as groups or clusters often obliterating the lumen by bulging into it. As already mentioned, plasma cell differentiation may be seen but these do not seem to have epitheliotropism.

As with lymphoma diagnosis in other sites, cytological evaluation of the suspicious cells is all important and is made easier if ultra-thin resin-embedded sections are available (Figs. 8–46 to 8–48). Many laboratories are now able to type suspicious cells using immunohistochemical methods even on paraffin sections, and this is beginning to take on a more important aspect. Perhaps in the not too distant future lymphoma typing will be based more upon which cell markers they carry rather than their morphological resemblance to cells that occur in normal lymphoid tissues. For the moment, however, a combination of these is proving extremely valuable. Tumours composed mainly of large bizarre cells without a tendency to form follicles behave more aggressively than those with cells exhibiting at least some tendency to differentiate towards similar cells in normal lymphoid tissue. A curious subtype of gastric lymphoma is one which by light microscopy appears as a signet ring cell lesion (Hernandez and Sheehan 1985). It is clearly important that a correct diagnosis is reached in such cases because of the much worse prognosis and the different therapeutic approach for signet ring cell adenocarcinoma.

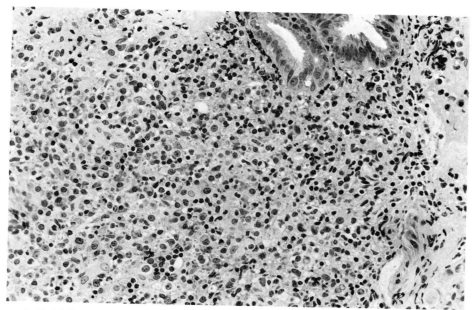

Figure 8–46. Malignant lymphoma of predominantly centroblastic type (H & E of resin section × 200).

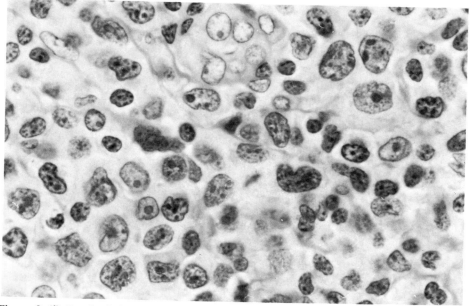

Figure 8–47. Detail of Figure 8–46. The majority of nuclei are large and irregular with multiple often peripheral nucleoli. A few immunoblasts with central nucleoli are also seen (H & E of resin section × 500).

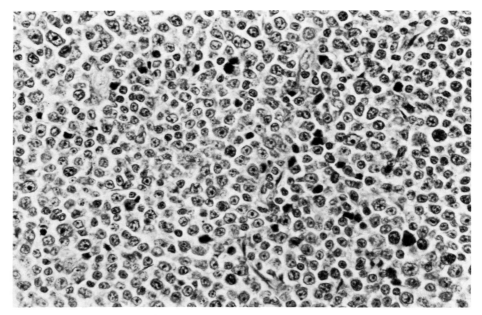

Figure 8–48. An immunoblastic sarcoma with a majority of large cells with prominent central and single nucleoli (H & E of resin section × 350).

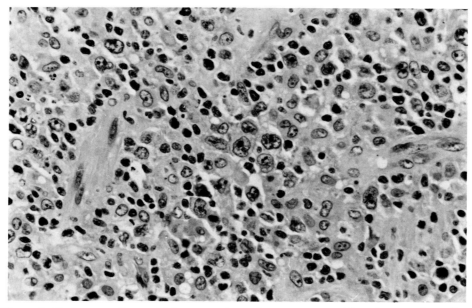

Figure 8–49. A true malignant histiocytoma. Apart from some normal lymphocytes, the malignant cells appear with bizarre irregular nuclei, frequent nucleoli and a prominent copious cytoplasm (H & E of resin section × 350).

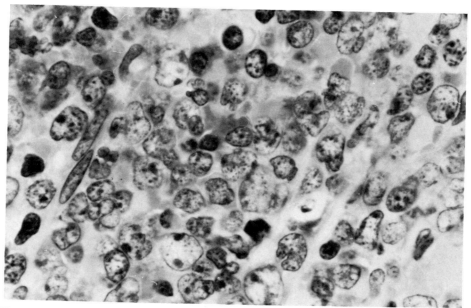

Figure 8–50. A malignant histiocytoma showing marked nuclear enlargement. The cytoplasm is less obvious than in Figure 8–49, but the tumour was typed histochemically (H & E resin section × 500).

Other forms of primary or secondary gastric lymphomas not of B cell origin seem to be uncommon. Hodgkin's disease, for example, is so rare that any such diagnosis should be seriously questioned. The problem with the remainder such as have been described in the past as histiocytic lymphomas, for example, (Isaacson et al 1979, Seo et al 1982) is that they were defined before the era of more specific immunohistochemical markers. As compared to B cell tumours, other primary gastric lymphomas deriving from other lymphoid cell lines appear to be quite uncommon. A malignant histiocytic tumour confirmed by histochemistry is illustrated in Figures 8–49 and 8–50.

OTHER TYPES OF GASTRITIS AND MISCELLANEOUS LESIONS

OTHER TYPES OF GASTRITIS

Eosinophilic Gastroenteritis

The stomach is virtually always involved in eosinophilic gastroenteritis, and a diagnosis can frequently be made in a gastric biopsy (Navab et al 1972, Katz, Goldman and Grand 1977). It is a disease affecting all age groups, from infancy to old age, which may also involve the oesophagus, the small intestine and occasionally the colon (Ashby, Appleton and Dawson 1964, Tedesco et al 1981, Matzinger and Daneman 1983, Zora et al 1984, Stringel et al 1984, Naylor and Pollet 1985, Moore et al 1986, Rumans and Lieberman 1987, Snyder et al 1987, Steele et al 1987). If mucosal involvement predominates, protein loss and malabsorption result, muscular involvement causes obstruction because of the attendant fibrosis and serosal disease is characterised by ascites (Klein et al 1970, Trounce and Tanner 1985). Mucosal ulceration and haemorrhage is reported infrequently (Lucak et al 1982). A peripheral blood eosinophilia is commonly present at some stage in the disease though not always (Kamal et al 1985, Van Rensberg, Keet and Adams 1986), and only about a quarter of the patients have a history of allergy. However, occasional cases of eosinophilic gastroenteritis seem to occur in the setting of the hypereosinophilic syndrome (Shah and Joglekar 1987). There are also claims based on immunohistochemical studies that in eosinophilic gastroenteritis there is an IgE mast cell mediated tissue reaction characterised by eosinophil degranulation (Oyaizu et al 1985, Keshavarzian et al 1985). A previously uncategorised subgroup is that associated with connective tissue diseases such as scleroderma, its variants and dermatomyositis (DeSchryver-Kecskemeti and Clouse 1984) The gastric lesion usually takes the form of thickening of the antrum and pylorus, but less commonly the whole stomach may be involved. Histologically, the diffuse form shows capillary and lymphatic dilatation of the mucosa and oedema of the lamina propria that pushes the gland tubules and crypts aside. There is always a conspicuous eosinophil polymorph leukocyte infiltration which varies in intensity from field to field and case to case. In addition it is usual to see occasional histiocytes, and these are sometimes multinucleate. Mucosal ulceration is distinctly uncommon, and in deep biopsies it becomes clear that it is the submucosa which is most heavily infiltrated (Fig. 9–1). It is usual also in this zone to find a degree of inflammatory fibrosis, and this is responsible for much of the thickening seen macroscopically. In addition to the tissue eosinophilia, IgE plasma cells are increased in number (Lucak et al 1982).

The disease usually responds dramatically to steroids, but this is not always so; fatal outcomes despite steroid therapy are recorded both in the adult (Tytgat et al 1976) and in childhood (Konrad and Meister 1979). It has been assumed that the disease has an allergic basis and constitutes a reaction to ingested antigenic material. Leinbach and Rubin (1970) carried out detailed investigations in a 23-year-old man in order to determine a possible aetiological role for specific antigens, but could only conclude that the disease was not a simple reversible allergic reaction to dietary substances. Rather, they postulated, it was a self-perpetuating process that may be symptomatically aggravated by different foods. Sherman and Cox (1982), however, describe a neonatal case apparently related to transplacental sensitisation of the colon by bovine milk antigens. The real situation is that the disease is incompletely understood and may be a manifestation of a variety of antigenic insults or allergic mechanisms.

It is of interest that some cases have been ascribed to the ingestion of the eggs or larvae of *Eustoma rotundatum*, which is now classified under the genus *Anisakis*, a parasite of the North Sea herring (Kuipers, Theil and Roskam 1960). It seems unlikely that this parasite is involved in all cases, but Watt et al (1979) also describe a case in Scotland due to the larvae of an *Anisakis* species and point out that several hundred cases of human infection by these larvae have been documented in Japan, Holland and North America. The disease seems to be acquired by eating raw, slightly salted or pickled sea fish and is probably that part of the broader spectrum of eosinophilic gastroenteritis in which a definite allergen has been identified.

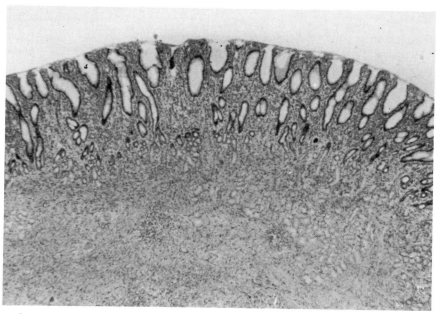

Figure 9–1. Pyloric mucosa in eosinophilic gastritis. The cellular infiltration and fibrosis is most marked in the submucosa (H & E × 60).

Inflammatory Fibroid Polyp

Before the two papers by Johnstone and Morson (1978a,b) the inflammatory fibroid polyp was widely regarded as a localised form of eosinophilic gastroenteritis, although as early as 1970 (Klein et al) doubt had been cast on their interrelationship. One of the reasons for confusion is that eosinophilic gastroenteritis can take the form of localised polypoidal disease (Bogomoletz 1984b). Inflammatory fibroid polyp, however, seems to differ in that it occurs in an older age group, an allergic history is usually absent and there is no blood eosinophilia. But they do have a similar distribution in the gut, and the fibroblastic tissue comprising their bulk is infiltrated by eosinophils, which, although in variable numbers, are a prominent feature in just over half of reported cases (LiVolsi and Perzin 1975, Blackshaw and Levison 1986). They frequently cause obstructive symptoms and occasionally result in intussusception (Winkler et al 1986). Suen and Burton (1979) also describe two other shared histological features in occasional cases, namely, necrotising eosinophil granulomas and vasculitis. They considered a relationship to other hypereosinophilic syndromes, allergic granulomatosis, and the angiitis of Churg and Strauss (1951) as well as polyarteritis nodosa. It is held by some that there are grounds for still posing the question of a possible relationship between the two conditions (Battin-Bertho et al 1987).

In biopsy tissues the lesion may or may not be ulcerated, but usually it is seen to be an essentially submucosal proliferation of vascular fibrous tissue with a sprinkling of lymphocytes and plasma cells and a variable number of eosinophil leukocytes. Although Shiner and Helwig (1984) have described the appearance as having a close resemblance to granulation tissue, Widgren and Pizzolato (1987) make a claim based on immunohistochemistry and electron microscopy that the main cellular component of this granulation tissue is the myofibroblast.

Granulomatous Lesions

It has been claimed that gastric biopsy will reveal granulomata in 10 per cent of patients with a confirmed diagnosis of systemic sarcoidosis, but who have no gastrointestinal symptoms (Palmer 1958). Infrequently, however, the stomach involvement produces a granulomatous and fibrotic rigid deformity of the pylorus and, as a consequence, the appropriate clinical picture of pyloric obstruction (Sirak 1954, Croxon, Chen and Davidson 1987). A less common form of presentation is upper gastrointestinal haemorrhage (Berens and Montes 1975, Fung, Foo and Lee 1975, Ona 1981, Chlumsky, Krtek and Chlumska 1985), and it can mimic peptic ulceration (Gallagher et al 1984) and Menetrier's disease (Chinitz et al 1985). When typical systemic sarcoidosis is present the diagnosis of gastric sarcoidosis can be based on finding typical granulomata in biopsy specimens (Figs. 9–2, 9–3, and 9–4). By themselves, however, granulomata might also denote gastric Crohn's disease, although in these circumstances it is likely that more marked diffuse cellular infiltration, lymphoid aggregates, oedema, fibrosis and ulceration would also be present, i.e., those histological features that help to characterise Crohn's disease elsewhere in the gastrointestinal tract.

Experience with rectal biopsy demonstrates that Crohn's involvement may show minimal diffuse mucosal infiltrate with scattered granulomata; a similar pattern of involvement has been described in the radiologically normal stomach (Korelitz et al 1981), and this makes histological distinction from sarcoidosis extremely difficult, if not impossible. Thus, if granulomata are found in a gastric biopsy,

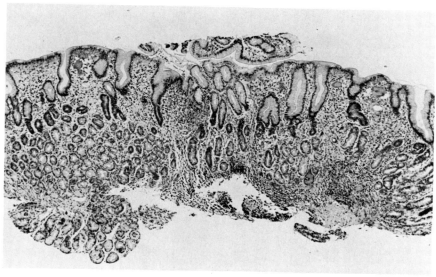

Figure 9–2. Pyloric biopsy in gastric sarcoidosis. There is a diffuse inflammatory cell infiltration with focal granulomata beneath the intact superficial epithelium (H & E × 35).

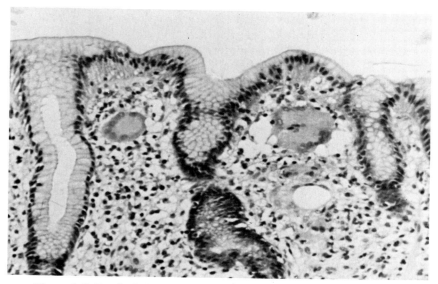

Figure 9–3. Detail of Figure 9–2 showing two granulomata (H & E × 105).

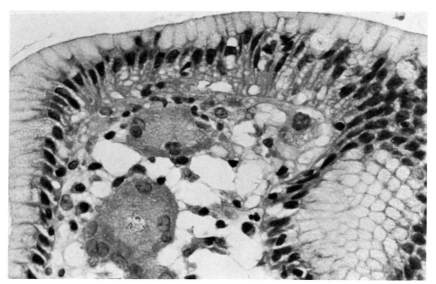

Figure 9–4. Detail of Figure 9–2 showing a Schaumann body in a giant cell (H & E × 210).

every effort should be made to differentiate between sarcoidosis and Crohn's disease because of the very different connotation the two diseases have. Consequently, full clinical and laboratory investigation is indicated and should include liver biopsy and perhaps lymph node biopsy. Differentiation even then may prove difficult because the two diseases may share many common features which include liver granulomata and a positive Kveim test, but granulomata in lymph nodes other than those draining areas involved by Crohn's disease have not been described.

On occasion giant cell granulomata are seen in the stomach wall in relation to food debris or other foreign bodies. In the usual circumstances there is an association with peptic ulceration, perforation, trauma or other obvious mechanical cause for the introduction of foreign material into the tissues. Sometimes, however, granulomata that show foreign material in close association with the giant cell reactions occur in mucosal biopsies without an apparent predisposing cause. Such "food granulomas" are probably the result of minor trauma to the mucosa, and as such have no great significance.

A granulomatous gastritis, unassociated with foreign body or with granulomatous involvement of other organs, has been called isolated granulomatous gastritis (Fahimi et al 1963). Although usually an adult disease, it has also been described in children (Hirsch et al 1989). In a personal case studied by the author it was an incidental finding in a gastrectomy specimen from a patient with a large bleeding peptic ulcer. The granulomatous gastritis was widespread, although the lesions tended to occupy the deep aspect of the mucosa (Figs. 9–5, 9–6). There was no evidence of systemic disease.

Other Forms of Gastritis or Infections

Tuberculous and syphilitic involvement of the stomach are rare. The necessity for a diagnosis of these conditions on gastric biopsy alone would hardly ever occur, but there could be difficulty in the differential diagnosis of tuberculosis and Crohn's disease in the absence of caseation necrosis. In tuberculosis, however,

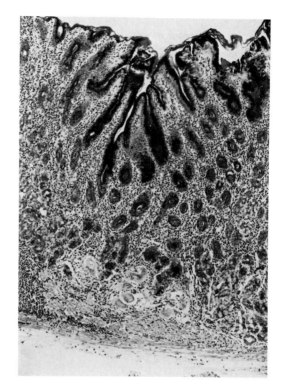

Figure 9–5. Isolated granulomatous gastritis. The giant cell granulomata are located near the muscularis mucosa. Note the coincident chronic atrophic gastritis. This was an incidental finding in a patient with a chronic peptic ulcer (H & E × 75).

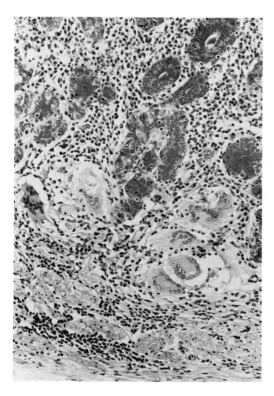

Figure 9–6. Detail of granulomata in Figure 9–5. (H & E × 120).

the more florid reaction, and the confluence of granulomata and their hyalinisation, would be helpful features. Misra et al (1982) have reviewed the literature on gastric tuberculosis and report a case presenting as a gastric ulcer, which is the usual clinical picture (Mathis, Dirschmid and Sutterlutti 1987). Subei et al (1987) describe a mass-like tuberculous lesion at the pylorus in a young man with no evidence of tuberculosis elsewhere.

In syphilitic gastropathy the mucosa is described as oedematous and friable with superficial discrete erosions (Reisman et al 1975). Biopsy revealed dense infiltration of the mucosa by mononuclear cells with a prominent plasma cell component. Neutrophils were also numerous, and in a Warthin-Starry preparation several spirochaetes were seen. Immunofluorescence preparations were also positive. A similar case of ulcero-infiltrative gastropathy was also described by Besses et al (1987).

Scott and Jenkins (1982) report a 20 per cent incidence of secondary monilial infection in gastric cancer and a 16 per cent incidence in gastric ulcer. The incidence reported by Gotlieb-Jensen and Andersen (1983) was somewhat higher at 36 per cent. The subject of *Candida* infection of peptic ulcers in oesophagus, stomach and duodenum is referred to in greater detail by Kalogeropoulos and Whitehead (1988). Primary gastric involvement, while unusual, does also occur and is usually, but not always, associated with debility or immune deprivation (Minoli, Terruzzi and Rossini 1979, Minoli et al 1982, Terruzzi and Minoli 1984).

Rarer forms of fungal colonisation of gastric ulcers are due to *Aspergillus fumigatus* (Smith 1969). In histoplasmosis gastric ulceration may occur as part of a generalised infection (Pinkerton and Iverson 1952). Primary gastric mucosal infection with mucormycosis that causes erosions and ulcers has also been described (Kahn 1963).

Cytomegalovirus inclusion disease usually occurs as an opportunistic infection. It is being diagnosed endoscopically with increasing frequency in patients with immunodeficiency or immunosuppressed states and malignancy (Kodama et al 1985, Iwasaki 1987, Spiller, Lovell and Silk 1988). Gastric involvement may be part of a generalised infection or it may be localised possibly due to secondary infection of a peptic ulcer (Andrade et al 1983). It is characterised by the presence of typical inclusions (see Fig. 6–6) in epithelial cells, endothelial cells and sometimes fibroblasts (Henson 1972, Allen et al 1981, Franzin, Muolo and Griminelli 1981, Strayer et al 1981, Iwasaki 1987).

Primary gastric actinomycosis is extremely rare, but Van Olmen et al (1984) describe a case presenting as a bleeding gastric tumour and review the literature. Other rare inflammatory lesions in which endoscopic examination and biopsy were considered to be of value are gastric anisakiasis (Hsiu et al 1986), emphysematous gastritis that followed acute pancreatitis (Bloodworth et al 1987) and localised phlegmonous gastritis (Aviles et al 1988).

MISCELLANEOUS

Gastric Xanthelasma (Xanthoma)

Gastric xanthelasma (Kimura 1969) may occur in any part of the stomach as rounded or oval, yellow or yellow-white macules or nodules between 1 and 5 mm in diameter. Histologically, they are usually superficial and are characterised by collections of large histiocytes with a clear cytoplasm and peripheral nucleus (Fig. 9–7). The cells tend to push the glandular elements aside. They contain neutral

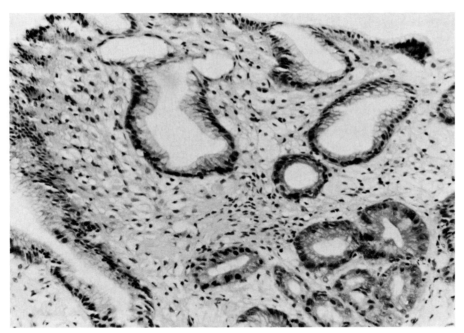

Figure 9–7. Gastric biopsy showing superficial aspect of an atrophic mucosa with pale histiocytes separating crypts and upper gland tubules. (H & E × 240).

fat and cholesterol but have no consistent relationship to blood lipid levels. Sometimes the collection of cells are multiple and they have been noted to disappear spontaneously (Mast et al 1976). There is some evidence that at least some of these lesions are related to previous ulceration or gastric surgery (Domellof et al 1977, Terruzzi et al 1980) and similar collections of cells occur in the region of healed chronic erosions (see Fig. 8–26). There would seem to be a particular relationship of xanthelasmas with forms of chronic gastritis and intestinal metaplasia (Moreto et al 1985). Coates et al (1986) report two cases in which severe gastric involvement by xanthelasmas disappeared with resolution of cholestasis and hypercholesterolemia, but as already stated, there is no relationship to blood cholesterol levels in the usual case.

Xanthelasmas become increasingly common with age whether associated with earlier surgery or not and are seen in approximately 60 per cent of all autopsies. Boger and Hort (1977) have shown in an electron microscope study that the lipid-laden cells can originate as smooth muscle cells as well as histiocytes. The importance of this lesion relates to the possibility of a misdiagnosis of signet ring carcinoma in ordinary H & E-stained slides (Drude et al 1982, Pieterse, Rowland and Labrooy 1985). The material within the histiocytes, however, can easily be shown to be PAS and Alcian blue-negative. In frozen sections the cells stain positively with oil red O or Sudan black.

Angiodysplasia

Similar endoscopic yellowish plaques have been described by Cocco et al (1969) in patients with pseudoxanthoma elasticum. Histologically, the lesions have an appearance similar to the other vascular lesions in this disease affecting primarily the submucosal vessels which show microaneurysms, intimal obliteration and dystrophic calcification (Berlyne 1960, Kundrotas et al 1988). The angiomatous lesions of Rendu-Osler disease have also been diagnosed in endoscopic biopsies (Ponsot et al 1983). Acquired angiodysplastic lesions of the stomach have also been described in gastroscopic biopsies (Bank et al 1983), and they have been attributed to cholesterol embolisation of the gastric mucosa due to aortic atheroma. They have been compared to the more commonly encountered colonic angiodys-plasia and basically consist of submucosal and mucosal capillary ectasia, sometimes involving draining veins. In the majority of cases, as in the colon, the aetiology appears obscure. Endoscopic descriptions of the lesions vary from hyperaemic mucosal spots to longitudinally arranged rugae converging on the pylorus, each containing dilated vessels which give an appearance resembling a watermelon (Jabbari et al 1984). Gastric angiodysplasia of this type has been described in association with chronic haemodialysis (Cunningham 1981), portal hypertension (Papazian et al 1986), and cirrhosis (Quintero et al 1987, Baxter and Dobbs 1988), but it occurs in their absence (Arendt et al 1987, Tung and Millar 1987).

Another increasingly recognised cause of gastric haemorrhage is so-called Dieulafoy's ulcer (Goldman 1964, Sarles et al 1984). This is basically a shallow ulcerated lesion related to an abnormal arterial or arteriovenous malformation of the submucosa frequently situated in the proximal stomach. Mower and Whitehead (1986) and Veldhuyzen van Zanten et al (1986) have reviewed the disease, and there is a report (Richter 1975) of actual endoscopic resection of the lesion.

Other Abnormalities

Gastric biopsy will reveal systemic amyloidosis (Filipe and Correia 1963), but it is generally held that rectal biopsy is technically easier and more likely to be

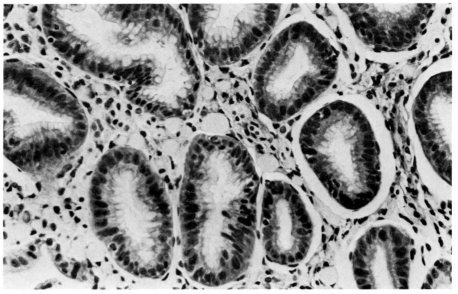

Figure 9–8. Gastric amyloidosis. The amyloid has an intertubular globular appearance. (H & E × 500).

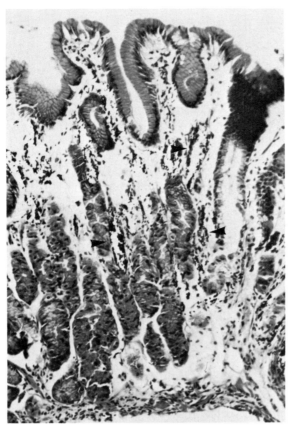

Figure 9–9. Gastric body mucosa with peritubular metastatic calcification (arrowheads) in hyperparathyroidism. (H & E × 150).

diagnostically helpful. In one study, however, evidence was produced from an autopsy examination that in primary amyloidosis and myeloma-associated disease, gastric biopsy would give a superior diagnostic yield (Yamada, Hatakeyama and Tsukagoshi 1985). However, this has been challenged (Ohno et al 1982), for it seems that gastric biopsy and rectal biopsy yield the same results. The deposition sometimes has a curious globular appearance (Fig. 9–8). Localised amyloid tumour of the stomach may also be diagnosed by biopsy (Ikeda and Murayama 1978, Balazs 1981). It is a lesion of some importance in that it mimics carcinoma grossly and may or may not occur in association with systemic amyloidosis. The chief cells will contain haemosiderin pigment in most patients with haemachromatosis (Joske, Finckh and Wood 1955), and gastric biopsy provides an alternative to liver biopsy if this is difficult or contraindicated. The gastric mucosa sometimes is the site of metastatic calcification (Fig. 9–9) in states of parathyroid hyperfunction.

With increasing use of hepatic arterial infusion chemotherapy for the treatment of metastatic colon cancer, there has been a recognition of its association with gastric ulceration. Biopsies from such ulcers may easily be mistaken for primary gastric carcinoma (Petras, Hart and Bukowski 1985). Features that indicate that the lesions are produced by the chemotherapy include the bizarre nature of the cellular atypia yet a low nuclear cytoplasmic ratio, few or no mitotic figures and relative preservation of mucosal architecture in the histologically abnormal areas (Figs. 9–10, 9–11). The more basal aspects of the glands appear to be involved

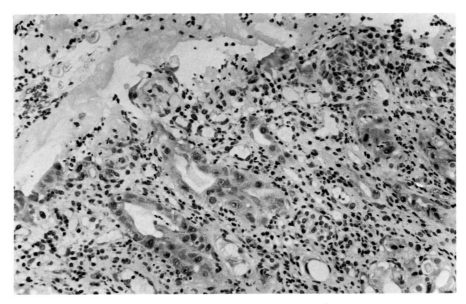

Figure 9–10. Gastric biopsy of base of an ulcer produced by hepatic intra-arterial infusion of mitomycin C and 5-fluorouracil. In the base of the ulcer there is marked nuclear pleomorphism, but the tubules, although deformed, have an overall preserved general architecture and an inflamed though normal lamina propria (H & E × 500).

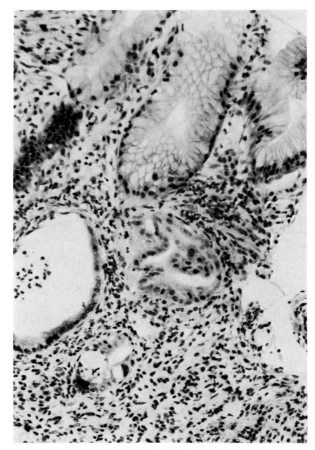

Figure 9–11. Ulcer edge from same patient as Figure 9–10. Note abnormal tubule forms and gross nuclear pleomorphism (H & E × 500).

maximally, and there may be radiation-like atypia in endothelial cells and fibroblasts.

Changes in the gastric mucosa may also result in graft-versus-host disease. The changes are often minimal and consist of single cell necrosis most likely to be seen in the foveolar region of the mucosa. The foveolae may be dilated and occasionally contain polymorphonuclear leukocytes (Snover et al 1985).

REFERENCES—SECTION II   GASTRIC BIOPSY

Aanestad O., Raknerud N., Aase S.T. and Narverud G. (1987) The Cronkhite-Canada syndrome. Acta Chirurgica Scandinavica *153*:143–145.

Allen J.I., Silvis S.E., Sumner H.W. and McClain C.J. (1981) Cytomegalic inclusion disease diagnosed endoscopically. Digestive Diseases and Sciences 26:133–135.

Andrada J.A. and Rose N.R. (1969) Experimental auto-immune gastritis in the Rhesus monkey. Clinical and Experimental Immunology *4*:293–310.

Andrade J. De S., Bambirra E.A., Lima G.F., Moreira E.F. and De Oliveira C.A. (1983) Gastric cytomegalic inclusion bodies diagnosed by histologic examination of endoscopic biopsies in patients with gastric ulcer. American Journal of Clinical Pathology 79:493–496.

Andrews G.R., Haneman B., Arnold B.J., Booth J.C. and Taylor K. (1967) Atrophic gastritis in the aged. Australasian Annals of Medicine *16*:230–235.

Arendt T., Barten M., Lakner V. and Arendt R. (1987) Diffuse gastric antral vascular ectasia: cause of chronic gastrointestinal blood loss. Endoscopy *19*:218–220.

Ashby B.S., Appleton P.J. and Dawson I. (1964) Eosinophilic granuloma of gastrointestinal tract caused by herring parasite Eustoma rotundatum. British Medical Journal *i*:1141–1145.

Assad R.T. and Eastwood G.L. (1980) Epithelial proliferation in human fundic mucosa after antrectomy and vagotomy. Gastroenterology 79:807–811.

Aukee S. and Krohn K. (1972) Occurrence and progression of gastritis in patients operated on for peptic ulcer. Scandinavian Journal of Gastroenterology 7:541–546.

Aviles J.F., Fernandez-Seara J., Barcena R., Domiinguez F., Fernandez C. and Ledo L. (1988) Localized phlegmonous gastritis: endoscopic view. Endoscopy 20:38–39.

Badenoch J., Evans J.R. and Richards W.C.D. (1957) The stomach in hypochromic anaemia. British Journal of Haematology *3*:175–185.

Baker A., Volberg F., Sumner T. and Moran R. (1986) Childhood Menetrier's disease: four new cases and discussion of the literature. Gastrointestinal Radiology *11*:131–134.

Balazs M. (1981) Amyloidosis of the stomach. Report of a case with ultrastructure. Virchows Archiv, A. Pathological Anatomy and Histology *391*:227–240.

Balfour D.C. (1922) Factors influencing the life expectancy of patients operated on for gastric ulcer. Annals of Surgery 76:405–408.

Bank S., Aftalion B., Anfang C., Altman H. and Wise L. (1983) Acquired angiodysplasia as a cause of gastric hemorrhage: a possible consequence of cholesterol embolization. American Journal of Gastroenterology 78:206–209.

Barthel J.S., Westblom T.U., Harvey A.D., Gonzalez F. and Everett E.D. (1988) Gastritis and campylobacter pylori in healthy, asymptomatic volunteers. Archives of Internal Medicine *148*:1149–1151.

Bartlett J.S. (1988) Campylobacter pylori: fact or fancy? Gastroenterology *94*:229–238.

Battin-Bertho R., Dauge M.C., Toublanc M., Grossin M., Marche C.I. and Bocquet L. (1987) Helwig's gastric pseudo-tumour. Report of three cases and review of the literature. Annals of Pathology 7:176–183.

Bauer T.W., Mendelsohn G., Humphrey R.L. and Mann R.B. (1982) Angioimmunoblastic lymphadenopathy progressing to immunoblastic lymphoma with prominent gastric involvement. Cancer 50:2089–2098.

Baxter J.N. and Dobbs B.R. (1988) Portal hypertensive gastropathy. Journal of Gastroenterology and Hepatology 3:635–644.

Bechi P., Amorosi A., Mazzanti R., Romagnoli P. and Tonelli L. (1987) Gastric histology and fasting bile reflux after partial gastrectomy. Gastroenterology 93:335–343.

Bedossa P., Lemaigre G. and Martin E.D. (1987a) Histochemical study of mucosubstances in carcinoma of the gastric remnant. Cancer *60*:2224–2227.

Bedossa P., Lemaigre G. and Martin E. (1987b) Fundic gland polyps and polyposis. Annales Pathologie 7:171–175.

Berens D.L. and Montes M. (1975) Gastric sarcoidosis. New York State Journal of Medicine *75*:1290–1293.

Berenson M.M., Sannella J. and Freston J.W. (1976) Menetrier's disease. Serial morphological, secretory, and serological observations. Gastroenterology 70:257–263.

Berkowitz D.M., Passaro E. Jr. and Isenberg J.I. (1977) Hypertrophic protein-losing gastropathy and vitiligo. Report of a second case. Americal Journal of Digestive Diseases 22:554–558.

Berlyne M. (1960) Pseudoxanthoma elasticum. Lancet 1:77–88.

Berry E.M., Ben-Dov Y. and Freund U. (1980) Spontaneous remission of protein-losing gastropathy associated with Menetrier's disease. Archives of Internal Medicine 140:99–100.

Berstad A., Alexander B., Weberg R., Serck-Hanssen A., Holland S. and Hirschowitz B.I. (1988) Antacids reduce campylobacter pylori colonization without healing the gastritis in patients with nonulcer dyspepsia and erosive prepyloric changes. Gastroenterology 95:619–624.

Berstad A. and Nesland A. (1987) Erosive prepyloric changes (EPC): A new entity. Scandinavian Journal of Gastroenterology 128:94–100.

Berthrong M. and Fajardo L.F. (1981) Radiation injury in surgical pathology. Part II Alimentary tract. American Journal of Surgical Pathology 5:153–178.

Besses C., Sans-Sabrafen J., Badia X., Rodriguez-Mendez F., Salord J.C. and Armengol J.R. (1987) Ulceroinfiltrative syphilitic gastropathy: silver stain diagnosis from biopsy specimen. American Journal of Gastroenterology 82:773–774.

Black W.C. and Haffner H.E. (1968) Diffuse hyperplasia of gastric argyrophil cells and multiple carcinoid tumours. An historical and ultrastuctural study. Cancer 21:1080–1099.

Blackburn E.K., Callendar S.T., Dacie J.V., Doll R., Girdwood R.H., Mollin D.L., Saracci R., Stafford J.L., Thompson R.B., Varadi S. and Wetherly-Mein G. (1968) Possible association between pernicious anaemia and leukaemia: a prospective study of 1625 patients with a note on the very high incidence of stomach cancer. International Journal of Cancer 3:163–170.

Blackshaw A.J. and Levison D.A. (1986) Eosinophilic infiltrates of the gastrointestinal tract. Journal of Clinical Pathology 39:1–7.

Blom H. (1984) Light-and electron-microscopy of normal and regenerating gastric mucosa with special reference to the parietal cells. Scandinavian Journal of Gastroenterology 105(Suppl):33–45.

Bloodworth L.L., Stevens P.E., Bury R.F., Arm J.P. and Rainford D.J. (1987) Emphysematous gastritis after acute pancreatitis. Gut 28:900–902.

Bloom R.A. (1981) Transient protein-losing enteropathy and enlarged gastric rugae. American Journal of Diseases of Children 135:29–33.

Bloom S.R. and Polak J.M. (1981) Gut Hormones. 2nd Edition. Edinburgh: Churchill Livingstone.

Bodner E., Pointner R. and Glaser K. (1988) Natural history of early gastric cancer. Lancet 2:631.

Boger A. and Hort W. (1977) The importance of smooth muscle cells in the development of foam cells in the gastric mucosa. An electron microscopic study. Virchows Archiv A. Pathological Anatomy and Histology 372:287–297.

Bogomoletz W.V. (1984a) Early gastric cancer. American Journal of Surgical Pathology 8:381–391.

Bogomoletz W.V. (1984b) Eosinophilic gastroenteritis: a complex disease entity. Survey of Digestive Diseases 2:85–91.

Bogomoletz W.V., Molas G., Potet F., Qizilbash A.H. and Barge J. (1985) Pathological features and mucin histochemistry of primary gastric stump carcinoma associated with gastritis cystica polyposa. American Journal of Surgical Pathology 9:401–410.

Bonney G.E., Elston R.E., Correa P., Haenszel W., Zavala D.E., Zarama G., Collazos T. and Cuello C. (1986) Genetic etiology of gastric carcinoma. Genetic Epidemiology 3:213–224.

Boon M.E., Kurver P.J.H., Baak J.P.A. and Thompson H.T. (1981) The application of morphometry in gastric cytological diagnosis. Virchows Archiv, A. Pathological Anatomy and Histology 393:159–164.

Borch K., Renvall H., Liedberg G. and Andersen B.N. (1986) Relations between circulating gastrin and endocrine cell proliferation in the atrophic gastric fundic mucosa. Scandinavian Journal of Gastroenterology 21:357–363.

Borchard F., Mittelstaedt A. and Kieker R. (1979) Incidence of epithelial dysplasia after partial gastric resection. Pathology, Research and Practice 164:282–293.

Bordi C., Ferrari C., D'Adda T., Pilato F., Carfagna G., Bertele A. and Missale G. (1986) Ultrastructural characterization of fundic endocrine cell hyperplasia associated with atrophic gastritis and hypergastrinaemia. Virchows Archiv, A. 409:335–347.

Bordi C. and Ravazzola M. (1979) Endocrine cells in the intestinal metaplasia of gastric mucosa. American Journal of Pathology 90:391–395.

Bordi C., Ravazzola M. and De Vita O. (1983) Pathology of endocrine cells in gastric mucosa. Annals of Pathology 3:19–28.

Boyd E.J.S., Hulks G., St.J. Thomas J., and McColl K.E.L. (1988) Hypertrophic gastritis associated with increased gastric mucosal prostaglandin E2 concentrations in a patient with the carcinoid syndrome. Gut 29:1270–1276.

Brooks A.M., Isenberg J. and Goldstein H. (1970) Giant thickening of the gastric mucosa with acid hyposecretion and protein-losing gastropathy. Gastroenterology 58:73–79.

Brooks J.J. and Enterline H.T. (1983) Gastric pseudolymphoma. Its three subtypes and relation to lymphoma. Cancer 51:476–486.

Brooks W.S., Wenger J. and Hersh T. (1975) Bile reflux gastritis. Analysis of fasting and postprandial gastric aspirates. American Journal of Gastroenterology 64:286–291.

Brousse N., Foldes C., Barge J., Molas G. and Potet F. (1983) Reliability of endoscopic biopsies in the diagnosis of malignant lymphomas of the stomach. Gastroenterologie Clinique et Biologique 7:145–149.

Brown R.C., Hardy G.J., Temperly J.M., Miloszewski K.J.A., Gowland G. and Losowsky M.S. (1981) Gastritis and cirrhosis: no association. Journal of Clinical Pathology *34*:744–748.

Burke J.S., Sheibani K., Nathwani B.N., Winberg C.D. and Rappaport H. (1987) Monoclonal small (well-differentiated) lymphocytic proliferations of the gastrointestinal tract resembling lymphoid hyperplasia: a neoplasm of uncertain malignant potential. Human Pathology *18*:1238–1245.

Burr M.L., Samloff I.M., Bates C.J. and Holliday R.M. (1987) Atrophic gastritis and vitamin C status in two towns with different stomach cancer death-rates. British Journal of Cancer *56*:163–167.

Byrnes D.J., Young J.D., Chisholm D.T. and Lazarus L. (1970) Serum gastrin in patients with peptic ulceration. British Medical Journal *ii*:626–629.

Calam J., Krasner N. and Haqqani M. (1982) Extensive gastrointestinal damage following a saline emetic. Digestive Diseases and Sciences *27*:936–940.

Carfagna G., Pilato F.P., Bordi C., Barsotti P. and Riva C. (1987) Solitary polypoid hamartoma of the oxyntic mucosa of the stomach. Pathology, Research and Practice *182*:326–330.

Celik C., Ettinger D. and Satchidanand S. (1984) Massive bleeding in hypertrophic gastropathy (Menetrier's disease) due to arterio-venous malformation. Journal of Medicine *15*:65–73.

Chakravorty R.C. and Schatzki P.F. (1975) Gastric cystic polyposis. American Journal of Digestive Disease *20*:981–989.

Chambers L.A. and Clark W.E. (1986) The endoscopic diagnosis of gastroesophageal malignancy. Acta Cytologica *30*:110–114.

Chanarin I. and James D. (1974) Humoral and cell-mediated intrinsic-factor antibody in pernicious anaemia. Lancet *i*:1078–1080.

Cheli R., Perasso A. and Giacosa A. (1983) Dyspepsia and chronic gastritis. Hepato-gastroenterology *30*:21–23.

Cheng J., Ritchie W.P. Jr. and Delaney J. (1969) Atrophic gastritis: an experimental model. Federation Proceedings *28*:513.

Chinitz M.A., Brandt L.J., Frank M.S., Frager D. and Sablay L. (1985) Symptomatic sarcoidosis of the stomach. Digestive Diseases and Sciences *30*:682–688.

Chlumsky J., Krtek V. and Chlumska A. (1985) Sarcoidosis of the stomach. Endoscopic diagnosis and possibilities of conservative treatment. Hepato-gastroenterology *32*:255–257.

Churg J. and Strauss L. (1951) Allergic granulomatosis, allergic angiitis and periarteritis nodosa. American Journal of Pathology *27*:277–294.

Clark C.G., Fresini A. and Gledhill T. (1985) Cancer following gastric surgery. British Journal of Surgery *72*:591–594.

Clarke A.C., Lee S.P. and Nicholson G.I. (1977) Gastritis varioliformis. American Journal of Gastroenterology *68*:599- 602.

Coates A.G., Nostrant T.T., Wilson J.A.P., Dobbins W.O. and Agha F.P. (1986) Gastric xanthomatosis and cholestasis. A causal relationship. Digestive Diseases and Sciences *31*:925–928.

Cocco A.E., Grayer D.I., Walker B.A. and Martyn L.J. (1969) The stomach in pseudoxanthoma elasticum. Journal of the American Medical Association *210*:2381–2382.

Cocking J.B. and Grech P. (1973) Pyloric reflux and the healing of gastric ulcers. Gut *14*:555–557.

Coghill N.F. (1960) The significance of gastritis. Postgraduate Medical Journal *36*:733–742.

Coghill N.F. (1969) Chronic idiopathic gastritis: cause and effect. In: Fifth Symposium on Advanced Medicine, p 14. Edited by Roger Williams. London: Pitman Medical.

Coghill N.F. and Williams A.W. (1958) Gastric mucosa in hypochromic anaemia. Proceedings of the Royal Society of Medicine *51*:464.

Correa P. (1980) The epidemiology and pathogenesis of chronic gastritis: three etiologic entities. Frontiers of Gastrointestinal Research *6*:98–108.

Correa P. (1982) Precursors of gastric and esophageal cancer. Cancer *50*:2554–2565.

Correa P. (1988) Chronic gastritis: a clinico-pathological classification. American Journal of Gastroenterology *83*:504–509.

Croft D.N. (1963) Aspirin and the exfoliation of gastric epithelial cells. Cytological and biochemical observations. British Medical Journal *ii*:897–901.

Cronkhite L.W. and Canada W.J. (1955) Generalized gastrointestinal polyposis; an unusual syndrome of polyposis, pigmentation, alopecia and onychotrophia. New England Journal of Medicine *252*:1011–1015.

Croxon S., Chen K. and Davidson A.R. (1987) Sarcoidosis of the stomach. Digestion *38*:193–196.

Cruveilhier J. (1862) Traite d'anatomie pathologique generale, p 484. Paris: Bailliere.

Cuello C., Lopez J., Correa P., Murray J., Zarama G. and Gordillo G. (1979) Histopathology of gastric dysplasias. Correlations with gastric juice chemistry. American Journal of Surgical Pathology *3*:491–500.

Cunningham J.T. (1981) Gastric telangiectasias in chronic hemodialysis patients: a report of six cases. Gastroenterology *81*:1131–1133.

Czerniak B., Herz F. and Koss L.G. (1987) DNA distribution patterns in early gastric carcinomas. Cancer *59*:113–117.

Daibo M., Itabashi M. and Hirota T. (1987) Malignant transformation of gastric hyperplastic polyps. American Journal of Gastroenterology *82*:1016–1025.

Daniel E.S., Ludwig S.L., Lewin K.J., Ruprecht R.M., Rajacich G.M. and Schwabe A.D. (1982) The

Cronkhite-Canada syndrome. An analysis of clinical and pathologic features and therapy in 55 patients. Medicine *61*:293–309.

Davenport H.W. (1967) Salicylate damage to the gastric mucosal barrier. New England Journal of Medicine *276*:1307–1312.

Davenport H.W. (1968) Destruction of gastric mucosal barrier by detergents and urea. Gastroenterology *54*:175–181.

Dawson I. (1970) The endocrine cells of the gastrointestinal tract. Histochemical Journal *2*:527–549.

De Aizpurua H.J., Cosgrove L.J., Ungar B. and Toh B-H. (1983) Autoantibodies cytotoxic to gastric parietal cells in serum of patients with pernicious anemia. New England Journal of Medicine *309*:625–629.

De Boer W.G.R.M., Forsyth A. and Nairn R.C. (1969) Gastric antigens in health and disease. Behaviour in early development, senescence, metaplasia and cancer. British Medical Journal *iii*:93–94.

Debray C., Hardouin J.P., Laumonier R., Housset P., Helie T.P. and Martin E. (1957) La gastrite ethylique sous le controle de la gastrobiopsie. Archives des maladies de appareil digestif et de la nutrition *46*:925–937.

Delaney J.P., Cheng J.W.B., Butler B.A. and Ritchie W.P. (1970) Gastric ulcer and regurgitation gastritis. Gut *11*:715–719.

DeSchryver-Kecskemeti K. and Clouse R.E. (1984) A previously unrecognized subgroup of 'eosinophilic gastroenteritis'. American Journal of Surgical Pathology *8*:171–180.

Deviere J., Buset M., Dumonceau J-M., Rickaert F. and Cremer M. (1989) Regression of Barrett's epithelium with Omeprazole. New England Journal of Medicine *320*:1497–1498.

Dewar P., Dixon M.F. and Johnston D. (1984) Bile reflux and degree of gastritis in patients with gastric ulcer: before and after operation. Journal of Surgical Research *37*:277–284.

Dinoso V.P. Jr., Chey W.Y., Braverman S.P., Rosen A.P., Ottenberg D. and Lorber S.H. (1972) Gastric secretion and gastric mucosal morphology in chronic alcoholics. Archives of Internal Medicine *130*:715–719.

Dixon M.F., O'Connor H.J., Axon A.T.R., King R.F.J.G. and Johnston D. (1986) Reflux gastritis: distinct histopathological entity? Journal of Clinical Pathology *39*:524–530.

Dixon M.F., Wyatt J.I., Burke D.A. and Rathbone B.J. (1988) Lymphocytic gastritis: relationship to campylobacter pylori infection. Journal of Pathology *154*:125–132.

Dommellof L., Eriksson S., Helander H.F. and Janunger K.-G. (1977) Lipid islands in the gastric mucosa after resection for benign ulcer disease. Gastroenterology *72*:14–18.

Dougherty St. H., Foster C.A. and Eisenberg M.M. (1982) Stomach cancer following gastric surgery for benign disease. Archives of Surgery *117*:294–297

Drude R.B., Balart L.A., Herrington J.P., Beckman E.N. and Burns T.W. (1982) Gastric xanthoma: histologic similarity to signet ring cell carcinoma. Journal of Clinical Gastroenterology *4*:217–221.

Duggan J.M., Dobson A.J., Johnson H. and Fahey P. (1986) Peptic ulcer and non-steroidal anti-inflammatory agents. Gut *27*:929–933.

Eastwood G.L.(1975) Effect of pH on bile salt injury to mouse gastric mucosa. A light and electron-microscopic study. Gastroenterology *68*:1456–1465.

Eckardt V.F., Willems D., Kanzler G., Remmele W., Bettendorf U. and Paulus W. (1984) Eighty months persistence of poorly differentiated early gastric cancer. Gastroenterology *87*:719–724.

Edwards F.C. and Coghill N.F. (1966) Aetiological factors in chronic atrophic gastritis. British Medical Journal *ii*:1409–1415.

Edwards F.C. and Edwards J.H. (1956) Tea drinking and gastritis. Lancet *ii*:543–545.

Elkeles A. (1964) Gastric ulcer in the aged and calcified atherosclerosis. American Journal of Roentgenology *91*:744–750.

Elsborg L., Anderson D., Myhre-Jansen O. and Bastrup-Madsen P. (1977) Gastric mucosal polyps in pernicious anaemia. Scandinavian Journal of Gastroenterology *12*:49–52.

Elster K. (1974) A new approach to the classification of gastric polyps. Endoscopy *6*:44–47.

Elster K. (1976) Histologic classification of gastric polyps. In: Current Topics in Pathology *63*:77–93. Edited by B.C. Morson. Heidelberg: Springer-Verlag.

Elster K., Carson W., Wild A., and Thomasko A. (1979) Evaluation of histological classification in early gastric cancer. (An analysis of 300 cases). Endoscopy *3*:203–206.

Elta G.H., Fawaz K.A., Dayal Y., McLean A.M., Phillips E., Bloom S.M., Paul R.E. and Kaplan M.M. (1983) Chronic erosive gastritis: a recently recognized disorder. Digestive Diseases and Sciences *28*:7–12.

Eras P., Goldstein M.J. and Sherlock P. (1972) Candida infection of the gastrointestinal tract. Medicine (Baltimore) *54*:367–379.

Evans D.M.D., Craven J.L., Murphy F. and Cleary B.K. (1978) Comparison of "early gastric cancer" in Britain and Japan. Gut *19*:1–9.

Faber K. (1935) Gastritis and its consequences. London: Oxford University Press.

Fahimi H.D.,Deren J.J., Gottlieb L.S. and Zamcheck N. (1963) Isolated granulomatous gastritis: its relationship to disseminated sarcoidosis and regional enteritis. Gastroenterology *45*:161–175.

Falkmer S. and Wilander E. (1989) The endocrine cell population. In: Gastrointestinal and Oesophageal Pathology. Edited by R. Whitehead. Edinburgh: Churchill Livingstone.

Farinati F., Cardin F., Di Mario F., Vianello F., Battaglia G., Arslan-Pagnini C., Cannizzaro R., Sava G.A., Rugge M. and Naccarato R. (1987) Early and advanced gastric cancer during follow-up of apparently benign gastric ulcer: significance of the presence of epithelial dysplasia. Journal of Surgical Oncology *36*:263–267.

Farini R., Leandro G., Farinati F., Di Mario F., Scalabrin G., Mazzucato B., Cecchetto A. and Naccarato R. (1981) Epithelial dysplasia in endoscopic gastric mucosal biopsies. Tumori 67:589–598.

Farrands P.A., Blake J.R.S., Ansell I.D., Cotton R.E. and Hardcastle J.D. (1983) Endoscopic review of patients who have had gastric surgery. British Medical Journal 286:755–758.

Farthing M.J.G., Fairclough P.D., Hegarty J.E., Swarbrick E.T. and Dawson A.M. (1981) Treatment of chronic erosive gastritis with prednisolone. Gut 22:759–762.

Ferrer-Roca O. (1982) Primary gastric plasmacytoma with massive intracytoplasmic crystalline inclusions. A case report. Cancer 50:755–759.

Filipe M.I. (1983) In: Histochemistry in Pathology. Edited by M.I. Filipe and B.D. Lake. New York: Churchill Livingstone, p. 128.

Filipe M.I. and Correia J.P. (1963) La valeur de la biopsie gastrique dans l' etude des lesions diffuses de l' estomac. Gastroenterologia 100:19–32.

Filipe M.I., Potet F., Bogomoletz W.V., Dawson P.A., Fabiani B., Chauveinc P., Fenzy A., Gazzard B., Goldfain D. and Zeegen R. (1985) Incomplete sulphomucin-secreting intestinal metaplasia for gastric cancer. Preliminary data from a prospective study from three centres. Gut 26:1319–1326.

Fitzgibbons P.L., Dooley C.P., Cohen H. and Appleman M.D. (1988) Prevalence of gastric metaplasia, inflammation, and campylobacter pylori in the duodenum of members of the normal population. American Journal of Clinical Pathology 90:711–714.

Flowers R.S., Kyle K. and Hoerr S.O. (1970) Post-operative hemorrhage from stress ulceration of the stomach and duodenum. American Journal of Surgery 119:632–639.

Fonde E.C. and Rodning C.B. (1986) Gastritis cystica profunda. American Journal of Gastroenterology 81:459–464.

Fontham E., Zavala D., Correa P., Rodriguez E., Hunter F., Haenszel W. and Tannenbaum S.R. (1986) Diet and chronic atrophic gastritis: a case control study. Journal of the National Cancer Institute 76:621–627.

Franzin G., Manfrini C., Musola R., Rodella S. and Fratton A. (1984) Chronic erosions of the stomach. Endoscopy 16:1–5.

Franzin G., Muolo A. and Griminelli T. (1981) Cytomegalovirus inclusions in the gastroduodenal mucosa of patients after renal transplantation. Gut 22:698–701.

Franzin G., Musola R., Zamboni G. and Manfrini C. (1985) Gastritis cystica polyposa: a possible precancerous lesion. Tumori 71:13–18.

Franzin G. and Novelli P. (1981) Gastritis cystica profunda. Histopathology 5:535–547.

Freeman K., Anthony P.P., Miller D.S. and Warin A.P. (1985) Cronkhite-Canada syndrome: a new hypothesis. Gut 26:531–536.

Freise J., Hofmann R., Gebel M. and Huchzermeyer H. (1979) Follow-up study of chronic gastric erosions. Endoscopy 1:13–17.

Frommer D.J., Carrick J., Lee A. and Hazell S.L. (1988) Acute presentation of campylobacter pylori gastritis. American Journal of Gastroenterology 83:1168–1171.

Fruin R.C., Littman M.S. and Littman A. (1963) Intragastric beta-irradiation with rutheniumrhodium 106 in patients with peptic ulcer and gastric neoplasm. Gastroenterology 45:34–42.

Fujita S. (1978) Biology of early gastric carcinoma. Pathology, Research and Practice 163:297–309.

Fukuda T., Ohnishi Y., Nishimaki T., Ohtani H. and Tachikawa S. (1988) Early gastric cancer of the small cell type. American Journal of Gastroenterology 83:1176–1179.

Fung W.P., Foo K.T. and Lee Y.S. (1975) Gastric sarcoidosis presenting with haematemesis. Medical Journal of Australia 2:47–49.

Gabreau T., Delage Y., Conte-Marti J. and Bodin F. (1982) Menetrier's disease with normal gastric acid secretion: report of a patient treated with Cimetidine. Gastroenterologie Clinique et Biologique 6:38–42.

Gad A. (1986) Erosions: a correlative endoscopic histopathologic multicenter study. Endoscopy 18:76–79.

Gallagher C.G., Lennon J.R. and Crowe J.P. (1987) Chronic erosive gastritis: a clinical study. American Journal of Gastroenterology 82:302–306.

Gallagher P., Harris M., Turnbull F.W.A. and Turner L. (1984) Gastric sarcoidosis. Journal of the Royal Society of Medicine 77:837–839.

Gazzard B.G. (1988) HIV disease and the gastroenterologist. Gut 29:1497–1505.

Gear M.W.L., Truelove S.C. and Whitehead R. (1971) Gastric ulcer and gastritis. Gut 12:639–645.

Gear M.W.L., Truelove S.C., Gwyn Williams D., Massarella G.R. and Boddington M.M. (1969) Gastric cancer simulating benign gastric ulcer. British Journal of Surgery 56:739–742.

Ghandur-Mnaymneh L., Paz J., Roldan E. and Cassady J. (1988) Dysplasia of nonmetaplastic gastric mucosa. American Journal of Surgical Pathology 12:96–114.

Giler S., Kadish U. and Urca I. (1976) Peroral staining method with toluidine blue as an aid in the diagnosis of malignant gastric lesions. American Journal of Gastroenterology 65:37–40.

Glass G.B. (1965) The natural history of gastric atrophy. A review of immunologic aspects and possible links to endogenous inhibitors of gastric secretion. American Journal of Digestive Diseases 10:376–398.

Glass G.B.J. (1977) Immunology of atrophic gastritis. New York State Journal of Medicine 77:1697–1706.

Glass G.B. and Ishimori A. (1961) Passage of serum albumin into the stomach. Its detection by paper electrophoresis of gastric juice in protein-losing gastropathies and gastric cancer. American Journal of Digestive Diseases 6:103–133.

Glass G.B., Speer F.D., Neiburgs H.E., Ishimori A., Jones E.L. Baker H., Schwartz S.A. and Smith R. (1960) Gastric atrophy, atrophic gastritis and gastric secretory failure. Correlative study by suction biopsy and exfoliative cytology of gastric mucosa, paper electrophoretic and secretory assays of gastric secretion and measurements of intestinal absorption and blood levels of vitamin B_{12}. Gastroenterology *39*:429–453.

Gledhill T., Leicester R.J., Addis B., Lightfoot N., Barnard J., Viney N., Darkin D. and Hunt R.H. (1985) Epidemic hypochlorhydria. British Medical Journal *290*:1383–1386.

Glober G., Pena A.S., Whitehead R., Gear M.W.L., Roca M., Kerrigan G. and Truelove S.C. (1972) A.B.O. blood groups, rhesus factor and intestinal metaplasia of the stomach. British Journal of Cancer *26*:420–422.

Goldgraber M.B., Rubin C.E., Palmer W.L., Dobson R.L. and Massey B.W. (1954) The early gastric response to irradiation, a serial biopsy study. Gastroenterology *27*:1–20.

Goldman H., French S. and Burbige E. (1981) Kulchitsky cell hyperplasia and multiple metastasizing carcinoids of the stomach. Cancer *47*:2620–2626.

Goldman H. and Ming S.C. (1968) Fine structure of intestinal metaplasia and adenocarcinoma of the human stomach. Laboratory Investigations *18*:203–210.

Goldman R.L. (1964) Submucosal arterial malformation ("aneurysm") of the stomach with fatal haemorrhage. Gastroenterology *46*:589–594.

Goldstein F., Kline T.S., Kline I.K., Thornton J.J., Abramson J. and Bell L. (1983) Early gastric cancer in a United States hospital. American Journal of Gastroenterology *78*:715–719.

Gonzalez-Crussi F. and Hackett R.L. (1966) Phlegmonous gastritis. Archives of Surgery *93*:990–995.

Gotlieb-Jensen K. and Andersen J. (1983) Occurrence of candida in gastric ulcers. Gastroenterology *85*:535–537.

Gottfried E.B., Korsten M.A. and Lieber C.S. (1978) Alcohol-induced gastric and duodenal lesions in man. American Journal of Gastroenterology *70*:587–592.

Graem N., Fischer A.B., Hastrup N. and Povlsen C.O. (1981) Mucosal changes of the Billroth II resected stomach. Acta Pathologica, Microbiologica et Immunologica Scandinavica, Section A *89*:227–234.

Graffner H. and Hesselvik M. (1987) Gastric pseudolymphoma. Acta Chirurgica Scandinavica *153*:471–472.

Graham D.Y. (1989) Campylobacter pylori and peptic ulcer disease. Gastroenterology *96*:615–625.

Graham D.Y., Agrawal N.M. and Roth S.H. (1988) Prevention of NSAID-induced gastric ulcer with Misoprostol: multicentre, double-blind, placebo-controlled trial. Lancet 2:1277–1280.

Graham D.Y. and Michaletz P.A. (1988) Should I search for campylobacter pylori in my patients? Much ado about not much? American Journal of Gastroenterology *83*:481–483.

Graham D.Y. and Smith J.L. (1986) Aspirin and the stomach. (Review). Annals of Internal Medicine *104*:390–398.

Green P.H.R., Fevre D.I., Barrett P.J., Hunt J.H., Gillespie P.E. and Nagy G.S. (1977) Chronic erosive (Verrucous) gastritis. A study of 108 patients. Endoscopy *9*:74–78.

Green P.H.R., O'Toole K.M., Weinberg L.M. and Goldfarb J.P. (1981) Early gastric cancer. Gastroenterology *81*:247–256.

Grigioni W.F., D'Errico A., Milani M., Villanacci V., Avellini C., Miglioli M., Mattioli S., Biasco G., Barbara L. and Possati L. (1984) Early gastric cancer. Clinico-pathological analysis of 125 cases of early gastric cancer (EGC). Acta Pathologica Japonica *34*:979–989.

Guardia, J., Mirada A., Moragas A., Armengol J.R. and Martinez-Vazquez J.M. (1980) Alpha chain disease of the stomach. Hepato-Gastroenterology *28*:238–239.

Halbert R.E. (1982) Peutz-Jeghers syndrome with metastasizing gastric adenocarcinoma (report of a case). Archives of Pathology and Laboratory Medicine *106*:517–520.

Halter F., Witzel L., Gretillat P.A., Scheurer U. and Keller M. (1977) Diagnostic value of biopsy, guided lavage, and brush cytology in esophagogastroscopy. American Journal of Digestive Diseases *22*:129–131.

Hamilton S.R. and Yardley J.H. (1980) Endoscopic biopsy diagnosis of aspirin-associated chronic gastric ulcers. Gastroenterology *78*:1178.

Haot J., Berger F., Andre C., Moulinier B., Mainguet P. and Lambert R. (1989) Lymphocytic gastritis versus varioliform gastritis. A historical series revisited. Journal of Pathology *158*:19–22.

Haot J., Hamichi L., Wallez L. and Mainguet P. (1988) Lymphocytic gastritis: a newly described entity: a retrospective endoscopic and histological study. Gut *29*:1258–1264.

Harvey B.C.H. (1907) A study of the structure of the gastric glands of dogs and the changes which they undergo after gastroenterostomy and occlusion of the pylorus. American Journal of Anatomy *6*:207–243.

Hatfield A.R.W., Slavin G., Segal A.W. and Levi A.J. (1975) Importance of the site of endoscopic gastric biopsy in ulcerating lesions of the stomach. Gut *16*:884–886.

Hattori T. (1985) Morphological range of hyperplastic polyps and carcinomas arising in hyperplastic polyps of the stomach. Journal of Clinical Pathology *38*:622–630.

Henson D. (1972) Cytomegalovirus inclusion bodies in the gastrointestinal tract. Archives of Pathology *93*:477–482.

Hermanek P. and Riemann J.F. (1982) The operated stomach: still a precancerous condition? Endoscopy *14*:113–114.

Hernandez J.A. and Sheehan W.W. (1985) Lymphomas of the mucosa-associated lymphoid tissue. Signet ring cell lymphomas presenting in mucosal lymphoid organs. Cancer *55*:592–597.

Hirsch B.Z., Whitington P.F., Kirschner B.S., Black D.D., Bostwick D.G. and Yousefzadeh D.K. (1989) Isolated granulomatous gastritis in an adolescent. Digestive Diseases and Sciences *34*:292–296.

Hoare A.M., Jones E.L., Alexander-Williams J. and Hawkins C.F. (1977) Symptomatic significance of gastric mucosal changes after surgery for peptic ulcer. Gut *18*:295–300.

Hodges J.R., Isaacson P. and Wright R. (1981) Diffuse enterochromaffin-like (ECL) cell hyperplasia and multiple gastric carcinoids: a complication of pernicious anaemia. Gut *22*:237–241.

Hoedemaeker P.J., Abels J., Wachters J.J., Adrends A. and Nieweg H.O. (1964) Investigations about the site of production of Castles' gastric intrinsic factor. Laboratory Investigation *13*:1394–1399.

Hoftiezer J.W., O'Laughlin J.C. and Ivey K.J. (1982) Effects of 24 hours of aspirin, Bufferin, paracetamol and placebo on normal human gastroduodenal mucosa. Gut *23*:692–697.

Hojgaard L., Matzen P. and Christoffersen P. (1987) Gastritis: a clinical entity? Scandinavian Journal of Gastroenterology *128*(suppl.):90–93.

Holt J.M., Gear M.W.L., and Warner G.T. (1970) The role of chronic blood loss in the pathogenesis of post gastrectomy iron deficiency anaemia. Gut *11*:847–850.

Honore L.H., Lewis A.S. and Ohara K.E. (1979) Gastritic glandularis et cystica profunda: report of 3 cases with discussion of etiology and pathogenesis. Digestive Diseases and Sciences *24*:48–52.

Houghton P.W.J., Mortensen N.J.McC., Thomas W.E.G., Cooper M.J., Morgan A.P. and Burton P. (1986) Intragastric bile acids and histological changes in gastric mucosa. British Journal of Surgery *73*:354–356.

Hsiu J-G., Gamsey A.J., Ives C.E., D'Amato N.A. and Hiller A.N. (1986) Gastric anisakiasis: report of a case with clinical, endoscopic, and histological findings. American Journal of Gastroenterology *81*:1185–1187.

Hyjek E. and Kelenyi G. (1982) Pseudolymphomas of the stomach: a lesion characterized by progressively tranformed germinal centres. Histopathology *6*:61–68.

Ida K., Hashimoto Y., Takeda S., Murakami K. and Kawai K. (1975) Endoscopic diagnosis of gastric cancer with dye scattering. American Journal of Gastroenterology *63*:316–320.

Ignatius J.A., Armstrong C.D. and Eversole S.L. (1970) Multiple diffuse cystic disease of the stomach in association with carcinoma. Gastroenterology *59*:610–614.

Iida F., Murata F. and Nagata T. (1978) Histochemical studies of mucosubstances in metaplastic epithelium of the stomach with special reference to the development of intestinal metaplasia. Histochemistry *56*:229–237.

Iida M., Yao T., Itoh H., Watanabe H., Matsui T., Iwashita A. and Fujishima M. (1988) Natural history of gastric adenomas in patients with familial adenomatosis coli/Gardner's syndrome. Cancer *61*:605–611.

Iida M., Yao T., Watanabe H., Imamura K., Fuyuno S. and Omae T. (1980) Spontaneous disappearance of fundic gland polyposis: report of three cases. Gastroenterology *79*:725–728.

Ikeda K. and Murayama K. (1978) A case of amyloid tumor of the stomach. Endoscopy *10*:54–58.

Ikkala E., Salmi H.J. and Siurala M. (1970) Gastric mucosa in iron deficiency anaemia. Results of a follow-up examination. Acta Haematologica *43*:228–231.

Ikkala E. and Siurala M. (1964) Gastric lesion in iron deficiency anaemia. Acta Haematologica *31*:313–324.

Imerslund O. (1960) Idiopathic chronic megaloblastic anaemia in children. Acta Paediatrica Supplement *119*:1–115.

Irvine W.J., Cullen D.R. and Mawhinney H. (1974) Natural history of autoimmune achlorhydric atrophic gastritis. A 1–15 year follow-up study. Lancet *ii*:482–485.

Isaacson P.G. and Spencer J. (1987) Malignant lymphoma of mucosa-associated lymphoid tissue. Histopathology *11*:445–462.

Isaacson P.G., Spencer J., and Finn T. (1986) Primary B-cell gastric lymphoma. Human Pathology *17*:72–82.

Isaacson P.G. and Wright D.H. (1983) Malignant lymphoma of mucosa-associated lymphoid tissue. Cancer *52*:1410–1416.

Isaacson P.G. and Wright D.H. (1984) Extranodal malignant lymphoma arising from mucosa-associated lymphoid tissue. Cancer *53*:2515–2524.

Isaacson P., Wright D.H., Judd M.A. and Mepham B.L. (1979) Primary gastrointestinal lymphomas. A classification of 66 cases. Cancer *43*:1805–1819.

Itsuno M., Watanabe H., Iwafuchi M., Ito S., Yanaihara N., Sato K., Kikuchi M. and Akiyama N. (1989) Multiple carcinoids and endocrine cell micronests in type A gastritis. Their morphology, histogenesis, and natural history. Cancer *63*:881–890.

Iwasaki T. (1987) Alimentary tract lesions in cytomegalovirus infection. Acta Pathologica Japonica *37*:549–565.

Jabbari M., Cherry R., Lough J.O., Daly D.S., Kinnear D.G., and Goresky C.A. (1984) Gastric antral vascular ectasia: the watermelon stomach. Gastroenterology *87*:1165–1170.

Jablokow V.R., Aranha G.V. and Reyes C.V. (1982) Gastric stomal polypoid hyperplasia: report of four cases. Journal of Surgical Oncology *19*:106–108.

Jarvinen H., Nyberg M. and Peltokallio P. (1983) Upper gastrointestinal tract polyps in familial adenomatosis coli. Gut *24*:333–339.

Jarvis L.R. and Whitehead R. (1980) Effect of nicotine on the morphology of the rat gastric mucosa. Gastroenterology *78*:1488–1494.

Jarvis L.R. and Whitehead R. (1985) Morphometric analysis of gastric dysplasia. Journal of Pathology *147*:133–138.

Jass J.R. (1983) A classification of gastric dysplasia. Histopathology 7:181–193.

Jass J.R. and Filipe M.I. (1979) A variant of intestinal metaplasia associated with gastric carcinoma: a histochemical study. Histopathology 3:191–199.

Jass J.R. and Filipe M.I. (1981) The mucin profiles of normal gastric mucosa, intestinal metaplasia and its variants and gastric carcinoma. Histochemical Journal 13:931–939.

Jeffries G.H. (1965) Recovery of gastric mucosal structure and function in pernicious anaemia during prednisolone therapy. Gastroenterology 48:371–378.

Jenkins D., Stephenson P.M. and Scott B.B. (1985) The Cronkhite-Canada syndrome: an ultrastructural study of pathogenesis. Journal of Clinical Pathology 38:271–276.

Johnson G.K., Soergel K.H., Hensley G.T., Dodds W.T. and Hogan W.J. (1972) Cronkhite-Canada: gastrointestinal pathophysiology and morphology. Gastroenterology 63:140–152.

Johnstone J.M. and Morson B.C. (1978a) Eosinophilic gastroenteritis. Histopathology 2:335–348.

Johnstone J.M. and Morson B.C. (1978b) Inflammatory fibroid polyp of the gastrointestinal tract. Histopathology 2:349–361.

Jones A.W., Kirk R.S. and Bloor K. (1970) The association between aneurysms of the abdominal aorta and peptic ulceration. Gut 11:679–684.

Joske R.A., Finckh E.S. and Wood I.J. (1955) Gastric biopsy: a study of 1,000 consecutive successful gastric biopsies. Quarterly Journal of Medicine 24:269–294.

Justrabo E., Guion L., Levillain P., Piard F. and Michiels R. (1987) Cystic glandular fundic polyps of the stomach. Report on 12 cases and review of the literature. Annals of Pathology 7:106–112.

Kahn L.B. (1963) Gastric mucormycosis: a report of a case with a review of the literature. South African Medical Journal 37:1265–1269.

Kalogeropoulos N.K. and Whitehead R. (1988) Campylobacter-like organisms and candida in peptic ulcers and similar lesions of the upper gastrointestinal tract: a study of 247 cases. Journal of Clinical Pathology 41:1093–1098.

Kamal M.F., Shaker K., Jaser N. and Leimoon B.A. (1985) Eosinophilic gastroenteritis with no peripheral eosinophilia. Annales Chirurgiae et Gynaecologiae 74:98–100.

Kamiya T., Morishita T., Asakura H., Munakata Y. and Miura S. (1981) Histoclinical long-standing follow-up study of hyperplastic polyps of the stomach. American Journal of Gastroenterology 75:275–281.

Karvonen A-L., Kekki M., Lehtola J., Sipponen P. and Ihamaki T. (1987) Prepyloric erosions: an entity of its own among erosive gastric lesions. Scandinavian Journal of Gastroenterology 22:1095–1101.

Karvonen A-L., Sipponen P., Lehtola J. and Ruokonen A. (1983) Gastric mucosal erosions. Scandinavian Journal of Gastroenterology 18:1051–1056.

Katayama Y., Kimura M. and Konn M. (1985) Cronkhite-Canada syndrome associated with a rectal cancer and adenomatous changes in colonic polyps. American Journal of Surgical Pathology 9:65–71.

Katz A.J., Goldman H. and Grand R.J. (1977) Gastric mucosal biopsy in eosinophilic (allergic) gastroenteritis. Gastroenterology 73:705–709.

Katz S., Klein M.S., Winawer S.J. and Sherlock P. (1973) Disseminated lymphoma involving the stomach. Correlation of endoscopy with directed cytology and biopsy. American Journal of Digestive Diseases 18:370–374.

Katzenstein A.L. and Maksem J. (1979) Candidal infection of gastric ulcers: histology, incidence, and clinical significance. American Journal of Clinical Pathology 71:137–141.

Kawai K., Shimamoto K., Misaki F., Murakami K. and Masuda M. (1970) Erosion of gastric mucosa: pathogenesis, incidence and classification of the erosive gastritis. Endoscopy 2:168–174.

Kaye M.D., Whorwell P.J. and Wright R. (1983) Gastric mucosal lymphocyte subpopulations in pernicious anemia and in normal stomach. Clinical Immunology and Immunopathology 28:431–440.

Kekki M., Hakkiluoto A. and Siurala M. (1976) Dynamics of atrophic gastritis in male and female subjects after partial gastric resection: an evaluation by stochastic analysis. Scandinavian Journal of Gastroenterology 11:597–601.

Kekki M., Saukkonen M., Sipponen P., Varis K. and Siurala M. (1980) Dynamics of chronic gastritis in the remnant after partial gastrectomy for duodenal ulcer. Scandinavian Journal of Gastroenterology 15:509–512.

Kekki M., Varis K., Pohjanpalo H., Isokoski M., Ihamaki T. and Siurala M. (1983) Course of antrum and body gastritis in pernicious anemia families. Digestive Diseases and Sciences 28:698–704.

Kekki M. and Villako K. (1981) Dynamic behaviour of gastritis in various populations and subpopulations. Annals of Clinical Research 13:119–122

Kekki M., Villako K., Tamm A. and Siurala M. (1977) Dynamics of antral and fundal gastritis in an Estonian rural population sample. Scandinavian Journal of Gastroenterology 12:321–324.

Kenny F.D., Dockerty M.B. and Waugh J.M. (1954) Giant hypertrophy of gastric mucosa; a clinical and pathological study. Cancer 7:671–681.

Keshavarzian A., Saverymuttu S.H., Tai P-C., Thompson M., Barter S., Spry C.J.F. and Chadwick V.S. (1985) Activated eosinophils in familial eosinophilic gastroenteritis. Gastroenterology 88:1041–1049.

Kimura K. (1969) Gastric xanthelasma. Archives of Pathology 87:110–117.

Klein N.C., Hargrove R.L., Sleisenger M.H. and Jeffries G.H. (1970) Eosinophilic gastroenteritis. Medicine 49:299–319.

Kliems G., Paquet K.J., Lindstaedt H. and Miederen S. (1979) Atrophic gastritis after Billroth I gastrectomy. Endoscopy 2:127–130.

Kodama T., Fukuda S., Takino T., Omori Y. and Oka T. (1985) Gastroduodenal cytomegalovirus infection after renal transplantation. Fiberscopic observations. Endoscopy 17:157–158.

Konrad E.A. and Meister P. (1979) Fatal eosinophilic gastroenterocolitis in a two-year-old child. Virchows Archiv A Pathological Anatomy and Histology 382:347–353.

Konturek S.J., Brzozowski T., Piastucki I., Dembinski A., Radecki T., Dembinska-Kiec A., Zmuda A. and Gregory H. (1981) Role of mucosal prostaglandins and DNA synthesis in gastric cyto- protection by luminal epidermal growth factor. Gut 22:927–932.

Korelitz B.I., Waye J.D., Kreuning J., Sommers S.C., Fein H.D., Beeber J. and Gelberg B.J. (1981) Crohn's disease in endoscopic biopsies of the gastric antrum and duodenum. The American Journal of Gastroenterology 76:103–109.

Korman M.G., Soveney C. and Hansky J. (1971) Serum gastrin in duodenal ulcer. 1. Basal levels and effect of food and atropine. Gut 12:899–902.

Korman M.G., Soveney C. and Hansky J. (1972) Gastrin studies in gastric ulcer. Gut 13:166–169.

Krag E. (1966) Enlarged gastric and duodenal rugae. The prognostic significance of the radiological findings of coarse mucosal folds in the stomach and duodenum. Acta Medica Scandinavica 179:343–348.

Kraut J.R., Powell R., Hruby M.A. and Lloyd-Still J.D. (1981) Menetrier's disease in childhood: report of two cases and a review of the literature. Journal of Pediatric Surgery 16:707–711.

Krentz K. and Gohrband G. (1976) Klinik und Verlauf gastraler erosionen. Medizinische Klinik 71:156–162.

Kristensen M. and Nilsson T. (1985) Mucus secretion in hypertrophic, hypersecretory, protein-losing gastropathy. American Journal of Gastroenterology 80:77–81.

Kuipers F.C., Theil P.H. van and Roskam E.T. (1960) Eosinophilic phlegmon of the small intestine caused by a worm not adapted to the human body. Nederlands Tijdshrift Voor Geneeskunde 104:422–427.

Kundrotas L., Novak J., Kremzier J., Meenaghan M. and Hassett J. (1988) Gastric bleeding in pseudoxanthoma elasticum. American Journal of Gastroenterology 83:868–872.

Lacy E.R. and Ito S. (1982) Microscopic analysis of ethanol damage in rat gastric mucosa after treatment with a prostaglandin. Gastroenterology 83:619–625.

Laine L. and Weinstein W.M. (1988a) Subepithelial hemorrhages and erosions of human stomach. Digestive Diseases and Sciences 33:490–503.

Laine L. and Weinstein W.M. (1988b) Histology of alcoholic hemorrhagic "gastritis": a prospective evaluation. Gastroenterology 94:1254–1262.

Lam S.K., Hui W.K.K., Ho J., Wong K.P., Rotter J.I. and Samloff I.M. (1983) Pachydermoperiostosis, hypertrophic gastropathy and peptic ulcer. Gastroenterology 84:834–839.

Lambert R., Andre C., Moulinier B. and Bugnon B. (1978) Diffuse varioliform gastritis. Digestion 17:159–167.

Lambert R., Moulinier B., Bugnon B. and Andre C. (1977) La gastrite hypertrophique superficielle (gastrite varioliforme). In: What's New in Endoscopy of the Upper Digestive Tract in Relation to Radiology and Surgery. Edited by M. Cremer. Brussels: Societe Belge d'Endoscopie Digestive.

Lancet (1989) Campylobacter pylori becomes Helicobacter pylori. ii:1019–1029.

Langhans P., Bues M. and Bunte H. (1984) Morphological changes in the operated stomach under the influence of duodenogastric reflux. Scandinavian Journal of Gastroenterology 19(suppl. 92):145–148.

Langman M.J.S. and Cooke A.R. (1976) Gastric and duodenal ulcer and their associated diseases. Lancet i:680–683.

Lanza F.L. (1984) Endoscopic studies of gastric and duodenal injury after the use of ibuprofen, aspirin and other nonsteroidal anti-inflammatory agents. American Journal of Medicine 77:19–24.

Larsen B., Tarp U. and Kristensen E. (1987) Familial giant hypertrophic gastritis (Menetrier's disease). Gut 28:1517–1521.

Lauren P. (1965) The two histological main types of gastric carcinoma; diffuse and so-called intestinal type carcinoma; an attempt at a histoclinical classification. Acta Pathologica Microbiologica et Immunologica Scandinavica, Section A 64:31–49.

Lawson H.H. (1988) Definition of gastroduodenal junction in healthy subjects. Journal of Clinical Pathology 41:393–396.

Lee R.G. and Burt R.W. (1986) The histopathology of fundic gland polyps of the stomach. American Journal of Clinical Pathology 86:498–503.

Lehnert T., Sternberg S.S., Sprossmann M. and DeCosse J.J. (1989) Early gastric cancer. American Journal of Surgery 157:202–207.

Leinbach G.E. and Rubin C.E. (1970) Eosinophilic gastroenteritis: a simple reaction to food allergens? Gastroenterology 59:874–889.

Lev R. (1966) The mucin histochemistry of normal and neoplastic gastric mucosa. Laboratory Investigations 14:2080–2100.

Lev R. and DeNucci T.D. (1989) Neoplastic Paneth cells in the stomach. Report of two cases and review of the literature. Archives of Pathology and Laboratory Medicine 113:129–133.

Levine J.S. and Allen R.H. (1985) Intrinsic factor within parietal cells of patients with juvenile pernicious anemia. Gastroenterology 88:1132–1136.

Lewin K.J., Dowling F., Wright J.P. and Taylor K.B. (1976) Gastric morphology and serum gastrin levels in pernicious anaemia. Gut *17*:551–560.

Lin H-J., Lee F-Y., Tsai Y-T., Lee S-D., Lin C-Y., Tsay S-H. and Chiang H. (1989) Alimentary tract and pancreas. A prospective evaluation of biopsy site in the diagnosis of gastric malignancy: the margin or the base? Journal of Gastroenterology and Hepatology *4*:137–141.

Lipkin M. (1981) Proliferation and differentiation of gastrointestinal cells in normal and diseased states. In: Physiology of the Gastrointestinal Tract. Edited by L.R. Johnson. New York: Raven Press, pp. 145–167.

Lipper S. and Kahn L.B. (1977) Superficial cystic gastritis with alopecia. A forme fruste of the Cronkhite-Canada syndrome. Archives of Pathology and Laboratory Medicine *101*:432–436.

Listrom M.B. and Fenoglio-Preiser C.M. (1987) Lymphatic distribution of the stomach in normal, inflammatory, hyperplastic, and neoplastic tissue. Gastroenterology *93*:506–514.

Littler E.R. and Gleibermann E. (1972) Gastritis cystica polyposa. Cancer *29*:205–209.

LiVolsi V.A. and Perzin K.H. (1975) Inflammatory pseudotumors (inflammatory fibrous polyps) of the small intestine. A clinicopathologic study. American Journal of Digestive Diseases *20*:325–336.

Loux H.A. and Zamcheck N. (1969) Cytological evidence for the long "quiescent" stage of gastric cancer in two patients with pernicious anaemia. Gastroenterology *57*:173–184.

Lucak B.K., Sansaricq C., Snyderman S.E., Greco M.A., Fazzini E.P. and Bazaz G.R. (1982) Disseminated ulcerations in allergic eosiniphilic gastroenterocolitis. American Journal of Gastroenterology *77*:248–252.

Lundegardh G., Adami H-O., Helmick C., Zack M. and Meirik O. (1988) Stomach cancer after partial gastrectomy for benign ulcer disease. New England Journal of Medicine *319*:195–200.

Lygidakis N.J. (1986) Histologic changes after elective surgery for duodenal ulcer. Acta Chirurgica Scandinavica *152*:139–144.

Macartney J.C., Camplejohn R.S. and Powell G. (1986) DNA flow cytometry of histological material from human gastric cancer. Journal of Pathology *148*:273–277.

MacDonald W.C. (1973) Correlation of mucosal histology and aspirin intake in chronic gastric ulcer. Gastroenterology *65*:381–389.

MacDonald W.C. and Rubin C.E. (1967) Gastric biopsy: a critical evaluation. Gastroenterology *53*:143–170.

McGuigan J.E. and Trudeau W.L. (1970) Serum gastrin concentrations in pernicious anaemia. New England Journal of Medicine *282*:358–361.

McIntyre R.L.E., Irani M.S. and Piris J. (1981) Histological study of the effects of three anti-inflammatory preparations on the gastric mucosa. Journal of Clinical Pathology *34*:836–842.

McNulty C.A.M., Dent J.C., Curry A., Uff J.S., Ford G.A., Gear M.W.L. and Wilkinson S.P. (1989) New spiral bacterium in gastric mucosa. Journal of Clinical Pathology *42*:585–591.

Magnus H.A. (1946) The pathology of simple gastritis. Journal of Pathology and Bacteriology *58*:431–439.

Magnus H.A. (1952) Gastritis. In: Modern Trends in Gastroenterology. First series. Edited by F.H. Jones. London: Butterworth, p. 323.

Magnus H.A. and Ungley C.C. (1938) The gastric lesion in pernicious anaemia. Lancet *i*:420–421.

Malfertheiner P. (1988) Role of infection in gastroduodenal pathology. Scandinavian Journal of Gastroenterology *23*(suppl. 142): 7–8.

Malhotra R. and Sheffield A. (1988) Cronkhite-Canada syndrome associated with colon carcinoma and adenomatous changes in C-C polyps. American Journal of Gastroenterology *83*:772–776.

Mann N.S. (1976) Bile-induced acute erosive gastritis. Its prevention by antacid, cholestyramine, and prostaglandin E_2. American Journal of Digestive Diseases *21*:89–92.

Marcheggiano A., Iannoni C., Agnello M., Paoluzi P. and Pallone F. (1987) Campylobacter-like organisms on the human gastric mucosa. Relation to type and extent of gastritis in different clinical groups. Gastroenterologie Clinique et Biologique *11*:376–381.

Marshall B.J. (1988) Should we now, routinely, be examining gastric biopsies for campylobacter pylori? American Journal of Gastroenterology *83*:479–481.

Marshall B.J., Armstrong J.A., McGechie D.B. and Glancy R.J. (1985) Attempt to fulfill Koch's postulates for pyloric campylobacter. Medical Journal of Australia *142*:436–444.

Mast A., Elewaut A., Mortier G., Quatacker J., Defloor E., Roels H. and Barbier F. (1976) Gastric xanthoma. American Journal of Gastroenterology *65*:311–317.

Mathis G., Dirschmid K. and Sutterlutti G. (1987) Tuberculous gastric ulcer. Endoscopy *19*:133–135.

Matzinger M.A. and Daneman A. (1983) Esophageal involvement in eosinophilic gastroenteritis. Pediatric Radiology *13*:35–38.

Meister H., Holubarsch C.H., Haverkamp O., Schlag P. and Herforth C.H. (1979) Gastritis, intestinal metaplasia and dysplasia versus benign ulcer in the duodenum and gastric carcinoma. Pathology, Research and Practice *164*:259–269.

Menetrier P. (1888) Des polyadenomes gastriques et de leurs rapports avec le cancer de l' estomac. Archives de Physiologie Normale et Pathologique *1*:32–55 and 236–262.

Metzger W.H., McAdam L., Bluestone R. and Guth P.H. (1976) Acute gastric mucosal injury during continuous or interrupted aspirin ingestion in humans. American Journal of Digestive Diseases *21*:963–968.

Miller T.A. (1987) Mechnisms of stress-related mucosal damage. American Journal of Medicine *83*(suppl. 6A):8–14.

Ming S-C. (1977) The classification and significance of gastric polyps. In: The Gastrointestinal Tract. Edited by J.H. Yardley, B.C. Mason, and M.R. Abell. International Academy of Pathology Monograph. Baltimore: Williams & Wilkins, *11*:149–175.

Ming S-C., Bajtai A., Correa P., Elster K., Jarvi O.H., Munoz N., Nagayo T. and Stemmerman G.N. (1984) Gastric dysplasia. Significance and pathologic criteria. Cancer *54*:1794–1801.

Mingazzini P., Carlei F., Malchiodi-Albedi F., Lezoche E., Covotta A., Speranza V., Polak J.M. (1984) Endocrine cells in intestinal metaplasia of the stomach. Journal of Pathology *144*:171–178.

Minoli G., Terruzi V., Butti G.C., Frigerio G. and Rossini A. (1982) Gastric candidiasis: an endoscopic and histological study in 26 patients. Gastrointestinal Endoscopy 28:59–61.

Minoli G., Terruzzi V., and Rossini A. (1979) Gastroduodenal Candidiasis occurring without underlying diseases (primary gastroduodenal candidiasis). Endoscopy *1*:18–22.

Misra R.C., Agarwal S.K., Prakash P., Saha M.M., and Gupta P.S. (1982) Gastric tuberculosis. Endoscopy *14*:235–237.

Mohri N. (1987) Primary gastric non-Hodgkin's lymphomas in Japan. Virchows Archiv (A) *411*:459–466.

Monroe L.E., Boughton G.A., and Sommers S.C. (1964) The association of gastric epithelial hyperplasia and cancer. Gastroenterology *46*:267–272.

Moore D., Lichtman S., Lentz J., Stringer D. and Sherman P. (1986) Eosinophilic gastroenteritis presenting in an adolescent with isolated colonic involvement. Gut 27:1219–1222.

Moreto M., Ojembarrena E., Zaballa M., Tanago J.G., Ibanez S. and Setien F. (1985) Retrospective endoscopic analysis of gastric xanthelasma in the non-operated stomach. Endoscopy *17*:210–211.

Morgan A.G.,McAdam W.A.F.,Pyrah R.D. and Tinsley E.G.F. (1976) Multiple recurring gastric erosions (aphthous ulcers) Gut *17*:633–639.

Mori K., Shinya H. and Wolff W.I. (1971) Polypoid reparative mucosal proliferation at the site of a healed gastric ulcer; sequential gastroscopic, radiological and histological observation. Gastroenterology *61*:523–529.

Mori M., Kitagawa S., Iida M., Sakurai T., Enjoji M., Sugimachi K. and Ooiwa T. (1987) Early carcinoma of the gastric cardia. Cancer *59*:1758–1766.

Morris A. and Nicholson G. (1987) Ingestion of campylobacter pyloridis causes gastritis and raised fasting gastric pH. American Journal of Gastroenterology *82*:192–199.

Morson B.C. (1955) Intestinal metaplasia of the gastric mucosa. British Journal of Cancer *9*:365–376.

Morson B.C., Sobin L.H., Grundmann E., Johansen A., Nagayo T. and Serck-Hanssen A. (1980). Precancerous conditions and epithelial dysplasia in the stomach. The Journal of Clinical Pathology *33*:711–721.

Mosbech J., and Videbaek A. (1950) Mortality from and risk of gastric carcinoma among patients with pernicious anaemia. British Medical Journal *ii*:390–394.

Mosimann F., Burris B., Diserens H., Fontolliet C., Loup P. and Mosimann R. (1981) Enterogastric reflux; experimental and clinical study. Scandinavian Journal of Gastroenterology *16*(suppl. 67):149–152.

Mosimann F., Sorgi M., Wolverson R.L., Donovan I.A., Fielding J.W.L., Harding L.K., Alexander-Williams J. and Thompson H. (1984) Gastric histology and its relationship to entero-gastric reflux after duodenal ulcer surgery. Scandinavian Journal of Gastroenterology *19*(suppl. 92):142–144.

Mountford R.A., Brown P., Salmon P.R., Alvarenga C., Neumann C.S. and Read A.E. (1980) Gastric cancer detection in gastric ulcer disease. Gut *21*:9–17.

Mower G.A. and Whitehead R. (1986) Gastric hemorrhage due to ruptured arteriovenous malformation (Dieulafoy's disease). Pathology *18*:54–57.

Mueller J., Kirchner T. and Mueller-Hermelink H.K. (1987) Gastric endocrine cell hyperplasia and carcinoid tumors in atrophic gastritis Type A. American Journal of Surgical Pathology *11*:909–917.

Muratani M., Nakamura T., Nakano G-I. and Mukawa K. (1989) Ultrastructural study of two subtypes of gastric adenoma. Journal of Clinical Pathology *42*:352–359.

Myhre M.J. and Isaacson P.G. (1987) Primary B-cell gastric lymphoma: a reassessment of its histogenesis. Journal of Pathology *152*:1–11.

Myren J., and Serck-Hanssen A. (1975) Gastroscopic observations related to bioptical histology in healthy medical students. Scandinavian Journal of Gastroenterology *10*:353–355.

Nagayo T. (1972) Histological diagnosis of biopsied gastric mucosa with special reference to that of borderline lesions. Gann Monographs in Cancer Research *11*:245–256.

Nakamura T. (1970) Pathohistologische Einteilung der Magenpolypen mit spezifischer Betrachtung ihrer malignen Entartung. Chirurg *41*:122–130.

Nakamura T. and Nakano G-I. (1985) Histopathological classification and malignant change in gastric polyps. Journal of Clinical Pathology *38*:754–764.

Nakanishi I., Kajikawa K., Migita S., Mai M., Akimoto R., and Mura T. (1982) Gastric plasmacytoma. An immunologic and immunohistochemical study. Cancer *49*:2025–2028.

Nardelli J., Bara J., Bosa B. and Burtin P. (1983) Intestinal metaplasia and carcinomas of the human stomach. The Journal of Histochemistry and Cytochemistry *31*:366–375.

Nasrallah S.M., Johnston G.S., Gadacz T.R. and Kim K.M. (1987) The significance of gastric bile reflux seen at endoscopy. Journal of Clinical Gastroenterology *9*:514–517.

Navab F., Kleinman M.S., Algazy K., Schenk E., and Turner M.D. (1972) Endoscopic diagnosis of eosinophilic gastritis. Gastrointestinal Endoscopy *19*:67–69.

Naylor A.R., and Pollet J.E. (1985) Eosinophilic colitis. Diseases of the Colon and Rectum *28*:615–618.

Nedenskov-Sorensen P., Bjorneklett A., Fausa O., Bukholm G., Aase S. and Jantzen E. (1988) Campylobacter pylori infection and its relation to chronic gastritis. Scandinavian Journal of Gastroenterology 23:867–874.

Nesland A.A. and Berstad A. (1985) Erosive prepyloric changes in persons with and without dyspepsia. Scandinavian Journal of Gastroenterology 20:222–228.

Nesland A.A., Berstad A. and Serck-Hanssen A. (1986) Histological findings in erosive prepyloric changes. Scandinavian Journal of Gastroenterology 21:239–245.

Nevin N.C., Eakins D., Clarke S.D. and Carson D.J.L. (1969) Acute phlegmonous gastritis. British Journal of Surgery 56:268–270.

Newbold K.M., MacDonald F. and Allum W.H. (1988) Undifferentiated columnar cells on the gastric interfoveolar crest: a previously undescribed observation. Journal of Pathology 155:311–316.

Niemela S., Karttunen T., Heikkila J. and Lehtola J. (1987) Characteristics of reflux gastritis. Scandinavian Journal of Gastroenterology 22:349–354.

Nonomura A., Ohta G., Ibata T., Shinozaki K., and Nishino T. (1980) Cronkhite-Canada syndrome associated with sigmoid cancer. Case report and review of 54 cases with the syndrome. Acta Pathologica Japonica 30:825–845.

O'Brien M.J., Burakoff R., Robbins E.A., Golding R.M., Zamcheck N. and Gottlieb L.S. (1985) Early gastric cancer. Clinicopathologic study. American Journal of Medicine 78:195–202.

Oehlert W., Keller P., Henke M., and Strauch M. (1975) Die Dysplasien der Magenschleimhaut. Deutsche Medicinische Wochenschrift 100:1950–1956.

Oehlert W., Keller P., Henke M., and Strauch M. (1979) Gastric mucosal dysplasia: What is their clinical significance? Frontiers of Gastrointestinal Research 4:173–182.

Offerhaus G.J.A., Huibregtse K., De Boer J., Verhoeven T., Van Olffen G.H., Van De Stadt J. and Tytgat G.N.J. (1984a) The operated stomach: a premalignant condition? Scandinavian Journal of Gastroenterology 19:521–524.

Offerhaus G.J.A., VD Stadt J., Huibregtse K. and Tytgat G.N.J. (1984b) Endoscopic screening for malignancy in the gastric remnant: the clinical significance of dysplasia in gastric mucosa. Journal of Clinical Pathology 37:748–754.

Ohno F., Numata Y., Yamano T., Suzuki M. and Miyoshi K. (1982) Gastroscopic biopsy of the stomach for the diagnosis of amyloidosis. Gastroenterologica Japonica 17:415–421.

Ohta H., Noguchi Y., Takagi K., Nishi M., Kajitani T. and Kato Y. (1987) Early gastric carcinoma with special reference to macroscopic classification. Cancer 60:1099–1106.

Oi M., Oshida K., and Sugimura S. (1959) The location of gastric ulcer. Gastroenterology 36:45–56.

Ona F.V. (1981) Gastric sarcoid. American Journal of Gastroenterology 75:286–288.

Ooi A., Nakanishi I. and Hashiba A. (1987) Gastric plasmacytoma: an early lesion diagnosed with the aid of immunoperoxidase and immunogold techniques. American Journal of Gastroenterology 82:572–578.

Orchard R., Reynolds K., Fox B., Andrews R., Parkins R.A. and Johnson A.G. (1977) Effect of lysolecithin on gastric mucosal structure and potential difference. Gut 18:457–461.

Ormiston M.C., Gear M.W.L. and Codling B.W. (1982) Five year follow-up study of gastritis. Journal of Clinical Pathology 35:757–760.

Ostertag H., and Georgii A. (1979) Early gastric cancer: A morphological study of 144 cases. Pathology, Research and Practice 164:294–315.

Ovaska J.T., Ekfors T.O., Havia T.V. and Kujari H.P. (1986) Endoscopic follow-up after resection for gastric or duodenal ulcer. Acta Chirurgica Scandinavica 152:289–295.

Overholt B.F., and Jeffries G.H. (1970) Hypertrophic, hypersecretory protein-losing gastropathy. Gastroenterology 58:80–87.

Owen D.A. (1986) Normal histology of the stomach. The American Journal of Surgical Pathology 10:48–61.

Oyaizu N., Uemura Y., Izumi H., Morii S., Nishi M. and Hioki K. (1985) Eosinophilic Gastroenteritis. Acta Pathologica Japonica 35:759–766.

Ozenc A.M., Ruacan S. and Aran O. (1988) Gastritis cystica polyposa. Archives of Surgery 123:372–373.

Palmer E.D. (1951) The morphologic consequences of acute exogenous (Staphylococcic) gastroenteritis on the gastric mucosa. Gastroenterology 19:462–475.

Palmer E.D. (1954) Gastritis:a revaluation. Medicine 33:199–290.

Palmer E.D. (1958) Note of silent sarcoidosis of the gastric mucosa. Journal of Laboratory and Clinical Medicine 52:231–234.

Papazian A., Braillon A., Dupas J.L., Sevenet F. and Capron J.P. (1986) Portal hypertensive gastric mucosa: an endoscopic study. Gut 27:1199–1203.

Parks T.G., Bussey H.J.R. and Lockhart-Mummery H.E. (1970) Familial polyposis coli associated with extra colonic abnormalities. Gut 11:323–329.

Parl F.F., Lev R., Thomas E. and Pitchumoni C.S. (1979) Histologic and morphometric study of chronic gastritis in alcoholic patients. Human Pathology 10:45–56.

Pastore G., Schiraldi G., Fera G., Sforza E., and Schiraldi O. (1976) A bioptic study of gastrointestinal mucosa in cholera patients during an epidemic in Southern Italy. Americal Journal of Digestive Diseases 21:613–617.

Pearse A.G.E., Couling I., Weavers B., and Friesen S. (1970) The endocrine polypeptide cells of the human stomach, duodenum and jejunum. Gut 11:649–658.

Peart A.G., Sivak M.V., Rankin G.B., Kish L.S. and Steck W.D. (1984) Spontaneous improvement of Cronkhite-Canada syndrome in a postpartum female. Digestive Diseases and Sciences 29:470–474.

Pemberton R.E. and Strand L.J. (1979) A review of upper- gastrointestinal effects of the newer nonsteroidal anti-inflammatory agents. Digestive Diseases and Sciences 24:53–64.

Petras R.E., Hart W.R. and Bukowski R.M. (1985) Gastric epithelial atypia associated with hepatic arterial infusion chemotherapy. Cancer 56:745–750.

Pickford I.R., Craven J.L., Hall R., Thomas G. and Stone W.D. (1984) Endoscopic examination of the gastric remnant 31–39 years after subtotal gastrectomy for peptic ulcer. Gut 25:393–397.

Pieterse A.S., Rowland R. and Labrooy J.T. (1985) Gastric xanthomas. Pathology 17:455–457.

Pinkerton H. and Iverson L. (1952) Histoplasmosis: Three fatal cases with disseminated sarcoid-like lesions. Archives of Internal Medicine 90:456–467.

Pointner R., Schwab G., Konigsrainer A., Bodner E. and Schmid K.W. (1988) Early cancer of the gastric remnant. Gut 29:298–301.

Ponsot P., Theodore C., Julien P.-E., Bard A., Molas G., Leymarios J. and Paolaggi J.-A. (1983) Angiodysplasies gastriques et maladie de Rendu-Osler. Gastroenterologie Clinique et Biologique 7:321–322.

Pounder R.E., Hunt R.H., Stekelman M., Miton-Thompson G.J., and Misiewicz J.J. (1976) Healing of gastric ulcer during treatment with cimetidine. Lancet i:337–339.

Price A.B. (1988) Histological aspects of campylobacter pylori colonisation and infection of gastric and duodenal mucosa. Scandinavian Journal of Gastroenterology 23(suppl. 142):21–24.

Pulimood B.M., Knudsen A., and Coghill N.F. (1976) Gastric mucosa after partial gastrectomy. Gut 17:463–470.

Queiroz D.M.M., Barbosa A.J.A., Mendes E.N., Rocha G.A., Cisalpino E.O., Lima G.F. and Oliveira C.A. (1988) Distribution of campylobacter pylori and gastritis in the stomach of patients with and without duodenal ulcer. American Journal of Gastroenterology 83:1368–1370.

Quintero E., Pique J.M., Bombi J.A., Bordas J.M., Sentis J., Elena M., Bosch J. and Rodes J. (1987) Gastric mucosal vascular ectasias causing bleeding in cirrhosis. Gastroenterology 93:1054–1061.

Rainsford K.D. and Willis C. (1982) Relationship of gastric mucosal damage induced in pigs by antiinflammatory drugs to their effects on prostaglandin production. Digestive Diseases and Sciences 27:624–638.

Ramesar K.C.R.B., Sanders D.S.A. and Hopwood D. (1987) Limited value of type III intestinal metaplasia in predicting risk of gastric carcinoma. Journal of Clinical Pathology 40:1287–1290.

Ramsey E.J., Carey K.V., Peterson W.L., Jackson J.J., Murphy F.K., Read N.W., Taylor K.B., Trier J.S. and Fordtran J.S. (1979) Epidemic gastritis with hypochlorhydria. Gastroenterology 76:1449–1457.

Rauws E.A.J., Langenberg W., Houthoff H.J., Zanen H.C. and Tytgat G.N.J. (1988) Campylobacter pyloris-associated chronic active antral gastritis. Gastroenterology 94:33–40.

Rees W.D.W. (1987) Mucus-bicarbonate barrier - shield or sieve. Gut 28:1553–1556.

Rees W.D.W. and Turnberg L.A. (1982) Mechanisms of gastric mucosal protection: a role for the 'mucus-bicarbonate' barrier. Clinical Science 62:343–348.

Reisman T.N., Leverett F.L., Hudson J.R., and Kalser M.H. (1975) Syphilitic gastropathy. American Journal of Digestive Diseases 20:588–593.

Richter R.M. (1975) Massive gastric haemorrhage from submucosal arterial malformation. American Journal of Gastroenterology 64:324–326.

Ritchie W.P. (1984) Alkaline reflux gastritis: a critical reappraisal. Gut 25:975–987.

Ritchie W.P. (1986) Alkaline reflux gastritis. Late results on a controlled trial of diagnosis and treatment. Annals of Surgery 203:537–544.

Ritchie W. Jr., and Delaney J. (1968) Gastric ulcer: an experimental model. Surgical Forum 19:312–313.

Roesch W. (1978) Erosions of the upper gastrointestinal tract. Clinics in Gastroenterology, Vol. 7:623–634.

Roesch W., Demling L., and Elster K. (1975) Is chronic gastritis a reversible process? Follow-up study of gastritis by step-wise biopsy. Acta Hepato-Gastroenterologia 22:252–255.

Roesch W. and Warnatz H. (1974) Immunfluoreszenzmikroskopische Untersuchungen bei Magenerosionen. In Fortschritte in der gastroenterologischen Endoskopie (Ed.) H. Lindner pp 194–251. Baden-Baden: Witzstrock.

Roth S.H. and Bennett R.E. (1987) Nonsteroidal anti-inflammatory drug gastropathy. Recognition and response. Archives of Internal Medicine 147:2093–2100.

Rubin W. (1969) Proliferation of endocrine-like (enterochromaffin) cells in atrophic gastric mucosa. Gastroenterology 57:641–648.

Rubin M., Tuthill R.J., Rosato E.F., and Cohen S. (1980) Cronkhite-Canada syndrome: report of an unusual case. Gastroenterology 79:737–741.

Rubio C.A. (1989) Paneth cell adenoma of the stomach. American Journal of Surgical Pathology 13:325–328.

Rubio C.A. and Kato Y. (1986) Ciliated metaplasia in the gastric mucosa. Studies on Japanese patients. Japanese Journal of Cancer Research (Gann) 77:282–286.

Rubio C.A. and Kato Y. (1987) Classification of vacuolated cells in the gastric mucosa. Journal of Surgical Oncology 34:128–132.

Rubio C.A. and Kato Y. (1988) Six types of intraepithelial vacuoles in the human gastric mucosa. Pathology, Research and Practice 183:321–325.

Rubio C.A., Kato Y., Sugano H. and Kitagawa T. (1987) Intestinal metaplasia of the stomach in Swedish and Japanese patients without ulcers or carcinoma. Japanese Journal of Cancer Research (Gann) 78:467–472.

Rubio C.A. and Serck-Hanssen A. (1986) Ciliated metaplasia in the gastric mucosa. II. In a European patient with gastric carcinoma. Pathology, Research and Practice 181:382–384.

Rubio C.A. and Slezak P. (1988) Foveolar cell vacuolization in operated stomachs. American Journal of Surgical Pathology 12:773–776.

Rumans M.C. and Lieberman D.A. (1987) Eosinophilic gastroenteritis presenting with biliary and duodenal obstruction. American Journal of Gastroenterology 82:775–778.

Russell D. McR., Bhathal P.S. and St. John D.J.B. (1983) Complete remission in Cronkhite-Canada syndrome. Gastroenterology 85:180–185.

Saffos R.O., and Rhatigan R.M. (1977) Benign (nonpolypoid) mucosal changes adjacent to carcinomas of the colon. A light microscopic study of 20 cases. Human Pathology 8:441–449.

Sakita T., Oguro Y., Takasu S., Fukutomi H., Miwa T., and Yoshimori M. (1971) Observations on the healing of ulcerations in early gastric cancer. Gastroenterology 60:835–844.

Saraga E-P., Gardiol D. and Costa J. (1987) Gastric dysplasia. A histological follow-up study. American Journal of Surgical Pathology 11:788–796.

Saraga P., Hurlimann J., and Ozzello L. (1981) Lymphomas and pseudolymphomas of the alimentary tract. An immunohistochemical study with clinicopathologic correlations. Human Pathology 12:713–723.

Sarles H.E., Schenkein J.P., Hecht R.M., Sanowski R.A. and Miller P. (1984) Dieulafoy's Ulcer: a rare cause of massive gastric hemorrhage in an 11-year-old girl: case report and literature review. American Journal of Gastroenterology 79:930–932.

Sasano N., Nakamuru K., Arai M., and Akazaki K. (1969) Ultrastructural cell patterns in human gastric carcinoma compared with non-neoplastic gastric mucosa - histogenetic analysis of carcinoma by mucin histochemistry. Journal of the National Cancer Institute 43:783–802.

Saukkonen M., Sipponen P., Varis K. and Siurala M. (1980) Morphological and dynamic behaviour of the gastric mucosa after partial gastrectomy with special reference to the gastroenterostomy area. Hepato-Gastroenterology 27:48–56.

Schade R.O.K. (1974) The borderline between benign and malignant lesions in the stomach. In: Early gastric cancer. E. Grundmann, H. Gruntze and S. Witte, Eds. Springer-Verlag, Berlin. pp 45–53.

Schafer L.W., Larson D.E., Melton III L.J., Higgins J.A. and Zinsmeister A.R. (1985) Risk of development of gastric carcinoma in patients with pernicious anemia: a population-based study in Rochester, Minnesota. Mayo Clinic Proceedings 60:444–448.

Scharschmidt B.F. (1977) The natural history of hypertrophic gastropathy (Menetrier's disease) Report of a case with 16 year follow-up and review of 120 cases from the literature. The American Journal of Medicine 63:644–652.

Schindler R. (1947) Gastritis. London, Heinemann.

Schmidt-Wilcke H.A., Haake U., and Riecken E.O. (1974) Investigations on the relationship between maximal acid output and parietal cells in gastric mucosal biopsies with special reference to duodenal ulcer. Acta Hepato-Gastroenterologica 21:297–302.

Schrumpf E., Serck-Hanssen A., Stadaas J., Aune S., Myren J., and Osnes M. (1977) Mucosal changes in the gastric stump 20–25 years after partial gastrectomy. Lancet 2:467–469.

Scott B.B., and Jenkins D. (1982) Gastro-oesophageal candidiasis. Gut 23:137–139.

Searcy R.M. and Malagelada J-R. (1984) Menetrier's disease and idiopathic hypertrophic gastropathy. Annals of Internal Medicine 100:565–570.

Seifert E., Butke H., Gail K., Elster K. and Cote S. (1979) Diagnosis of early gastric cancer. American Journal of Gastroenterology 71:563–567.

Seo I.S., Binkley W.B., Warner T.F.C.S., and Warfel K.A. (1982) A combined morphologic and immunologic approach to the diagnosis of gastrointestinal lymphomas. I. Malignant lymphoma of the stomach (A clinicopathologic study of 22 cases) Cancer 49:493–501.

Seppala K., Lehtola J., and Siurala M. (1976) The possible precancerous significance of abnormal cells in gastric cytology specimens: a follow-up study of 545 patients. Scandinavian Journal of Gastroenterology 11:513–515.

Sethi P., Banerjee A.K., Jones D.M., Eldridge J. and Hollanders D. (1987) Gastritis and gastric campylobacter-like organisms in patients without peptic ulcer. Postgraduate Medical Journal 63:543–545.

Shah A.M. and Joglekar M. (1987) Eosinophilic colitis as a complication of the hypereosinophilic syndrome. Postgraduate Medical Journal 63:485–487.

Sherman M.P., and Cox K.L. (1982) Neonatal eosinophilic colitis. The Journal of Pediatrics 100:587–589.

Shimer G.R. and Helwig E.B. (1984) Inflammatory fibroid polyps of the intestine. American Journal of Clinical Pathology 81:708–714.

Shiner M., and Doniach I. (1957) A study of x-ray negative dyspepsia with reference to histologic changes in the gastric mucosa. Gastroenterology 32:313–324.

Shousha S., Keen C. and Parkins R.A. (1989) Gastric metaplasia and campylobacter pylori infection of duodenum in patients with chronic renal failure. Journal of Clinical Pathology 42:348–351.

Shuster L.D., Cox G., Bhatia P. and Miner P.B. (1989) Gastric mucosal nodules due to cytomegalovirus infection. Digestive Diseases and Sciences 34:103–107.

Silen W. (1985) Pathogenetic factors in erosive gastritis. American Journal of Medicine 79(suppl. 2C):45–48.

Silen W. (1987) The clinical problem of stress ulcers. Clinical and Investigative Medicine 10:270–274.

Silva S. and Filipe M.I. (1986) Intestinal metaplasia and its variants in the gastric mucosa of Portuguese subjects: a comparative analysis of biopsy and gastrectomy material. Human Pathology 17:988–995.

Sirak H.D. (1954) Boeck's sarcoid of the stomach simulating linitis plastica: report of a case and comparison with twelve recorded cases. Archives of Surgery 69:769–776.

Siurala M., and Salmi H.J. (1971) Long-term follow-up of subjects with superficial gastritis or a normal gastric mucosa. Scandinavian Journal of Gastroenterology 6:459–463.

Siurala M., and Seppala K. (1960) Atrophic gastritis as a possible precursor of gastric carcinoma and pernicious anaemia. Results of follow-up examinations. Acta Medica Scandinavica 166:455–474.

Siurala M., Sipponen P. and Kekki M. (1985) Chronic gastritis: dynamic and clinical aspects. Scandinavian Journal of Gastroenterology 20(suppl. 109):69–76.

Sjoblom S-M., Sipponen P., Karronen S-L. and Jarvinen H.J. (1989) Mucosal argyrophil endocrine cells in pernicious anaemia and upper gastrointestinal carcinoid tumours. Journal of Clinical Pathology 42:371–377.

Skillman J.J., and Silen W. (1972) Stress ulcers. Lancet 2:1303–1306.

Skinner J.M., Heenan P.J., and Whitehead R. (1975) Atrophic gastritis in gastrectomy specimens. British Journal of Surgery 62:23–25.

Smith J.M.B. (1969) Mycoses of the alimentary tract. Gut 10:1035–1040.

Snover D.C., Weisdorf S.A., Vercellotti G.M., Rank B., Hutton S. and McGlave P. (1985) A histopathologic study of gastric and small intestinal graft-versus-host disease following allogeneic bone marrow transplantation. Human Pathology 16:387–392.

Snyder J.D., Rosenblum N., Wershil B., Goldman H. and Winter H.S. (1987) Pyloric stenosis and eosinophilic gastroenteritis in infants. Journal of Pediatric Gastroenterology and Nutrition 6:543–547.

Spiller R.C., Lovell D. and Silk D.B.A. (1988) Adult acquired cytomegalovirus infection with gastric and duodenal ulceration. Gut 29:1109–1111.

Spinelli P., Lo Gullo C. and Pizzetti P. (1980) Endoscopic diagnosis of gastric lymphomas. Endoscopy 12:211–214.

Stalsberg H., and Taksdal S. (1971) Stomach cancer following gastric surgery for benign conditions. Lancet ii:1175–1177.

Stamm B. and Saremaslani P. (1989) Coincidence of fundic glandular hyperplasia and carcinoma of the stomach. Cancer 63:354–359.

Steele R.J.C., Mok S.D., Crofts T.J. and Li A.K.C. (1987) Two cases of eosinophilic enteritis presenting as large bowel perforation and small bowel haemorrhage. Australian and New Zealand Journal of Surgery 57:335–336.

Stemmermann G.N. (1967) Comparative study of histochemical patterns in non-neoplastic and neoplastic gastric epithelium. A study of Japanese in Hawaii. Journal of the National Cancer Institute 39:375–382.

Stemmermann G.N. and Hayashi T. (1979) Hyperplastic polyps of the gastric mucosa adjacent to gastroenterostomy stomas. American Journal of Clinical Pathology 71:341–345.

Stillman A.E., Sieber O., Manthei U., and Pinnas J. (1981) Transient protein-losing enteropathy and enlarged gastric rugae in childhood. American Journal of Diseases of Children 135:29–33.

Strayer D.S., Phillips G.B., Barker K.H., Winokur T., and DeSchryver-Kecskemeti K. (1981) Gastric cyomegalovirus infection in bone marrow transplant patients. Cancer 48:1478–1483.

Strickland R.G., Bhathal P.S., Korman M.G., and Hansky J. (1971) Serum gastrin and the antral mucosa in atrophic gastritis. British Medical Journal iv:451–453.

Strickland R.G., Fisher J.M., Lewin K., and Taylor K.B. (1973) The response to prednisolone in atrophic gastritis: a possible effect on non-intrinsic factor-mediated vitamin B_{12} absorption. Gut 14:13–19.

Strickland R.G., and Mackay I.R. (1973) A reappraisal of the nature and significance of chronic atrophic gastritis. Americal Journal of Digestive Diseases 18:426–440.

Stringel G., Mercer S., Sharpe D., Shipman R. and Jimenez C. (1984) Eosinophilic Gastroenteritis. Canadian Journal of Surgery 27:182–183.

Subei I., Attar B., Schmitt G. and Levendoglu H. (1987) Primary gastric tuberculosis: a case report and literature review. American Journal of Gastroenterology 82:769–772.

Suen K.C., and Burton J.D. (1979) The spectrum of eosinophilic infiltration of the gastrointestinal tract and its relationship to other disorders of angiitis and granulomatosis. Human Pathology 10:31–43.

Sugihara K., Muto T., Kamiya J., Konishi F., Sawada T., and Morioka Y. (1982) Gardner's syndrome associated with periampullary carcinoma, duodenal and gastric adenomatosis. Report of a case. Diseases of the Colon and Rectum 25:766–771.

Sutton D.R., Baird I.M., Stewart J.S., and Coghill N.F. (1970) 'Free' iron loss in atrophic gastritis, post-gastrectomy states, and adult coeliac disease. Lancet ii:387–389.

Suzuki S., Suzuki H., Endo M., Takemoto T., Kondo T., and Nakayama K. (1973) Endoscopic dyeing method for diagnosis of early cancer and intestinal metaplasia of the stomach. Endoscopy 5:124–129.

Takaki K. (1986) Lymphoid follicles appearing in gastric mucosa, especially in reactive lymphoid hyperplasia and malignant lymphoma. Acta Pathologica Japonica 36:1627–1641.

Talley N.J., Cameron A.J., Shorter R.G., Zinsmeister A.R. and Phillips S.F. (1988) Campylobacter pylori and Barrett's esophagus. Mayo Clinic Proceedings *63*:1176–1180.

Talley N.J. and Phillips S.F. (1988) Non-ulcer dyspepsia: potential causes and pathophysiology. Annals of Internal Medicine *108*:865–879.

Tarpila S., Telkka A., and Siurala M. (1969) Ultrastructure of various metaplasias of the stomach. Acta Pathologica et Microbiologica Scandinavica 77:187–195.

Tatsuta M., and Okuda S. (1975) Location, healing, and recurrence of gastric ulcers in relation to fundal gastritis. Gastroenterology *69*:897–902.

Tatsuta M., Okuda S., Tamura H., and Taniguchi H. (1982) Endoscopic diagnosis of early gastric cancer by the endoscopic Congo red-methylene blue test. Cancer *50*:2956–2960.

Tedesco F.J.,Huckaby C.B.,Hamby-Allen M. and Ewing G.C. (1981) Eosinophilic ileocolitis. Expanding spectrum of eosinophilic gastroenteritis. Digestive Diseases and Sciences 26: 943–948.

Terruzzi, V., Minoli G., Butti G.C., and Rossini A. (1980) Gastric lipid islands in the gastric stump and in non-operated stomach. Endoscopy *12*:58–62.

Terruzzi, V. and Minoli G. (1984) Gastric candidiasis revisited. Gastrointestinal Endoscopy *30*:268–269.

Tokunaga O., Watanabe T. and Morimatsu M. (1987) Pseudolymphoma of the stomach. Cancer *59*:1320–1327.

Tomenius J. (1950) Instrument for gastrobiopsies. Gastroenterology *15*:498–504.

Tominaga K. (1975) Distribution of parietal cells in the antral mucosa of human stomachs. Gastroenterology *69*:1201–1207.

Torikata C., Mukai M. and Kawakita H. (1989) Ultrastructure of metaplastic ciliated cells in human stomach. Virchows Archiv (A) *414*:113–119.

Torikata C., Mukai M., Kawakita H. and Kageyama K. (1986) Ciliated cells in human metaplastic gastric mucosa. A proposal of a new term: Ciliated metaplasia. Proceedings of the XIth International Congress on Electron Microscopy, Kyoto 1986; pp 3549–3550.

Tosi P., Luzi P., Baak J.P.A., Miracco C., Vindigni C., Lio R. and Barbini P. (1987) Gastric dysplasia: a stereological and morphometrical assessment. Journal of Pathology *152*:83–94.

Totten J., Burns H.J.G. and Kay A.W. (1983) Time of onset of carcinoma of the stomach following surgical treatment of duodenal ulcer. Surgery, Gynecology and Obstetrics *157*:431–433.

Trounce J.Q. and Tanner M.S. (1985) Eosinophilic gastroenteritis. Archives of Disease in Childhood *60*:1186–1188.

Tung K.T. and Millar A.B. (1987) Gastric angiodysplasia - a missed cause of gastrointestinal bleeding. Postgraduate Medical Journal *63*:865–866.

Tytgat G.N., Grijm R., Dekker W., and Den Hartog N.A. (1976) Fatal eosinophilic enteritis. Gastroenterology *71*:479–483.

Uibo R. and Salupere V. (1981) Immunology of chronic gastritis. Annals of Clinical Research *13*:130–132.

Utsunomiya J., Maki T., Iwama T., Matsunaga Y., Ichikawa T., Shimomura T., Hamaguchi E., and Aoki N. (1974) Gastric lesion of familial polyposis coli. Cancer *34*:745–754.

Van den Heule B., Van Kerkem C., and Heimann R. (1979) Benign and malignant lymphoid lesions of the stomach. A histological reappraisal in the light of the Kiel classification for non-Hodgkin's lymphomas. Histopathology *3*:309–320.

Van Olmen G., Larmuseau M.F., Geboes K., Rutgeerts P., Penninckx F. and Vantrappen G. (1984) Primary gastric actinomycosis: a case report and review of the literature. American Journal of Gastroenterology *79*:512–516.

Van Rensburg L.C.J., Keet A.C. and Adams G. (1986) Eosinophilic granuloma of the stomach. Journal of Surgical Oncology *31*:143–147.

Varis K. (1981) Family behaviour of chronic gastritis. Annals of Clinical Research *13*:123–129.

Veldhuyzen van Zanten S.J.O., Bartelsman J.F.W.M., Schipper M.E.I. and Tytgat G.N.J. (1986) Recurrent massive haematemesis from Dieulafoy vascular malformations - a review of 101 cases. Gut *27*:213–222.

Vendelboe M. and Jespersen J. (1981) Hypertrophic protein- losing gastritis (Menetrier's disease) treated with Cimetidine. Acta Medica Scandinavica *209*:125–127.

Voigt J.-J., Cassigneul J., Pradere M., Vinel J.-P., Carballido M. and Guiu M. (1983) Cystic glandular fundic polyps of the stomach. Gastroenterologie Clinique et Biologique 7:171–176.

Walker F.B. (1981) Spontaneous remission in hypertrophic gastropathy (Menetrier's disease). Southern Medical Journal *74*:1273–1276.

Watanabe A., Nagashima H., and Motoi M. (1979) Familial juvenile polyposis of the stomach. Gastroenterology *77*:148–151.

Watanabe H., Enjoji M., Yao T., and Ohsato K. (1978) Gastric lesions in familial adenomatosis coli. Human Pathology 9:269–283.

Watt I.A., McLean N.R., Girdwood R.W.A., Kissen L.H., and Fyfe A.H.B. (1979) Eosinophilic gastroenteritis associated with a larval anisakine nematode. The Lancet 2:893–894.

Watt P.C.H., Sloan J.M. and Kennedy T.L. (1983) Changes in gastric mucosa after vagotomy and gastrojejunostomy for duodenal ulcer. British Medical Journal *287*:1407–1410.

Watt P.C.H., Sloan J.M., Spencer A. and Kennedy T.L. (1983) Histology of the postoperative stomach before and after diversion of bile. British Medical Journal *287*:1410–1412.

Wattel W. and Geuze J.J. (1978) The cells of the rat gastric groove and cardia. An ultrastructural and carbohydrate histochemical study, with special reference to the fibrillovesicular cells. Cell and Tissue Research *186*:375–391.

White R.M., Levine M.S., Enterline H.T. and Laufer I. (1985) Early gastric cancer. Recent experience. Radiology *155*:25–27.

Whitehead R., Truelove S.C., and Gear M.W. (1972) The histological diagnosis of chronic gastritis in fibreoptic gastroscope biopsy specimens. Journal of Clinical Pathology *25*:1–11.

Widgren S. and Pizzolato G.P. (1987) Inflammatory fibroid polyp of the gastrointestinal tract: possible origin in myofibroblasts? Ann Pathol *7*:184–192.

Wilander E. (1981) Achylia and the development of gastric carcinoids. Virchows Archiv, A. Pathological Anatomy and Histology, *394*:151–160.

Williams A.W. (1956) The effects of alcohol on gastric mucosa. British Medical Journal i:256–259.

Winkler H., Zelikovski A., Gutman H., Mor C. and Reiss R. (1986) Inflammatory fibroid polyp of the jejunum causing intussusception. American Journal of Gastroenterology *81*:598–601.

Witzel L., Halter F., Gretillat P.A., Scheurer U., and Keller M. (1976) Evaluation of specific value of endoscopic biopsies and brush cytology for malignancies of the oesophagus and stomach. Gut *17*:375–377.

Wolf J.A., Jr. and Spjut H.J. (1981) Focal lymphoid hyperplasia of the stomach preceding gastric lymphoma: Case report and review of the literature. Cancer *48*:2518–2523.

Wood I.J., Doig R.K., Motteram R., and Hughes A. (1949) Gastric biopsy: report on 55 biopsies using new flexible gastric biopsy tubes. Lancet i:18–21.

Wright R., Whitehead R., Wangel A.G., Salem S.N., and Schiller K.F.R. (1966) Autoantibodies and microscopic appearances of gastric mucosa. Lancet i:618–621.

Wyatt J.I. and Dixon M.F. (1988) Chronic gastritis - a pathogenetic approach. Journal of Pathology *154*:113–124.

Yamada M., Hatakeyama S. and Tsukagoshi H. (1985) Gastrointestinal amyloid deposition in AL (primary or myeloma-associated) and AA (secondary) amyloidosis. Human Pathology *16*:1206–1211.

Yeomans N.D. (1976) Electron microscopic study of the the repair of aspirin-induced gastric erosions. American Journal of Digestive Diseases *21*:533–541.

Zollinger R.M., and Moore F.T. (1968) Zollinger-Ellison syndrome comes of age. Journal of the American Medical Association *204*:361–365.

Zora J.A., O'Connell E.J., Sachs M.I. and Hoffman A.D. (1984) Eosinophilic gastroenteritis: a case report and review of the literature. Annals of Allergy *53*:45–47.

Small-Intestinal Biopsy

Chapter

NORMAL APPEARANCES IN SMALL-INTESTINAL BIOPSY SPECIMENS

10

Classical normal appearances will be seen only in sections cut at right angles to the plane of the muscularis mucosa. Oblique sections produce a variable combination of two principal features, i.e., cross-sectioning of glands and cross-sectioning of villi. With technical care it is usually possible to produce correctly oriented sections, but an experienced pathologist generally can assess sections that are suboptimal in this respect. A possible source of misinterpretation is the presence of artefacts. A potential cause is the trauma of the suction used at biopsy. The superficial epithelium at the tips of villi may be lifted to produce subepithelial blebs (Fig. 10–1), or on occasion the villous tips are denuded. In volunteers, ethanol ingested in quantities equivalent to moderate drinking seems to increase the incidence of this type of artefact (Millan et al 1980). In rats it has been shown that alcohol temporarily destabilises the intercellular junction of the epithelium (Draper et al 1983), which could play a part in the production of this type of lesion. There is also some evidence that chronic ethanol ingestion in the rat reduces enterocyte turnover rates (Mazzanti and Jenkins 1987).

This type of damage may also result from rough handling once the specimen has been obtained. Attempts to unroll a specimen in order to lay it flat or to remove adherent surface mucin so that a better dissecting microscope view can be obtained should be made with great care or avoided altogether. Sometimes tissue fluid or even blood appears under the surface epithelium and must be differentiated from oedema fluid or meaningful haemorrhage. These artefacts are not significantly hard for trained histopathologists to interpret because they are common to biopsy material from other areas. Clearly, however, every effort should be made to avoid them so that all possible information can be extracted from these tissue samples.

The mucosa of the small intestine has the same structure everywhere along its length: finger-like villi project from a simple gland layer that lies on a muscularis mucosa (Fig. 10–2). The villi are covered by a columnar epithelium that has a distinct PAS-positive brush border. Sometimes in good preparations occasional minute PAS-positive granules, which probably are lysosomes, can be seen in the apical cytoplasm, and the faintly positive membranes of the Golgi apparatus just above the nucleus are visible. The villi are between three and five times as long as the simple crypt-like glands that take origin at their bases to dip into the lamina

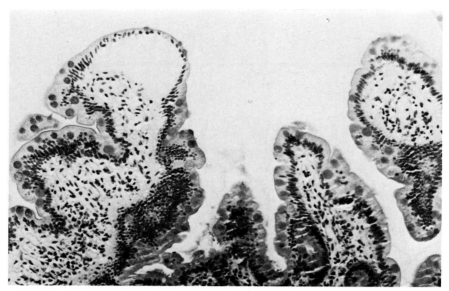

Figure 10–1. Small-intestinal suction biopsy showing a traumatic subepithelial bleb (H & E × 250).

propria. The villous epithelium is continuous with that lining the crypts, but the latter has a less distinct brush border; whereas mitotic figures are frequently seen in the crypt epithelium, they are never present in that covering the villi. The crypt epithelium is the regenerative zone, and by a process of migration is responsible for new cell types both in the crypts and on the villous processes, the effete absorptive cells being lost from the villous tips.

At the base of the glands Paneth cells are present. It is surprising that the functional significance of such a distinctive cell type should still be in doubt. Although goblet cells and Paneth cells probably have a common precursor cell and cells intermediate between the two occur (Montero and Erlandsen 1978), the

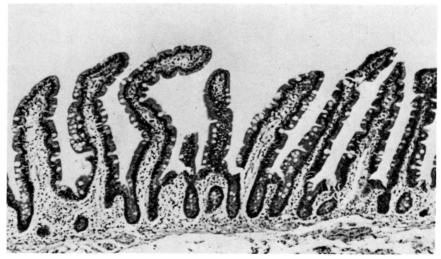

Figure 10–2. Jejunal biopsy finger-like villi and a gland layer supported by a muscularis mucosa. Goblet cells, which appear as empty circular spaces, are obvious (H & E × 100).

Paneth cells usually do not migrate upwards onto the villi. Sandow and Whitehead (1979) and Trier and Madara (1981) have extensively reviewed the subject of Paneth cell structure and function, and more recently Mathan, Hughes and Whitehead (1987) have studied their morphogenesis by immunocytochemical electron microscopy. In humans it appears that the cells arise away from the base of the crypts and migrate towards the base as they mature. Also scattered about in the crypts there are occasional enterochromaffin cells. These are only part of a much larger system of endocrine cells, the function of which has attracted a substantial body of research. Reviews by Rayford, Miller and Thompson (1976a, b), Buffa et al (1978), Buchan and Polak (1980), Solcia et al (1980), Bloom and Polak (1981), Sjolund et al (1983) and Falkmer and Wilander (1989) are testament to the seemingly ever-increasing complexity of the gut-associated endocrine system and the wide variety of tumours that they can give rise to (Chejfec et al 1988).

PAS-positive goblet cells are seen both in the glands and among the surface absorptive cells, but they progressively decrease in number towards the villous tip where they are scattered among the epithelial cells. Often appearing within a vacuole, which is probably a shrinkage artefact, an occasional intraepithelial lymphocyte is usually observed; these were designated "theliolymphocyte" by Fichtelius, Yunis and Good (1968). This is often shortened to "theliocyte," and, in fact, these cells lie in the spaces between the epithelial cells after having passed through the basement membrane. They occur in a ratio of one for every six epithelial cells and form an integral part of the gut-associated lymphoid tissue along with the immunocytes of the lamina propria, the solitary lymphoid follicles, Peyer's patches and mesenteric lymph nodes. There is recent evidence that in humans the number of lymphoid follicles in the large intestine has been grossly underestimated, Langman and Rowland (1986) having shown that there is an average density of 18.4 per cm^2 in the caecum, 15 per cm^2 in the colon and as many as 25.4 per cm^2 in the rectum. This is far in excess of the 5 per cm^2 accepted as normal since the early study by Dukes and Bussey (1926).

Intraepithelial lymphocytes, or theliocytes, have been studied in detail in animals in an effort to establish their functional significance. In humans, Bartnick et al (1980), using a technique for producing isolates of lymphoid cells from intestinal mucosa, claimed that the theliocyte population contained approximately equal proportions of T, B and null cells. Selby, Janossy and Jewell (1981), however, using frozen sections and lymphocyte antibodies in an immunofluorescent study, found that over 95 per cent of theliocytes were T cells and this is in keeping with the results of earlier observations in experimental animals. Human intestinal intraepithelial lymphocytes, their origin and putative functions in relation to overall lymphoepithelial interactions and the mucosal immune system, have been recently reviewed (Dobbins 1986, Brandtzaeg et al 1988).

Both in crypts and on villi a further cell type can by recognised by electron microscopy. It is called the caveolated cell or tuft cell (Nabeyama and Leblond, 1974). It is pear-shaped with a narrow apex bearing long microvilli whose filamentous cores extend deep into the apical cytoplasm. Among the filaments are the caveoli, which appear as irregular vesicles occasionally in continuity with the apical plasma membrane. The function of these cells, which are also found in the stomach and colon, is unknown. In the ileum a further cell type occurs. This is known as the M cell and is also only recognisable at electron microscopy. They are always located overlying Peyer's patches and other lymphoid follicles (Owen and Nemanic, 1978). The surface of the cell has low anastomosing convolutions, and its cytoplasm is attenuated around several lymphocytes although it maintains intercellular adhesion with neighbouring enterocytes. Owen (1977) has demonstrated the M cell's capacity for macromolecular protein uptake, using horseradish peroxidase as a tracer. This would allow the cells to function in the mechanisms for antigen absorption and processing.

In ordinary preparations the core of the villi and the rest of the lamina propria, i.e., that area between the crypts bounded externally by the muscularis mucosa, appear as delicate loose connective tissue infiltrated by a small number of lymphocytes and occasional plasma cells, eosinophils, mast cells and histiocytes. The importance of using the correct fixative, i.e., Carnoy's, in any study of mast cells in jejunal biopsies has been stressed by Strobel, Busuttil and Ferguson (1983). The villi also contain a central blind-ending lacteal which is usually collapsed and often only recognisable as a parallel double row of flat endothelial nuclei in the villous core. A capillary plexus lying beneath the basement membrane is more obvious, and the smooth muscle cells that extend upwards from the muscularis mucosa can be recognised as they surround the central lacteal passing to the very tip of the villous process.

This basic structure is subject to some minor variations in different parts of the small intestine. The normal proximal duodenum has shorter and broader villi that frequently show an increased number of stunted and leaf-shaped or branching forms when compared with the jejunum (Fig. 10–3). Brunner's glands, tradition-ally thought to be localised to the duodenum, have a marked variation of distribution often extending to the jejunum, particularly in children (Landboe-Christensen 1944). They occur on both sides of and between the elements of the muscularis mucosa, which thus appears split. Rarely, small groups of glands occur within the superficial epithelium (Fig. 10–4). Hyperplasia or undue prominence of Brunner's glands is often associated with obvious villous stunting. In the region of the duodenal papilla the villi are also short and stubby and biopsies not infrequently include mucus glands and smooth muscle related to the termination of the duct system and mixing valve (see later). As the ileum is approached (Fig. 10–5), the ratio of goblet cells to absorptive cells increases, and the villi tend to become slightly broader and shorter than in the jejunum. Lymphoid aggregates

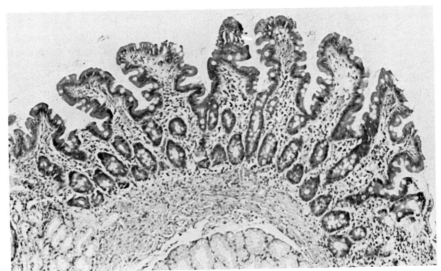

Figure 10–3. Duodenal biopsy. The villi are shorter and broader and some forms are irregular. Note the Brunner's glands (H & E × 75).

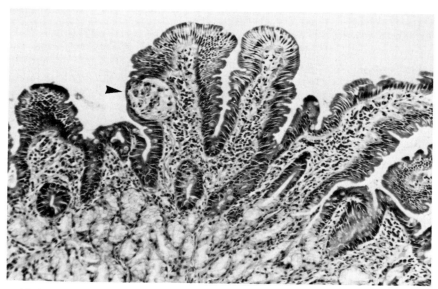

Figure 10–4. Duodenal biopsy. A small group of Brunner's glands (arrowhead) is present within the epithelium (H & E × 225).

that split the muscularis mucosae, being thus partially mucosal and partially submucosal, often show a central germinal centre. They increase in number in the more distal parts of the small intestine as solitary follicles, but also in confluence in the ileum as Peyer's patches. Villi overlying lymphoid areas are often stubby or absent.

Villous architecture is determined in part by the depth of tissue obtained at biopsy. When the muscularis mucosa is present the villi are taller, slimmer, and lie more closely together than when this tethering layer is absent. Without a muscularis mucosa and a measure of mucosal stretching due to too much handling

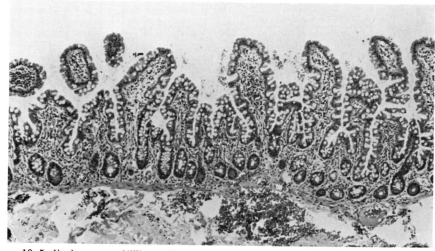

Figure 10–5. Ileal mucosa. Villi are slightly shorter and broader than in the jejunum and goblet cells are more obvious (H & E × 140).

of the biopsy, the appearance produced, with broad-based, widely separated villi, can be distinctly abnormal (Fig. 10–6). It is also claimed that villi are shorter on the crests of mucosal folds than in the less exposed valleys between, and that increased trauma in the former site is the cause (Creamer 1967). This presupposes that such mucosal folds as may be seen at necropsy or in surgical specimens are fixed structures and reflect the living state. If the contours of the mucosal surface are constantly changing during life, as seems likely, this observation is probably an artefact possibly related to a terminal contracture of the bowel musculature.

Detailed morphological studies of small bowel mucosal morphology in an entirely normal group, as opposed to a control group of patients not overtly suffering from gastrointestinal disease, are rare, but it would appear that villous morphology varies in different ethnic groups. When compared with biopsies from English or North Americans the villi of the Thai (Sprinz et al 1962), Africans (Banwell, Hutt and Tunnicliffe 1964), Indians (Baker et al 1962), South Vietnamese (Colwell et al 1968), Haitians (Brunser, Eidelman and Klipstein 1970) and Arabs (Shiner and Pearson 1981) are shorter, thicker and have an increased proportion of leaf-shaped forms and short ridges, and the lamina propria contains proportionately more inflammatory cells. In the past there has been controversy as to whether these are true racial variations or simply reflections of altered intraluminal environment due to different standards of health and hygiene.

There is no doubt that alterations of gut flora in experimental animals have a profound effect on villous shape (Creamer 1967, King and Toskes 1979). In humans, also, a range of jejunal mucosal abnormalities has been described in patients with parasitic infestations (Magalhaes, Trevisan and Pereira 1975), and the mild variations in small intestinal morphology that occur with age in infants under five years have been ascribed to the changing bacterial colonisation of the intestinal lumen (Walker-Smith 1972). The tendency for shorter villi and longer crypts to occur in children has been verified in a morphologic study by Penna et al (1981), but there is no evidence based upon a morphometric study that the jejunal mucosal morphology varies in adult life; in particular no reduction of surface area occurs with increasing age (Corazza et al 1986).

In a group of 21 volunteers from a normal population of British Caucasians,

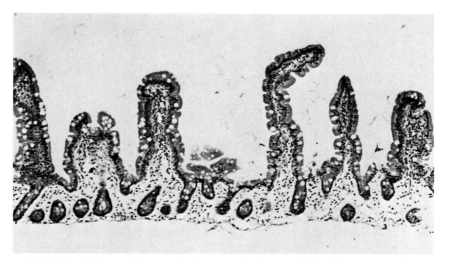

Figure 10–6. Jejunal biopsy. The muscularis mucosa is absent, and the villi are more widely separated and appear somewhat shortened (H & E × 75).

jejunal biopsies showed finger-like villi as the sole or predominant villous feature (Pena, Truelove and Whitehead 1973). Fourteen of these showed one or more leaf-shaped villi, which can be defined as two or three finger-like villi fused side by side. Three specimens showed, in addition to fingers and leaves, a small number of short ridges. Ridges dimensionally resemble two or three leaves fused side by side. In the study of normal jejunal biopsies made by Burhol and Myren (1968), the histological appearances were divided into groups I and II. Group I had predominantly long and slender villi without an increased cellular infiltration of the lamina propria, and group II had predominantly branched and fused villi also without increased cellular infiltration. These authors did not appear to have examined serial sections. In the normal cases examined by Pena et al it was not possible to make a similar subdivision. Each biopsy specimen was examined in step serial sections, and appearances corresponding to groups I and II of Burhol and Myren were seen in different levels. In all specimens most villi were tall, slender and finger-like, but all also showed a proportion of bifid (Fig. 10–7) and occasional trifid forms and a few fused or tongue-shaped villi with occasional mucosal bridges (Fig. 10–8). It is obvious that in any investigation involving morphology, anatomical and pathological variation will be minimised by standardising the biopsy site. It is the usual practice to secure jejunal biopsies, for example, from a point just distal to the ligament of Treitz under radiological control. Duodenal biopsies are being taken under direct vision using fibreoptic instruments and, again, can be accurately located in relation to the anatomical landmarks. Comparisons should be made only with normal as opposed to "control"

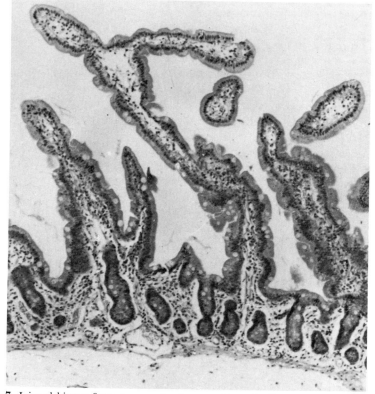

Figure 10–7. Jejunal biopsy from a normal volunteer. Central villous process showing bifurcation (H & E × 128).

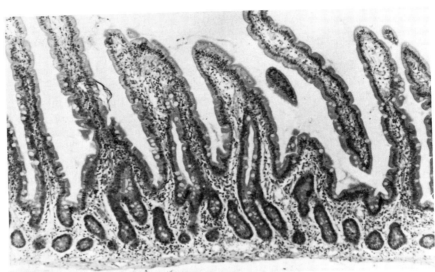

Figure 10–8. Jejunal biopsy from a normal volunteer. Fusion of villous tips and formation of mucosal bridges (H & E × 150).

groups, and these should be selected from the same ethnic and environmental background as the test cases.

Even when all these criteria are fulfilled and there is meticulous care in the technical handling of the material, minor villous abnormalities still cause difficulties in interpretation. It is for this reason that several attempts were made to replace subjective by more objective quantitative observations (Rubin et al 1960, Thurlbeck, Benson and Dudley 1960, Madanagopolan, Shiner and Rowe 1965, Stewart et al 1967, and many others). However, they were only partially successful because of the lack of proper normal control series and poor selection of abnormal material; e.g., Thurlbeck, Benson and Dudley (1960) compared tissue obtained at necropsy, at laparotomy, and by tube biopsy, all at unspecified sites. In addition, the methods used are open to criticism; e.g., the use of intersecting lines to assess villous surface area (Madanagopolan, Shiner and Rowe 1965) without relating this to volume results in gross underestimates if there is any degree of villous separation due to an absent muscularis mucosa or a stretching artefact. Measurements of villous height and depth of glands are only approximate, since in the majority of biopsies most of the villi are bent over to some degree. The point at which a villus ends and a crypt begins cannot be standardised, and when there is a severe degree of total villous atrophy it becomes impossible. Accurate measurement of epithelial cell height in the normal is feasible, but on the surface epithelium of a flat mucosa of severe gluten-sensitive enteropathy it becomes virtually impossible because of the palisading of cells and the irregularity of basement membranes and brush border.

It is doubtful if these rather insensitive quantitative methods give any better idea of minor morphological changes than a simple visual assessment by an experienced interpreter, and some workers (Rubin and Dobbins 1965) have thus resorted to "the method of blind review." The complexity of a mathematically accurate method of quantitation of the small intestine is described by Hennig (1956). He shows that in order to obtain absolutely accurate information the mucosa must be sectioned and quantitated in three different planes, and the method includes a very large number of observations, so that its value for easy application to human jejunal biopsy tissue is limited.

Dunnill and Whitehead (1972), however, devised a simple method of quantitating the surface area to volume ratio in jejunal biopsies. This method, based on the combined point-counting principle (Chaukley 1943) for volume determination with the linear intercept principles (Short 1950) for surface area measurement, is free from the errors of earlier simple methods and, although it does not give absolute information, it allows a relative comparison of one biopsy with another. A template of 15 lines of equal length (Fig. 10–9) is drawn according to the specifications of Weibel (1963) in such a way that each line joins the vertices of a regular hexagonal point network. Weibel states that this avoids bias and allows for an even distribution. The jejunal biopsy specimen to be examined is projected on a Leitz projector fitted with a xenon lamp onto the template (Fig. 10–10). The magnification is kept constant and the section is cast at random onto the template. On each occasion the number of times, c, the lines cut the mucosal surface and the number of end points of the lines, h, that fall on the tissue above, but not including the muscularis mucosae, are counted. The greater the number of fields cast on the template the more accurate will be the final result, but in practice it was found to be sufficient if the value for h was about 200. If the biopsy is large it is possible to superimpose the grid on more than one field in a single section; if this is so it is usually sufficient to make counts on two or three sections. For small biopsy specimens a larger number of serial sections must be examined, perhaps six or eight. If l is the length of the line used, the ratio $c{:}lh$ will give an index of the complexity of the villous pattern and of the surface to volume ratio. It is important that the length of the line used always be stated in order that the ratio $c{:}lh$ can be compared between different centres of investigation. Provided the magnification is also kept constant during the examination, the mean number of hits per field on the mucosa, h, for each specimen will be proportional to the mucosal volume. It is thus possible to compare not only the state of the villi, but also the mucosal volumes between specimens.

In this way an assessment of the efficacy of treatment in sequential follow-up studies (Pena et al 1972, Pena, Truelove and Whitehead 1972) can be carried out, and an easy comparison made of information arising in different centres of study. In more recent times there have been several attempts to apply morphological techniques for the measurement of other histological components. The sources

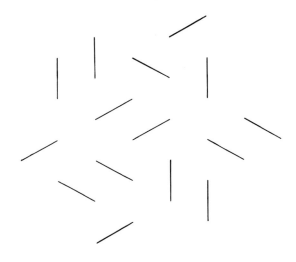

Figure 10–9. The template of 15 lines of equal length drawn according to Weibel (1963).

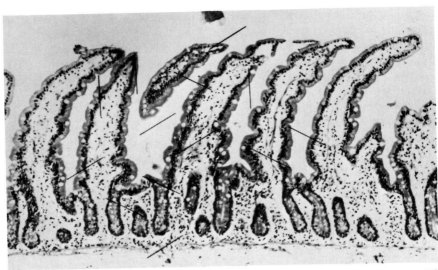

Figure 10–10. The template in Figure 10–9 superimposed on a normal jejunal biopsy. The end points of the lines lying on the mucosa are counted as hits. The places where the lines cut the mucosal surface are counted as cuts (H & E × 150).

of inaccuracy and the rationale for acceptable methods are discussed by Skinner and Whitehead (1976). With increasingly sophisticated computerised image analysis systems such as described by Slavin et al (1980), minor abnormalities in jejunal morphology can now be routinely objectively measured. Even with the method of Dunnill and Whitehead (1972) significant subjective interobserver variation has been convincingly demonstrated (Corazza et al 1982). There have also been applications of morphometric techniques in the determination of numbers of lamina propria cell types (Dhesi et al 1984). The principles involved in mathematically accurate determination are outlined by Skinner and Whitehead (1976). A comprehensive publication by Aherne and Dunnill (1982) is recommended to those wishing to employ a variety of morphometric methods in the study of small intestinal diseases, but it is of interest that Corazza et al (1985), who compared computer-aided microscopy, linear measurement and stereology in the assessment of jejunal biopsy specimens, concluded that the latter technique, employing a simple eye-piece graticule, was the method of choice.

SMALL-INTESTINAL BIOPSY IN DISEASE

11

The preservation of the morphological form of the small-intestinal mucosa is the result of a balance between the rate of cell loss from the villous surface and the rate of cell production in the crypts. There is some experimental evidence that this is controlled by a feed-back mechanism operating from the surface to the crypts (Galjaard, van der Meer-Fieggen and Giesen 1972, Rijke et al 1976). Williamson (1982) summarised the situation concerning the many factors involved in the maintenance of small-intestinal morphology. Acceleration of cell renewal, for example, is triggered by a variety of stimuli. Notably, intestinal resection and hyperphagia both result in an increase in the small-intestinal mucosal volume. Jejunal bypass causes overall mucosal hyperplasia and can even result in changes in the type of mucins produced (Olubuyide et al 1984). The importance of oral food intake in maintaining intestinal mucosal morphology has been demonstrated in humans (Biasco et al 1984). Alkaline phosphatase activity is increased locally and produces a rise in serum levels following intestinal resection (Delgado et al 1986). Not surprisingly hypophagia or deprival of the mucosa of contact with the luminal contents results in a decrease in its mass. The trophic effects are mediated in part by bile and pancreatic juice (Hauer-Jensen et al 1988), but there are numerous and complex neurovascular and humoral influences, the precise nature of which is yet to be determined.

The other aspects of small bowel morphology such as the lamina propria lymphoid tissue, the lacteal system and the Brunner's gland are also known to be dependent for their form and maintenance on equally complex controlling systems. The range of abnormalities that results when these controls are disturbed by disease processes is very wide. Nevertheless, because of functional physiological differences and the pathology that ensues when they are compromised by disease, abnormalities in the small-intestinal mucosa are best considered on a regional basis.

BIOPSIES FROM THE DUODENAL BULB

Bulbitis

Biopsy specimens taken from the proximal duodenum, in that part known as the bulb, frequently show villous abnormalities, even allowing for the increased number of leaf-shaped forms and short ridges that are normal in this zone.

Inflammatory infiltration and other morphological abnormalities are also encountered fairly commonly. Abnormalities in the duodenal bulb may but do not necessarily reflect what the remainder of the upper small intestine is like. It was because of this that the practice of precisely located jejunal biopsy arose for the investigation of malabsorption states. However, this was before the era of fibreoptic endoscopes; with their increased use and the facility to biopsy the more distal parts of the duodenum, it became plain that there was often no necessity to biopsy the small intestine in the investigation of malabsorptive and other states at a site beyond the ligament of Treitz (see later).

Because the duodenal bulb is the usual site of duodenal ulcer disease, the inflammatory lesion that precedes this is known as bulbitis or ulcer-associated duodenitis. One of the difficulties in defining the criteria for diagnosing significant bulbitis is the quite wide variations seen in biopsies from this site. These consist of simple excess of plasma cells and lymphocytes in the lamina propria through a range comprising increasing inflammatory infiltrate and progressive villous deformity and atrophy (Figs. 11–1 to 11–6). The surface epithelium shows degenerative changes and loses its characteristic appearance, assuming a flatter simple type, with nuclear hyperchromasia, cytoplasmic basophilia and sometimes a syncytial appearance (Fig. 11–7). Frank metaplasia to a surface gastric epithelium is seen, as are all apparent stages in between (Fig. 11–8).

Sometimes a more acute inflammatory cell component is superimposed on the lymphocyte and plasma cell population, and the picture is one of acute disease superimposed on chronic disease. Surface erosions (Figs. 11–9, 11–10) produced when the loss of superficial epithelium exceeds the regenerative process of repair are seen in the most severe stage. From the pathologists' point of view there is every indication that the changes constitute a readily recognisable lesion. The precise significance of these changes, however, has been the subject of a variety of interpretations. One of the difficulties has been the failure to recognise that the theliocytes and the other white cells of the lamina propria, as part of the gut-

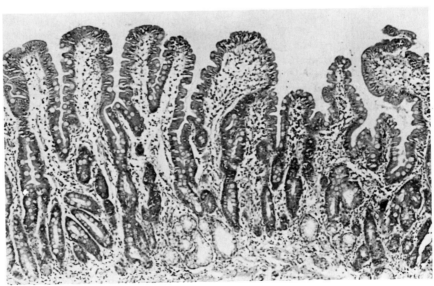

Figure 11–1. Duodenal biopsies (Figs. 11–1 to 11–6) showing progressive increase in inflammatory changes with distortion and effacement of villous processes. Brunner's glands on the luminal side of the muscularis mucosa become more obvious (H & E × 140).

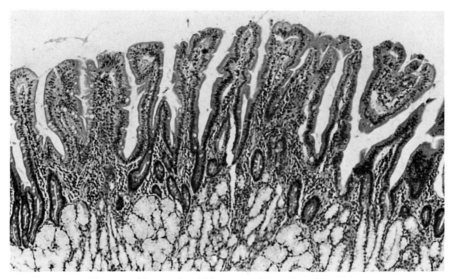

Figure 11–2. Duodenal biopsy specimen. See Figure 11–1.

associated lymphoid tissue, may react as part of the whole system when the stimulus to react occurs in a site distant from the duodenum. This may occur in viral, bacterial or parasitic infections or in other circumstances of antigenic stimulation such as protein intolerance or when the duodenum is involved in a specific disease process such as Crohn's disease.

The duodenum may also exhibit changes in cellularity of the lamina propria as the result of its involvement in a "field" change due to lesions in neighbouring organs, e.g., stomach, pancreas or bile ducts. Lev et al (1980) have shown, for example, that mononuclear cell counts in duodenal biopsies are elevated in the presence of chronic gastritis. When these considerations are made there can be little doubt that "duodenitis" or "non-specific duodenitis," as first described by Baudin (1837), exists as a specific entity. Konjetzny (1924) recognised duodenitis in the mucosa adjacent to duodenal ulcer, and MacCarty (1924) showed that

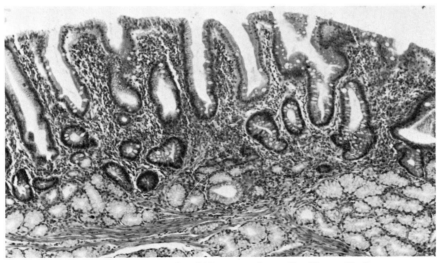

Figure 11–3. Duodenal biopsy specimen. See Figure 11–1.

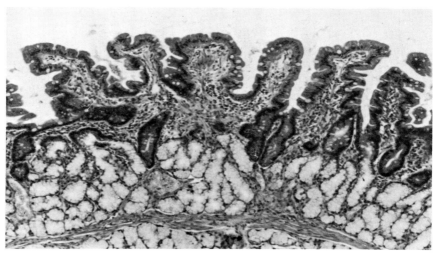

Figure 11–4. Duodenal biopsy specimen. See Figure 11–1.

identical appearances were sometimes seen in operation specimens from patients with typical duodenal ulcer history, but no ulcer. Thus it was that a relationship between this form of duodenitis, or bulbitis, and duodenal ulcer was proposed (Judd and Nagel 1927). With the advent of flexible tube biopsy procedures the evidence of a diathesis comprising hyperchlorhydria and proximal duodenitis proceeding to duodenal ulcer (Rhodes 1964, Beck et al 1965, Rhodes et al 1968, Gear and Dobbins 1969, Whitehead, Roca and Truelove 1972, Cotton et al 1973, Thomson et al 1977, Paoluzi et al 1982, Schmitz-Moormann et al 1984, Jenkins et al 1985, Scott et al 1985, Sircus 1985, Venables 1985) has been strengthened.

Other workers, however (Doniach and Shiner 1957, Aronson and Norfleet 1962, Gear and Dobbins 1969, Cheli, Aste and Ciancamerla 1973, Gregg and

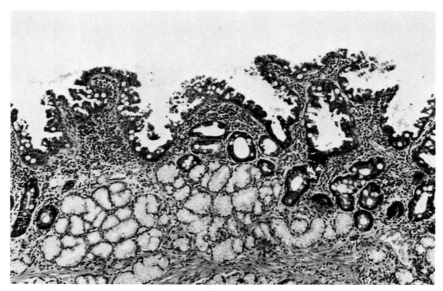

Figure 11–5. Duodenal biopsy specimen. See Figure 11–1.

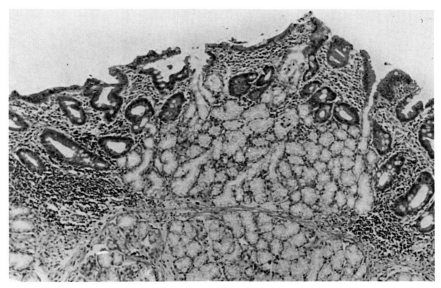

Figure 11–6. Duodenal biopsy specimen. See Figure 11–1.

Garabedian 1974, Gelzayd, Biederman and Gelfand 1975, Cheli 1985, Lawson 1987), regard duodenitis as a lesion, not closely related to duodenal ulcer, which may or may not have clinical manifestations. These discordant results are due to a variety of factors. In earlier studies cases were selected on the basis of radiological findings, and biopsies were blind and localised fluoroscopically. Since the use of fibreoptic instruments, cases have been selected on directly viewed mucosal appearances. Nevertheless, there has been no standardisation as to the endoscopic appearance of duodenitis, and different authors may be studying different groups

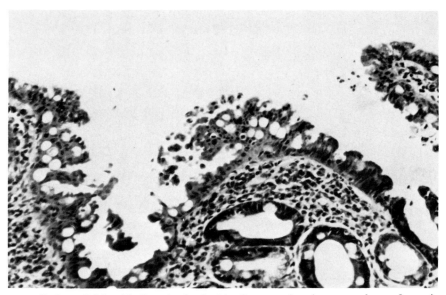

Figure 11–7. Superficial epithelium in duodenitis. Degenerative changes and transformation into syncytial masses (H & E × 300).

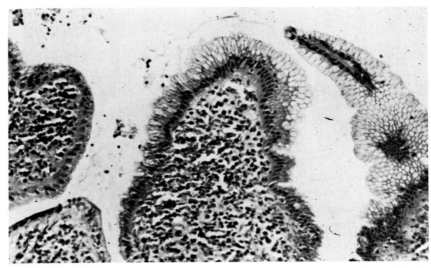

Figure 11–8. Superficial epithelium in duodenitis. Stages of progressive metaplasia visible from left to right. Process on right is covered by almost normal gastric superficial epithelium (H & E × 300).

of patients. It is becoming plain, however, that a reddened duodenal mucosa is not necessarily inflamed, but that the appearances are likely to be the result of vasomotor phenomena. Different authors have also used different histological criteria in defining duodenitis, and there is clearly a need to adopt a uniform classification. To this end and based upon more than 700 biopsies, a grading of histological features seen in duodenal biopsies was proposed by Whitehead et al (1975) and is now modified in the light of further experience (Table 11–1). Each main histological parameter of the mucosa is considered in turn.

(a) *Villous processes*: The villous processes of the duodenum, as already noted, are less regular and shorter than those in the jejunum and tend to be even more stubby or absent over lymphoid follicles or prominent mucosal Brunner's glands. There is, however, a progressive villous obliteration that is related to increasing inflammation of the mucosa, and in its severest form this leads to a flat mucosal surface.

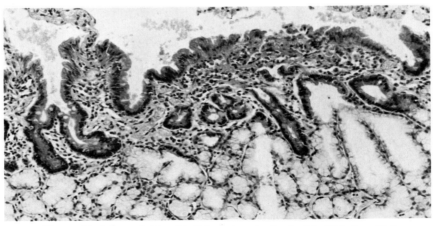

Figure 11–9. Superficial epithelial erosions in duodenitis (H & E × 210).

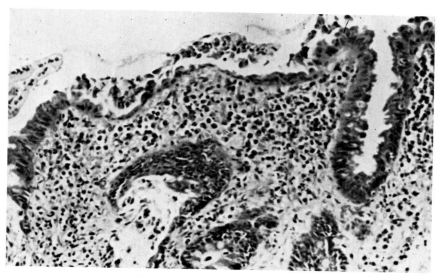

Figure 11–10. Same as Figure 11–9.

(b) *Superficial epithelium*: The superficial epithelium may appear flatter than normal and show nuclear hyperchromasia and increased basophilia of the diminished cytoplasm. The brush border becomes progressively less distinct, and the cells may come to appear stratified with nuclei at different levels. Sometimes bud-like syncytial masses are formed that project from the surface. The increased cellularity of the epithelium is associated with occasional mitotic figures and is added to by an increase in the number of intraepithelial lymphocytes and invading polymorphs. When polymorph invasion is marked, epithelial erosions also occur. These epithelial changes clearly reflect a change in mucosal dynamics and cell turnover. Mitotic activity in the crypts is increased and the tendency for immature cells to occupy the surface is apparent with a decrease in the goblet cell population. Another distinctive superficial epithelial feature is metaplastic transformation focally or more widespread into an epithelium of gastric surface mucin-secreting type. This change is most easily appreciated in the section stained by the PAS technique. It is commonest in the more severe degrees of inflammation (White-head, Roca and Truelove 1972), but with increasing experience it has been

Table 11–1. Histological Grading of Duodenitis (Bulbitis)

Grade of Change	Distinguishing Histological Features		General Histological Features
0	normal		
1	superficial epithelium and general morphology normal; increased cellularity of lamina propria	increasing cellularity of lamina propria and loss of the villous pattern	neutrophil polymorph infiltration + or −
2	abnormality of the surface epithelium		gastric superficial epithelial metaplasia + or −
3	erosion of the surface epithelium		

appreciated that focal areas may be present when inflammation is relatively slight or even absent.

(c) *Crypts*: The crypts are involved in the inflammatory degenerative and regenerative changes described above only in the most severe examples of duodenitis. The ducts of Brunner's glands may also be involved as they enter the base of the crypts, but as most of the glands are beneath muscularis mucosa, they themselves are usually spared. Sometimes, however, glands also occur internal to and among the fibres of the muscularis mucosa, so that they may also be involved.

(d) *Lamina propria*: The lamina propria shows a variable increase in inflammatory cells including lymphocytes, plasma cells and polymorphs. Neutrophil polymorphs occur in increased numbers, especially in the more severe grades of epithelial damage, and may be accompanied by vascular dilatation and oedema. Lymphoid aggregates occur normally in approximately 20 per cent of normal duodenal biopsies, but in duodenitis they are seen in increased numbers.

The least severe degree of recognisable change is designated grade 1. There are no significant alterations in general morphology, and the superficial epithelium is normal in height but may contain an excess of lymphocytes. The principal histological feature is an excessive cellularity of the lamina propria with or without lymphoid aggregates. It is obvious that there will be some difficulty in differentiating those biopsies with a minimal increase of cells from those which are normal, and with increasing experience it is becoming apparent that this type of abnormality may constitute the upper end of the normal range.

Grade 2 is the next grade of severity that can be recognised. In this, in addition to increased cellularity of the lamina propria, the critical feature is abnormalities of the superficial epithelium. Sometimes there is also deformity of the villous architecture with shortening of the processes, but it is the superficial epithelial changes that are used to grade the biopsy.

The most severe, or grade 3, change is characterised by the critical feature of erosion of the abnormal epithelium. This is invariably associated with complete effacement and loss of the villous processes and the heaviest degree of inflammatory cell infiltration.

When there is a polymorph component in the inflammatory infiltrate it may be associated with vascular dilatation and some oedema. The presence of polymorphs can be recorded as a separate feature because, although it is usually found in the severe group, this is not always so, and it might be of significance in terms of activity of the inflammatory process, as has been suggested to be the case in chronic gastritis (Whitehead 1973). It should be noted that the blood vessel changes that accompany acute inflammation, namely, dilation and congestion, are notoriously difficult to assess in histological preparations unless polymorph margination is seen. Dilation may well disappear during the fixation procedure and subsequent tissue processing with its attendant tissue shrinkage. As a consequence, there is poor correlation between histological inflammation and erythema seen at endoscopy (MacKinnon, Willing and Whitehead 1982). Reddening with erosion and petechiae, however, correlate well with severe histological duodenitis.

The presence of gastric surface epithelial metaplasia should also be recorded. It is important to realise that this is an entity distinct from gastric heterotopia, which occurs as slightly raised isolated islands of gastric mucosa composed of both superficial epithelium, crypts and specialised glands, usually containing parietal cells, but occasionally also chief cells (see Fig. 14–21). The capacity of this ectopic mucosa to secrete acid has been demonstrated at endoscopy by using Congo red after pentagastrin stimulation (Ikeda et al 1982), and it is perhaps not so rare as was once thought. Shousha, Spiller and Parkins (1983) found it in 10 per cent of duodenal biopsies from patients with dyspepsia. Another fact that requires emphasis is that the pyloro-duodenal junction is frequently not well demarcated. Biopsies from the transitional zone can easily be misinterpreted as duodenal mucosa showing gastric metaplasia and vice versa. This probably accounts in part for the very high incidence of "gastric metaplasia" reported in a normal population by Kreuning et al (1978). Indeed, if gastric surface epithelium is seen in the absence of significant duodenal inflammation, the biopsy site is probably from a broader than usual transitional zone between pylorus and duodenum. Gastric metaplasia is extensive only in biopsies that show a severe grade of duodenitis. Focal areas can also be seen in grade 2 and, rarely, grade 1 change, but hardly ever if the biopsy is entirely normal. It is rarely seen except in the first part of the duodenum. Johansen and Hansen (1973) and Patrick, Denham and Forrest (1974) have shown that there is a statistically significant correlation between prevalence of metaplasia and gastric acid ouput. Indeed, it can be induced in cats by stimulating hypersecretion of hydrochloric acid (Rhodes 1964). The metaplastic epithelium has the same histochemical profile as the identical epithelium in the stomach (Johansen 1974). It has been suggested that it is important as one of the pathophysiological mechanisms involved in the recurrence of duodenal ulcer (Hara et al 1988). This is of interest in view of the as yet unproven view that colonisation of the metaplastic epithelium by *Campylobacter pylori* is related to a mucosal defence weakness and the genesis of duodenal ulcer (Goodwin 1988).

This grading of duodenal change was shown to be accurate by Whitehead et al (1975) by comparing the results of subjective examination of duodenal biopsies with those obtained by two morphometric methods. One method estimated the surface to volume ratio of the mucosa, and the other the number of cells in the lamina propria. By the use of this or similar classifications it is becoming increasingly plain that changes of grade 2 or 3 are a significant cause of duodenal ulcer-like symptoms. Grade 1 change that corresponds to the "interstitial duoden-itis" of Cheli, Aste and Ciancamerla (1973) is likely to represent a variation of normal or a lesion associated with neighbouring pathology or be the result of a generalised stimulation of the gut-associated immune system. It has been reported to exist in normal volunteers (Roca, Truelove and Whitehead 1975). The consensus view of an international gathering of gastroenterologists was that severe duodenal change corresponding to grades 2 and 3 is indeed part of the peptic ulcer diathesis (Walan 1981); the consistent coexistence of grades 2 and 3 duodenitis in the duodenal bulb of duodenal ulcer patients supports this view (Paoluzi et al 1982, Hasan et al 1983).

Brunner's Gland Hyperplasia

Some patients with the clinical picture of non-ulcer dyspepsia and duodenal ulcer disease have radiological evidence of coarse duodenal folds, and in the past it was postulated that this may be due to Brunner's gland hyperplasia. There are obvious difficulties in assessing Brunner's gland mass in endoscopic biopsies, but in some studies it was claimed that Brunner's gland hyperplasia may well be associated with duodenitis (Maratka et al 1979). Even before this, in an autopsy study (Feyrter 1934), enlargement of Brunner's glands was classified as circum-scribed nodular hyperplasia, diffuse nodular hyperplasia, and adenomatous hy-perplasia. It is not clear why the first form was not regarded as an earlier stage of the third. Ten years later, Landboe-Christensen (1944) claimed that Brunner's gland hyperplasia was almost always associated with signs of inflammation, lymphoid hyperplasia or scarring of the duodenum. This suggested that there is an association between duodenitis, previous ulceration and Brunner's gland hyperplasia, and these findings are perhaps more significant when it is realised that cases with obvious ulcers or larger scars were excluded from the study. Cases showing hyperplasia of Brunner's glands that did not have evidence of inflammation or ulceration were also observed, and thus evidence for two varieties of Brunner's gland enlargement, i.e., focal and diffuse, strengthened. At the present time most workers recognise a diffuse form associated with duodenitis or duodenal ulcer and a localised form presenting as a tumour. The latter has been called a Brunneroma (Bastlein et al 1988) and is regarded as an adenoma (Major and Brandt 1976, Nakanishi et al 1984), whereas others argue that it is a hamartoma (Skellenger et al 1983, Rufenacht et al 1986).

The author has experience of one case of Brunner's gland enlargement gross enough to present as pyloric obstruction and a multiple duodenal polyposis on radiological examination. The extent of the lesion would almost certainly not have been revealed by endoscopic biopsy, and only became apparent when an open surgical biopsy was examined subsequently. This not only showed the Brunner's gland nature of the polypoidal lesions but also a diffuse duodenitis and superficial gastric epithelial metaplasia. Thus in some instances a diffuse nodular Brunner's hyperplasia associated with duodenitis may well give rise to more massive focal hyperplasia/adenoma; this would parallel the situation that occurs in other glandular tissues. Certainly the diffuse multinodular lesion would appear to be more common. Franzin et al (1985), for example, describe 206 cases in association with hyperacidity of which more than 80 per cent had coexistent duodenitis. These authors have stressed that a biopsy indication of Brunner's hyperplasia in these circumstances is for the glands to appear consistently extending up to the surface mucosa, which is frequently avillous and flattened (Fig. 11–11). There is some

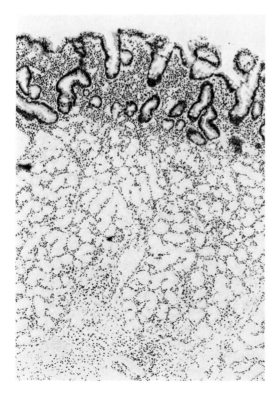

Figure 11–11. Duodenitis with a prominent extension of Brunner's glands well into the lamina propria above the muscularis, which is seen at the very bottom of the field (H & E × 75).

evidence that the nodular duodenitis that is frequently seen in patients with end stage renal disease (Zukerman et al 1983, Mangla, Pereira and Bhargava 1985) is often characterised by Brunner's gland hyperplasia (Paimela et al 1984). In Feyrter's autopsy study already referred to, 55 per cent of cases showing Brunner's hyperplasia had had uraemia. On a physiological note, a reactive hyperplasia of Brunner's glands driven by hyperchlorhydria would be explicable on the basis of its neutralising bicarbonate secretion and the production of urogastrone, an inhibitor of gastric secretion (Stolte, Schwabe and Prestle 1981).

Lymphoid Hyperplasia

Hyperplasia of the mucosal lymphoid elements of itself may be so marked as to cause irregularity of the duodenal mucosa, and this should be clearly evident in a duodenal biopsy specimen. This type of lymphoid hyperplasia is distinct from that associated with gamma globulin abnormalities (see Chapter 14), and it is almost always associated with the changes of duodenitis, so that at least sometimes it is probably similar to that which occurs in the stomach affected by chronic gastritis or the colon in chronic ulcerative colitis. Why it occurs in some cases and not in others that otherwise show the same morphological features is not known. Apart from Brunner's gland hyperplasia some of the nodular appearances seen in uraemic patients also seem to be due to lymphoid nodular hyperplasia as part of the coexistent duodenitis (Zukerman et al 1983). Some cases of duodenal lymphoid hyperplasia, however, are not associated with any significant inflammatory features of duodenitis, and one assumes that they represent reactive phenomena triggered by a different mechanism such as a viral infection.

BIOPSIES BEYOND THE BULB

The duodenum is being biopsied more and more frequently in circumstances other than when duodenitis or peptic ulcer is present. Most endoscopists can produce biopsies from well into the third part of the duodenum and beyond. Mucosal irregularities often sampled prove to be ectopic gastric body mucosa or isolated lymphoid nodules.

Most islands of ectopic gastric body mucosa are small and barely raised but some are frankly polypoidal (Tsadilas 1984, Tsubone et al 1984, Kundrotas et al 1985). It is claimed that sometimes such islands of gastric mucosa show hyperplastic change and give rise to polyps similar to the lesions that occur in the stomach (Rosch and Hoer 1983). Franzin, Novelli and Fratton (1983) also describe a hyperplastic polyp with characteristics similar to the common lesion of the colon, with villi and crypts lined by serrated hyperplastic epithelium. In this author's experience this type of hyperplastic polyp is not all that uncommon. They are composed of irregular villous or cystic formations covered by simple cuboidal epithelium that shows a variable degree of gastric superficial epithelial metaplasia and residual small bowel type epithelium usually with scanty goblet cells. Not infrequently some Brunner's glands are incorporated and half-way stages between Brunner's type gland cells, undifferentiated crypt cells, and gastric epithelial mucous cells can be seen. These lesions are almost certainly the result of a hyperplastic response to mucosal injury or an erosion, which is sometimes also revealed in the biopsy. The lamina propria in relation to these hyperplastic polyps is frequently inflamed (Figs. 11–12 to 11–17).

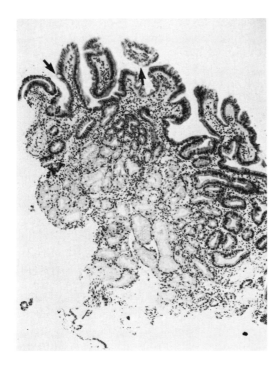

Figure 11–12. Hyperplastic duodenal polyp. Note the branched irregular mucosal projections covered by metaplastic epithelium with only scattered goblet cells (arrows) and the irregular configuration of the Brunner's glands (H & E × 75).

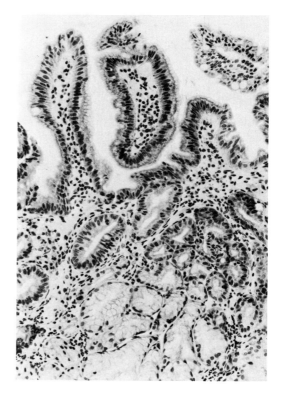

Figure 11–13. Showing the character of the gastric superficial epithelial metaplasia and the residual goblet cells (arrowed in Figure 11–12) (H & E × 300).

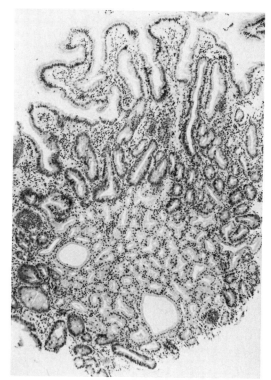

Figure 11–14. Hyperplastic duodenal polyp. The Brunner's gland component shows a focal cystic change (H & E × 75).

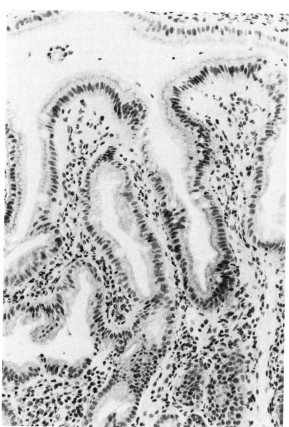

Figure 11–15. Detail of Figure 11–14. The epithelium varies between small intestinal type and gastric superficial epithelial type and there are interspersed goblet cells (H & E × 300).

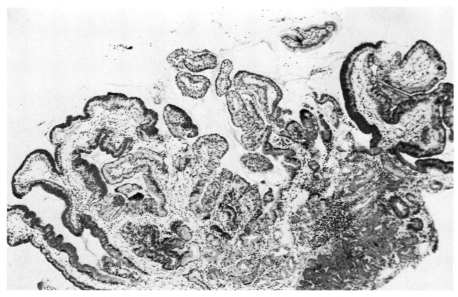

Figure 11–16. Hyperplastic duodenal polyp with only a minor Brunner's gland component. The configuration is quite bizarre and bears no resemblance to normal duodenum. The gastric metaplasia is widespread and easily seen in this PAS preparation (PAS × 75).

More rarely, small lymphangiomas (Salata et al 1984), haemangiomas or vascular hamartomas are recognised. Duodenal varices (Nakayama et al 1983, Gushurst and Lesesne 1984, Sukigara et al 1987) and Dieulafoy's aneurysm (McClave et al 1988) are all described, but only rarely are vascular lesions biopsied (Fig. 11–18).

With the increasing use of endoscopy in the investigation of jaundice an increasing range of lesions of the papilla are being seen. Small villous adenomas

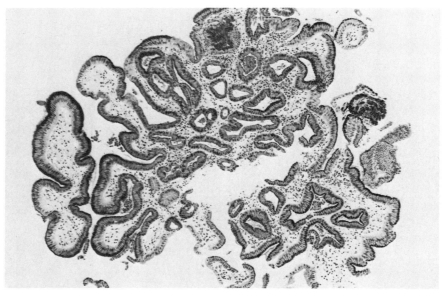

Figure 11–17. This hyperplastic polyp could easily be misinterpreted as tubulovillous adenoma, but the epithelium although metaplastic (shown to best effect at left) is not in any way dysplastic (PAS × 75).

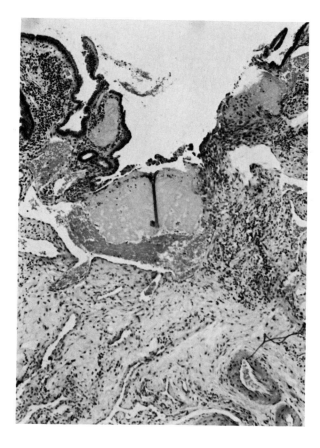

Figure 11–18. A small submucosal vascular abnormality of predominantly cavernous type. The superficial duodenal mucosa has eroded and caused significant haemorrhage (H & E × 150).

or early carcinomas that are most commonly located at this site cause few problems in interpretation (Figs. 11–19 to 11–21) because they are essentially similar to their much more common colonic counterparts (Blackman and Nash 1985). When the adenomatous change involves the duct system in the region of the ampulla

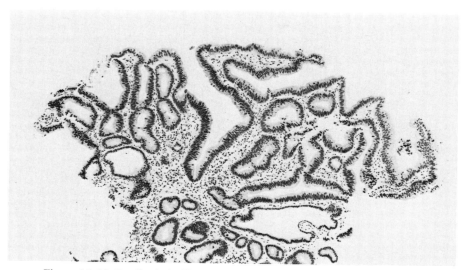

Figure 11–19. Small tubulovillous adenoma of duodenal papilla (H & E × 75).

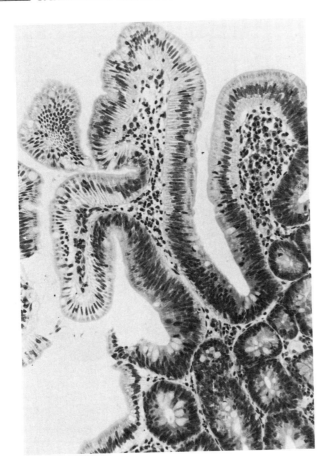

Figure 11–20. Detail of Figure 11–19. The dysplastic nature of the epithelium is clearly different from that of metaplastic polyps (compare with Figures 11–13 and 11–15).

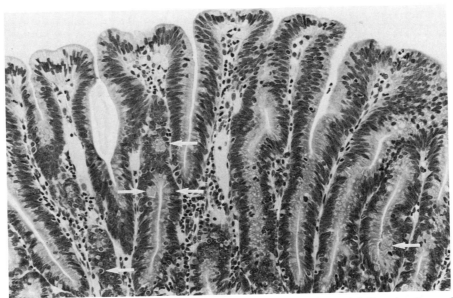

Figure 11–21. Mainly villous adenoma of duodenum. This lesion has a rich Paneth cell population visible even in an H & E preparation (arrows) (H & E × 400).

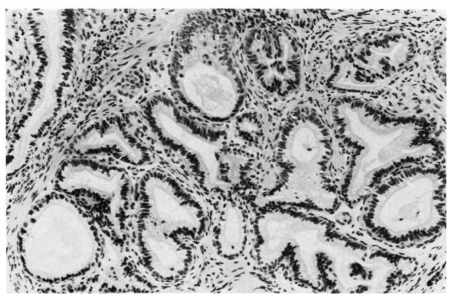

Figure 11–22. Adenomatous change involving the duct system and epithelial elements of the mixing valve at the ampulla. The atypical glandular formations are surrounded by normal smooth muscle elements (H & E × 350).

the abnormal glands have a very close relationship to the muscle bundles in that region, and this can make differentiation between adenoma and adenocarcinoma quite difficult. One has eventually to rely on cytological features and the absence of convincing desmoplasia in order to resolve this (Fig. 11–22). In a similar fashion, regenerative and reactive changes that occur in the epithelium of the collecting tubules of the ampullary valve can cause similar problems in interpretation, and the same guidelines are advocated in reaching a diagnosis (Figs. 11–23, 11–24). Sometimes, however, a small biopsy of a larger villous lesion may not reveal the malignant nature in another area of the same lesion (Ryan, Schapiro and Warshaw 1986). There is now common acceptance that carcinomas of the ampullary region arise, as in the colon, through an adenoma-carcinoma sequence (Talbot et al 1988) and some examples are notably rich in Paneth cells (London et al 1988). Adenomas seem to be especially common in patients with familial adenomatous polyposis and have been shown to be regularly accompanied by conspicuous argyrophil and argentaffin endocrine cell populations (Morgensen, Bulow and Hage 1989a,b). There is some evidence that the risk of malignancy in these duodenal adenomas may be as high as that for their colonic counterpart. Mixed glandular and carcinoid differentiation is also occasionally seen in tumours arising in nonpolyposis patients (Jones, Griffith and West 1989).

The interpretation of other biopsies from the ampullary region in the investigation of jaundice can be more difficult. This is due in part to the complexity of the glands, muscle bundles and epithelial folds that make up the mixing valve at this end of the duct system. Stones passed cause inflammatory fibrosis and regenerative epithelial changes that can exhibit quite marked atypia suspicious of invasive malignancy, especially because of their close relationship to the muscle bundles in the vicinity. Malformations or hamartomas of this area are also occasionally seen (Fig. 11–25), and no doubt, with increasing numbers of biopsies of the area, dysplasia and the earlier lesions of malignancy will be identified.

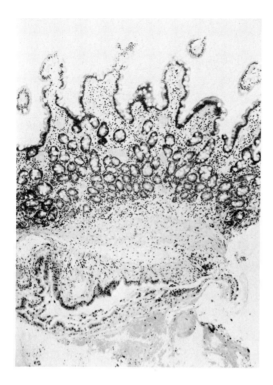

Figure 11–23. Duodenal biopsy in the region of the papilla, following an episode of biliary colic. Note the duct-like structures beneath the muscularis (H & E × 125).

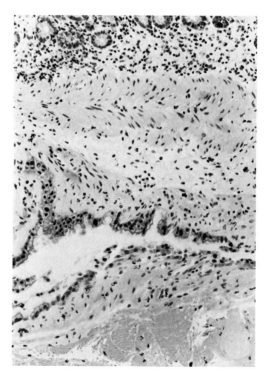

Figure 11–24. Detail of Figure 11–23. The duct lining cells exhibit reactive atypia. Note the normal appearance of the surrounding smooth muscle (H & E × 400).

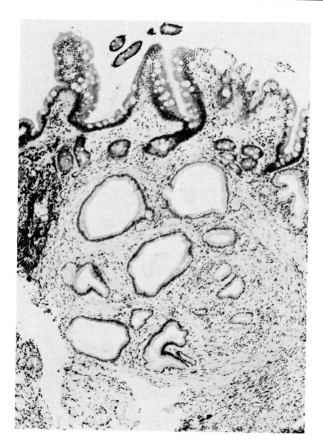

Figure 11–25. Biopsy excision of a small duodenal nodule that is clearly a small hamartoma of pancreatic or bile ducts (H & E × 1250).

Biopsies beyond the papilla are now used in most centres in the evaluation of malabsorption and other lesions for which jejunal mucosa was once preferred. This is discussed in further detail in the section on the lesion of villous atrophy. Duodenal biopsy may also reveal diagnostic information in Crohn's disease, amyloidosis, giardiasis, storage diseases, etc. As far as Crohn's disease is concerned, it is argued that the biopsies are too small for there to be a significant diagnostic yield. In the absence of granulomas a spectrum of rather non-specific findings may occur (Schuffler and Chaffee 1979), but these can be of importance in diagnosis when seen in the context of other clinical, radiological, endoscopic and biopsy findings. As in the stomach, ulceration and gross epithelial atypia in duodenal biopsies, easily misinterpreted as malignant, are being increasingly described in patients receiving hepatic arterial infusion chemotherapy (Schuger et al 1988).

DUODENAL BIOPSY IN THE INVESTIGATION OF MALABSORPTION

The last five years have seen general acceptance of utilisation of the distal duodenal biopsy in the investigation of malabsorption (Mee et al 1985, Achkar et al 1986, Sanfilippo et al 1986). The changes that occur in the bulb in peptic ulcer disease in association with hyperchlorhydria do not affect the distal duodenum except in rare instances of hypergastrinaemia such as in the Zollinger-Ellison syndrome. Furthermore, it is possible to suspect coeliac disease by the endoscopic appearances alone. Brocchi et al (1988) describe markedly decreased or absent duodenal Kerckring's folds and recommend biopsy when this sign is present, even if the patient has minimal transient or seemingly unrelated symptomatology.

Detailed morphological observations coupled with an increasing knowledge of cell turnover have resulted in the recognition of two types of villous atrophy: one associated with hyperplasia of the crypts and one with hypoplasia of the crypts.

Crypt Hyperplastic Villous Atrophy

In this type the villi are atrophic or absent, but the overall thickness of the mucosa is normal or only slightly decreased and the crypts are clearly hyperplastic and elongated. The absorptive epithelium shows a variable degree of damage manifested by an apparent increase in intraepithelial lymphocytes between the surface cells, which themselves may show hyperchromasia and palisading of nuclei, which often appear pyknotic. There is blurring of the cytoplasmic boundaries so that in PAS preparations the normally distinct brush borders of the enterocytes appear frayed and ragged. Since the paper by Ferguson and Murray (1971) it is frequently stated that the number of theliocytes per unit of epithelium in the coeliac mucosa is increased. Indeed it has been credited with diagnostic importance (Holmes et al 1974, Lancaster-Smith et al 1976a). This increase, however, is a function of the method of their quantitation in that the coeliac lesion is character-ised by a marked decrease in epithelial surface per unit length of muscularis mucosa. If expressed as number per unit length of mucosa, a normal number will appear, therefore, as an increase. If quantitated per unit of muscularis mucosa that is not altered by the disease process, it has been convincingly shown that the number of intraepithelial lymphocytes is either normal (Guix, Skinner and Whitehead 1979) or slightly decreased (Marsh 1980, Corazza, Frazzoni and Gasbarrini 1984). Thus the role of intraepithelial lymphocytes is still very much a matter of dispute (Marsh 1985), perhaps due to claims based upon faulty methodology.

It is claimed that blast transformation and an increased mitotic rate occur in the intraepithelial lymphocytes in coeliac disease (Marsh 1982, Marsh and Haeney 1983) and that this can be used to differentiate a coeliac mucosa from a flat mucosa due to other causes. The method of determining the mitotic index in each specimen necessitates observation of lymphocyte metaphase figures in a population of 3,000 epithelial cells located between the mouths of crypts. The claim is made that an index in excess of 0.2 per cent is indicative of gluten-sensitive enteropathy and excludes other causes of a flat mucosa, namely, immu-nodeficiency, lymphoma or Crohn's disease. It has not been this author's experi-ence that this diagnostic criterion is useful in practice. Firstly, lymphocyte mitoses are clearly uncommon, and, secondly, their certain recognition is difficult in ordinary paraffin sections because the heaped and palisaded superficial epithelium contains a large proportion of degenerating cells with pyknotic nuclei. Thirdly, at light microscopy level it is unclear how it can be ascertained that in a flat mucosa a mitotic figure is located in a lymphocyte as opposed to an epithelial cell at the top of a crypt which itself is not in the plane of sectioning.

Marsh also advocates the counting of only metaphase-anaphase figures and this is a further restriction of the method. Resin-embedded semi-thin sections lend themselves better to this type of examination, but the pursuit of this diagnostic phenomenon is probably not justified on the evidence. Ferguson and Ziegler

(1986) have claimed that the presence of intraepithelial lymphocyte mitoses is a non-specific phenomenon that can be seen when the jejunal mucosa is otherwise normal. Nevertheless, the role of the intraepithelial lymphocytes is the subject of continued debate. It is claimed that subjects who do not have coeliac disease but who have raised alpha-gliadin antibody titres also have raised intraepithelial lymphocyte counts (O'Farrelly et al 1987). The lymphocytes are known to be T cells of both suppressor/cytotoxic and helper/inducer type and supposedly increase significantly in number in treated coeliacs subjected to a gluten challenge (Freedman et al 1987). However, since they tend to return to normal levels on gluten exclusion, it has been suggested that these changes are the result of a stimulation of the mucosal immune mechanisms and do not imply a primary pathogenetic role (Kelly et al 1987). Moreover, epithelial lymphocyte numbers in rectal mucosa have been said to increase in treated coeliacs following instillation of gluten enemas (Austin and Dobbins 1988). There is also some evidence that an adenovirus protein may have a role in the pathogenesis of coeliac disease and that there is immunological cross reactivity between antigens shared by the virus and alpha-gliadins (Kagnoff et al 1987).

The lamina propria contains an increased number of lymphocytes, plasma cells, some eosinophils, histiocytes and mast cells. Whether mucosal mast cells in coeliac disease are increased or decreased has been the subject of dispute, even in quantitative studies (Strobel, Busuttil and Ferguson 1983, Kosnai et al 1984). Marsh and Hinde (1985), however, have concluded that there is an increase in mast cells, eosinophils and basophils that is gluten dependent and probably the result of a cell-mediated effector mechanism concerned in the pathogenesis of the disease. A similar claim has been made not only for eosinophils and basophils, but also for neutrophils (Hallgren et al 1989). The crypts contain an increased number of cells in mitosis. Paneth cells and enterochromaffin cells, which normally are also found in the crypts, may appear numerically increased. This was substantiated by Polak et al (1973), Challacombe and Robertson (1977) and Sjolund et al (1979). Wheeler and Challacombe (1984) showed that the enterochromaffin cells were producing mainly serotonin. Further, Pietroletti et al (1986) have demonstrated that the increase in endocrine cells demonstrated by a chromagranin monoclonal antibody is abolished by successful treatment with a gluten-free diet. In about one third of cases with severe changes, collagen deposition may be seen immediately beneath the surface epithelium (this is referred to in some detail later).

In its severest form this type of villous atrophy is seen par excellence in gluten-sensitive enteropathy, and in the untreated case the mucosa shows either a severe degree of villous effacement or is virtually devoid of villous processes altogether (Figs. 11–26, 11–27). It appears to be the direct result of ingestion of gluten in the diet and a toxic action on the mucosa that results in increased cell loss from the villous surface (Croft, Loehry and Creamer 1968, Pink, Croft and Creamer 1970). Similar appearances are produced by chronic trauma to small-intestinal mucosa in abnormal situations, e.g., in jejunum transplanted as an artificial oesophagus (personal observation), at ileostomy stomas, in urinary ileal conduits or immediately neighbouring areas of ulceration. It has been produced experimentally by the repeated instillation of acid into the jejunum of dogs (Townley, Cass and Anderson 1964) and in jejunum explanted to the anterior abdominal wall in rats (Loehry and Grace 1974). Wright et al (1973a,b) and Watson, Appleton and Wright (1982) have shown a threefold expansion of the mass of proliferating and maturing cells with a halving of the cell cycle time, resulting in a sixfold increase in the crypt cell production rate. Coupled with a pathologically rapid cell

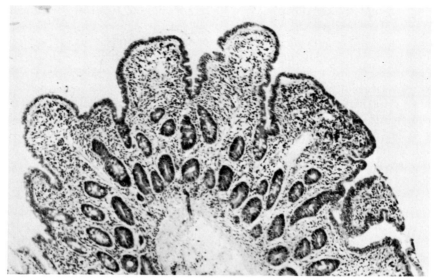

Figure 11–26. Jejunal mucosa in severe untreated gluten-sensitive enteropathy. Degree of villous atrophy corresponding to "convoluted mucosa" seen in the dissecting microscope (H & E × 100).

loss from the mucosal surface this forms the basis of the change in mucosal morphology.

In previous descriptive accounts of this type of mucosal lesion the terms "partial villous atrophy" and "subtotal villous atrophy" (Doniach and Shiner 1957) have been used and are still in common use. They correspond roughly to the dissecting microscopic appearances of convoluted and flat types respectively (Fig. 11–28 A,B,C,D). In practice, however, there is a continuum of appearances, from normal to a completely flat-surfaced mucosa without villous projections. This is paralleled stereoscopically by an increasing number of leaf-shaped villi, short then long ridges, which anastomose, form convolutions and become progressively lower, sometimes passing through a mosaic phase, to end up finally completely flat. It is

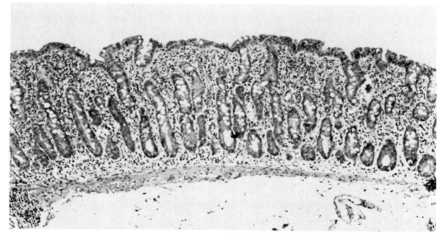

Figure 11–27. Jejunal mucosa in severe untreated gluten-sensitive enteropathy. Degree of villous atrophy corresponding to the flat or mosaic type seen in the dissecting microscope (H & E × 100).

clear that the two descriptive terms do not satisfactorily cover the possible histological range. A better but not ideal terminology, therefore, is "crypt hyperplasia with total villous atrophy" when there are no villous projections from the surface, and "mild, moderate or severe partial villous atrophy" when there are. Assessment of partial villous atrophy will be best accomplished, however, by the simple quantitative method already outlined.

There is a long list of case reports of disease states said to be associated with a jejunal mucosal lesion identical to that in untreated gluten-sensitive enteropathy (childhood and adult coeliac disease), i.e., crypt hyperplasia with total or severe partial villous atrophy. In coeliac disease the causal agent has been identified. There is a disparity between the histological findings and the degree of malabsorption of individual dietary factors. This accounts for the diverse clinical presentations of the disease, not the least of which is an apparent onset in adult life. Usually there is a clinical improvement on gluten withdrawal, and the jejunal mucosa reverts to normal both morphologically (Pollack et al 1970) and histochemically (Riecken 1970). However, the degree of clinical improvement may not parallel the improvement in mucosal appearances (Kumar et al 1979). More specifically, if there is a subsequent gluten challenge, damage to the mucosa is reestablished, and within a few hours of the dose, changes can be seen by electron microscopy and by immunocyte counts, suggestive of an immune reaction (Shiner and Shmerling 1970, Shiner 1973, Holmes et al 1974, Lancaster-Smith et al 1976a,b, Baklien, Brandtzaeg and Fausa 1977). This is especially true if toxic fractions of gluten are used in challenge experiments (Dissanayake et al 1973, Anand et al 1981). Further evidence for a role of the immune system in mucosal injury in this condition is provided by the depleted circulating thymus-dependent lymphocytes in coeliacs, which return to normal after dietary gluten exclusion (O'Donoghue et al 1976).

It is perhaps of some importance, therefore, that prednisolone administered to coeliac patients has the same effect on the mucosa as gluten withdrawal (Wall et al 1970). Nevertheless, doubt is raised as to the role of B cells in the pathogenesis of coeliac disease by the occurrence of gluten-sensitive enteropathy in hypogammaglobulinaemia (Webster et al 1981). Thus, as Kelly et al (1987) indicate, many of the immune phenomena observed in this intriguing disease may be secondary. Davidson and Bridges (1988) recently analysed the aetiological possibilities and have argued a strong case for investigating a possible fault in the intraluminal phase of the in-vivo processing of dietary gluten.

A group of cases with otherwise identical morphological lesions to those in adult coeliac disease apparently fail to respond to gluten withdrawal, and when the patient has also had another disease at the same time it has been implied that the malabsorption is secondary to this disease. Failure of a clinical response is not an adequate criterion for assessing gluten sensitivity. A clinical response is difficult to assess, because when it does occur it can be extremely variable. Failure of a morphological response of the mucosa is a much more objective measurement, although this too is extremely variable, especially in adults. Kluge et al (1982), for example, failed to achieve a complete restitution of the mucosa in any of 18 patients on a strict gluten diet, although in an analysis of their study only 3 of these gave no history of occasional lapses. However, in a similar study (Bardella et al 1985) a quarter of their rebiopsied cases had mild partial villous atrophy even when the diet was strictly controlled.

The longer that the disease state has been present the more likely it is that secondary factors may be having an additional effect. Some secondary factors, for example, vitamin deficiency or protein depletion, may be the direct result of the

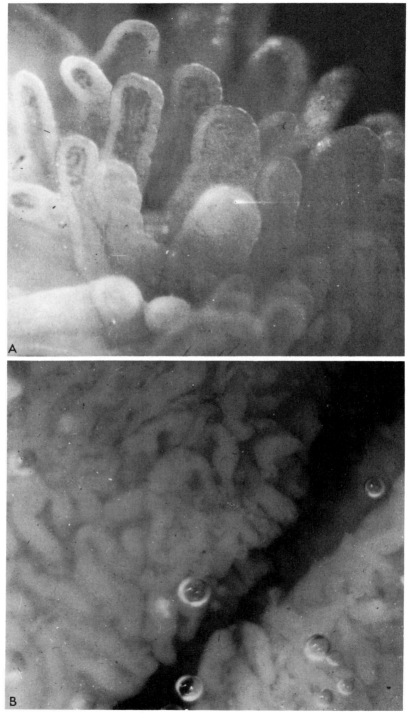

Figure 11–28. Dissecting microscope appearances. Jejunal biopsies showing **(A)** normal, **(B)** convoluted, **(C)** mosaic and **(D)** flat biopsies.

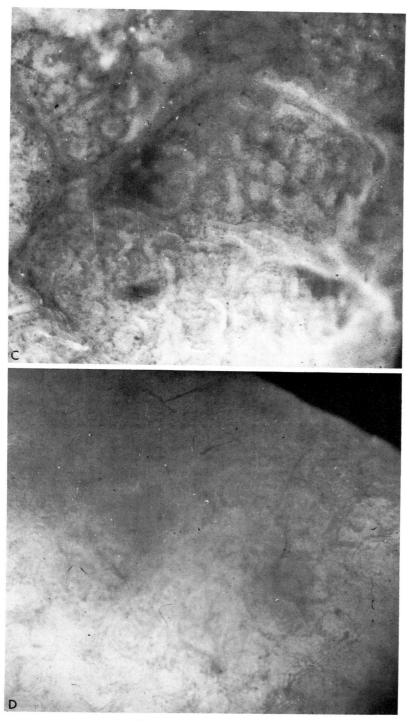

Figure 11–28 *Continued.*

malabsorption syndrome itself, but there may be many others. It is not surprising that gluten withdrawal results in a much slower recovery of the mucosa when the disease has been untreated for many years, and in general the longer it has gone untreated the slower is the response once treatment is instituted, although age at time of diagnosis does not seem to be a factor (Dissanayake, Truelove and Whitehead 1974). However, it is claimed that challenge in some childhood cases, by using a normal diet, may not provoke severe morphological changes even after weeks or months (Lebenthal and Branski 1981), and it is suggested that susceptibility to gluten damage may vary in severity between individuals and in the same individual with time (McNeish 1980). This is highlighted by the report of Paerregaard et al (1988), who showed that in some cases of adults with coeliac disease, even with a flat mucosa and evidence of biochemical malabsorption, there was no evidence of clinical disease or growth retardation. These patients had been treated in early childhood for presumed gluten sensitivity but had not been biopsied. Variation in susceptibility to mucosal damage and malabsorption is thus well established, and thus, perhaps surprisingly, healthy siblings of coeliac patients do not show mucosal sensitivity to damage by diets containing large supplements of gluten (Polanco et al 1987).

The situation concerning gluten sensitivity and response to gluten exclusion is far from clear in view of the findings that in adults mucosal recovery may be incomplete after even as long as four years on a gluten-free diet (Grefte et al 1988). The quality of the gluten-free control is, however, a factor difficult to ascertain, especially in adults, and the failure of some patients to respond is often due to an inadvertent or unadmitted gluten ingestion (Pink and Creamer 1967). Some children who seem to be progressing satisfactorily on a gluten-free diet often exhibit mucosal abnormalities on biopsy (Congdon et al 1981), and this is more common in adults (Kluge et al 1982). Relatively small quantities of gluten can produce marked mucosal change, and it probably requires only a weekly lapse to perpetuate the mucosal damage. Consequently, for a proper diagnosis sequential morphological studies should be performed during a strict period of gluten withdrawal, preferably in a hospitalised patient, and this should be followed by a gluten challenge. Until a better and simpler method is available this should be the minimum requirement for a strict diagnosis of gluten-sensitive enteropathy before a patient, especially a child, is subjected to a lifelong gluten-free diet. Only when such a method is employed will it be possible to categorise other forms of enteropathy and so determine if indeed some cases are aetiologically independent of gluten. Holmes et al (1974) have suggested that mucosal lamina propria cell counts may prove of value in the accurate diagnosis of gluten-sensitive enteropathy, but Macromichalis et al (1976) have found considerable overlap of lamina propria cell counts in patients with coeliac disease, cow's milk protein intolerance, giardiasis and "intractable diarrhoea." The value of theliocyte counts and theliocyte mitosis has already been referred to in this regard.

It is pertinent that the malabsorption syndrome so often associated with dermatitis herpetiformis has been shown to be of gluten-sensitive type (Marks et al 1968). In fact evidence is at hand that all patients given a big enough gluten load will develop small-intestinal mucosal abnormalities (Reunala et al 1984, Andersson et al 1984, Kosnai et al 1986, Ferguson, Blackwell and Barnetson 1987). Further, if a sufficient number of biopsies are examined, almost all cases of dermatitis herpetiformis will show some intestinal mucosal abnormalities (Brow et al 1971). This implication of a patchy distribution of the abnormality led to multiple biopsy studies in coeliac disease, and a degree of patchiness was observed in these also (Scott and Losowsky 1976). Variation in the degree of damage in coeliacs is slight, however, although the degree of abnormality decreases as one proceeds distally down the bowel. Degrees of gluten sensitivity, as exhibited in patients with dermatitis herpetiformis, may thus suggest a possible reason that some coeliacs present in childhood and others apparently in adult life. The remission that seems to occur in the teens might also suggest a varying sensitivity, although Weir and Hourihane (1974) showed persistent flat mucosa even in teenagers who had wholly remitted clinically. The acquisition of gluten sensitivity, e.g., following gastroenteritis, has also been postulated, and transient gluten sensitivity is also described (see postinfective malabsorption). The author has personal experience of one female patient, aged 28, with a flat mucosa and proven gluten sensitivity by strict criteria, who had been investigated for iron deficiency anaemia two years previously, and was found to have a normal jejunal biopsy. An almost identical case has been reported by Egan-Mitchell, Fottrell and McNicholl (1981) but in a much younger patient. In patients with recurrent aphthous stomatitis but no evidence of malabsorption it is not unusual to find mild small bowel morphological abnormalities, and some 16 per cent have been shown to have reversible gluten-sensitive villous atrophy (Veloso and Saleiro 1987).

Similarly, those cases of malabsorption in diabetes that have a coeliac-like mucosal lesion are gluten-sensitive (Rubin and Dobbins 1965). The coeliac-like mucosal atrophy seen occasionally in patients with carcinoma outside the bowel (Creamer 1964) has also been shown in some cases to be gluten sensitive (Pollack et al 1970). The concurrence of gluten-sensitive enteropathy with inflammatory bowel disease (Gillberg, Dotevall and Ahren 1982) is probably more common than previously suspected. Of 42 patients with coeliac disease who underwent rectal biopsy, 14 had inflammation of varying degrees of severity and in 3 it was compatible with a diagnosis of ulcerative colitis. Further, the diarrhoea in these 3 cases persisted despite a gluten-free diet (Breen et al 1987). An association between coeliac disease and systemic sarcoidosis has also been claimed (Douglas et al 1984). Primary biliary cirrhosis coincident with coeliac disease (Olsson, Kagevi and Rydberg 1982) is also well documented. In recent years it has become evident that the group of patients with malabsorption syndrome and a jejunal lesion typical of that seen in coeliac disease who are not gluten sensitive is certainly very much smaller than earlier papers (e.g., Cooke et al 1963) have suggested. Critical diagnostic tests in the future may reduce this number even further, but it seems likely that gluten-induced damage over a long period or of a severe degree may reach a state from which recovery is impossible. This would certainly seem to apply to those cases of longstanding gluten-sensitive enteropathy that go on to develop malignant lymphoma (see later).

There is an even longer list of conditions said to be associated with minor degrees of crypt hyperplastic villous atrophy (Rubin and Dobbins 1965, Whitehead 1968b). Poor histological technique, inexperienced interpretation and lack of proper controls account for many of the reports that have led to conflicting results and much controversy. Marks and Shuster (1970), for example, have shown that the so-called mucosal abnormalities described in association with eczema, psoriasis and rosacea are fictitious. Until evaluated in much more critical fashion, the previously reported non-gluten sensitive jejunal abnormalities said to be associated with cirrhosis of the liver other than the primary biliary type, postgastrectomy states, iron deficiency anaemia, scleroderma, neomycin administration, Crohn's disease not involving the site of small bowel biopsy or neighbouring bowel, ulcerative colitis, chronic pancreatitis and sarcoidosis must remain the subject of doubt. The validity of the observations of villous abnormalities in various gener-alised virus infections (Sheehy, Artenstein and Green 1964) must also be questioned until reinvestigated in a more critical manner using sequential biopsies during and after recovery from the illness. Soltoft and Soeberg (1972a), however, have shown an increase in cells containing the immunoglobulins A and D in the lamina propria of patients with viral hepatitis when compared with normal controls. The authors did not follow up these patients in an attempt to show reversal to normal on recovery from the illness. The jejunal mucosal morphology in more specific gastroenteritides will be referred to under postinfective malabsorption syndrome.

Schlossberg et al (1984) describe a case of crypt hyperplastic villous atrophy that resulted in diarrhoea in a patient with relapsing secondary syphilis. Although the lamina propria contained an excess of plasma cells, spirochaetes were not demonstrated. The mucosal morphology returned to normal following therapy and the symptoms subsided.

In tropical sprue the morphological abnormality varies from "normal" to "very abnormal" (Baker and Mathan 1970), bearing in mind that the "normal" has to be defined with reference to the local population. Brunser, Eidelman and Klipstein (1970) have shown, for example, that in rural Haitians there are no qualitative differences in jejunal morphology between those with and those without tropical sprue, but in the former the changes were more severe. With a few exceptions the most severe lesion is a crypt hyperplastic partial villous atrophy (Fig. 11–29) with chronic inflammatory cell infiltration of the lamina propria and surface epithelial changes similar to, but milder than, those seen in gluten-sensitive enteropathy. Schenk, Samloff and Klipstein (1965) have claimed that when frozen sections of biopsy tissue in both tropical sprue and gluten-sensitive enteropathy are stained with oil red O, the appearances in tropical sprue are distinctive. Neutral lipid is said to be found in the epithelial cell cytoplasm and in the basement membrane in tropical sprue, but only in the supranuclear cytoplasm of epithelial cells in gluten-sensitive enteropathy. Electron microscopy studies suggest faults in fat transport (Mathan, Mathan and Baker 1975), but this cannot be regarded as specific for tropical sprue. In practice, since total villous atrophy seldom if ever occurs in tropical sprue, differentiation from untreated coeliac disease causes little difficulty.

Sequential biopsy studies after treatment with vitamin B_{12} or folic acid (Swanson, Wheby and Bayless 1966) show somewhat variable results, although it is perhaps

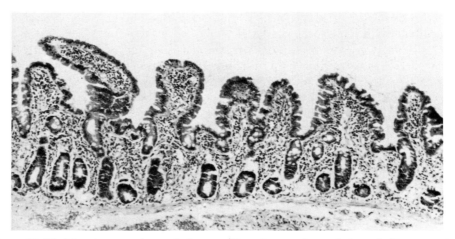

Figure 11–29. Jejunal mucosa in tropical sprue. There is crypt hyperplasia and villous atrophy (H & E × 75).

pertinent that both agents produce maximum effect in the cases with the severest mucosal lesions. Guerra, Wheby and Bayless (1965) demonstrated marked histological improvement after tetracycline therapy, and over half of their cases had already shown resistance to folic acid and vitamin B_{12}. This introduced the possibility of an infectious aetiology, and Tomkins, Drasar and James (1975) have isolated enterobacteria from cases of tropical sprue and shown that after specific treatment with tetracycline, which eliminated the organisms, there was a clinical and biochemical cure. Klipstein and Schenk (1975) tested the enterotoxins of certain coliform organisms isolated from tropical sprue patients for their effects on the ileal mucosa of rats. They showed a direct toxic effect manifested as a mucosal damage similar to that in tropical sprue, and it was independent of the presence or absence of the organisms themselves. Upper-intestinal colonisation by enterobacteria, which is so frequent in sprue, could be responsible for mucosal damage via an enterotoxin-induced or other cytopathic effect. In addition, Baker et al (1982) describe sprue patients with a chronic enterocyte infection by coronavirus. Both phenomena are compatible with the view that the syndrome has a complex aetiology involving several agents. This is expressed in an editorial review of tropical malabsorption by Tomkins (1981), who concludes that it is unlikely that a single "sprue agent" will be found that is common to all cases in different parts of the world. Whatever these agents are it appears that they produce their effect on the mucosa via a direct action on the epithelium rather than on the lymphoid tissue, which nevertheless appears to be involved in a cell mediated immune reaction. This was the conclusion reached by Marsh, Mathan and Mathan (1983), who showed that the epithelial changes characterised more critically in a further study (Mathan, Ponniah and Mathan 1986) actually precede the changes in the epithelial lymphoid population. This view would be in accord with the hypothesis that initial enterocyte damage and resultant release of enteroglucagon cause a slowing of intestinal transit and further bacterial overgrowth which perpetuates the initial injury. This cycle of events with its consequent folic acid deficiency would explain the favourable response to antibiotics, particularly if folic acid supplements are also used (Cook 1984).

There are further conditions with which crypt hyperplastic villous atrophy is associated. Ament and Rubin (1972) describe a case in which soy protein ingestion was associated with a rapidly developing jejunal mucosal lesion indistinguishable from that seen in gluten-sensitive enteropathy. Some infants have a milk protein intolerance (Fontaine and Navarro 1975, Shiner et al 1975), and Walker-Smith (1978) has shown that acute symptoms can be precipitated by challenging with milk after a period of milk exclusion and that the morphology of the jejunal mucosa is adversely affected (Vitoria, Camarero and Solaguren 1979, de Sousa et al 1986). Jejunal biopsy may show obvious villous atrophy (Fig. 11–30). Shiner, Ballard and Smith (1975) demonstrated that following milk challenge, there is also evidence of deposition of IgG and complement on basement membranes and connective tissue, and a degranulation of mast cells with increase in the number of IgM plasma cells in the lamina propria. These findings were interpreted as indicative of several simultaneous immune reactions occurring in the intestinal mucosa. In a quantitative study Maluenda et al (1984) claimed that the principal change seen in cow's milk sensitivity enteropathy is increase in intraepithelial eosinophils, but not of those in the lamina propria. There was also a decrease in overall mucosal thickness during active disease despite milk withdrawal, and this returned to normal when the condition resolved. The authors concluded that in this condition there is a limitation of the capacity of crypt cells to respond and compensate for the loss of villous epithelium. One of the characteristics of the

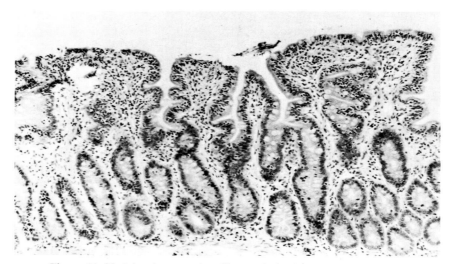

Figure 11–30. Jejunal mucosa in milk protein intolerance (H & E × 180).

mucosal lesion in cow's milk protein intolerance is said to be its patchy distribution (Variend, Phillips and Walker-Smith 1984), although this is difficult to explain unless the intolerance is secondary to focal damage produced by another agent. Of interest in this regard is the demonstration of rotavirus particles in the epithelial cells in some cases (Phillips et al 1985). There is now evidence that other infections not uncommonly precede cow's milk protein, soy protein and other intolerance states in infants (Iyngkaran et al 1988a, Iyngkaran et al 1989). Cow's milk intolerance or sensitivity may manifest itself by primarily involving other parts of the gastrointestinal tract such as the stomach and upper duodenum (Coello-Ramirez and Larossa-Hara 1984) or the colon (see later). Although cow's milk protein intolerance is normally a self-limited condition lasting a few months or a year, there is a likelihood that these patients retain an atopic tendency throughout childhood (Businco et al 1985). Vitoria et al (1982) have also described an essentially similar enteropathy associated with the ingestion of fish, rice and chicken protein.

Unlike gluten enteropathy all these protein-intolerant states are transient, and this is true even in the rare event of combined cow's milk protein and gluten-induced enteropathy (Watt, Pincott and Harries 1983). There is some evidence that in gluten-sensitive enteropathy, coexistent dietary soy protein sensitivity may adversely influence the response to gluten withdrawal (Haeney et al 1982). It is thus becoming clear that diet may have a very significant role in the clinical course and management of protein intolerance states that not infrequently follow gastroenteritis in infancy (Iyngkaran et al 1988a,b).

In view of the experimental evidence of mucosal damage to the jejunum of dogs following the instillation of acid (Townley, Cass and Anderson 1964), it is not surprising that patchy jejunal atrophy and microulceration are described in Zollinger-Ellison syndrome with hyperchlorhydria (Singleton, Kern and Waddell 1965). The mucosa, however, shows a much more obvious polymorphonuclear leukocytic infiltrate than is seen in the coeliac lesion. There are also some severe degenerative changes in the surface epithelium, which may show erosions and almost invariably exhibit superficial gastric epithelial metaplasia or so-called antralisation with the acquisition of pyloric type mucous glands. However, extensive villous atrophy may be present in some cases, and Kingham, Levison and Fairclough (1981) describe two patients with Zollinger-Ellison syndrome who presented with steatorrhoea and who responded to treatment with histamine$_2$ antagonists. In the stasis, or blind loop, syndrome there is bacterial colonisation of parts of the small intestine where normally there is only a transient population. Sometimes the mucosa related to this abnormal bacterial proliferation will show morphological changes. This is usually patchy in distribution and of only moderate severity, i.e., a crypt hyperplasia with slight to moderate villous atrophy. The small intestinal mucosa will also show a villous atrophy in association with mural infiltration by malignancy (see Fig. 12–6). Whether this is also related to stasis caused by mechanical interference, secondary to the infiltration, or due to lymphatic obstruction or both is not known.

Postinfective Malabsorption Syndrome

Both bacterial and viral gastroenteritis are known to cause reversible small intestinal mucosal damage (Burke, Kerry and Anderson 1965, Soltoft and Soeberg 1972b, Davidson and Barnes 1979, Ulshen and Rollo 1980), but small bowel biopsy plays little, if any, part in diagnosis or management. The mucosa, however, shows crypt hyperplastic villous atrophy and cellular infiltration of the lamina propria, which is usually only of mild or moderate severity, although of 31 cases described by Barnes and Townley (1973) 5 had severe mucosal lesions comparable to those seen in gluten-sensitive enteropathy. One of the characteristics of the infective lesions is their more obviously acute inflammatory nature. One may see hyperaemia and oedema with polymorph margination of capillaries. Polymorphs can also be seen traversing the epithelium of the crypts to form so-called crypt abscesses. In adults the acute lesion is not as marked, and Montgomery et al (1973), describing 13 adult cases, stressed the absence of severe mucosal lesions and the similarity of the clinical features to tropical sprue. Walker-Smith (1970) has described an infant who appeared to develop typical biopsy-positive gluten-sensitive enteropathy following an episode of *Salmonella* enteritis. After a dramatic response to a gluten-free diet, which was continued for one year, he was given a normal diet, and a subsequent biopsy proved to be normal. It should be pointed out, however, that the gluten-free diet may well have coincided with the recovery phase of the intestinal infection and that the question of transient gluten intolerance is still an open one.

Postinfective malabsorption syndromes may be preceded by bacterial or viral gastroenteritis. Patients give a clear history of gastroenteritis of acute onset and typical symptomatology. In contrast to the usual course of events, the diarrhoea continues, weight loss occurs and on investigation a malabsorption syndrome has clearly developed. Jejunal biopsy usually shows crypt hyperplasia and partial villous atrophy of mild to moderate degree (Fig. 11–31). There is a striking increase in round cells of lymphocyte and plasma cell type in the lamina propria and an apparent increase of those in the intraepithelial zone. Histiocytes sometimes containing haematoxylphilic debris in their cytoplasm may also be seen, and the whole appearance of the mucosa is distinctly abnormal. Montgomery and Shearer (1974) have drawn particular attention to the similarity of the cell population in the mucosal lesion to that seen in gluten-sensitive enteropathy and tropical sprue. Indeed, when folic acid deficiency is the main clinical feature, such cases are reported as acute nontropical or temperate sprue (Drummond and Montgomery 1970). Why reaction to an infection should take this form in some persons and

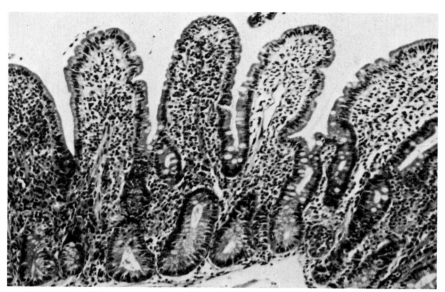

Figure 11–31. Jejunal biopsy appearance in postinfective malabsorption. Note the heavy inflammatory infiltrate in the lamina propria (H & E × 175).

not others is not known, of course, but it is tempting to postulate that it is related to subtle differences in individual immune mechanisms. Clearly the condition needs further study.

Halliday, Edimeades and Shepherd (1982) in a prospective analysis of 32 cases of postenteritis diarrhoea in children identified in just over half persisting pathogenic agents, carbohydrate intolerance or milk protein intolerance. In the remainder no significant cause for persisting diarrhoea could be ascertained. There is some evidence that selective deficiency of IgA plasma cells in the lamina propria may determine a susceptibility to gastroenteritis in patients with protein-energy malnutrition (Green and Heyworth 1980).

Intractable (Protracted) Diarrhoea of Early Infancy

Most of the chronic diarrhoeas in infancy can be diagnosed with precision, they are short-lived and can be managed effectively. Avery et al (1968) characterised a subgroup in patients less than three months of age in which the diarrhoea was without apparent cause, refractory to treatment and frequently fatal. In a biopsy study Rossi et al (1980) established that the condition was usually associated with a mucosal abnormality. Total villous atrophy with crypt hyperplasia was described by Stern, Gruttner and Krumback (1980), while Davidson et al (1978) and Fisher, Boyle and Holtzapple (1981) have reported cases with villous atrophy and crypt hypoplasia. In the large series published by Candy et al (1981) both types of lesions were observed. Shwachman et al (1973) had earlier commented on the striking eosinophil infiltration of the lamina propria in some patients and the occasional presence of lymphangiectasia. With the advent of intravenous alimentation fewer cases end in death and complete recovery is possible. The true nature of this condition is unknown, but both Davidson et al and Candy et al described a tendency for cases to occur on a familial basis. Booth et al (1982) described an association with severe combined immunodeficiency and drew attention to the presence of large PAS-positive macrophages in the jejunal mucosa in such cases.

By the early 1980s it was becoming apparent that this clinical entity was probably the manifestation of several different forms of mucosal injury. An initial mucosal insult and resultant malnutrition could then cause disturbances in immune function and sensitisation to ingested proteins, making the mucosa susceptible to further damage. Thus the morphological appearances of the small intestinal mucosa could be expected to vary, and it has been claimed that there is often a disparity between the clinical course of the illness and the biopsy findings (Orenstein 1986, Goldgar and Vanderhoof 1986). Nevertheless, there seem to be emerging at least two recognisable morphological subgroups within the spectrum of changes seen in this condition.

The first of these has been called microvillous inclusion disease. These patients have persistent intractable diarrhoea from birth or shortly afterwards. There is evidence that the diarrhoea is secretory (Candy et al 1981) and at least some cases are inherited in an autosomal recessive manner (Davidson et al 1978, Howard et al 1981). The mucosa is hypoplastic with stunted villi and no elongation of the crypts; inflammatory changes are not a feature. Electron microscopic examination reveals relatively normal crypts, but surface cells are shorter, have few stunted microvilli, increased lysosomal and cytolysosomal bodies and characteristic membrane bound bodies containing obvious microvilli. These mucosal microvillous involutions are regarded as the diagnostic feature of this condition (Phillips et al 1985). In colonic mucosa that otherwise appears normal these typical inclusions may also be seen. It seems that the intestinal mucosa is inherently abnormal in this disease, and oral feeding after birth precipitates a secretory diarrhoea that is usually fatal. The condition can also be demonstrated by ordinary light microscopy using a histochemical method for alkaline phosphatase. The brush border inclusions, strongly positive for this enzyme, can be clearly visualised in the apical enterocyte cytoplasm (Lake 1988).

Other forms of intractable diarrhoea of infancy form a larger group than those due to microvillous inclusion disease. These usually have a later onset outside the neonatal period, but generally within the first few months of life. The small bowel biopsy in these cases is somewhat variable, which accounts for the earlier reports already mentioned in which both crypt hyperplastic and crypt hypoplastic villous atrophy were described. In some patients, however, the enteropathy may have an autoimmune basis, and circulating antibodies to gut enterocytes have been demonstrated (Walker-Smith et al 1982, Savage et al 1985); thus a second variant can be defined. The jejunal morphology is said to vary from near normal to one which is completely flat. Mirakian et al (1986) have proposed that a positive test for enterocyte antibody is diagnostic for this condition and a persisting high titre indicates a poor prognosis.

Currently it would seem that the categorisation of intractable diarrhoea is evolving. Kanof et al (1987), for example, describe a case of secretory diarrhoea from birth. There was histological evidence of both acute and chronic inflammation of the small bowel, an avillous mucosa and submucosal fibrosis. Of interest, however, was concomitant involvement by the inflammatory and fibrosing process in the colon. It is possible therefore that microvillous inclusion disease and the autoimmune variety of the intractable diarrhoea of childhood are the first two of several possible definable subgroups. Certainly the morphological appearances seen show a good deal of variation from case to case (Figs. 11–32 to 11–34 and 11–35 to 11–37). A variety of degrees of villous atrophy, crypt hyperplasia and hypoplasia, some or no inflammatory component, increase or decrease in goblet cells and a range of ultrastructural abnormalities are all described (Fagundes-Neto et al 1985, Orenstein 1986). This disorder clearly presents a challenge for further research.

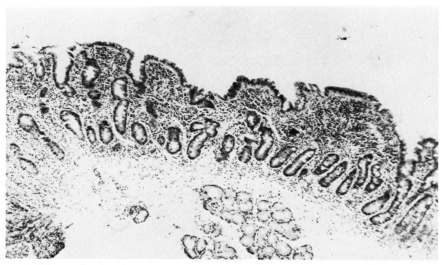

Figure 11–32. Duodenal endoscopic biopsy in intractable diarrhoea in a child aged three months. The first biopsy shows partial villous atrophy with slight crypt hyperplasia (H & E × 70).

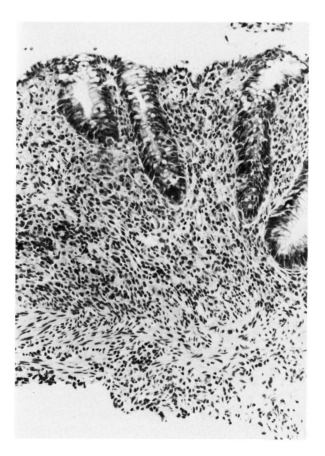

Figure 11–33. Follow-up biopsy two weeks after that in Figure 11–32. The infiltrate is now more dense, villi are absent and the crypts hypoplastic (H & E × 250).

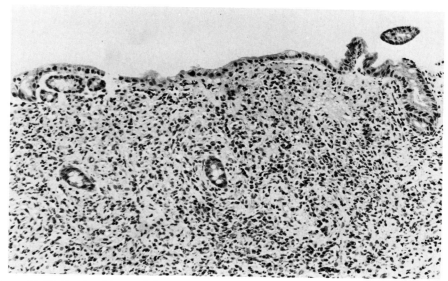

Figure 11–34. Further biopsy of the same case as in Figures 11–32 and 11–33. The avillous mucosa now has virtually no crypts. The patient later died (H & E × 250).

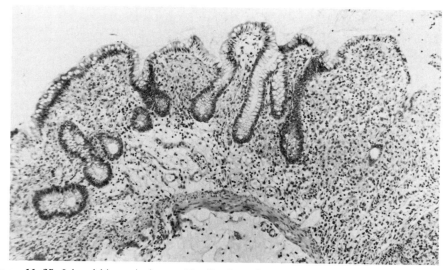

Figure 11–35. Jejunal biopsy in intractable diarrhoea from a one month old child. The lamina is expanded by oedema and cellular infiltrate but the villi and crypts are atrophic. Note the superficial epithelium is not greatly abnormal (H & E × 250).

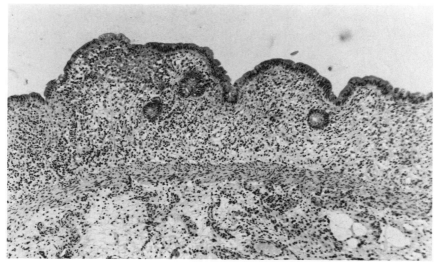

Figure 11–36. Further biopsy one week later. Even more atrophy and increased cellularity of the lamina propria are evident. The superficial epithelium is now more abnormal (H & E × 250).

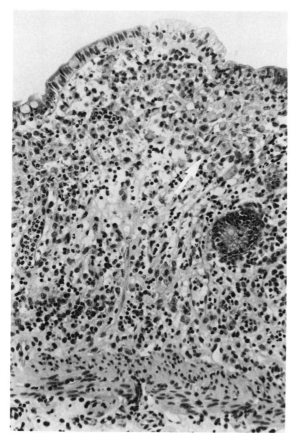

Figure 11–37. Detail of Figure 11–36. The lamina propria is occupied by a very prominent histiocyte population, especially noticeable nearer the lumen (arrow) (H & E × 500).

Crypt Hypoplastic Villous Atrophy

This lesion hitherto has not received a great deal of attention. It is characterised by shortening of the crypts, which show a reduced mitotic rate and a varying degree of villous atrophy, so that the overall thickness of the mucosa is decreased. Creamer (1967) was the first to draw attention to it, and the lesion has been likened to hypoplastic anaemia in that a decreased cell production, rather than an increased loss, seems to be involved. It appears, however, that a simple hypoplasia of the crypts may not be the full explanation, since experimental reduction of the crypt mitotic rate in humans with methotrexate (Trier 1962) did not produce villous abnormalities. Moreover, the appearance in both animals and humans following irradiation, which produces reduction of the crypt cell mitosis rate and a collapse of the villous architecture (Wiernik, Shorter and Creamer 1962, Wiernik 1966), is not identical to crypt hypoplastic villous atrophy. It is, nevertheless, clear that manoeuvres that decrease cell turnover (Creamer 1967) in the small intestine may greatly influence villous shape and crypt length, and the closest approximation to crypt hypoplastic villous atrophy as it occurs in humans is seen in Rhesus monkeys after protein malnutrition (Deo and Ramalingaswami 1965).

Malnutrition in children, however, may result in a jejunal lesion similar to that in gluten-sensitive enteropathy (Shiner, Redmond and Hansen 1973). One might expect a crypt hypoplastic villous atrophy such as occurs in hypophagic animals (Robinson 1972), but it is likely that lesions seen in kwashiorkor are multifactorial in aetiology. Green and Heyworth (1980), for example, have shown a decrease in IgA plasma cells of the lamina propria in children with protein-energy malnutrition and this might predispose to recurrent infection and alteration in villous morphology secondary to inflammatory damage to the mucosa.

Crypt hypoplasia and villous atrophy in association with intractable diarrhoea of infancy have already been referred to, but it should be noted that normal or hyperplastic crypts and villous atrophy are the more usual lesions.

In adults, crypt hypoplastic villous atrophy has been described in association with malignancy (Creamer 1964), Paneth cell deficiency (Pink and Creamer, 1967) and in hypopituitarism (Riecken 1970) and is seen in some cases of coeliac disease at a time when they no longer respond to a gluten-free diet (Fig. 11–38).

It has been demonstrated that the jejunal mucosa shows a varying degree of

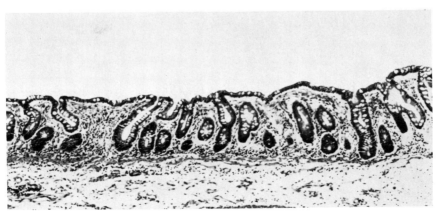

Figure 11–38. Jejunal mucosa showing crypt hypoplastic villous atrophy associated with malabsorption not responding to a gluten-free diet (H & E × 70).

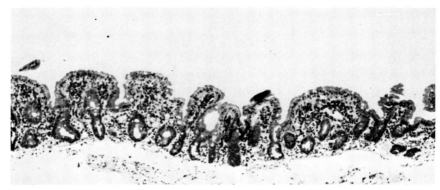

Figure 11–39. Jejunal mucosa in untreated pernicious anaemia showing crypt hypoplastic villous atrophy (H & E × 70).

crypt-hypoplastic villous atrophy in untreated pernicious anaemia (Fig. 11–39) (Pena et al 1972). The crypt and superficial epithelial cells show typical megalocytic changes (Foroozan and Trier 1967) characterised by large round and pale nuclei (Fig. 11–40). The superficial epithelium may otherwise appear relatively normal, but, in the more severely affected, slight nuclear palisading, distortion of the cells and lack of definition of the brush border in PAS preparations are seen. Mitotic figures are decreased in number and there are fewer Paneth cells, which often are poorly granulated. The lamina propria shows a mixed inflammatory infiltrate of varying density with a high lymphocytic preponderance. In some cases the inflammatory infiltrate is more marked (Fig. 11–41), and another abnormality occasionally observed consists of colonies of bacteria within the lumen, but the significance of this is not known. All the observed changes revert to normal if vitamin B_{12} (Figs. 11–42, 11–43) is given, and in treated pernicious anaemia the changes are absent. It is tempting to assume that the hypoplastic villous appearance

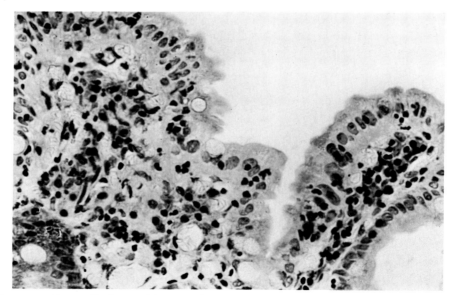

Figure 11–40. Detail of superficial epithelium in Figure 11–39. The nuclei vary in size and are "megalocytic" in type (H & E × 350).

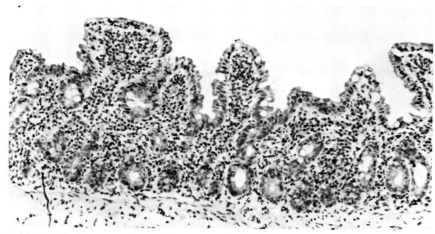

Figure 11–41. Jejunal mucosa in pernicious anaemia showing heavy cellular infiltration of the lamina propria (H & E × 140).

is related to the disturbances of deoxyribonucleic acid metabolism induced by vitamin B_{12} deficiency.

Such an explanation might account for some of the cases of crypt hypoplastic villous atrophy seen in malignancy, and it is of interest that in Creamer's case 5 (1964) there was a carcinoma of the stomach, although vitamin B_{12} levels were not measured, and in case 4, which was associated with carcinoma of the bronchus, there was vitamin B_{12} deficiency. It is known that the latter is often present in some cases of coeliac disease. Because vitamin B_{12} is absorbed in the ileum it is not surprising that Stewart et al (1967) have shown a better correlation between abnormality of vitamin B_{12} absorption and ileal, rather than jejunal, mucosal atrophy. Ileal involvement is more common in the severe or longstanding untreated disease, and a delayed poor quality response to gluten withdrawal may in part be due to the vitamin B_{12} deficiency, which tends to produce crypt hypoplasia.

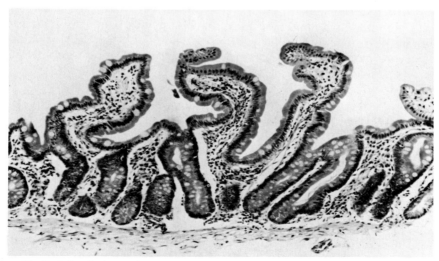

Figure 11–42. Jejunal mucosa in same patient as in Figure 11–39 one week after treatment with vitamin B_{12} (H & E × 105).

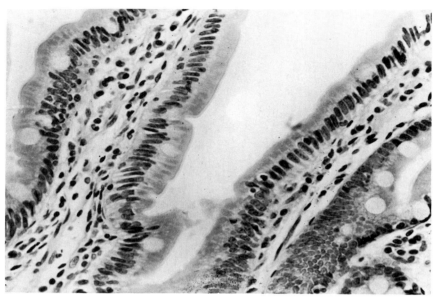

Figure 11–43. Detail of Figure 11–42 showing reversion of nuclear appearance to normal; compare with Figure 11–40 (H & E × 350).

In addition to the superficial absorptive cells, proliferative activity of the crypt cells also gives rise to Paneth cells and goblet cells. A crypt hypoplasia induced by vitamin B_{12} deficiency might thus result in Paneth cell deficiency, and this could have secondary deleterious effects on the mucosa, Creamer (1967) having postulated a sustentacular role for the Paneth cell, its secretions helping to support the rest of the mucosa.

Swanson and Thomassen (1965) describe a tendency towards "atrophy" of the mucosa in severe tropical sprue. This is associated with a fall in the mitosis count and a decrease in crypt length and number of argentaffin cells. Whatever the agent primarily responsible for the mucosal damage in coeliac disease, tropical sprue or any other malabsorption syndrome, when the disorder is well established one or more additional factors may begin to influence the morphology of the mucosa. The situation is clearly complex; Davidson and Townley (1977) described four infants with nutritional folic acid deficiency who showed villous shortening in the jejunal biopsy but elongation of the crypts. The enterocytes showed macrocytic characteristics.

Other Abnormalities

It is likely that villous atrophy will be shown to occur not only in association with crypt hyperplasia and hypoplasia but also with all stages between. An unusual association with villous atrophy is the generalised growth failure that occurs in the syndrome accompanied by ring chromosome 15 (Kosztolanyi and Pap 1986). Pinkerton et al (1982) reported a fall in crypt mitotic index and degenerative changes in Paneth cells and crypt enterocytes following methotrexate therapy for childhood leukaemia. These changes have also been seen following the administration of other chemotherapeutic agents in both animals and humans (Moore 1984, Cunningham et al 1985). The question of whether they can induce villous atrophy is not settled. Nevertheless, it is sensible that the overall mucosal structure seen in such circumstances will depend on the balance between cell loss and cell production so that one might expect that villous atrophy could occur. It is claimed that fat stains may be an aid in the interpretation of minor degrees of villous atrophy (Variend et al 1984). Fine granular fat globules are seen in surface cells in both normal and abnormal mucosa, but deep mucosal fat is seen in normal mucosa. Large fat globules, however, are seen only in surface cells in coeliac mucosa and cow's milk protein enteropathy and this may relate to the degree of villous atrophy. However, in cow's milk sensitivity large globules were also present in the surface cells even when the villous atrophy was minimal. Similarly, an increased cell proliferation in the crypts and a normal rate of surface loss would be expected to result in villous hypertrophy. Gleeson et al (1970) have described villous enlargement in humans occurring in association with a renal tumour. Villous hypertrophy has also been reported as the result of a pancreatic glucagon-oma (Jones et al 1983, Stevens et al 1984).

Mucosal hyperplasia is well recognised in experimental animals (Dowling 1967, Fenyo et al 1976, Obertop et al 1977), and it occurs in humans following jejunal resection or jejunoileal bypass operations for intractable obesity (Solhaug 1976). It is also well recognised that experimental hyperthyroidism in animals results in intestinal villous hyperplasia (Wall et al 1970) and that hypothyroidism has the reverse effect (Blanes et al 1977). The author, however, knows of no reports of villous alterations in thyroid disease in humans.

ILEAL BIOPSY

In gastroenterological practice the ileum is rarely preferentially biopsied with the expectation of a diagnostic yield. It is clearly possible to obtain tissue via an ileostomy stoma, and biopsies are not infrequently obtained through the ileo-caecal valve at colonoscopy.

Most of the pathological processes that may affect the small intestinal mucosa diffusely along its length, e.g., Whipple's disease, the storage diseases, lymphangiectasia, will be diagnosed with greater facility in upper intestinal biopsy tissue. Some pathological processes, however, are characteristically located at the terminal ileum or ileo-caecal region. Consequently, on occasion, a tissue diagnosis of Crohn's disease can be made in an ileal biopsy by finding epithelioid granulomata when colonic mucosal tissues are unproductive. Indeed, Coremans et al (1984) claim ileoscopy and biopsy as a very valuable procedure in the diagnosis of ileal disease. Even ileoscopic removal of inflammatory polyps has been described in Crohn's disease (Corless et al 1984). However, biopsy of other lesions may also reveal characteristic features. It is possible, for example, that the typical sulphur granules composed of colonies of *Actinomycosis* organisms may be seen, although it is usually diagnosed in resection specimens (Mahant et al 1983). The same could be said to apply to the recognition of the tissue reaction in ileo-caecal tuberculosis and the demonstration of acid-fast bacilli. Lesions of *Yersinia enterocolitica* infections of the ileo-caecal region may also rarely provide diagnostic biopsy tissue (Fig. 11–44). Characteristically, pathology has been described in resection specimens (Gleason and Patterson 1982), and biopsy of the aphthoid ulcers that occur in hyperplastic lymphoid follicles might reveal the typical central microabscess and peripheral palisade of histiocytes. However, some difficulty would be experienced in differentiating these appearances from Crohn's disease if epithelioid granulomata were absent. Sometimes amoebic infection occurs as a mass lesion in the ileo-caecal region, but in chronic cases vegetative organisms are few and likely to be deep seated. It is nevertheless possible that a colonoscopic ileal or ileo-caecal biopsy

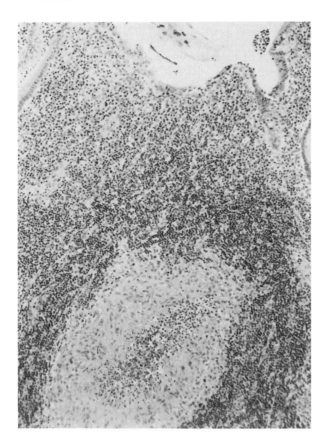

Figure 11–44. Biopsy of terminal ileal ulceration in *Yersinia* infection. Note the granuloma with central necrosis (H & E × 300).

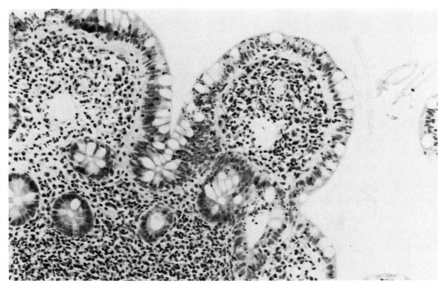

Figure 11–45. Ileal mucosa in a patient investigated for diarrhoea. Subsequent investigation indicated a salmonella infection. Note the mild acute enteritis with polymorph invasion of the surface epithelium (H & E × 500).

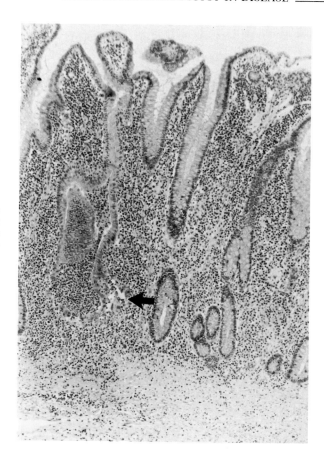

Figure 11–46. Ileal biopsy from a case of stomal ileitis in an ulcerative colitis patient. Note the marked inflammation and crypt abscess formation (arrow) (H & E × 200).

would prove diagnostic. Rarely an ileal biopsy shows evidence of acute inflammation in patients being investigated for diarrhoea, and presumably sometimes this is due to infection (Fig. 11–45).

In the mucosa of ileal reservoirs constructed in the treatment of colonic diseases such as familial adenomatous polyposis and ulcerative colitis, a variety of pathological changes have been observed. Chronic inflammation and varying degrees of villous atrophy are common. Pyloric metaplasia of the pouch is less common as is acute inflammation and ulceration or "pouchitis," which more commonly occurs in association with ulcerative colitis (Fig. 11–46). There appears to be no relationship between the presence of backwash ileitis and the subsequent complication of pouchitis in ulcerative colitis patients treated by ileal pouch anal anastomosis (Gustavsson, Weiland and Kelly 1987). Furthermore, in histochemical studies there is a change from small to large bowel mucin type (Shepherd et al 1987a). Johnson and White (1988) describe not only colonic metaplasia but the formation of adenomatous polyps. Seemingly even metaplastic colonic mucosa in such patients is prone to neoplastic change. In ileal mucosa chronically exposed to urine in reservoirs created following total cystectomy, changes vary from villous blunting and crypt hyperplasia to more severe atrophy of both villi and crypts, decreased epithelial height and even ulceration (Hockenstrom et al 1986).

Halphen et al (1989) describe a curious case of idiopathic villous atrophy of the ileum. The proximal half of the small intestine was quite normal. Accompanying the ileal lesion there was a vascular abnormality consisting of mucosal and submucosal glomeruloid collections of capillaries that contained occasional hyaline thrombi.

12

LYMPHOMA IN COELIAC DISEASE, UNRESPONSIVE, COLLAGENOUS AND ULCERATIVE COELIAC DISEASE, MEDITERRANEAN LYMPHOMA

LYMPHOMA IN COELIAC DISEASE

The association of abdominal lymphadenopathy and steatorrhoea has long been recognised and has been extensively reviewed (Kent 1964, Eidelman, Parkins and Rubin 1966). There seems no doubt that a generalised lymphoma with involvement of the bowel and/or abdominal lymph nodes can be associated with steatorrhoea (Sleisenger, Almy and Barr 1953), and that at least in some areas the mucosa shows the same histological lesion as in gluten-sensitive enteropathy (Selby and Gallagher 1979). This is probably non-specific, for a flat coeliac-like mucosa is sometimes, but not always, also seen in the intestine when there is lymphatic infiltration by other forms of malignancy (Figs. 12–1 to 12–3). Nevertheless, the view has been expressed that because of the marked variation in the clinical manifestations of gluten-sensitive enteropathy, the development of lymphoma may cause the patient to present for the first time with malabsorption (Cooper, Holmes and Cooke 1982). If there is still some doubt that primary abdominal lymphoma can cause mucosal atrophy and a malabsorption, there can be no doubt that longstanding gluten-sensitive enteropathy may be complicated by bowel or abdominal lymph node sarcoma (Austad et al 1967, Harris et al 1967, Swinson et al 1983). This was characterised as a reticulosarcoma by Whitehead (1968a), but in today's terminology this would be inclusive of any large cell lymphoma. The characterisation of this lesion in terms of actual subtype has been the subject of debate, and various claims have been made according to the methods used for typing the cells. Taylor (1976) included a number of the cases originally examined by Whitehead in a study that aimed to determine whether or not the cells of these lymphomas had surface immunoglobulins. All were positive and it was thought to indicate that the tumour possibly originated in B-type lymphocytes. This was of interest because of the claim that the development of the lymphoma could be traced to the cellular elements of the lamina propria of the bowel wall and the

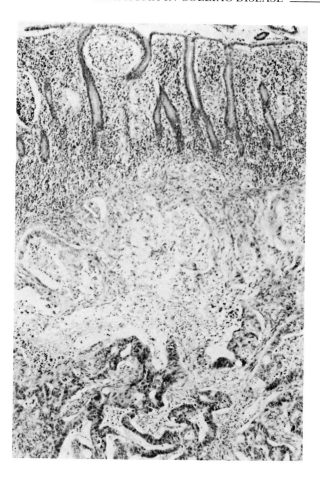

Figure 12–1. Flat jejunal mucosa overlying an infiltrating adenocarcinoma of colonic origin (H & E × 75).

regional lymph nodes and emerged through a stage of progressive hyperplasia (Whitehead 1968a). This process was seemingly characterised by a deterioration in the clinical picture, associated with recurrence of diarrhoea and a reversal of the response to gluten withdrawal, fever, weight loss, abdominal pain, and finger clubbing. In some cases there was a sustained rise in serum IgA levels, which occurred independently of whether there were disturbances in immunogobulins (Hobbs et al 1969) before the gluten-free diet was instituted earlier in the disease. Interestingly enough, two cases of lymphadenopathy associated with coeliac disease that regressed on a gluten exclusion diet have been described (Simmonds and Rosenthal 1981). The account of the histological appearances was unfortunately poor and so it is difficult to know if the lymphadenopathy was comparable to the progressive hyperplasia described by Whitehead (1968a), but it raised the possible reversibility of the condition should early diagnosis and treatment be instituted. Kavin (1981) describes a patient with coeliac disease complicated by non-specific ulceration of the small and large intestine and pronounced non-specific mesenteric lymphoid hyperplasia. The concept of a malignancy arising in hyperplasia is not new, because the neoplastic process is generally accepted as being a gradual stepwise alteration in the genome. Nevertheless, some part of the apparent lymphoid hyperplasia could conceivably be the result of a reactive infiltrate stimulated by the emerging malignant cells such as is postulated in Hodgkin's lymphoma. It is of interest that in a retrospective electron microscopic examination

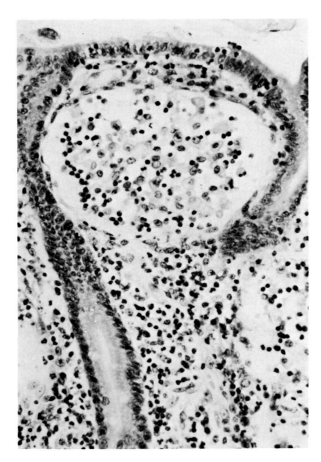

Figure 12–2. Detail of Figure 12–1. The epithelial surface is not greatly abnormal and there is a dilated lacteal centrally containing lymphocytes and histiocytes, which is an indication of lymphatic obstruction by the tumour infiltration (H & E × 600).

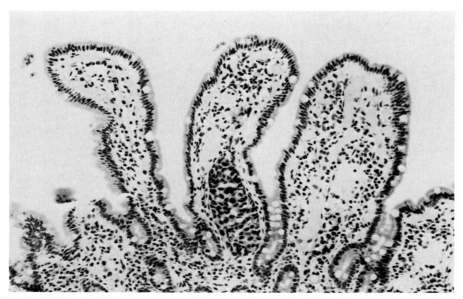

Figure 12–3. Duodenal mucosa with extensive lacteal permeation by malignant melanoma cells (H & E × 200).

of five patients with presumed coeliac disease who had a fatal outcome and in three who had a terminal lymphoma, occasional abnormal cells with features suspicious of malignancy were described (Horowitz and Shiner 1981).

Isaacson and Wright (1978) and Isaacson (1981) outlined claims that the lesion was a malignant histiocytosis based upon polyclonality of the cells for immuno-globulins and their possession of markers for histiocytes, particularly alpha-1-antitrypsin. Other workers did not support this claim (Otto et al 1981) and classified the tumour as of B lymphocyte origin and of immunoblastic type. That the lesion was a malignant histiocytosis prevailed for some time, owing to the insistence of Isaacson and coworkers (Isaacson et al 1982). However, there was evidence that malignant large cell lymphomas could be polyclonal (Curran and Jones 1979, Robinson et al 1980, Warnke et al 1980), and clonal switch from IgM to IgG synthesis by lymphoma has been described (Gordon and Smith 1980). On general grounds it seemed reasonable that the gene derepression, which occurs as part of the malignant process, could account for many of the apparently contradictory phenomena observed in these tumours, especially since by ordinary standards they appear poorly differentiated. Whereas a well-differentiated B cell tumour composed of plasma cells might predictably be monoclonal, a poorly differentiated B cell tumour might be polyclonal, and similar arguments could easily explain the loss or the acquisition of other proteins such as alpha-1-antitrypsin, which might lead to argument as to the histiocytic nature of the cells. However, despite having classified the tumour as malignant histiocytosis, Isaacson et al (1985) provided evidence for a T cell origin based upon their reaction with monoclonal antibodies against T lymphoid cell lines and a rearrangement of genes for the beta chain of the T-cell antigen receptor. Despite this and arguably to the detriment of the subject, this tumour was still being referred to as malignant histiocytosis long after 1985 (Mead et al 1987, Spencer et al 1989). There is evidence for a T cell origin from some workers (Loughran, Kadin and Deeg 1986, Spencer et al 1988), but others suggest that it is more likely a centroblastic B cell tumour (Nash, Gradwell and Day 1986), and some authors (Van der Valk, Lindeman and Meijer 1988) believe that the lymphoma complicating coeliac disease might be B cell, T cell or of histiocytic phenotype. It seems likely, as is being appreciated more widely in tumour biology generally, that the more that tumours are examined by increasing numbers of different antibodies the more diverse does their antigen expression become apparent. This probably reflects only the different degrees of alteration of the genome that are integral to the neoplastic process and underlines the claim that, increasingly, phenotyping needs to be based upon the use of large panels of antisera so that patterns rather than single antigen expression can be recognised (Norton and Isaacson 1989a,b). The one aspect of this lesion that is clear is its very malignant character and the fact that in coeliac patients it may arise not only in the small bowel in multifocal fashion (Freeman and Chiu 1986a) and related nodes, but elsewhere in the gastrointestinal tract, including the stomach (Roehrkasse et al 1986).

From a diagnostic point of view the jejunal biopsy may show features that together with the clinical and biochemical abnormalities allow a diagnosis to be strongly suspected. The usual finding is a flat mucosa with total villous atrophy and crypt hyperplasia that exhibits an obviously dense cellular infiltrate of the lamina propria (Fig. 12–4). The mucosa may be slightly thicker than normal, but it is the infiltrate that may be of diagnostic importance (Figure 12–5). Especially in those cases with an increased serum IgA there is a plasma cell component in obvious excess of that seen in an ordinary coeliac mucosa. Most plasma cells are in no way cytologically abnormal, and they occur in the company of lymphocytes

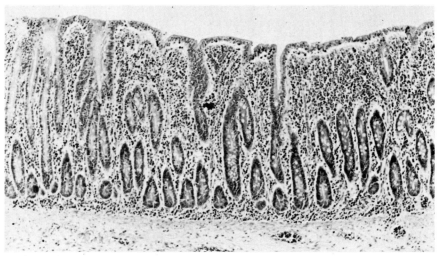

Figure 12–4. Jejunal biopsy in longstanding gluten-sensitive enteropathy in the stage of "progressive hyperplasia." Note the elongated crypts, total villous atrophy and extremely dense cellular infiltrate in the lamina propria (H & E × 75).

and eosinophils. Eosinophils are always more obvious in the deeper layers of the lamina and may be very conspicuous, so that they constitute a striking feature of the histological picture (Shepherd et al 1987a). A variable number of abnormal cells suspected of being malignant because of their cytological features may be found only with difficulty early in the course of this complication of coeliac disease. This has been confirmed by Isaacson (1980), who advocates that multiple biopsies are indicated and that serial section of the tissues should be obtained. Later the collections of cells are obvious and show a range of abnormality varying from

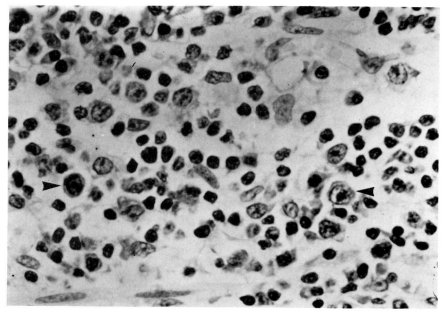

Figure 12–5. Detail of cellular infiltrate in Figure 12–4. Large lymphoid cells are obvious and some appear abnormal (arrowheads) (H & E × 450).

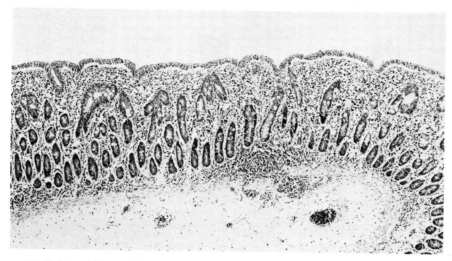

Figure 12–6. Jejunal biopsy in longstanding gluten-sensitive enteropathy in the stage of progressive hyperplasia. Note extension of the infiltrate through the muscularis mucosa (H & E × 75).

enlarged normal to frankly atypical and malignant. A characteristic feature is the tendency for these malignant cells to invade the epithelium of glands in small groups. It is these cells that subsequently increase in number at the expense of other cell types to produce the sarcomatous appearance. At this stage or even earlier in the disease, surface ulceration may occur, not only in the jejunum, but also in other areas of the gastrointestinal tract. The cellular infiltrate often extends below the muscularis mucosa, a feature that may be of value in biopsy material (Fig. 12–6). This infiltrate is frequently composed of cells similar to those in the non-malignant areas of the bowel, especially early in the disease when the frankly malignant cells are hard to find. Later, however, there is a clear malignant infiltration of the deeper aspects of the bowel mucosa.

The time that elapses between the stage of progressive hyperplasia and the development of sarcoma seems to vary between a few months and many years— in the cases seen by the author the longest was eight years. There is no doubt that many patients die in the phase of progressive hyperplasia from perforation of ulcers or intercurrent infection. In the case described by Kavin (1981) already referred to death followed an episode of intravascular coagulation. Infections are not infrequently of fungal type and probably reflect a disturbed immunological state, as postulated by Hobbs et al (1969). A suggestion that poor dietary control might increase the incidence of sarcoma was at first not substantiated by Holmes et al (1976). These authors reviewed all their 292 patients with coeliac disease and found that of the 43 deaths one third were due to "reticulosarcoma." After a longer follow-up, however, Holmes et al (1989) have now reported that a gluten-free diet does protect not only against lymphoma but also against other malignancies to which coeliac patients seem prone, e.g., cancers of the mouth, pharynx and oesophagus. An association between coeliac disease, splenic atrophy and cavitation of enlarged mesenteric nodes has been described (Matuchansky et al 1984). The so-called cavitation is in fact a hyalin or necrotic central area with peripheral nodal remains that are often hyperplastic. The association of splenic atrophy and small bowel lymphoma in coeliacs is well recognised (O'Grady, Stevens and McCarthy 1985), and a case of lymphoma, splenic atrophy and lymph node cavitation is also on record (Freeman and Chiu 1986b). One cannot help but postulate that these are all manifestations of the complex immune disturbance involved in longstanding gluten-sensitive enteropathy that involves lymphoid hyperplasia and subsequent atrophy or progression to sarcoma.

UNRESPONSIVE COELIAC DISEASE, MUCOSAL COLLAGENISATION AND ULCERATION

Weinstein et al (1970) described a case with typical jejunal morphology showing an initial response to dietary gluten exclusion, but subsequent relapse. This was followed by a steady deterioration despite a rigid gluten-free regime, and was associated with severe jejunal mucosal atrophy and deposition of collagen in the immediately subepithelial zone of the lamina propria. These authors called this lesion "collagenous sprue" and thought it was possibly a new and distinct entity. It seems more likely that it represents an end stage of gluten-sensitive enteropathy at a time when the mucosa can no longer respond to gluten exclusion.

Deposition of collagen under the enterocyte basement membrane in fact is not uncommon in mucosal biopsies showing severe partial or total villous atrophy, having been commented upon in some of the earliest observations on the jejunal morphology associated with steatorrhoea (Cooke et al 1963, Hourihane 1963). In this author's experience it is extremely rare in young children with gluten-sensitive enteropathy and is seen only in adults, especially those with a long history of disease (Fig. 12–7). Sometimes it is barely perceptible, other times obvious, and in sequential biopsies it may be seen to progress (Figs. 12–8, 12–9). When collagen deposition is marked, the mucosa shows a crypt hypoplastic appearance and sometimes Paneth cell deficiency, but the latter is not invariable. However, one thing common to all these cases is the much worse prognosis when compared to uncomplicated gluten-sensitive enteropathy. This was the conclusion of Bossart et al (1975), who, in a large series of 146 coeliac patients, noted subepithelial collagen in 36 per cent and concluded that although its presence when severe might indicate a poor prognosis, it did not represent a separate clinical entity.

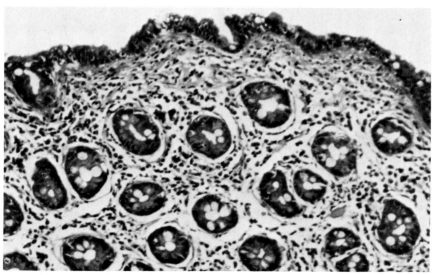

Figure 12–7. Jejunal biopsy in longstanding gluten-sensitive enteropathy. There is a thin layer of subepithelial collagen (H & E × 245).

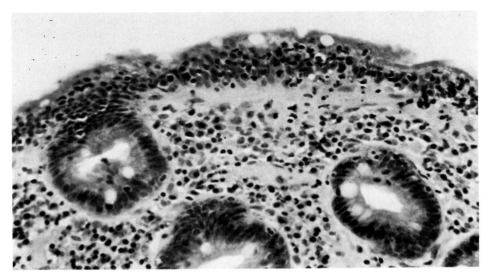

Figure 12–8. Progression (Figs. 12–8 and 12–9) in the deposition of subepithelial collagen in the jejunal mucosa of a patient with gluten-sensitive enteropathy who gradually became resistant to treatment. The biopsy in Figure 12–8 was taken three months before that in Figure 12–9 (H & E × 280).

Some cases give a clear history of gluten-sensitive disease becoming refractory, but others are unresponsive to gluten-exclusion diets at the time they present. This does not necessarily mean that they are fundamentally different. If, as many believe, gluten-sensitive enteropathy is an immune-mediated disease, one can draw an analogy with Hashimoto's disease of the thyroid. Low-grade non-goitrous Hashimoto's disease may first present as hypothyroidism at a time when the autoimmune process is no longer active and the thyroid is a tiny fibrous remnant showing marked epithelial atrophy. Low-grade or subclinical gluten-sensitive

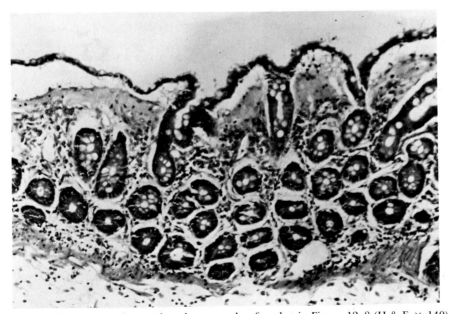

Figure 12–9. Biopsy specimen taken three months after that in Figure 12–8 (H & E × 140).

disease likewise may first present at a time when the mucosa is so atrophic that it can no longer respond to gluten-exclusion diets. Whatever the aetiology, ulceration may supervene and when it does there is usually a fatal outcome, for, although evidence of healing may be seen in surgical or autopsy material, the ulceration is always recurrent.

An interesting association of collagenous colitis (see later) and severe partial duodenal villous atrophy with subepithelial collagen deposition has also been described (Eckstein, Dowsett and Riley 1988). It is probably too early to speculate that there is some form of relationship between collagenous colitis and gluten-sensitive enteropathy.

Some cases referred to as chronic ulcerative jejunitis (Bayless et al 1967, Jeffries, Steinberg and Sleisenger 1968, Moritz, Moran and Patterson 1971, Gouffier et al 1977) are also considered by some to be related to coeliac disease, although the position is far from clear. While it is plain that ulceration can occur in proven coeliac disease (Thompson 1976), it is less certain whether chronic ulcerative jejunitis exists as a separate entity comparable to non-specific ileal ulceration in patients who do not have coeliac disease or some other primary disease, e.g., a vasculitis. One of the four cases described by Jeffries, Steinberg and Sleisenger (1968) developed a "reticulosarcoma" of the bowel and elsewhere after the excision of an ulcerated segment of small bowel.

The case reported by Barry, Morris and Read (1970) associated with hyperglobulinaemia and the cases of Hourihane and Weir (1970) with focal intestinal lymphoma, although not gluten sensitive at the time of presentation, tempt one to the view that these and similar cases represent an end stage in a complex immune-mediated disease. This is manifested by a failure to maintain the structure of the intestinal mucosa and leads to ulceration and, as in other immune-mediated disease of long standing, sarcoma may develop. The view that ulceration is always a manifestation of early lymphoma development is held by Isaacson (1980), but Kavin (1981) describes a case in which the ulceration seems to have occurred at the stage of lymphoid hyperplasia. This author has experience of similar cases in which at presentation the patient has a flat mucosa with a dense lymphoplasmacytic infiltrate that is not cytologically malignant (Figs. 12–10, 12–11). There are multiple ulcers of the mucosa and the lesion is non-responsive to a gluten-free diet. It could be argued that this represents a clinical presentation of occult gluten-sensitive enteropathy due to ulceration at a time when the disease is no longer responsive to gluten exclusion. However, Robertson et al (1983) in a study of eight cases conclude that small bowel ulceration of this type is a spectrum of disorders with an inconsistent relationship to gluten sensitivity and small intestinal lymphoma; Jewell (1983) reaches the same conclusion.

However, it is only in sequential jejunal biopsies over many years in all patients with proven coeliac disease, and in particular those with a recent change in clinical picture, that early diagnosis of these conditions will be possible and a better understanding of the exact relationships between gluten-sensitive enteropathy, so-called chronic ulcerative jejunitis, and intestinal lymphoma complicating steatorrhoea will be gained. It seems possible that at least some of these cases are more closely related to immunoproliferative small intestinal disease (IPSID) (see later). The doubts that some have of the relationship of these lymphomas to preexisting coeliac disease has also led them to suggest that it is the lymphoma that causes the mucosal changes (Hall et al 1988). Thus the term "enteropathy-associated T cell lymphoma" is sometimes used to describe such lesions (Isaacson and Spencer 1987).

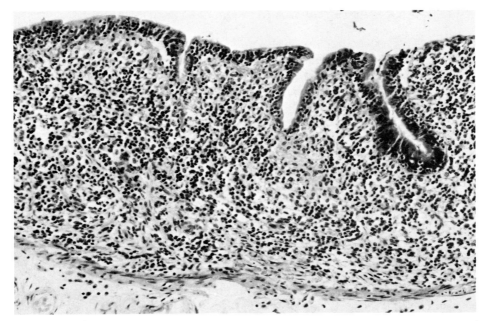

Figure 12–10. Jejunal biopsy in a patient non-responsive to a gluten exclusion diet at time of presentation. Multiple mucosal ulcers were also present. Note the density of the infiltrate (H & E × 150).

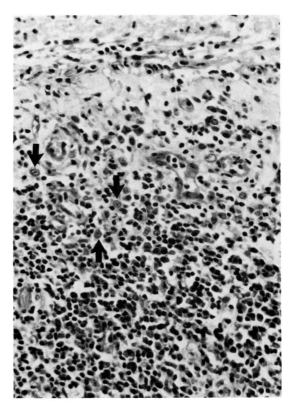

Figure 12–11. Detail of base of an ulcer in the same case depicted in Figure 12–10. Apart from lymphocytes and plasma cells there are scattered immunoblasts with central nucleoli (arrows), but no definitive indications of malignancy (H & E × 500).

MEDITERRANEAN LYMPHOMA (ALPHA-CHAIN DISEASE)

Non-Ashkenazi Jews and Israeli Arabs were shown to be particularly prone to the development of a primary small-intestinal and regional node lymphoma associated with a malabsorption syndrome (Eidelman, Parkins and Rubin 1966). The disease was characterised not only by the youth of the patients but also by the more or less diffuse nature of the intestinal involvement. Later it became clear that the disease also occurred in many other parts of the world. In a publication of five new cases and a review of previous literature, Doe et al (1972) commented that it was seen not only in the Middle East and North Africa but also in Colombia, Argentina, Cambodia, South Africa, Bangladesh, Greece, Pakistan and Iran; however, it is still extremely rare in Western countries.

It has been suggested that intestinal infection, possibly parasitic, may be the common factor in these patients, providing a stimulus for the excessive proliferation of IgA synthesising plasma cells (Seligmann, Mihaesco and Frangione 1971). Doe et al (1972) used electron microscopy to confirm that most cells in the infiltrate were plasma cells, but in one of their cases the cells were intermediate between plasma cells and lymphocytes. The cytoplasmic features were typical of the former, but the nuclei typical of the latter. In another ultrastructural study (Crow and Asselah 1984), the early stages of the disease were found to be characterised by immature plasma cells while later the cells had immunoblastic features. In some of the patients reported, excessive amounts of the heavy chains of immunoglobulin IgA have been identified in the blood, urine and intestinal juice (Rambaud et al 1968, Doe et al 1972). The condition has thus come to be known as alpha-chain disease and does not appear to be related to gluten-sensitive enteropathy. Further evidence (Brouet et al 1977) confirmed that the condition is basically an immunoblastic lymphoma and that a proportion of cases are associated with specific globulin synthesis and secretion. In some cases the same pathology is not accompanied by secretion of IgA heavy chains, and the term immunoproliferative small-intestinal disease (IPSID) was coined (World Health Organisation Meeting Report 1976). However, the alpha chain may be present in jejunal juice or at a cellular level even if it does not circulate (Hibi et al 1982, Rambaud et al 1983, Asselah et al 1983, Salem et al 1987). Khojasteh, Haghshenass and Haghighi (1983) have claimed that the production of the alpha heavy chain protein is more likely to occur in the earlier, better differentiated stages of the disease, although Gilinsky et al (1985) concluded that not all cases of IPSID either elaborate detectable alpha heavy chain or evolve into a lymphoma. McDonald et al (1985) describe a similar group of cases whose clinical course was characterised by intestinal pseudo-obstruction. Galian et al (1977) recognise three stages in its development: Stage A is morphologically plasmacytic; Stage C an immunoblastic sarcoma; and Stage B a transitional stage between A and C. All stages arise from the same clone of cells, but the development of the stages is not synchronous for the different sites of involvement. The authors therefore propose a staging laparotomy in order to determine the best form of treatment. The importance of jejunal biopsy in the diagnosis of this disorder is stressed (Nasr et al 1976, Helmy 1980), and areas involved show a dense cellular infiltrate of the lamina propria with cells distinctly plasmacytic or less characteristically so, and sometimes appearing as large undifferentiated cells. These cells may dominate the histological picture, especially late in the course of the disease. The villous pattern is also abnormal, but this is probably secondary to the cellular infiltration. It takes the form of shortening of villi, which appear bloated and deformed, and the epithelial abnormalities seen in gluten-sensitive enteropathy are usually absent. The cellular infiltrate is so

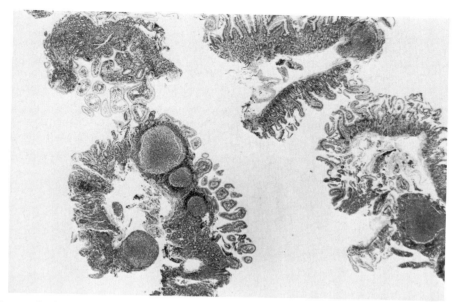

Figure 12–12. Multiple distal duodenal biopsies showing clear evidence of a nodular lymphoid lesion (H & E × 50).

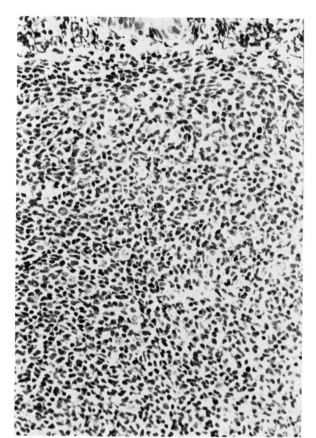

Figure 12–13. Detail of lymphoid nodules showing atypical morphology of the malignant lymphoid cells (H & E × 500).

dense that it also alters the crypt pattern, tending to push them farther apart. In the later stages the villous pattern is lost more or less completely as the lamina becomes packed with cellular elements. Although recovery following treatment is described (Manousos et al 1974, Doe 1975, Gilinsky, Chaimowitz and Van Staden 1986), complete or prolonged remissions probably occur only in the early plasmacytic stage of the disease (Galian et al 1977, Monges et al 1975, 1980). The diagnostic value of upper intestinal fibreoptic endoscopy in this disease has already been demonstrated (Halphen et al 1986). A quite distinct condition is multiple lymphomatous polyposis (Figs. 12–12, 12–13). This is another B cell neoplasm that has also been diagnosed by endoscopic biopsy (Fernandes, Amato and Goldfinger 1985, Stessens et al 1986).

PARASITIC DISEASES

13

GIARDIASIS

Although there is some controversy over the actual pathogenicity of *Giardia lamblia*, it has long been recognised that a heavy infestation can cause disturbance of intestinal function (Petersen 1972, Raizman 1976). When there are sufficient organisms to be seen in a jejunal biopsy specimen, infestation can be presumed to be heavy, and under such circumstances the organisms are capable of producing both diarrhoea and malabsorption. Population groups who are not normally exposed to infection may exhibit an illness of epidemic proportions on first contact with the organism (Lancet 1974), and giardiasis is a well-recognised complication of hypogammaglobulinaemia (Webster 1980). Kamath and Murugasu (1974), in a study comparing four different methods of identifying *Giardia*, found examination of biopsy impression smears to be superior to stool examination, duodenal aspiration examination and examination of processed and sectioned jejunal biopsy. Eastham, Douglas and Watson (1976), however, found biopsy examination to be superior to examination of mucosal imprint. Individual expertise in recognising the organisms in either preparation probably plays a part in the success rate. A technique applied to tissue sections utilising the immunoperoxidase method and specific antisera has also been utilized (Fleck, Hames and Warhurst 1985). The further evaluation of an immunofluorescent test is indicated, using patients' sera and *Giardia lamblia* cysts as antigen (Ridley and Ridley 1976).

In ordinary H & E preparations the vegetative forms appear as grey, flattened, pear-shaped structures (Fig. 13–1), bilaterally symmetrical and 10 to 18 μm in length. The organism has two nuclei that can be identified at light microscope level when seen "en face." Eight flagellae are arranged in pairs, and ventrally the organism has a sucking disc, but these and others of its finer structures can be appreciated only by electron microscopy (Fig. 13–2). Claims that the protozoon can invade the surface epithelium (Morecki and Parker 1967) and the lamina propria (Brandborg et al 1967) have not been substantiated by other workers, and this invasion has never been seen by the author in human or in experimental animal material, despite a careful search in serial preparations stained by the method advocated by Brandborg et al or in material examined by electron microscopy.

The latest claim purporting to have demonstrated mucosal invasion is by Saha and Ghosh (1977). A careful appraisal of their illustrations does not reveal convincing proof. Two of the photomicrographs show parasites in close proximity to discharging goblet cells and this has been misinterpreted as evidence of invasion. Indeed, in one of these instances the collapsed goblet cell is identified as an

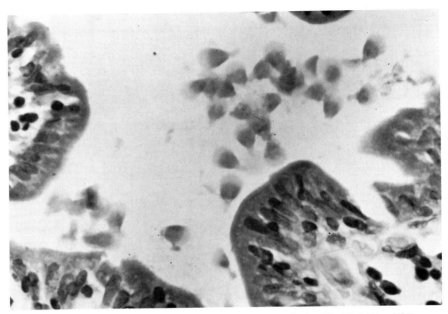

Figure 13–1. Jejunal biopsy showing vegetative *Giardia lamblia* (H & E × 525).

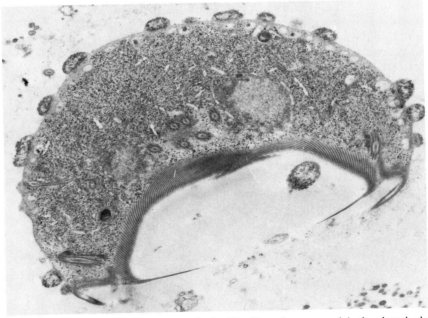

Figure 13–2. Electron micrograph of *Giardia lamblia*. Note the two nuclei, the dorsal phagocytic vesicles and the ventral sucking disc with which the organism probably attaches itself to the microvillous layer (× 7000).

intramucosal parasite, and a further parasite tail-on to the discharging mucin is identified as being in the process of entering the track made by the first. It is pertinent that the authors find no tissue reaction to the so-called invasive *Giardia*, and their interpretation is regarded by this author as fanciful. However, remnants of *Giardia muris* have been described in macrophages within Peyer's patches in a mouse experimental model of giardiasis (Owen, Allen and Stevens 1981).

Even in the heaviest of infestations the jejunal mucosa shows only a minimal degree of villous atrophy of crypt hyperplastic type, with a slight but definite increase in inflammatory cells in the lamina (Fig. 13–3). A high proportion of these are often eosinophil polymorphs. In a quantitative study Wright and Tomkins (1978) were able to show a correlation between decrease in surface area and impairment of absorptive functions. If *Giardia* are seen in association with a villous atrophy comparable to that in untreated gluten-sensitive enteropathy, a coexisting pathology should be suspected (see Chapter 14), although rarely does it occur. Rosekrans, Lindeman and Meijer (1981) have stressed that increased numbers of IgA, as opposed to IgM plasma cells that occur in coeliac disease, are of differential diagnostic importance.

Several theories have been postulated to explain how *Giardia* exert their deleterious effect on the intestinal mucosa. It has been suggested that they damage the microvilli of absorptive epithelial cells of the mucosa (Balazs and Szatloczky 1978), or that there is a significant nutritional competition between host and parasite. The evidence for the view that *Giardia* cause actual damage to the epithelial cells is not convincing (Owen, Nemanic and Stevens 1979), but when present in large numbers the organisms may cause a mechanical blockade of the mucosa (Barbieri et al 1970). The parasite attaches itself to the microvillous surface of the absorptive cells via its ventral suction disc, and feeds through its dorsal surface. As the microvillous layer is the site of most of the digestive enzymes, it is entirely feasible that in heavy infestation enough of the microvillous layer of the small intestine is covered by parasites to prevent interaction of digestive enzymes and luminal substrate.

The mechanism of malabsorption in giardiasis has also been studied by Tandon

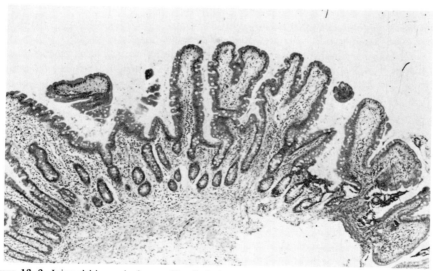

Figure 13–3. Jejunal biopsy in heavy *Giardia* infestation. There is slight villous atrophy with crypt hyperplasia. Giardia are just visible in the intervillous spaces (H & E × 75).

et al (1977), who showed that steatorrhoea and D-xylose malabsorption in infected patients was significantly correlated with evidence of jejunal bacterial overgrowth, and that the malabsorption was related to bile-salt deconjugation as in the stagnant loop syndrome (Gorbach and Tabaqchali 1969). Anand et al (1980), using an experimental model in rats, concluded that *Giardia* trophozoites in some way interfere with the active transport mechanisms of the enterocytes, and Gillon, Thamery and Ferguson (1982) in another mouse model postulate a direct toxic or irritant effect of the parasite on the brush border of the enterocyte.

In a review of the pathogenesis of the diarrhoea and malabsorption secondary to giardiasis, Halliday and Farthing (1986) list the mucosal damage, bacterial overgrowth and both bile-salt uptake and deconjugation by the organism as the important factors. More recently, however, Inge, Edson and Farthing (1988) have demonstrated that *Giardia* possess a surface membrane mannose binding lectin. There are appropriate binding sites on intestinal epithelial cells, at least in the rat, and having attached to the cells, the *Giardia* are set to interfere with the cells' function.

HOOKWORM DISEASE

Ankylostomiasis is caused by two hookworms, *Ankylostoma duodenale* and *Necator americanus*. The adult worm lives in the intestine, and the eggs that are passed develop in soil into infective filariform larvae. These invade the venous system by penetrating the skin and lodge in the lungs. They then migrate via the trachea and oesophagus to the intestine where they mature into adults, attaching themselves to the mucosa where each worm consumes as much as 0.5 ml of blood daily (Meyers, Naefie and Connor 1976). In developing countries it is a fairly common infestation. Chavalittamrong and Jirapinyo (1984), for example, found infestation in 2 per cent of a paediatric population investigated for diarrhoea in Thailand.

In addition to causing iron deficiency anaemia, it is claimed that hookworm infestation can also result in a malabsorption syndrome with steatorrhoea (Sheehy et al 1962). Disturbance of small-intestinal function probably occurs only with an extremely heavy infestation. It is only in this group that morphological abnormalities occur. In the author's personal material these have consisted of crypt hyperplasia and mild to moderate villous atrophy characterised by stunted, branched, and leaf-shaped villi and few ridges. Exactly how much of this abnormality is related to the infestation and how much is simply a reflection of, for example, racial variation will be determined only on follow-up studies on patients who have been successfully treated. Occasionally one observes circular spaces in the mucosa (Fig. 13–4) that represent the channels in which the adult worms lie, and there may be erosions of the superficial epithelium that are presumably the sites where the worms attach themselves to the mucosa via their mouth parts. In the lamina propria it is usual to see an increase in inflammatory cells, and particularly in relation to the circular channels and erosions there is often a conspicuous eosinophil leukocyte element.

STRONGYLOIDIASIS

Strongyloides stercoralis has a life cycle similar to the hookworm, but the eggs hatch in the bowel and some undergo a metamorphosis into infective larvae and penetrate the gut wall so that an endogenous cycle is established. This is called

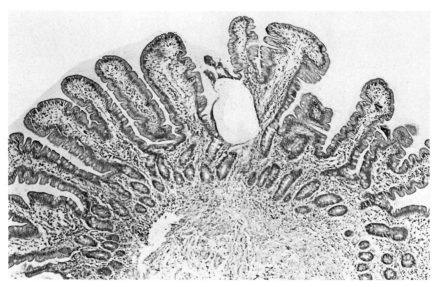

Figure 13–4. Jejunal biopsy in heavy hookworm infestation. Note the cellular infiltrate, mild villous atrophy and crypt hyperplasia, and the obvious circular channel in the mucosa (H & E × 75).

autoinfestation and accounts for the persistence of the parasite, even when the patient has left the area where the infestation was acquired, and also for the hyperinfestation syndrome.

Diarrhoea and malabsorption syndrome are not infrequent complications of *Strongyloides stercoralis* infestation, although it is more usually symptomless (de Paola, Dias and da Silva 1962). The infestation invariably results in a transient duodenojejunitis, but rarely the whole bowel may be involved in severe cases due to autoinfection; an uncommon complication is paralytic ileus (Cookson et al 1972). Secondary gram-negative septicaemia and *Escherichia coli* meningitis have also been described (Smallman et al 1986). A jejunal biopsy may reveal crypt hyperplasia and a varying degree of villous atrophy associated with an inflammatory infiltrate of the lamina propria. Distortion of crypts and erosions of the epithelium can be clearly related to the presence of adult worms, rhabditiform larvae, and ova (Figs. 13–5 to 13–7). The ova characteristically embed themselves in the crypt walls, and within the lumen of the crypts the larval forms can be seen. The jejunal morphology would appear to be the direct result of the presence of parasites, since in treated cases the villous pattern returns to normal (Bras et al 1964). Da Costa (1971) has shown a high turnover rate of intestinal epithelial cells in this condition. Hyperinfection with *Strongyloides stercoralis* may also occur in states of altered immunity such as malignant lymphoma (Adam et al 1973). Humans are the main host for *Strongyloides stercoralis*; a second species, *Strongyloides fulleborni*, is a natural parasite of monkeys, humans being secondarily infected. *Strongyloides fulleborni* more commonly affects human infants than adults.

CAPILLARIASIS

Whalen et al (1969) have described an infestation in humans of epidemic proportions by a species of the roundworm *Capillaria*. Occurring in the Philippines, the disease took the form of severe painful diarrhoea associated with protein-

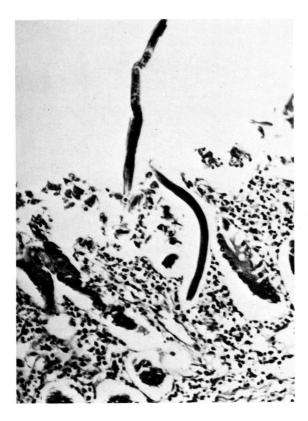

Figure 13–5. Strongyloidiasis. Adult worms (H & E × 120).

losing enteropathy and malabsorption. Jejunal biopsies showed moderate to severe mucosal abnormalities with villous atrophy and inflammatory infiltration of the lamina propria. These changes, however, were no more marked than in controls. In about half the cases examined *Capillaria* worms were found to have penetrated beneath the superficial mucosa. In postmortem material on one of the original epidemic cases, which has been made available to me by Professor Marcial-Rojas of the Puerto Rico Medical School, eggs were found after a search within the small-intestinal crypts, but in contrast to those in strongyloidiasis they did not appear to embed themselves in the mucosa (Fig. 13–8).

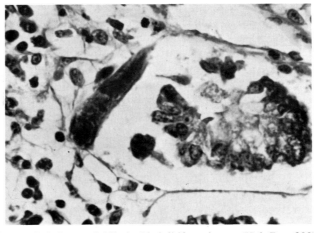

Figure 13–6. Strongyloidiasis. Rhabditiform larvae (H & E × 300).

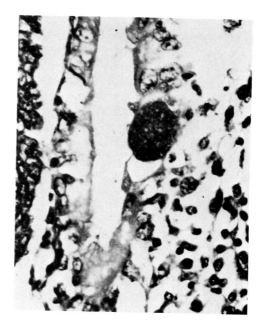

Figure 13–7. Strongyloidiasis. Eggs in jejunal mucosa (H & E × 300).

COCCIDIOSIS

Reviewing the literature and describing six new cases, Brandborg, Goldberg and Breidenbach (1970) produced evidence that human infection with the protozoan *Isospora belli* may produce diarrhoea and steatorrhoea. There is a simple direct transmission cycle in humans, but a related organism producing a similar

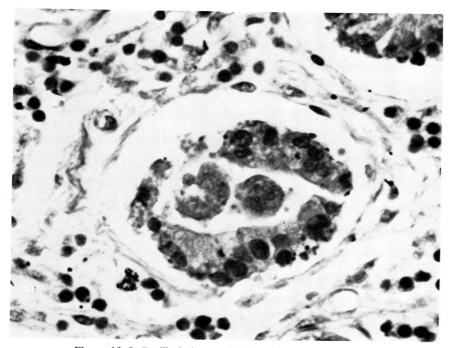

Figure 13–8. Capillariasis: eggs in jejunal crypt (H & E × 375).

illness, *Isospora hominis*, has man as the definitive host and the cow or pig as obligative intermediate hosts (Knight and Wright 1978). The jejunal biopsy changes apparently vary from slight villous abnormality with clubbing to a flat mucosa with an increased cellular infiltrate of the lamina propria. Parasites in all stages of endogenous development are observed within the epithelial cells and rarely in the lamina propria and submucosa. Ingested oocysts penetrate the epithelial cells and undergo progressive cyclical development. Recognition of the merozoites, schizonts and gametocytes is facilitated using a combination of staining procedures, including Giemsa, in addition to H & E. In a guinea pig model of the disease the cellular localisation and the structural analysis of the absorptive cell-parasite membrane interactions have been described in detail in an electron microscopic study (Marcial and Madara 1986). The authors also state that, in the guinea pig at least, although *cryptosporidia* are confined to the apex of absorptive cells in the region of Peyer's patches, they can be seen in macrophages subjacent to overlying M cells. This suggests that cryptosporidial antigens may be sampled by the lymphoid cells in these sites.

Human coccidiosis has hitherto been considered rare, but it may be responsible for many cases of undiagnosed malabsorption. However, there is a distinct possibility that the parasitisation in some cases is coincidental. For example, Henry, Bird and Doe (1974) reported a single case of coccidiosis arising in association with alpha-chain disease. The organisms were identified by electron microscopy and occurred within the epithelial cell cytoplasm.

Human infection with a related organism in the coccidia group, *Cryptosporidium*, has also been recorded (Nime et al 1976), and sometimes it has occurred as a complicaton of hypogammaglobulinaemia (Meisel et al 1976, Lasser, Lewin and Ryning 1979). Weinstein et al (1981) describe coexistent cryptosporidiosis and cytomegalovirus infection. Tzipori et al (1982) have transferred cryptosporidiosis from an adult human to newborn lambs, using faecal extracts. Current et al (1983) have claimed that infection of immunocompetent humans with *Cryptosporidium* may be more common then hitherto suspected, especially for those in contact with infected animals. A case is made for the screening of all patients with acute diarrhoea for the organism (Biggs et al 1987); in developing countries *Cryptosporidium* appears to be a major pathogen being isolated from 13.5 per cent of children hospitalised for diarrhoea (Sallon et al 1988). The incidence in countries with a higher standard of living, however, is very low, and the disease seems to be limited largely to the immunocompromised (Marshall et al 1987). At light microscope level the organism appears as round or oval bodies, 2–3 μ in diameter applied to the surface of the epithelial cells. They are weakly basophilic in H & E preparations and are better demonstrated in Giemsa preparations. A periodic acid–Schiff stain will demonstrate the cyst wall. At electron microscopy the organism appears to be incorporated into the apex of the cell and is covered by the surface membrane. In this site various stages in the life cycle of the parasite can be recognised (Bird and Smith 1980).

SCHISTOSOMIASIS

There are sporadic reports of schistosomal (*Schistosoma mansoni*) involvement of the upper small intestine (Sadek 1965, Sherif 1970). The organism most likely to affect the small intestine is *Schistosoma japonicum*. Ova and a secondary inflammatory infiltration occur in the mucosa (Contractor et al 1988), but whether these changes are always or ever associated with malabsorption seems not to have been ascertained. The jejunal mucosa has been examined in detail in 100 patients with schistosomiasis (Castro et al 1971). Light microscopy sections and mucosal crush preparations for the identification of schistosomal elements showed that the villous pattern did not differ from that seen in a comparable control group. It also revealed that the mucosal crush preparations were superior to routine histological section procedures in the study of involvement of the small intestine in schistosomiasis. Jejunal biopsy specimens are poor indicators of schistosomal infestation in patients excreting eggs (Halstead, Sheir and Raasch 1969), although occasional cases are recorded (Witham and Mosser 1979) when upper small bowel biopsy has shown eggs when they were not found in the faeces.

LEISHMANIASIS

In a study of jejunal function and morphology in visceral leishmaniasis, Muigai et al (1983) described mucosal abnormalities. In heavy infestation crypt hyperplasia and partial villous atrophy were seen, but the striking feature was the presence of parasites, both free and within histiocytes in the lamina propria, especially in the tips of villi. They were also seen in the submucosa.

14

MISCELLANEOUS CONDITIONS

IMMUNE DEFICIENCY

The morphological abnormalities that may occur in the jejunum of patients with immune deficiency syndromes are reviewed by Doe (1979) and Ament (1985). These are distinct from the wide range of morphological abnormalities that may be associated with lymphopenia and low levels of gamma globulin and albumin due to excessive loss from the intestine or urinary tract (Waldmann 1970). Sometimes serum IgG is low when IgA and IgM are normal, which reflects its considerably slower rate of synthesis. Small bowel biopsy may prove helpful in the diagnosis of these latter states if the lesion is diffuse or if it involves a sufficient length of the small intestine. In intestinal lymphangiectasia and Whipple's disease, for example, the biopsy will show typical features (see later), and the low levels of IgM (Hobbs and Hepner 1968) and IgA (Crabbe and Heremans 1967) that can occur in gluten-sensitive enteropathy will be associated with the morphological abnormalities that are usual for that condition. Malignancy, especially the lymphomas and myeloma, may decrease the competency of the immune mechanism, as may steroid and cytotoxic therapy. Whenever this occurs, the gastrointestinal tract is likely to be the site of lesions produced by an increased susceptibility to infections by a wide spectrum of pathogens, bacterial, fungal and viral. Small bowel biopsy may be helpful in the diagnosis of these.

Diarrhoea and malabsorption syndrome can complicate primary hypogammaglobulinaemia of both congenital and acquired type (Barandun, Riva and Spengler 1968), but their severity can vary from case to case. This may be in part due to the variation that occurs between local concentrations of immunoglobulin and those circulating in the serum. Another factor is the compensatory expansion in secretory IgM capacity in some patients (Nagura, Kohler and Brown 1979). The classification of the immunodeficiencies given by Good et al (1968) has been expanded considerably, and there are increasing reports of gastrointestinal disturbances associated with immunological deficiency in the paediatric age group.

B Lymphocyte Abnormalities

In infantile X-linked hypogammaglobulinaemia (Bruton type), small intestinal biopsy usually shows only sparsity or absence of lamina propria plasma cells (Fudenberg et al 1970). Villous architecture is usually normal, but Rhee et al

(1975) have described a case with villous atrophy and intramucosal bacteria. In X-linked immunodeficiency with elevated or normal IgM apart from oesophageal candidiasis, intestinal cryptosporidiosis is described (Vanderhoof et al 1977). Ament (1985) also records moderate to severe crypt hyperplastic villous atrophy in immunodeficiency associated with hyperglobulinaemia. There was a noticeable increase in lamina propria plasma cells, and rotavirus infection was the putative cause. Common variable hypogammaglobulinaemia is usually sporadic, but some familial cases appear to be inherited in an autosomal recessive manner. Small intestinal abnormalities in this condition are not uncommon. Some have abnormality of brush border enzymes comparable to those that occur in the tropical malabsorption syndrome (Dawson et al 1986). A minority show crypt hyperplastic villous atrophy and may have a severe coexistent *Giardia lamblia* infestation. *Giardia* infestation is fairly common in the absence of villous changes but may be associated with dissaccharidase deficiencies. When villous abnormality and giardiasis coexist, an improvement in villous architecture is said to follow specific anti-*Giardia* therapy (Ament and Rubin 1972). In those with a serious mucosal lesion comparable to that seen in coeliac disease, it is only rarely responsive to a gluten exclusion diet (Frexinos et al 1979). Webster et al (1981), however, describe another such case with relapse of the mucosal lesion following gluten challenge. Whatever the state of the villous pattern in this condition the lamina propria contains few or no plasma cells, the predominant cell type being a small lymphocyte (Fig. 14–1). Nodular lymphoid hyperplasia also occurs in a proportion of these patients (see later).

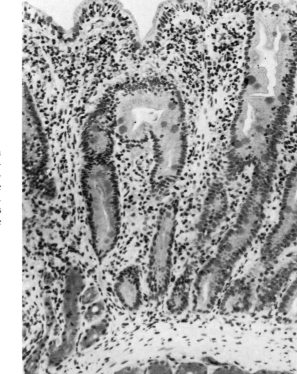

Figure 14–1. Duodenal biopsy in a patient with acquired hypogamma-globulinaemia. There is crypt hyperplastic villous atrophy and an absence of plasma cells in the lamina propria. Note that the superficial epithelium is relatively normal. No *Giardia* were present (H & E × 250).

In selective IgA deficiency, which is the commonest primary immunodeficiency in humans, the majority of patients suffer no significant disability. This may reflect that the lack of IgA is compensated by an increase in secretory IgM, although in some cases serum levels of IgA may not reflect either the mucosal levels or its functional capacity. Diarrhoea and steatorrhoea are the commonest intestinal manifestations and may be due to cow's milk intolerance, disaccharidase deficiency, giardiasis or gluten-sensitive enteropathy. The frequency of coeliac disease in selective IgA deficiency is some ten times that in the population at large. The mucosal lesion is identical to that seen in the usual form of the disease, except that IgA-containing cells, as demonstrated by immunohistochemical methods, are absent or few in number. It has been suggested that in the absence of local IgA, bowel antigens enter the intestine unimpeded and thus predispose to the acquisition of gluten sensitivity.

In transient IgA deficiency and isolated secretory piece deficiency, diarrhoea is a frequent complication, probably as a result of intestinal infection. It could be predicted that the mucosa in such circumstances would show non-specific inflammatory changes and villous atrophy. In a study conducted by Perlmutter et al (1985) some 50 per cent of 55 infants with low IgG levels and chronic diarrhoea showed a crypt hyperplastic villous atrophy varying from mild to severe.

T Lymphocyte Abnormalities

In congenital thymic aplasia (Di George syndrome) the lamina propria of the small intestine is devoid of all lymphoid cells (Dubois et al 1970), and any follicular collections are atrophic and have no germinal centres. Diarrhoea may occur but is rarely severe and sometimes is due to lactose deficiency (Ament, Ochs and Davis 1973).

In chronic mucocutaneous candidiasis no distinctive intestinal lesion is described, but oesophageal involvement may lead to strictures.

Combined B and T Lymphocyte Abnormalities

In infants suffering from severe combined immunodeficiency both T and B lymphocyte function is compromised. The jejunal mucosa may reveal stunting of villi and oedema of the lamina propria, but the striking feature is the presence of PAS-positive macrophages in the lamina propria (Doe 1979). They are not unlike the macrophages also seen in Waldenstrom's macroglobulinaemia (see later). Death results early from respiratory tract infection and malnutrition.

Diarrhoea and malabsorption may be a clinical feature in Nezelof's syndrome, ataxia telangiectasia, the short-limbed dwarfism syndrome, and the Wiskott-Aldrich syndrome, but the morphological basis for this is not known.

Chronic Granulomatous Disease

In this disease there is an inherited defect of neutrophil and macrophage function so that they are unable to kill catalase-positive organisms. Diarrhoea and steatorrhoea occur commonly, and intestinal biopsy shows a normal villous structure with PAS-positive macrophages at the tips of villi. Ament and Ochs (1973) also record the presence of lipofuscin in some of the macrophages and note that there is a generalised reticulo-endothelial hyperplasia in this disease.

Nodular Lymphoid Hyperplasia

Hypogammaglobulinaemia and nodular lymphoid hyperplasia, first described in detail by Hermans et al (1966), are characterised by a very low or absent IgA and IgM and a decreased IgG. There is a susceptibility to infections, particularly in the respiratory tract; diarrhoea, which may or may not be associated with steatorrhoea; and nodular hyperplasia of the lymphoid elements of the small and sometimes the large intestine. The small intestine also invariably harbours the parasite *Giardia lamblia*. Ajdukiewicz, Youngs and Bouchier (1972), describing a patient, also reviewed the literature on this condition, which up to the time of their report contained 22 other cases. The jejunal biopsy specimen (Figs. 14–2 and 14–3) may show a nodular mucosal appearance visible to the naked eye. The nodules vary between 1 and 4 mm, and histologically are composed of normal immature cells and scattered pale histiocytes containing nuclear debris. The case illustrated here did not reveal an increased mitotic rate in the follicles, although this was reported by Hermans et al (1966). The margin of the germinal centre is characterised by an abrupt edge next to a very thin layer of compressed small lymphocytes. Beyond the follicles the cellular component of the lamina propria shows a virtual absence of plasma cells, but a very painstaking search may reveal occasional examples. Although not reported by Hermans et al in their material, the lamina propria shows a patchy and slight increase in eosinophil polymorphonuclear leukocytes. The villous pattern remains basically normal except over the follicles, where the villi are stunted or absent (as is usual even over normal follicles), and even in the biopsy tissues most cases show numerous vegetative *Giardia lamblia*, both in relation to the surface epithelium and in the crypts.

It has been postulated (Webster et al 1977) that nodular lymphoid hyperplasia is a secondary phenomenon in association with hypogammaglobulinaemia and represents a local immune response to antigens originating in the gut lumen. Macroscopically similar lymphoid hyperplasia also occurs in the small intestine unassociated with hypogammaglobulinaemia. It is probably a reactive phenomenon and has been seen by the author associated with caecal carcinoma. In infants,

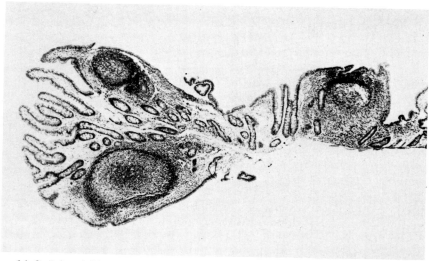

Figure 14–2. Jejunal biopsy, nodular lymphoid hyperplasia with hypogammaglobulinaemia (H & E × 43).

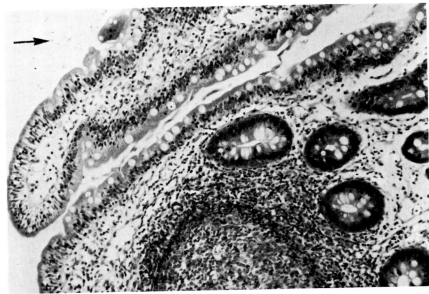

Figure 14–3. Detail of Figure 14–2. Note the germinal centre, its clean-cut margin bounded by small lymphocytes and *Giardia* (arrow) just discernible in the intervillous space (H & E × 175).

Atwell, Bunge and Wright (1985) have ascribed its occurrence to echovirus and adenovirus infection. Shaw and Hennigar (1974) describe its occurrence as a non-specific benign entity and in association with lymphoma in other parts of the lymphoid system.

As more cases are described it is becoming clear that nodular lymphoid hyperplasia is not a distinct clinical entity. As a benign condition it is seen as an apparent reaction to small-intestinal malignant lymphoma in the absence of hypogammaglobulinaemia (Matuchansky et al 1980) or in association with it (Lamers et al 1980) and in patients with coexistent giardiasis who have normal immunoglobulins (Ward et al 1983). It is to be distinguished from malignant lymphoid polyposis, which is a true lymphoma of B cells (Isaacson, MacLennan and Subbuswamy 1984, Isaacson 1985, Zuckerman et al 1986).

Waldenstrom's Macroglobulinaemia

Diarrhoea and steatorrhoea are uncommon manifestations of Waldenstrom's macroglobulinaemia. Cabrera, de la Pava and Pickren (1964) reported an infiltration of the lamina propria by large foamy histiocytes in Waldenstrom's macroglobulinaemia. Some of the cells showed PAS positivity, and similar homogeneous material giving the same staining reaction was also seen in the lamina propria, both in an extracellular situation and distending the lymphatics (Fig. 14–4). Villous abnormalities when present are slight and they appear as simple deformities secondary to the infiltration. The tips of villi often are most severely involved and this imparts a club-like appearance. The material has been shown by immunofluorescence stains to be monoclonal IgM macroglobulin (Pruzanski et al 1973). It also stains for fat (Brandt et al 1981), which suggests that its presence may interfere with the absorption of fat so that it is held up in the lamina propria before entering the lymphatics. Hoang et al (1985) describe a case with the additional feature of lymphangiectasia to which they ascribed a coexistent protein-losing enteropathy.

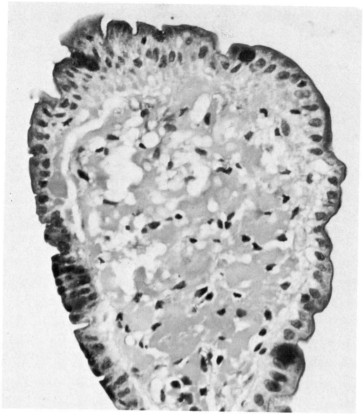

Figure 14–4. Jejunal mucosa in Waldenström's macroglobulinaemia. The lamina propria is filled with PAS-positive immunoglobin (PAS × 550).

ACANTHOCYTOSIS (A-BETA-LIPOPROTEINAEMIA, BASSEN-KORNZWEIG SYNDROME)

This is a syndrome (Bassen and Kornzweig 1950) comprising acanthocytosis of red cells, retinitis pigmentosa, central nervous system manifestations, absence of beta-lipoproteins, and steatorrhoea. The jejunal biopsy shows no significant abnormality in villous shape, but the absorptive cells of the superficial epithelium show typical vacuolation of the apical cytoplasm (Salt et al 1960, Lamy et al 1962). This is seen even in the fasting state and is known to be due to accumulation of lipid (Figs. 14–5 to 14–7). Dobbins (1966) has shown in an electron microscopic study that, in this syndrome, free fatty acids and monoglycerides enter the absorptive cell and are re-esterified in normal fashion. However, the Golgi vacuoles do not subsequently become distended with lipid, nor is there chylomicron formation, and the re-esterified lipid accumulates in the cells to be seen as apical vacuolation in light microscope preparations. These findings support the concept that the absorptive defect is concerned with the exit of fat from the absorptive cell, and that this is the result of impaired chylomicron formation with which beta-lipoproteins are intimately concerned (Isselbacher et al 1964).

Treatment with low-fat diets does not significantly alter the histological appearances (Greenwood 1976). Although the disease is generally fatal in childhood, Lazaro et al (1986) describe a male patient 29 years of age. There is some evidence

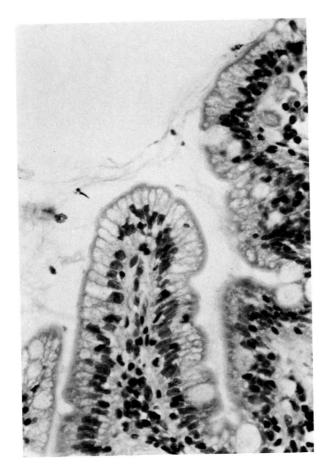

Figure 14–5. Jejunal biopsy in A-beta-lipoproteinaemia. There is a normal villous pattern, but the enterocytes appear vacuolated (H & E × 300).

Figure 14–6. Detail of absorptive epithelium. Note normal brush border and vacuolated apical cytoplasm. Occasional cells show nuclear reversion (arrow) (H & E × 500).

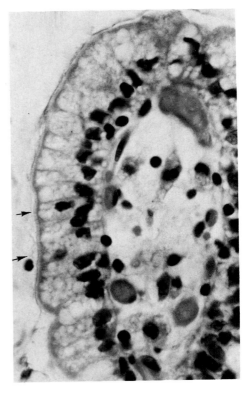

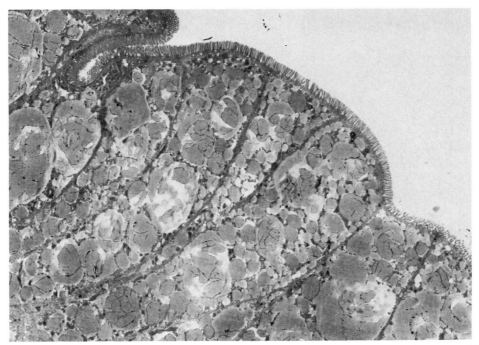

Figure 14–7. Electron micrograph of the apical cytoplasm of the enterocytes showing neutral fat accumulation. There are artefacts due to prior formalin fixation (× 4580).

(Scott, Miller and Losowsky 1979) that there may be a broader spectrum of beta-lipoprotein abnormality than hitherto appreciated. Lesser degrees of the beta-lipoprotein deficiency may be associated with milder and less complete forms of the disease. For example, steatorrhoea with fat-filled enterocytes is also a classic feature of homozygous hypobetalipoproteinaemia (Cottrill et al 1974). There is an absence of apolipoprotein B in their plasma and it cannot be demonstrated histochemically in small-intestinal absorptive cells (Herbert et al 1982, Green et al 1982). A similar clinical syndrome with fat-filled enterocytes, decreased plasma apolipoprotein B and apolipoprotein A–1, but with increased enterocyte apolipoprotein B, is described by Roy et al (1987). This recessively transmitted condition thus differs from abetalipoproteinaemia and the homozygous form of hypobetalipoproteinaemia but is also caused by a defect in the final assembly of chylomicrons or in the mechanism by which they leave the enterocyte.

WHIPPLE'S DISEASE

Except for the PAS positivity of the macrophages and recent electron microscopic observations, little has been added to the morphological descriptions of this condition since it was first described by Whipple (1907). However, it is now well known that it is a systemic disease and apart from the gastrointestinal tract may have manifestations due to involvement of the joints, skin, nervous system, eye, skeletal muscle, heart, serosal membranes, lung, kidney, liver, spleen and lymph nodes (Feldman 1986, Fleming, Wiesner and Shorter 1988). The small intestine is always involved, and biopsy is the method of choice as a diagnostic procedure (Hendrix and Yardley 1970). The dissecting microscope reveals several low,

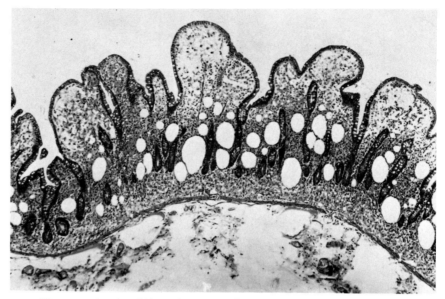

Figure 14–8. Jejunal biopsy in untreated Whipple's disease (H & E × 75).

bulging, bloated villi of white or yellow appearance. Histologically the villous pattern is distorted by a mucosal infiltrate of large macrophages (Fig. 14–8) with a basophilic stippled cytoplasm. The macrophages surround empty spaces and are PAS-positive diastase-resistant (Fig. 14–9), which is due to cytoplasmic inclusions of rods and granules. Similar particles also occur outside the macrophages lying free in the lamina propria. In preparations stained for iron, macrophages containing haemosiderin are frequently located deep in the lamina propria, and the muscularis mucosal cells may contain lipofuscin.

Electron microscopic studies (Watson and Haubrich 1969, Silva, Macedo and

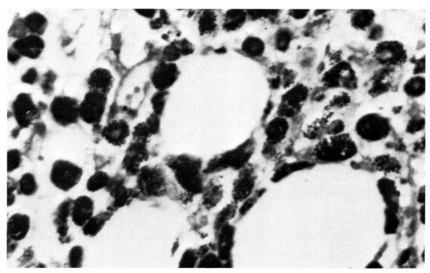

Figure 14–9. Whipple's disease. PAS-positive macrophages surround the empty spaces. Occasional granules appear to be extracellular (PAS × 600).

Nunes 1985) have confirmed Whipple's original suggestion that the basophilic macrophages might contain organisms. These appear as bacilliform bodies that may be seen in the lumen of the bowel in between the epithelial cells, and in and between macrophages in the mucosa and submucosa. In addition to more or less well-preserved intracellular forms there are others within lysosomes that show various stages of intracellular digestion. There are also granular and membranous dense bodies that represent the end products of this digestion and which are the counterpart of the PAS-positive granules seen with the light microscope. Dobbins and Kawanishi (1981) in a more extensive study also describe the bacilli in epithelial cells, lymphatic and capillary endothelium, polymorphs, plasma cells, lymphocytes and mast cells. Degranulation of mast cells has been described as a prominent feature in Whipple's disease, and it is suggested that there may be cooperation between macrophage and mast cell in the defence against Whipple's bacillus (Veloso and Saleiro 1982).

Dobbins and Kawanishi also stressed the unique nature of the outer membrane external to the cell wall of the organism and expressed the view that this may be related to difficulty in culturing the organism in vitro. Indeed, attempts to culture the organisms in Whipple's disease have not given any consistent results to date. Bacteria recognised include *Klebsiella, Haemophilus, Nocardia, Corynebacterium* and several strains of *Streptococcus*, some of which have shown cell wall deficiency. Evans and Ali (1985) used immunohistochemistry to demonstrate the presence of a rhamnose polysaccharide antigen in Whipple's bacilli. It is known that this sugar is found in many bacterial polysaccharides, notably those in streptococci, lactobacilli, shigella and corynebacteria. Gupta et al (1986) have also demonstrated that the reaction between circulating antibodies and the characteristic material in Whipple's macrophages can be blocked by rhamnose. It has been postulated, therefore, that more than one organism may be responsible and that there is a basic immunological defect in the patient. Dobbins (1981) argues the case for an abnormality in the cellular immune system, and Kwitko et al (1980) favour an underlying defect in intestinal antigen exclusion. Earlier workers (Tytgat et al 1977, Clancy et al 1975), however, had demonstrated a return to normal of the decreased cell-mediated immunity that was present before treatment had been given, and this has been further substantiated (Veloso et al 1981). Together with the apparent antigenic similarity of the agent in three different cases of Whipple's disease described by Keren et al (1976), the evidence so far seems to favour a previous claim by Charache et al (1966) that organisms with an unusual cell wall are responsible and that any immunologic deficit is secondary, although there is clearly scope for further investigation. Antibiotic therapy is effective in treatment and the disease is no longer inevitably fatal.

The circular spaces in the lamina propria and elsewhere in the other tissues involved contain neutral fat, but exactly how they form is in dispute. Some believe that they are dilated lymphatics, but others deny this, pointing out that the spaces are not lined by endothelium, but by macrophages. Endothelium, however, has the capacity to convert into macrophages, but lymphatic obstruction has not been demonstrated and there seems to be no good reason why fat should accumulate in dilated lymphatic spaces. The reason for the presence of the lipid deposits is that they form as the result of a disturbance in fat absorption, but this hardly explains why they are also seen in sites other than the bowel and mesenteric nodes.

The changes that occur in the mucosa following antibiotic treatment have been reported in detail by Maizel, Ruffin and Dobbins (1970) and Denholm, Mills and More (1981). The gradual disappearance of the organisms and PAS-positive

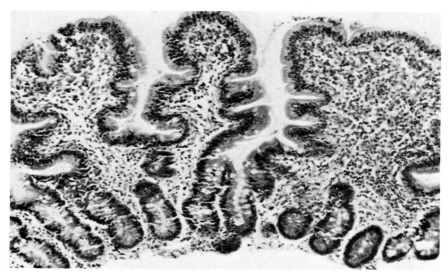

Figure 14–10. Jejunal mucosa in Whipple's disease showing partial recovery of villous pattern with fewer macrophages and absence of fat spaces (H & E × 150).

macrophages (Figs. 14–10, 14–11) and the slow return of the mucosa to normal are further evidence that the various features of the disease are in fact manifestations of an infection. In times such as these, antibiotics are widely used, often in repeated regimes of treatment for a variety of disease states. Under these conditions, the classical clinicopathological picture of Whipple's disease may be modified, and this should be borne constantly in mind if the diagnosis is not to be missed (Figs. 14–12, 14–13). Atypical forms certainly exist, and the case described by Moorthy, Nolley and Hermos (1977) in which intestinal lesions were minimal bears this out. A morphological feature in treated Whipple's disease not stressed by other authors was reported by Oliva et al (1972). They described

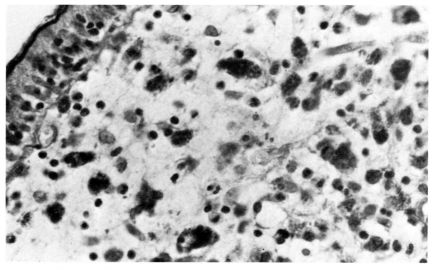

Figure 14–11. Treated Whipple's disease showing marked decrease in PAS-positive histiocytes (PAS × 800).

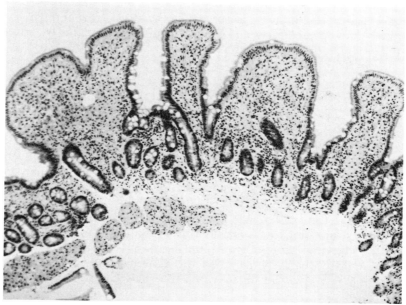

Figure 14–12. Jejunal mucosa in a patient who had received several courses of antibiotics over the years for bronchiectasis. Note the virtual absence of lipid spaces (H & E × 75).

lympho-histiocytic granulomata in the lamina propria. Centrally there is a necrotic cell, probably a degenerate histiocyte, and this is surrounded by a cuff of lymphocytes. These granulomata were seen when the jejunal biopsy was otherwise almost normal after nearly ten years of intermittent antibiotic therapy. Babaryka, Thorn and Langer (1979) have also described sarcoid-like epithelioid granulomata

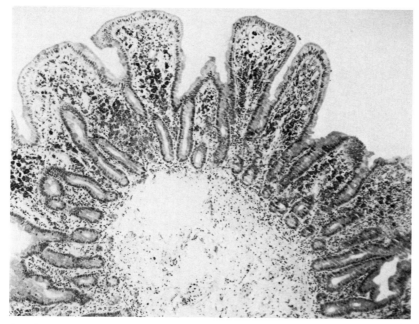

Figure 14–13. Same case as in Figure 14–12. A diagnosis of Whipple's disease modified by previous therapy was made after a PAS stain was performed (PAS × 75).

in an untreated case of Whipple's disease. Sometimes a sarcoid-like systemic disease proves to be Whipple's disease when the typical bacilliform bodies are demonstrated in non-caseating granulomas in the lymph nodes or other tissues affected (Cho et al 1984, Wilcox et al 1987).

INTESTINAL LYMPHANGIECTASIA

Small bowel biopsy plays an important role in the diagnosis of protein-losing enteropathy, since many of the 70 or more conditions associated with protein loss from the gastrointestinal tract may be associated with morphological abnormalities. Among these are coeliac disease, tropical sprue, hookworm infestation, giardiasis, Crohn's disease, and numerous other inflammatory and neoplastic lesions (for a comprehensive list see Waldmann 1970). More recently recognised and morphologically distinct is the condition of intestinal lymphangiectasia, which usually involves the small intestine and sometimes the large. It is unusual for lymphangiectasia to be confined to the large intestine only (Asakura et al 1986). This designation should probably be reserved for those cases showing villi with oedematous tips, imparting to the mucosa a pebble-like appearance as seen in the dissecting microscope. Histologically, there is oedema of the lamina propria, submucosa, and the absorptive cells of the surface epithelium. The latter is said to push the nucleus away from its basal position towards the luminal surface (Mistilis, Skyring and Stephen 1965), an appearance, however, also seen in relation to the suction trauma of biopsy. The mucosal lymphatics within the tips of the villi are dilated (Fig. 14–14), but the villi are only slightly distorted, and there is no villous atrophy. The lamina propria contains foamy macrophages and an

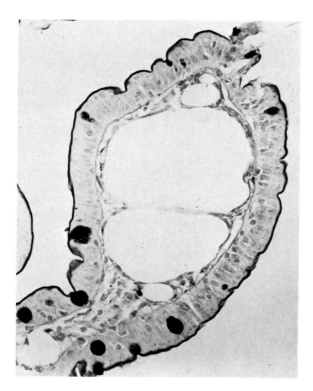

Figure 14–14. Jejunal biopsy in intestinal lymphangiectasia. Bloated villous tip with dilated lymphatic vessels (PAS × 280).

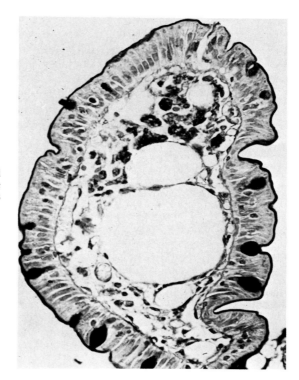

Figure 14–15. Jejunal biopsy in intestinal lymphangiectasia to show PAS-positive macrophages around the lymphatic spaces (PAS × 280).

occasional multinucleated giant cell, and the macrophages, which are only weakly PAS-positive (Fig. 14–15), also contain neutral fat. Fat as chylomicrons can also be demonstrated between epithelial cells and in the lamina propria, and there is dilatation of the interepithelial cell spaces—especially noticeable at electron microscopy (Asakura et al 1981, Bujanover et al 1981, Riemann and Schmidt 1981).

The intestinal lymphatic dilatation is frequently part of a more widespread congenital abnormality. Pomerantz and Waldmann (1963) and Mistilis, Skyring and Stephen (1965) have shown ectasia of some and absence of other lymphatics in lower extremity lymphangiograms in patients with intestinal lymphangiectasia. Intestinal lymphangiectasia should always be suspected in childhood or adolescent onset of bilateral leg oedema (Gallo-Van Ess, Strasburger and Turetsky 1986). A generalised lymphangiectasia involving intestine, lung, and lymph nodes was accompanied by thymic hypoplasia in the case described by Sorensen et al (1985). It is also claimed that any lymphatic obstruction, whether due to malignancy, fibrosis (Rubin and Dobbins 1965, Belaiche et al 1980) or simply to congestive cardiac failure (Waldmann 1970), may produce a similar picture. Lymphangiectasia is said to occur in Behçet's disease (Asakura et al 1973), but the illustrations in this paper are far from convincing, and an electron microscopic abnormality that they describe was present in only one of 16 cases. None of the patients had hypoproteinaemia. The coexistence of intestinal lymphangiectasia and the nephrotic syndrome (de Sousa et al 1968) also requires further investigation, but the association with macroglobulinaemia (Harris, Burton and Scarffe 1983) seems more than fortuitous. The increased viscosity of the lymph consequent on its high IgM content may be important in the pathogenesis. Bolton, Cotter and Losowsky (1986) also describe an association with impaired neutrophil function, and the condition has been reported as a consequence of combined radiotherapy and chemotherapy (Rao, Dundas and Holdsworth 1987).

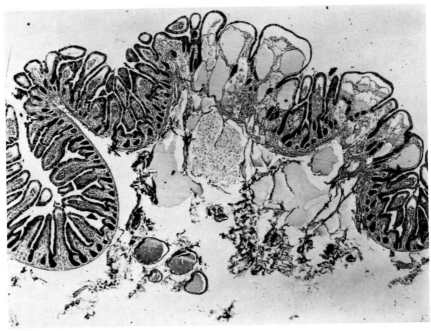

Figure 14–16. Lymphangiectatic cyst in jejunum. Large irregular spaces distort the villous pattern and contain coagulated lymph and macrophages. The villi adjacent to the lesion are normal (PAS × 17).

Intestinal lymphangiectasia must be distinguished from the entity of lymphangiectatic cysts (Shilken, Zerman and Blackwell 1968), which usually have no clinical significance. These occur particularly in the jejunum in some 20 per cent of necropsies, usually in patients over the age of 55 (Aase and Gundersen 1983). They are up to 1 cm in diameter and often multiple, and may be biopsied during life (Fig. 14–16). The dilated lymphatic spaces are large and irregular in shape and they usually affect the submucosa. Sometimes the villi are involved, but, in contrast to lymphangiectasia, several adjacent villi appear distorted by large and irregular lymphatic spaces, whereas their neighbours are entirely normal. There may be lipid-containing histiocytes, found not in the lamina propria but within the lymphatic spaces. The spaces frequently contain pink inspissated lymph rich in neutral fat. A further contrast with diffuse intestinal lymphangiectasia is that lipofuscinosis is not seen.

ALLERGIC GASTROENTEROPATHY AND FOOD ALLERGY

A condition that requires more precise definition is that of allergic gastroenteropathy (Waldmann et al 1967). These authors described a protein-losing enteropathy occurring in children who also showed anaemia, eosinophilia and growth retardation. The jejunum had a normal villous architecture or minor abnormalities, but there was an eosinophilic infiltration in the lamina propria. Sometimes there was associated asthma, eczema and rhinitis. An allergy to ingested milk protein was suggested and further claims for such an entity are made by Businco et al (1985) and Challacombe, Wheeler and Campbell (1986). One of the problems is to decide where in the spectrum of food allergy in general the condition of allergic gastroenteropathy as a specific entity occurs. Certainly urticarial reactions, oedema, eczema and asthmatic attacks may be precipitated by certain foodstuffs (Walker-Smith 1978, Lancet 1979). Van Spreeuwel et al (1984) also claim that allergy to foodstuff may be reflected in an increase in IgE plasma cells in the mucosa of the upper gastrointestinal tract. The relationship of so-called allergic gastroenteropathy to milk protein intolerance needs clarification. The evidence suggests they are related but that they possibly differ in magnitude. Advances in immunology in the last few years, and a greater understanding of the immediate hypersensitivity reaction, have opened up a new and vast field for further investigation. It could be suggested, for example, that the effects of parasitic infestations, the mechanisms of some causes of protein-losing enteropathy and such disease entities as pylorospasm, colonic spasm, "idiopathic" diarrhoea and proctitis, nausea and upper abdominal pain are all mediated through the mechanism of local anaphylaxis. The morphological features of hyperaemia, oedema, eosinophil leukocyte and lymphocyte infiltration and degranulation of basophils need only be transient, and biopsy examination carried out when major symptoms have subsided would be normal.

The problem of allergic gastroenteropathy was put into perspective by the report of Cooper et al (1980) describing eight adult patients with abdominal pain and diarrhoea. The only abnormality in jejunal morphology was an increase in plasma cells and a decrease in lymphocytes in the lamina propria and an increase in intraepithelial lymphocytes. These patients had their symptomatology dramatically relieved by a gluten-free diet, but there was a return of symptoms when gluten was reintroduced. The problem of food allergy is probably greater in children and often involves several food substances in the same patients. The jejunal biopsy is usually reported as normal (Minford, MacDonald and Littlewood 1982). Not only are there abdominal symptoms, but eczema, urticaria and oedema may occur, as well as asthma. There is some evidence that patients with eczema and food allergy have an abnormally increased molecular permeability of their bowel wall (Jackson et al 1981). It is thus of interest that atopic children without gastrointestinal symptoms often show eosinophil infiltration and minor villous abnormalities when subjected to jejunal biopsy (Kokkonen, Simila and Herva 1980). In both children with mucosal abnormalities in cow's milk protein intolerance and in adults with a variety of food allergies, Rosekrans et al (1980) claim to show an increase in lamina propria IgE containing plasma cells. More research for a morphological or physiological basis to allergic reaction in relation to food substances is clearly needed. Kikindjanin et al (1985), for example, describe a case of recurrent urticaria and diarrhoea in which impaired intestinal mucosal immunity could be implicated.

LIPOFUSCINOSIS

In any case of hypoalbuminaemia the muscularis mucosa and occasional histiocytes in the lamina propria and submucosa of the jejunal biopsy may show lipofuscin pigmentation (Fig. 14–17). It is probably found in these sites only when pigmentation of other smooth muscle is fairly heavy. The muscularis propria of the bowel wall usually is heavily infiltrated, so much so that the bowel is obviously discoloured macroscopically and the condition is sometimes called brown-bowel syndrome. The pigment is PAS-positive and autofluorescent in ultraviolet light, can be stained by Sudan black, and is usually acid-fast with Ziehl-Neelsen's stain.

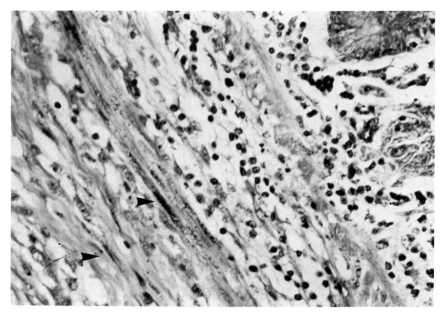

Figure 14–17. Jejunal biopsy in hypoalbuminaemia due to gluten-sensitive enteropathy. The muscularis mucosal cells contain lipofuscin pigment (arrowheads) (H & E × 300).

The significance of the pigmentation is not fully understood, but it is thought to be related to vitamin E deficiency (Ansanelli and Lane 1957, Tofler, Hukill and Spiro 1963, Binder et al 1965, Hosler, Kimmel and Moeller 1982), and to hypoalbuminaemia (Richards 1959). In human jejunal biopsy material, when lipofuscin pigmentation is seen, hypoalbuminaemia is almost always present; this is probably explained by the very close interrelationship that exists between vitamin E and protein metabolism (Fox 1967). Lipofuscin production is thought to be the result of a progressive oxidation of various cellular constituents (Lancet 1970), and it is seen in a variety of body tissues as a normal concomitant of ageing. Deficiency of a potent antioxidant such as vitamin E might well be expected, therefore, to contribute to an accelerated and excessive production of this pigment. Cases are recorded of disappearance of the pigment following vitamin E supplements (Lee and Nicholson 1976). Foster (1979) in an ultrastructural study compared the abnormalities in smooth muscle with skeletal muscle changes in myopathies of mitochondrial origin and proposed that lipofuscinosis be considered a smooth muscle myopathy. These mitochondrial changes seen by electron microscopy have been confirmed (Horn et al 1985). However, in most instances the condition appears to be secondary to a systemic disease, sometimes in the bowel itself (Gallager 1980), and there is doubt as to whether the pigmentation interferes significantly with muscle function (Stamp and Evans 1987).

DISACCHARIDASE DEFICIENCIES

In isolated disaccharidase deficiency no detectable abnormality of the jejunal mucosa can be demonstrated in the light microscope or by conventional electron microscopy. Where there are morphological abnormalities in the jejunal biopsies, all the disaccharidases measured, i.e., lactase, maltose and sucrose, are depressed compared with the normal. Results of estimating villous surface area by relating it to volume indicate that depression of disaccharidase levels is a sensitive index of decrease in villous surface area, i.e., villous atrophy. For example, the depression of enzymes in the jejunal mucosa in pernicious anaemia is much less than untreated coeliac disease. Moreover, in coeliac disease during treatment by gluten-exclusion diet, the enzyme level corresponds closely with the degree of persistent villous atrophy, only returning to normal when the villous pattern is normal (Pena at al 1972, Pena, Truelove and Whitehead 1972). In an electron microscopic study Phillips et al (1980) have shown that in secondary disaccharidase deficiency there is a correlation between enzyme levels and the surface area of the microvilli. This is indeed what one might predict, since the enzymes are located in that site. Of some interest is the fact that it has been shown that disaccharidases can be demonstrated at light microscopy in resin-embedded sections, whereas in the past frozen sections were advocated (Hand 1987).

RADIATION INJURY

This is dealt with more fully in the section dealing with irradiation colitis (Chapter 17). The small intestine, however, is more sensitive than the colon to the effects of irradiation, but from external sources it receives rather better protection from the body wall. The lesions parallel those described in the colon, with an early phase of mucosal degeneration followed by recovery, and later more chronic reaction with persistent ulceration, scarring and fistula formation. In the acute phase, the features of which have been described by Trier and Browning (1966), a reduction in crypt mitoses is the first change, and then cell damage becomes evident. The dividing cells in the crypts are most severely affected and are shed into the lumen. The decreased production of cells results in shortening of both crypts and villi, and Paneth cells are reduced in number. The goblet cells and absorptive cells are shorter than normal, and there may be an increase in nuclear size and abnormalities of shape. Lymphocytes in the lamina propria disappear, and plasma cells appear increased in number. An infiltrate of polymorphs in response to cell damage occurs, and cell debris and neutrophils occupy some of the crypts. These changes take place in the three weeks after exposure and will revert to normal if exposure ceases over the next two weeks. Late changes develop and cause symptoms any time between two months and 20 years after exposure. In some instances the chronic changes are responsible for malabsorption (Tankel, Clark and Lee 1965), which probably has a varied aetiology. In the event of strictures and intestinal stasis the defect has the same cause as other stagnant loop syndromes and is related to bacterial colonisation of the bowel. This leads to disturbances in bile-salt deconjugation and the deleterious effect that this has on fat absorption (Tabaqchali and Booth 1970). Malabsorption, however, may also be related to residual mucosal damage, and changes may be seen in small-intestinal biopsy material. The features of old irradiation injury that may be seen include a varying degree of villous atrophy, in the extreme case so severe as to produce a flat mucosa. There may also be an increase in round cells in the lamina propria, but a striking feature is the fibrosis that can occur in this zone (Fig. 14–18). This is often accompanied by hypoplasia and distortion due to atrophy of the crypts, and in the submucosa typical small vessel hyalinisation will be present.

STORAGE DISEASES

Owing to an increasing sophistication of biochemical and electron microscope technology, there is a rapidly growing list of inborn errors of metabolism that

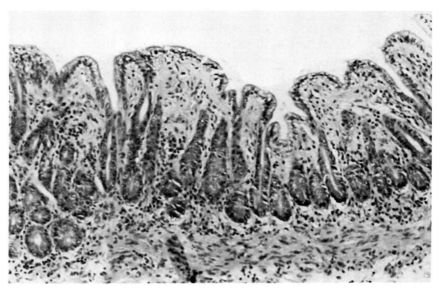

Figure 14–18. Jejunal mucosa showing villous atrophy and fibrosis of the lamina propria due to irradiation (H & E × 113).

result in the excessive formation and storage of a number of different substances. Usually the genetic disorder results in excessive accumulation of a normal metabolite owing to a defect in an enzyme involved in its metabolism, or there is similar accumulation of an abnormal substance produced as the result of the unsuccessful operation of an alternative biochemical pathway. The enzymes involved are frequently lysosomal, and the disorders are sometimes collectively known as lysosomal storage disorders. They have been grouped together according to certain similarities, which in the past have been described under such headings as "glycogen storage diseases" or "glycogenoses," the "lipoidoses" and the "mucopolysaccharidoses," according to the group of macromolecular substances that accumulate. These storage abnormalities are responsible for the distention and vacuolation of affected cells, and different combinations of tissue and organ involvement have allowed reasonably specific clinical subgroups to be defined. These are the subject of a comprehensive review by Glew et al (1985), who classify lysosomal storage disease into the sphingolipidoses, glycoproteinoses, mucolipidoses, mucopolysaccharidoses and others such as cystinosis, Pompe's disease, Wolman's disease and cholesterol ester storage disease. Not all these subtypes are associated with involvement of the gastrointestinal tract, but when it is involved the abnormality may be recognised in biopsy tissues. When there is colonic involvement a rectal biopsy is obviously preferred, but small bowel involvement interferes with function and may lead to a small biopsy procedure. There is a modern trend, however, for biochemical determination of the diagnosis of lysosomal storage disease in samples of chorionic villi obtained early in pregnancy (Kerr 1984). This allows termination of pregnancy and thus avoids the birth of infants with devastating physical and mental defects for which there is currently no therapy.

Malabsorption is rarely due to small-intestinal involvement in Fabry's disease, an X-linked disorder of lipid metabolism caused by a deficiency of ceramide trihexosidase. Flynn et al (1972) report a case with jejunal biopsy appearances characterised by a normal villous pattern, but with abnormalities of the blood vessels, submucosal neurones and muscularis mucosa. The neurones were enlarged and vacuolated and stained positively with Sudan black and Luxol fast blue, and the blood vessels and muscularis mucosa contained birefringent deposits of sudanophilic, Luxol-fast-blue–positive material. This material is the sphingolipid ceramide trihexose, and in an electron microscope study O'Brien et al (1982) ascribe the diarrhoea that may occur in these cases to secondary intestinal bacterial overgrowth. This is the consequence of stasis secondary to the neural and muscle deposits. Indeed, Sheth et al (1981) noted a high frequency of gastrointestinal symptoms in the 50 patients in their series. Ganglion cell involvement also occurs in Niemann-Pick disease. Dinari et al (1980) also describe lipid-filled histiocytes in the lamina propria in jejunal biopsies in this condition and suggest the intestinal involvement is more frequent than hitherto recognised in the type A disease. Involvement of the lamina propria by histiocytes swollen with lipid is recognised in small as well as large intestine in cholesterol ester storage disease, Tangier disease and Wolman's disease. Dincsoy et al (1984) also describe non-birefringent autofluorescent granules within histiocytes in the duodenum in cholesterol ester storage disease. Electron microscopic changes have been described by Partin and Schubert (1969) and Tylki-Szymanska et al (1987). It is likely that as this group of diseases becomes more frequently recognised and investigated, intestinal involvement will be described more commonly.

CYSTINOSIS

Morecki, Paunier and Hamilton (1968) reported changes in jejunal biopsy tissues in a case of cystinosis. In ordinary H & E sections of formalin-fixed, paraffin-embedded material no abnormalities were present, but in 1 μ sections of epoxy resin-embedded material, changes were present that were later confirmed by electron microscopy. Angular spaces corresponding to the shape of cystine crystals were prominent in the lamina propria and located in an intracellular site within histiocytes. A proportion of the surface absorptive cells contained vacuoles. Some of these were small and basally situated in a subnuclear position, but others were large and appeared in a supranuclear site in the region of the Golgi apparatus.

ACRODERMATITIS ENTEROPATHICA

This is a rare familial disorder with autosomal recessive inheritance. Chronic dermatitis of the oro-anal regions and the extremities, along with baldness, are associated with diarrhoea and failure to thrive. No consistent abnormality of the jejunal mucosa is seen with light microscopy. Electron microscopy, however, reveals abnormal inclusion bodies in the Paneth cells. These resemble abnormal granules but could represent lysosomes, although they have been shown to be acid-phosphatase–negative. In view of the high zinc content of normal Paneth cells and the response of this disease to zinc therapy, it has been postulated that a Paneth cell abnormality is concerned in its aetiology. Bohane et al (1977), however, have examined the Paneth cells before and after treatment and shown that the lysosome-like inclusions or altered granules disappear following therapy. Accordingly, the authors claim that Paneth cell abnormalities could well be due to a primary zinc deficiency.

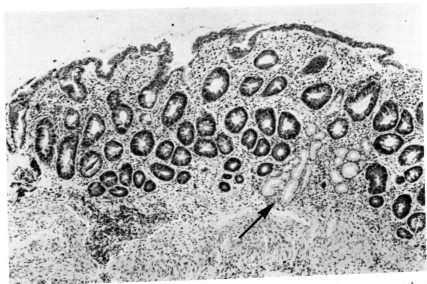

Figure 14–19. Jejunal biopsy near ulceration due to Crohn's disease. There are crypt hyperplasia and villous atrophy with pyloric gland metaplasia (arrow) (H & E × 75).

METAPLASIA

The intestinal crypts on occasion may be replaced by simple mucous glands of pyloric type (Fig. 14–19). These always occur above the muscularis mucosa, and because of this the change is often referred to as pyloric gland metaplasia rather than Brunner's gland metaplasia. It is simply a manifestation of the marked metaplastic potential of the epithelium of the gastrointestinal tract as a whole.

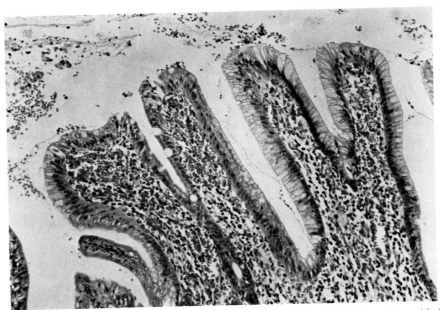

Figure 14–20. Jejunal biopsy near ulceration due to Crohn's disease. The absorptive epithelium is largely replaced by metaplastic gastric superficial epithelium (H & E × 375).

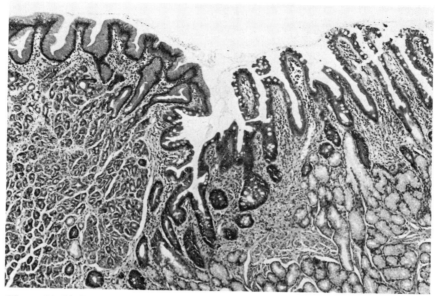

Figure 14–21. Ectopic gastric mucosa (left) in the duodenum (right) (H & E × 38).

This metaplasia rarely, if ever, occurs unless there is or has been ulceration in the vicinity, and this is clearly of diagnostic importance when seen in jejunal or other small-intestinal biopsy material.

As already mentioned under the section dealing with the duodenum, the superficial epithelium of the small intestine undergoes metaplasia to a type that is typical of the superficial gastric epithelium (Fig. 14–20). It is seen in the duodenum or jejunum in conditions of high gastric acid secretion (James 1964, Rhodes 1964), but like pyloric metaplasia it may also appear near areas of ulceration, and both are particularly frequent as part of the histological spectrum of Crohn's disease of the small intestine. It is an easy matter to distinguish these appearances from those seen when true heterotopic gastric mucosa (Fig. 14–21) occurs in the small intestine.

HAEMOSIDERIN PIGMENTATION

Not infrequently the lamina propria in the tips of villi will contain groups of macrophages filled with haemosiderin granules (Fig. 14–22). This occurs normally, but is much more frequent after oral or parenteral iron administration. In transfusional haemosiderosis the appearances are accentuated, and sometimes pigmented macrophages appear to be traversing the epithelium. The epithelial cells themselves do not contain iron, in contrast to the appearances in haemochromatosis (Astaldi, Meardi and Lisino 1966). In addition to the epithelial haemosiderin, the pattern of distribution of the pigment macrophages is also different. In haemochromatosis they tend to be more diffusely scattered throughout the lamina propria and around vessels, a distribution similar to that shown by the iron-containing macrophages in Whipple's disease.

PSEUDOMELANOSIS DUODENI

Since its recognition in the early days of fibreoptic endoscopy (Bisordi and Kleinman 1976), there have been several case reports of this curious pigmentation

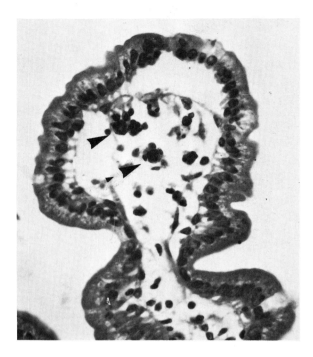

Figure 14–22. Jejunal villous tip containing macrophages (arrowheads) filled with haemosiderin (Perls × 500).

of the duodenal mucosa. It affects the bulb and often the second part also. The mucosa has a speckled dark-brown or black appearance, which is due to pigment accumulation in the lysosomes of lamina propria macrophages at the tips of the villi (Fig. 14–23). The pigment has been analysed by electron probe analysis and shown to contain both iron and sulphur as ferric sulphide (Pounder et al 1982, Kang et al 1987, Rex and Jersild 1988). It usually, but not always, stains positively with Perl's and the PAS method and occasionally with Masson Fontana, as does

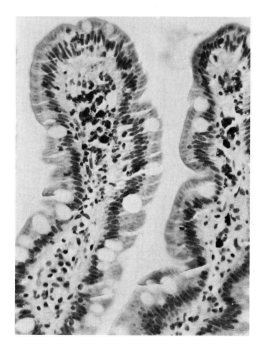

Figure 14–23. Duodenal appearance in pseudomelanosis. The pigment is much more prominent and blacker than the brown colour of haemosiderin pigmentation in routine H & E sections (H & E × 500).

true melanin. The condition has been ascribed to the ingestion of a variety of drugs, and there is an association with hypertension and renal failure. It is apparently more common in black females but has been described in Orientals and whites (Yamase, Norris and Gillies 1985, Gupta and Weinstock 1986, Lee, O'Donnell and Keren 1987, Castellano et al 1988, Kuo and Wu 1988, Lin et al 1988 and West 1988).

MEASLES GIANT CELLS AND CYTOMEGALOVIRUS INCLUSIONS

Giant cells may occur in the jejunal mucosa during the prodromal phase of measles as they may in other lymphoid tissues, and thus can be seen on occasions in biopsy tissues from all areas of the gastrointestinal tract. Watson and Parkin (1970) illustrate these cells as an incidental finding in a patient who was biopsied as part of the investigation for a malabsorption syndrome. The patient was found to have a typical flat mucosa characteristic of gluten-sensitive enteropathy but also had measles giant cells in the lamina propria. The rash ensued four days after the biopsy was taken.

Cytomegalovirus inclusions in the epithelial cells of the stomach have already been mentioned. The increasing number of patients receiving immunosuppressive therapy has led to an increase in secondary cytomegalovirus infection in adults, and involvement of the gastrointestinal tract is common (Henson 1972). Primary cytomegalovirus infection of the small bowel is distinctly uncommon (Dent et al 1975). The typical inclusions are intranuclear and separated from the nuclear membrane by a clear halo. Less frequently, PAS-positive intracytoplasmic inclusions occur. Inclusions may be located in lamina propria fibroblasts and capillary endothelial cells as well as the epithelial cells.

GRANULOMATA

The significance of granulomata in jejunal biopsy material poses the same problem as when they occur in other areas of the gastrointestinal tract. As already outlined in the section on gastric sarcoidosis, granulomata will usually prove to be a manifestation of generalised sarcoidosis, of Crohn's disease, or of some other chronic granulomatous disease, e.g., tuberculosis. Hermos et al (1970) have reported two patients in whom the diagnosis of Crohn's disease of the upper small intestine was verified by finding granulomata in peroral duodenal biopsy specimens. Rarely, however, one finds granulomata in biopsies that are otherwise normal (Fig. 14–24) or sometimes in biopsies showing the apparently unrelated lesions of gluten-sensitive enteropathy (Fig. 14–25). Their presence in these circumstances defies adequate explanation, although Bjorneklett et al (1977) describe disappearance of the granulomata in response to gluten exclusion in a similar case.

HISTOPLASMOSIS

Involvement of the gastrointestinal tract in this fungal disease is discussed in more detail in Chapter 17. Predominant involvement of the small intestine, although rare, does occur, and a jejunal biopsy diagnosis is thus possible. Some-

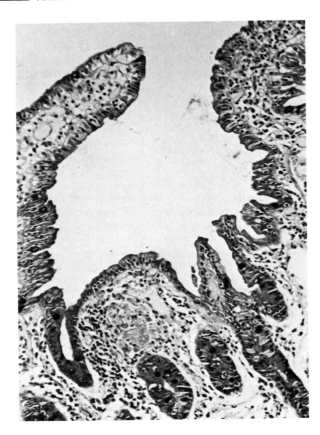

Figure 14–24. Jejunal biopsy normal except for epithelioid and giant cell granuloma in the lamina propria (H & E × 280).

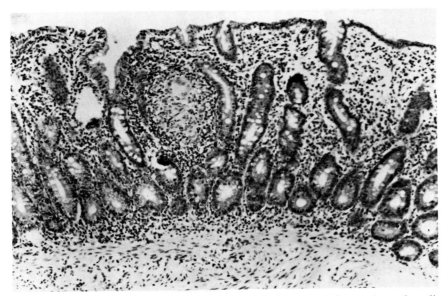

Figure 14–25. Jejunal biopsy in a patient who subsequently responded to a gluten-free diet. The mucosa shows a crypt hyperplastic type of villous atrophy with an epithelioid and giant cell granuloma in the lamina propria (H & E × 105).

times a malabsorption syndrome results (Orchard, Luparello and Brunskill 1979) or a protein-losing enteropathy (Bank et al 1965). In a single case seen by the author, diagnosis was a simple matter once the condition was considered. There was total villous atrophy and lateral separation of the crypts due to an inflammatory infiltrate and the presence of typical histiocytes containing the organisms, which displayed a pronounced PAS-positive capsule (Figs. 14–26, 14–27).

MASTOCYTOSIS

The literature concerning mastocytosis and mast cell involvement of the small intestine is reviewed by Scott, Hardy and Losowsky (1975). They describe an additional case and discuss its relationship to gluten-sensitive enteropathy, which appears to be more than fortuitous. In addition to mast cell infiltration of the lamina propria there may be a crypt hyperplastic villous atrophy that reverts to normal following gluten exclusion. Blunting and shortening of villi with crypt hyperplasia, however, may be seen in mastocytosis of the jejunum in the absence of gluten sensitivity (Belcon et al 1980, Braverman, Dollberg and Shiner 1985). Cases with a simple increase in lamina propria mast cells and otherwise normal jejunal morphology are also described (Reisberg and Oyakawa 1987). The whole subject of gastrointestinal dysfunction in mastocytosis, including hyperchlorhydria and either duodenitis or duodenal ulcer, is reviewed by Cherner et al (1988).

HISTIOCYTOSIS X

Keeling and Harries (1973) reported an infant with unequivocal evidence of intestinal malabsorption associated with histiocytic involvement of the small intestinal lamina propria. They also examined autopsy tissues from another 11 fatal cases that revealed small intestinal involvement in almost 50 per cent.

MYELOID METAPLASIA

Rarely the gut is the site of extramedullary haematopoiesis. Schreibman et al (1988) describe small bowel involvement in a patient with myelofibrosis.

SYPHILITIC ENTERITIS

Syphilitic involvement of the gastrointestinal tract usually involves the rectum. Schlossberg et al (1984) describe a seemingly unique example of symptomatic small bowel relapsing secondary syphilis characterised by partial villous atrophy, crypt hyperplasia and pronounced plasma cell infiltration of the lamina propria. The mucosa returned to normal following two months of antisyphilitic therapy.

EFFECT OF CYTOTOXIC DRUGS

In humans (Cunningham et al 1985) and experimental animals (Moore 1984) cytotoxic drugs used in the therapy of cancer have been shown to cause damage to intestinal crypt cells. Although mature epithelium is unaffected, immature cells

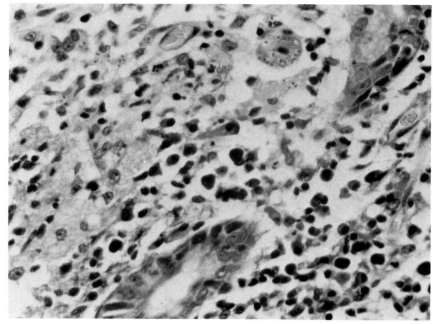

Figure 14–26. Jejunal involvement in histoplasmosis. Pale foamy histiocytes, some with rounded cytoplasmic inclusions (H & E × 450).

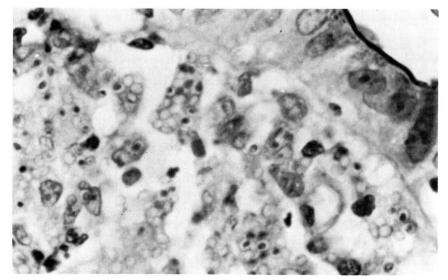

Figure 14–27. Detail of histiocytes to show numerous encapsulated yeast forms of histoplasmosis (PAS × 850).

in the crypts show vacuolation at light microscopy, which at electron microscopy were seen to be due to large secondary lysosomes containing partially degraded fragments of damaged crypt cells.

INFANTILE SYSTEMIC HYALINOSIS

Hyaline material is deposited in skin, gastrointestinal tract, adrenals, bladder, skeletal muscles, thymus, parathyroids and other sites in this presumed autosomal recessive disease. The hyaline is characteristically laid down in lamina propria and submucosa of the stomach and intestine. It leads to intractable diarrhoea and malabsorption and is usually fatal within the first two years of life (Landing and Nodorra 1986).

ATHEROMATOUS EMBOLI

Rarely, small-intestinal biopsy will reveal evidence of small vessel embolisation by atheromatous material. Socinski et al (1984) describe a patient diagnosed on jejunal biopsy who presented with diarrhoea.

REFERENCES—SECTION III
SMALL-INTESTINAL BIOPSY

Aase S. and Gundersen R. (1983) Submucous lymphatic cysts of the small intestine. Acta Pathologica, Microbiologica et Immunologica Scandinavica *91*:191–194.

Achkar E., Carey W.D., Petras R., Sivak M.V. and Revta R. (1986) Comparison of suction capsule and endoscopic biopsy of small bowel mucosa. Gastrointestinal Endoscopy *32*:278–281.

Adam M., Morgan O., Persaud C. and Gibbs W.N. (1973) Hyperinfection syndrome with strongyloides stercoralis in malignant lymphoma. British Medical Journal *1*:264–266.

Aherne W.A. and Dunnill M.S. (1982) Morphometry. London: Edward Arnold.

Ajdukiewicz A.B., Youngs G.R. and Bouchier I.A.D. (1972) Nodular lymphoid hypoplasia with hypogammaglobulinaemia. Gut *13*:589–595.

Ament M.E. (1985) Immunodeficiency syndromes of the gut. Scandinavian Journal of Gastroenterology *20*(Suppl. 114):127–135.

Ament M.E. and Ochs H. (1973) Gastrointestinal manifestations of chronic granulomatous disease. New England Journal of Medicine *288*:382–387.

Ament M.E., Ochs H.D. and Davis S.D. (1973) Structure and function of the gastrointestinal tract in primary immunodeficiency syndromes. Medicine (Baltimore) *52*:227–248.

Ament M.E. and Rubin C.E. (1972) Soy protein: another cause of the flat intestinal lesion. Gastroenterology *62*:227–234.

Anand B.S., Kumar M., Chakravarti R.N., Sehgal A.K. and Chhuttani P.N. (1980) Pathogenesis of malabsorption in Giardia infection: an experimental study in rats. Transactions of the Royal Society of Tropical Medicine and Hygiene *74*:565–569.

Anand B.S., Piris J., Jerrome D.W., Offord R.E. and Truelove S.C. (1981) The timing of histological damage following a single challenge with gluten in treated coeliac disease. Quarterly Journal of Medicine *197*:83–94.

Andersson H., Bjorkman A-C., Gillberg R., Kastrup W., Mobacken H. and Stockbrugger R. (1984) Influence of the amount of dietary gluten on gastrointestinal morphology and function in dermatitis herpetiformis. Human Nutrition: Clinical Nutrition *38C*:279–285.

Ansanelli V. Jr. and Lane N. (1957) Lipochrome (ceroid) pigmentation of the small intestine. Annals of Surgery *146*:117–123.

Aronson A.R. and Norfleet R.G. (1962) The duodenal mucosa in peptic ulcer disease: a clinical pathological correlation. American Journal of Digestive Diseases *7*:506–514.

Asakura H., Miura S., Morishita T., Aiso S., Tanaka T., Kitahora T., Tsuchiya M., Enomoto Y. and Watanabe Y. (1981) Endoscopic and histopathological study on primary and secondary intestinal lymphangiectasia. Digestive Diseases and Sciences *26*:312–320.

Asakura H., Morita A., Morishita T., Tsuchiya M., Watanabe Y. and Enomoto Y. (1973) Histopathological and electron microscopic studies of lymphangiectasia of the small intestine in Behcet's disease. Gut *14*:196–203.

Asakura H., Tsuchiya M., Katoh S., Kobayashi K., Yonei Y., Yoshida T., Hamada Y., Miura S., Morita A., Kuramochi S. and Teramoto T. (1986) Pathological findings of lymphangiectasia of the large intestine in a patient with protein-losing enteropathy. Gastroenterology *91*:719–724.

Asselah F., Slavin G., Sowter G. and Asselah H. (1983) Immunoproliferative small intestinal disease in Algerians. I. Light microscopic and immunochemical studies. Cancer *52*:227–237.

Astaldi G., Meardi G. and Lisino T. (1966) The iron content of jejunal mucosa obtained by Crosby's biopsy in haemochromatosis and haemosiderosis. Blood *28*:70–82.

Atwell J.D., Burge D. and Wright D. (1985) Nodular lymphoid hyperplasia of the intestinal tract in infancy and childhood. Journal of Pediatric Surgery *20*:25–29.

Austad W.I., Cornes J.S., Gough K.R., McCarthy C.F. and Read A.E. (1967) Steatorrhea and malignant lymphoma. American Journal of Digestive Diseases *12*:475–490.

Austin L.L. and Dobbins W.O. (1988) Studies of the rectal mucosa in coeliac sprue: the intraepithelial lymphocyte. Gut *29*:200–205

Avery G.B., Villavicencio O., Lilly J.R. and Randolph J.G. (1968) Intractable diarrhea in early infancy. Pediatrics *41*:712–722.

Babaryka I., Thorn L. and Langer E. (1979) Epithelioid cell granulomata in the mucosa of the small intestine in Whipple's disease. Virchows Archiv. A Pathological Anatomy and Histology *382*:227–235.

Baker S.J. and Mathan V.I. (1970) In Modern Trends in Gastroenterology. Volume 4. Edited by W.I. Card and B. Creamer. London: Butterworth, p. 198.

Baker S.J., Ignatius M., Mathan V.I., Vaish S.K. and Chacko C.C. (1962) Intestinal biopsy, p. 184. Edited by G.E. Wolstenholme and M.P. Cameron (Study group No. 14). London: Ciba Foundation.

Baker S.J., Mathan M., Mathan V.I., Jesudoss S. and Swaminathan S.P. (1982) Chronic enterocyte infection with coronavirus. One possible cause of the syndrome of tropical sprue? Digestive Diseases and Sciences *27*:1039–1043.

Baklien K., Brandtzaeg P. and Fausa O. (1977) Immunoglobulins in jejunal mucosa and serum from patients with adult coeliac disease. Scandinavian Journal of Gastroenterology *12*:149–159.

Balazs M. and Szatloczky E. (1978) Electron microscopic examination of the mucosa of the small intestine in infection due to giardia lamblia. Pathology Research and Practice *163*:251–260.

Bank S., Trey C., Gans I., Marks I.N. and Groll A. (1965) Histoplasmosis of the small bowel with "giant" intestinal villi and secondary protein-losing enteropathy. American Journal of Medicine *39*:492–504.

Banwell J.G., Hutt M.S.R. and Tunnicliffe R. (1964) Observations on jejunal biopsy in Ugandan Africans. East African Medical Journal *41*:46–54.

Barandun D., Riva G. and Spengler G.A. (1968) Immunological deficiency diseases in man. Birth defects: Original Article Series IV, 1, p. 40. Edited by D. Bergsma and R.A. Good, New York: The National Foundation–March of Dimes.

Barbieri D., de Brito T., Hoshino S., Nasciemento O.B., Martins-Campos J.V., Quarentei G. and Marcondes E. (1970) Giardiasis in childhood. Absorption tests and biochemistry, histochemistry, light, and electron microscopy of jejunal mucosa. Archives of Disease in Childhood *45*:466–472.

Bardella M.T., Molteni N., Quatrini M., Velio P., Ranzi T. and Bianchi P.A. (1985) Clinical, biochemical and histological abnormalities in adult celiac patients on gluten-free diet. Gastroenterologie Clinique et Biologique *9*:787–789.

Barnes G.L. and Townley R.R.W. (1973) Duodenal mucosal damage in 31 infants with gastroenteritis. Archives of Diseases in Childhood *48*:343–349.

Barry R.E., Morris J.S. and Read A.E.A. (1970) A case of small intestinal mucosal atrophy. Gut *11*:743–747.

Bartnick W., ReMine S.G., Chiba M., Thayer W.R. and Shorter R.G. (1980) Isolation and characterization of colonic intraepithelial and lamina proprial lymphocytes. Gastroenterology *78*:976–985.

Bassen F.A. and Kornzweig A.L. (1950) Malformation of the erythrocytes in a case of atypical retinitis pigmentosa. Blood *5*:381–387.

Bastlein Ch., Decking R., Voeth Ch. and Ottenjann R. (1988) Giant Brunneroma of the duodenum. Endoscopy *20*:154–155.

Baudin J.B. (1837) M.D. thesis, University of Paris. Cited by Ostow J.D., Resnick R.H. (1959) Annals of Internal Medicine *51*:1303.

Bayless T.M., Kapelowitz R.F., Shelley W.M., Ballinger W.F. and Hendrix T.R. (1967) Intestinal ulceration: a complication of coeliac disease. New England Journal of Medicine *276*:996–1002.

Beck I.T., Kahn D.S., Lacerte M., Solymar J., Callegarini U. and Geokas M.C. (1965) Chronic duodenitis. Gut *6*:376–383.

Belaiche J., Vesin P., Chaumette M.T., Julien M. and Cattan D. (1980) Lymphangiectasies intestinales et fibrose des ganglions mesenteriques. Gastroenterologie Clinique et Biologique *4*:52–58.

Belcon M.C., Collins S.M., Castelli M.F. and Qizilbash A.H. (1980) Gastrointestinal hemorrhage in mastocytosis. Cancer Medical Association Journal *122*:311–314.

Biasco G., Callegari C., Lami F., Minarini A., Miglioli M. and Barbara L. (1984). Intestinal morphological changes during oral refeeding in a patient previously treated with total parenteral nutrition for small bowel resection. Americal Journal of Gastroenterology *79*:585–588.

Biggs B-A., Megna R., Wickremesinghe S. and Dwyer B. (1987) Human infection with Cryptosporidium spp.: results of a 24-month survey. Medical Journal of Australia *147*:175–177.

Binder H.J., Herting D.C., Hurst V., Finch S.C. and Spiro H.M. (1965) Tocopherol deficiency in man. New England Journal of Medicine *273*:1289–1297.

Bird R.G. and Smith M.D. (1980) Cryptosporidiosis in man: parasite life cycle and fine structure pathology. Journal of Pathology *132*:217–233.

Bisordi W.M. and Kleinman M.S. (1976) Melanosis duodeni. Gastrointestinal Endoscopy *23*:37–38.

Bjorneklett A., Fausa O., Refsum S.B., Torsvik H. and Sigstad H. (1977) Jejunal villous atrophy and granulomatous inflammation responding to gluten-free diet. Gut *18*:814–816.

Blackman E. and Nash S.V. (1985) Diagnosis of duodenal and ampullary epithelial neoplasms by endoscopic biopsy. Human Pathology *16*:901–910.

Blanes A., Martinez A., Bujan J., Ramon Y., Cajal S. and Carballido S.M. (1977) Intestinal mucosal changes following induced hypothyroidism in the developing rat. Virchows Archiv: A Pathological Anatomy and Histology *375*:233–239.

Bloom S.R. and Polak J.M. (Eds) (1981) Gut Hormones. London: Churchill Livingstone.

Bohane T.D., Cutz E., Hamilton J.R. and Gall D.G. (1977) Acrodermatitis enteropathica, zinc, and the Paneth cell. A case report with family studies. Gastroenterology *73*:587–592.

Bolton R.P., Cotter K.L. and Losowsky M.S. (1986) Impaired neutrophil function in intestinal lymphangiectasia. Journal of Clinical Pathology *39*:876–880.

Booth I.W., Chrystie I.L., Levinsky R.J., Marshall W.C., Pincott J. and Harries J.T. (1982) Protracted diarrhoea, immunodeficiency and viruses. European Journal of Pediatrics *138*:271–272.

Bossart R., Henry K., Booth C.C. and Doe W.F. (1975) Subepithelial collagen in intestinal malabsorption. Gut *16*:18–22.

Brandborg L.L., Goldberg S.B. and Breidenbach W.C. (1970) Human coccidiosis: a possible cause of malabsorption. New England Journal of Medicine *283*:1306–1313.

Brandborg L.L., Tankersley C.B., Gottlieb S., Barancik M. and Sartor V.E. (1967) Histological demonstration of mucosal invasion by Giardia lamblia in man. Gastroenterology *52*:143–150.

Brandt L.J., Davidoff A., Bernstein L.H., Biempica L., Rindfleisch B. and Goldstein M.L. (1981) Small intestinal involvement in Waldenstrom's macroglobulinemia. Case report and review of the literature. Digestive Diseases and Sciences *26*:174–180.

Brandtzaeg P., Sollid L.M., Thrane P.S., Kvale D., Bjerke K., Scott H., Kett K. and Rognum T.O. (1988) Lymphoepithelial interactions in the mucosal immune system. Gut *29*:1116–1130.

Bras G., Richards R.C., Irvine R.A., Milner P.F.A. and Ragbeer M.M.S. (1964) Infection with Strongyloides stercoralis in Jamaica. Lancet *2*:1257–1260.

Braverman D.Z., Dollberg L. and Shiner M. (1985) Clinical, histological and electron microscopic study of mast cell disease of the small bowel. American Journal of Gastroenterology *80*:30–37.

Breen E.G., Coughlan G., Connolly C.E., Stevens F.M. and McCarthy C.F. (1987) Coeliac proctitis. Scandinavian Journal of Gastroenterology *22*:471–477.

Brocchi E., Corazza G., Caletti G., Treggiari E.A., Barbara L. and Gasbarrini G. (1988) Endoscopic demonstration of loss of duodenal folds in the diagnosis of celiac disease. New England Journal of Medicine *319*:741–744.

Brouet J.C., Mason D.Y., Danon F., Preud'homme J.L., Seligmann M., Reyes F., Navab F., Galian A., Rene E. and Rambaud J.C. (1977) Alpha-chain disease: evidence for common clonal origin of intestinal immunoblastic lymphoma and plasmacytic proliferation. Lancet *1*:861.

Brow J.R., Parker F., Weinstein W.M. and Rubin C.E. (1971) The small intestinal mucosa in dermatitis herpetiformis. 1. Severity and distribution of the small intestinal lesion and associated malabsorption. Gastroenterology *60*:355–361.

Brunser O., Eidelman S. and Klipstein F.A. (1970) Intestinal morphology in rural Haitians. A comparison between overt tropical sprue and asymptomatic subjects. Gastroenterology *58*:655–668.

Buchan A.M.J. and Polak J.M. (1980) The classification of the human gastroenteropancreatic endocrine cells. Investigative and Cell Pathology *3*:51–71.

Buffa R., Capella C., Fontana P., Usellini L. and Solcia E. (1978) Types of endocrine cells in the human colon and rectum. Cell and Tissue Research *192*:227–240.

Bujanover Y., Liebman W.M., Goodman J.R. and Thaler M.M. (1981) Primary intestinal lymphangiectasia. Case Report with radiological and ultrastructural study. Digestion *21*:107–114.

Burhol P.G. and Myren T. (1968) Jejunal biospy findings in healthy young men. Scandinavian Journal of Gastroenterology *3*:346–350.

Burke V., Kerry K.R. and Anderson C.M. (1965) The relationship of dietary lactose to refractory diarrhoea in infancy. Australian Paediatric Journal *1*:147–152.

Businco L., Benincori N., Cantani A., Tacconi L. and Picarazzi A. (1985) Chronic diarrhea due to cow's milk allergy. A 4 to 10 year follow-up study. Annals of Allergy *55*:844–847.

Cabrera A., de la Pava S. and Pickren J.W. (1964) Intestinal localisation of Waldenstrom's disease. Archives of Internal Medicine *114*:399–407.

Candy D.C.A., Larcher C.F., Cameron D.J.S., Norman A.P., Tripp J.H., Milla P., Pincott J.R. and Harries J.T. (1981) Lethal familial protracted diarrhea. Archives of Disease in Childhood *56*:15–23.

Castellano G., Canga F., Lopez I., Colina F., Gutierrez J., Costa R. and Solis-Herruzo J.A. (1988) Pseudomelanosis of the duodenum. Journal of Clinical Gastroenterology *10*:150–154.

Castro L., de P., Dani R., Alvarenga R.J., Chamone D. de A.F. and de Oliveira C.A. (1971) A peroral biopsy study of the jejunum in human schistosomiasis mansoni. Review of the Institute of Tropical Medicine, Sao Paulo *13*:103–109.

Challacombe D.N. and Robertson K. (1977) Enterochromaffin cells in the duodenal mucosa of children with coeliac disease. Gut *18*:373–376.

Challacombe D.N., Wheeler E.E. and Campbell P.E. (1986) Morphometric studies and eosinophil cell counts in the duodenal mucosa of children with chronic nonspecific diarrhoea and cow's milk allergy. Journal of Pediatric Gastroenterology and Nutrition *5*:887–891.

Charache P., Bayless T.M., Shelley W.M. and Hendrix T.R. (1966) Atypical bacteria in Whipple's disease. Transactions of the Association of American Physicians *79*:399–408.

Chaukley H.W. (1943) Method for the quantitative morphological analysis of tissues. Journal of the National Cancer Institute *4*:47–53.

Chavalittamrong B. and Jirapinyo P. (1984) Intestinal parasites in pediatric patients with diarrhoeal diseases in Bangkok. Southeast Asian Journal of Tropical Medicine and Public Health *15*:385–388.

Chejfec G., Falkmer S., Askensten U., Grimelius L. and Gould V.E. (1988) Neuroendocrine tumours of the gastrointestinal tract. Pathology, Research and Practice *183*:143–154.

Cheli R. (1985) Is duodenitis always a peptic disease? American Journal of Gastroenterology *80*:442–444.

Cheli R., Aste H. and Ciancamerla G. (1973). Histological follow-up of duodenitis. Endoscopy *5*:135–139.

Cherner J.A., Jensen R.T., Dubois A., O'Dorisio T.M., Gardner J.D. and Metcalfe D.D. (1988) Gastrointestinal dysfunction in systemic mastocytosis. Gastroenterology *95*:657–667.

Cho C., Linscheer W.G., Hirschkorn M.A. and Ashutosh K. (1984) Sarcoidlike granulomas as an early manifestation of Whipple's disease. Gastroenterology *87*:941–947.

Clancy R.L., Tomkins W.A.F., Muckle T.J., Richardson H. and Rawls W.E. (1975) Isolation and characterization of an aetiological agent in Whipple's disease. British Medical Journal *3*:568–570.

Coello-Ramirez P. and Larrosa-Haro A. (1984) Gastrointestinal occult hemorrhage and gastroduodenitis in cow's milk protein intolerance. Journal of Pediatric Gastroenterology and Nutrition *3*:215–218.

Colwell E.J., Welsh J.D., Legters L.J. and Proctor R.F. (1968) Jejunal morphological characteristics in South Vietnamese residents. Journal of the American Medical Association *206*:2273–2276.

Congdon P., Mason M.K., Smith S., Crollick A., Steel A. and Littlewood J. (1981) Small-bowel mucosa in asymptomatic children with celiac disease. Mucosal changes with gluten-free diets. American Journal of Diseases in Children *135*:118–121.

Contractor Q.Q., Benson L., Schulz T.B., Contractor T.Q. and Kasturi N. (1988) Duodenal involvement in Schistosoma mansoni infection. Gut *29*:1011–1012.

Cook G.C. (1984) Aetiology and pathogenesis of postinfective tropical malabsorption (tropical sprue). (Occasional Survey) Lancet *i*:721–723.

Cooke W.T., Fone D.J., Cox E.V., Meynell M.J. and Gaddie R. (1963) Adult coeliac disease. Gut *4*:279–291.

Cookson J.B., Montgomery R.D., Morgan H.V. and Tudor R.W. (1972) Fatal paralytic ileus due to strongyloidiasis. British Medical Journal *4*:771–772.

Cooper B.T., Holmes G.K.T. and Cooke W.T. (1982) Lymphoma risk in coeliac disease of later life. Digestion *23*:89–92.

Cooper B.T., Holmes G.K.T., Ferguson R., Thompson R.A., Allan R.N. and Cooke W.T. (1980) Gluten-sensitive diarrhea without evidence of celiac disease. Gastroenterology *79*:801–806.

Corazza G.R., Bonvicini F., Franzzoni M., Gatto M. and Gasbarrini G. (1982) Observer variation in assessment of jejunal biopsy specimens. Gastroenterology *83*:1217–1222.

Corazza G.R., Franzzoni M., Dixon M.F. and Gasbarrini G. (1985) Quantitative assessment of the mucosal architecture of jejunal biopsy specimens: a comparison between linear measurement, stereology, and computer aided microscopy. Journal of Clinical Pathology *38*:765–770.

Corazza G.R., Franzzoni M. and Gasbarrini G. (1984) Jejunal intraepithelial lymphocytes in coeliac disease: are they increased or decreased? Gut *25*:158–162.

Corazza G.R., Franzzoni M., Gatto M.R.A. and Gasbarrini G. (1986) Ageing and small-bowel mucosa: a morphometric study. Gerontology *32*:60–65.

Coremans G., Rutgeerts P., Geboes K., Van den Oord J., Ponette E. and Vantrappen G. (1984) The value of ileoscopy with biopsy in the diagnosis of intestinal Crohn's disease. Gastrointestinal Endoscopy *30*:167–172.

Corless J.K., Tedesco F.J., Griffin J.W. and Panish J.K. (1984) Giant ileal inflammatory polyps in Crohn's disease. Gastrointestinal Endoscopy *30*:352–354.

Cotton P.B., Price A.B., Tighe J.R. and Beales J.S.M. (1973) Preliminary evaluation of duodenitis by endoscopy and biopsy. British Medical Journal *3*:430–433.

Cottrill C., Glueck C.J., Lauba V., Millet F., Pupprione D. and Brown M.V. (1974) Familial homozygous hypobetalipoproteinemia. Metabolism *23*:779–791.

Crabbe P.A. and Heremans J.F. (1967) Selective IgA deficiency with steatorrhea. American Journal of Medicine *42*:319–326.

Creamer B. (1964) Malignancy and the small intestinal mucosa. British Medical Journal *2*:1435–1436.

Creamer B. (1967) The turnover of the epithelium of the small intestine. British Medical Bulletin *23*:226–230.

Croft D.N., Loehry C.A. and Creamer B. (1968) Small bowel cell loss and weight loss in the coeliac syndrome. Lancet *ii*:68–70.

Crow J. and Asselah F. (1984) Immunoproliferative small intestinal disease in Algerians. Cancer *54*:1908–1913.

Cunningham D., Morgan R.J., Mills P.R., Nelson L.M., Toner P.G., Soukop M., McArdle C.S. and Russell R.I. (1985) Functional and structural changes of the human proximal small intestine after cytotoxic therapy. Journal of Clinical Pathology *38*:265–270.

Curran R.C. and Jones E.L. (1979) Non-Hodgkin's lymphomas: An immunohistochemical and histological study. Journal of Pathology *129*:179–190.

Current W.L., Reese N.C., Ernst J.V., Bailey W.S., Heyman M.B. and Weinstein W.M. (1983) Human cryptosporidiosis in immunocompetent and immunodeficient persons. The New England Journal of Medicine *308*:1252–1257.

Da Costa L.R. (1971) Small intestinal cell turnover in patients with parasitic infections. British Medical Journal *3*:281–283.

Davidson A.G.F. and Bridges M.A. (1988) Coeliac disease: an analysis of aetiological possibilities and re-evaluation of the enzymopathic hypothesis. Medical Hypotheses *26*:155–160.

Davidson G.P. and Barnes G.L. (1979) Structural and functional abnormalities of the small intestine in infants and young children with rotavirus enteritis. Acta Paediatrica Scandinavica *68*:181–186.

Davidson G.P., Cutz E., Hamilton J.R. and Gall D.G. (1978) Familial enteropathy: a syndrome of protracted diarrhea from birth, failure to thrive, and hypoplastic villus atrophy. Gastroenterology *75*:783–790.

Davidson G.P. and Townley R.R.W. (1977) Structural and functional abnormalities of the small intestine due to nutritional folic acid deficiency in infancy. Journal of Paediatrics *90*:590–594.

Dawson J., Bryant M.G., Bloom S.R. and Peters T.J. (1986) Jejunal mucosal enzyme activities, regulatory peptides and organelle pathology of the enteropathy of common variable immunodefiency. Gut *27*:273–277.

Delgado M.J., Moreno J., Murillo M.L., Bolufer J. and Lopez-Campos J.L. (1986) Histophysiologic aspects of the remnant intestine of rats subjected to partial resection of the small intestine. Revista Espanola de Fisiologia *42*:205–212.

Denholm R.B., Mills P.R. and More I.A.R. (1981) Electron microscopy in the long-term follow-up of Whipple's disease. American Journal of Surgical Pathology *5*:507–516.

Dent D.M., Duys P.J., Bird A.R. and Birkenstock W.E. (1975) Cytomegalic virus infection of bowel in adults. South African Medical Journal *49*:669–672.

Deo M.G. and Ramalingaswami V. (1965) Reaction of the small intestine to induced protein malnutrition in Rhesus monkeys: a study of cell population kinetics in the jejunum. Gastroenterology *49*:150–157.

de Paola D., Dias L.B. and da Silva J.R. (1962) Enteritis due to strongyloides stercoralis. A report of five fatal cases. American Journal of Digestive Diseases 7:1086–1098.

de Sousa J.S., da Silva A., Pereira M.V., Soares J. and Ramalho P.M. (1986) Cow's milk protein-sensitive enteropathy: number and timing of biopsies for diagnosis. Journal of Pediatric Gastroenterology and Nutrition *5*:207–209.

de Sousa J.S., Guerreiro O., Cunha A. and Araujo J. (1968) Association of nephrotic syndrome with intestinal lymphangiectasia. Archives of Disease in Childhood *43*:245–248.

Dhesi I., Marsh M.N., Kelly C. and Crowe P. (1984) Morphometric analysis of small intestinal mucosa. Virchows Archiv (A) *403*:173–180.

Dinari G., Rosenbach Y., Grunebaum M., Zahavi I., Alpert G. and Nitzan M. (1980) Gastrointestinal manifestations of Neimann-Pick disease. Enzyme 25:407–412.

Dincsoy H.P., Rolfes D.B., McGraw C.A. and Schubert W.K. (1984) Cholesterol ester storage disease and mesenteric lipodystrophy. American Journal of Clinical Pathology *81*:263–269.

Dissanayake A.S., Truelove S.C., Offord R.E. and Whitehead R. (1973) Nature of toxic component of wheat gluten in coeliac disease. Lancet *ii*:709–710.

Dissanayake A.S., Truelove S.C. and Whitehead R. (1974) Jejunal mucosal recovery in coeliac disease in relation to adherence to a gluten free diet. Quarterly Journal of Medicine *170*:161–185.

Dobbins W.O. III (1966) An ultrastructural study of the intestinal mucosa in congenital B-lipoprotein deficiency with particular emphasis upon the intestinal absorptive cell. Gastroenterology *50*:195–210.

Dobbins W.O. III (1981) Is there an immune deficit in Whipple's disease? Digestive Diseases and Sciences 26:247–252.

Dobbins W.O. III (1986) Human intestinal intraepithelial lymphocytes. Gut 27:972–985.

Dobbins W.O. III and Kawanishi H. (1981) Bacillary characteristics in Whipple's disease: an electron microscopic study. Gastroenterology 80:1468–1475.

Doe W.F. (1975) Alpha chain disease. Clinicopathological features and relationship to so-called Mediterranean lymphoma. British Journal of Cancer *31*(Suppl. II):350–355.

Doe W.F. (1979) An overview of intestinal immunity and malabsorption. The American Journal of Medicine 67:1077–1084

Doe W.F., Henry K., Hobbs J.R., Avery Jones F., Dent C.E. and Booth C.C. (1972) Five cases of alpha chain disease. Gut *13*:947–957.

Doniach D. and Shiner M. (1957) Duodenal and jejunal biopsies. Gastroenterology *33*:71–86.

Douglas J.G., Gillon J., Logan R.F.A., Grant I.W.B. and Crompton G.K. (1984) Sarcoidosis and coeliac disease: an association. Lancet *ii*:13–14.

Dowling R.H. (1967) Compensatory changes in intestinal absorption. British Medical Bulletin *23*:275–278.

Draper L.R., Gyure L.A., Hall J.G. and Robertson D. (1983) Effect of alcohol on the integrity of the intestinal epithelium. Gut *24*:399–404.

Drummond M.B. and Montgomery R.D. (1970) Acute sprue in Britain. British Medical Journal 2:340–341.

Dubois R.S., Roy C.C., Fulginiti V.A., Merrill D.A. and Murray R.L. (1970) Disaccharidase deficiency in children with immunologic deficits. Journal of Pediatrics 76:337.

Dukes C. and Bussey H.J.R. (1926) The number of lymphoid follicles of the human large intestine. Journal of Pathology and Bacteriology 29:111–116.

Dunnill M.S. and Whitehead R. (1972) A method for the quantitation of small intestinal biopsy specimens. Journal of Clinical Pathology 25:243–246.

Eastham E.J., Douglas A.P. and Watson A.J. (1976) Diagnosis of giardia lamblia infection as a cause of diarrhoea. Lancet *ii*:950–951.

Eckstein R.P., Dowsett J.F. and Riley J.W. (1988) Collagenous enterocolitis: a case of collagenous colitis with involvement of the small intestine. American Journal of Gastroenterology *83*:767–771.

Eidelman S., Parkins R.A. and Rubin C.E. (1966) Abdominal lymphoma presenting as malabsorption. Medicine (Baltimore) *45*:111–137.

Egan-Mitchell B., Fottrell P.F. and McNicholl B. (1981) Early or pre-coeliac mucosa: development of gluten enteropathy. Gut 22:65–69.

Evans D.J. and Ali M.H. (1985) Immunocytochemistry in the diagnosis of Whipple's disease. Journal of Clinical Pathology *38*:372–374.

Fagundes-Neto U., Wehba J., Viaro T., Machado N.L. and Patricio F.R. (1985) Protracted diarrhea in infancy: clinical aspects and ultrastructural analysis of the small intestine. Journal of Pediatric Gastroenterology and Nutrition *4*:714–722.

Feldman M. (1986) Whipple's Disease. (Southern Internal Medicine Conference). American Journal of Medical Sciences *291*:56–67.

Fenyo G., Hallberg D., Soda M. and Roos K.A. (1976) Morphological changes in the small intestine following jejuno-ileal shunt in parenterally fed rats. Scandinavian Journal of Gastroenterology *11*:635–640.

Ferguson A., Blackwell J.N. and Barnetson R. St. C. (1987) Effects of additional dietary gluten on the small-intestinal mucosa of volunteers and of patients with dermatitis herpetiformis. Scandinavian Journal of Gastroenterology 22:543–549.

Ferguson A. and Murray D. (1971) Quantitation of intraepithelial lymphocytes in human jejunum. Gut *12*:988–994.

Ferguson A. and Ziegler K. (1986) Intraepithelial lymphocyte mitosis in a jejunal biopsy correlates with intraepithelial lymphocyte count, irrespective of diagnosis. Gut *27*:675–679.

Fernandes B.J., Amato D. and Goldfinger M. (1985) Diffuse lymphomatous polyposis of the gastrointestinal tract. Gastroenterology *88*:1267–1270.

Feyrter F. (1934) Uber Wucherungen der Brunnerschen Drusen. Virchows Archiv (A) *293*:509–520.

Fichtelius K.E., Yunis J.E. and Good R.A. (1968) Occurrence of lymphocytes within the gut epithelium of normal and neonatally thymectomised mice. Proceedings of the Society for Experimental Biology *128*:185–188.

Fisher S.E., Boyle J.T. and Holtzapple P. (1981) Chronic protracted diarrhoea and jejunal atrophy in an infant. Cimetidine-associated stimulation of jejunal mucosal growth. Digestive Diseases and Sciences *26*:181–186.

Fleck S.L., Hames S.E. and Warhurst D.C. (1985) Detection of Giardia in human jejunum by immunoperoxidase method. Specific and non-specific results. Transactions of the Royal Society of Tropical and Medical Hygiene *79*:110–113.

Fleming J.L., Wiesner R.H. and Shorter R.G. (1988) Whipple's disease: clinical, biochemical and histopathologic features and assessment of treatment of 29 patients. Mayo Clinic Proceedings *63*:539–551.

Flynn D.M., Lake B.D., Boothby D.B. and Young E.P. (1972) Gut lesions in Fabry's disease without a rash. Archives of Disease in Childhood *47*:26–33.

Fontaine J.L. and Navarro J. (1975) Small intestinal biopsy in cow's milk protein allergy in infancy. Archives of Disease in Childhood *50*:357–362.

Foroozan P. and Trier J.S. (1967) Mucosa of the small intestine in pernicious anaemia. New England Journal of Medicine *277*:553–559.

Foster C.S. (1979) The brown bowel syndrome: a possible smooth muscle mitochondrial myopathy? Histopathology *3*:1–17.

Fox B. (1967) Lipofuscinosis of the gastrointestinal tract in man. Journal of Clinical Pathology *20*:806–813.

Franzin G., Musola R., Ghidini O., Manfrini C. and Fratton A. (1985) Nodular hyperplasia of Brunner's glands. Gastrointestinal Endoscopy *31*:374–378.

Franzin G., Novelli P. and Fratton A. (1983). Hyperplastic and metaplastic polyps of the duodenum. Gastrointestinal Endoscopy *29*:140–142.

Fraser G.M., Pitman R.G., Lawrie J.H., Smith G.M.R., Forest A.P.M. and Rhodes J. (1964) The significance of the radiological findings of coarse mucosal folds in the duodenum. Lancet *ii*:979–982.

Freedman A.R., Macartney J.C., Nelufer J.M. and Ciclitira P.J. (1987) Timing of infiltration of T lymphocytes induced by gluten into the small intestine in coeliac disease. Journal of Clinical Pathology *40*:741–745.

Freeman H.J. and Chiu B.K. (1986a) Multifocal small bowel lymphoma and latent celiac sprue. Gastroenterology *90*:1992–1997.

Freeman H.J. and Chiu B.K. (1986b) Small bowel malignant lymphoma complicating celiac sprue and the mesenteric lymph node cavitation syndrome. Gastroenterology *90*:2008–2012.

Frexinos J., Pudebat M., Duffaut M., Rumeau J-L. and Arlet P. (1979) Hypogammaglobulemie globale et atrophie villositaire sensible au regime sans gluten. Gastroenterologie Clinique et Biologique *8*:893–898.

Fudenberg H.H., Good R.A., Hitzig W., Kunkel H.G., Roitt I.M., Rosen F.S., Rowe D.S., Seligmann M. and Soothill J.R. (1970) Classification of the primary immunodeficiencies: W.H.O. recommendation. New England Journal of Medicine *283*:656.

Galian A., Lecestre M-J., Scott J., Bognel C., Matuchansky C. and Rambaud J-C. (1977) Pathological study of alpha-chain disease with special emphasis on evolution. Cancer *39*:2081–2101.

Galjaard H., van der Meer-Fieggen W. and Giesen J. (1972) Feedback control by functional villus cells on cell proliferation and maturation in intestinal epithelium. Experimental Cell Research *73*:197–207.

Gallager R.L. (1980) Intestinal ceroid deposition: "Brown bowel syndrome." A light and electron microscopic study. Virchows Archiv (A) *389*:143–151.

Gallo-Van Ess D.M., Strasburger V.C. and Turetsky R.A. (1986) Intestinal lymphangiectasia in an adolescent. Journal of Adolescent Health Care *7*:259–264.

Gear E.V. and Dobbins W.O. (1969) The histologic spectrum of proximal duodenal biopsy in adult males. The American Journal of Medical Science *257*:90–99.

Gelzayd E.A., Biederman M.A. and Gelfand D.W. (1975) Changing concepts of duodenitis. American Journal of Gastroenterology *64*:213–216.

Gilinsky N.H., Chaimowitz G. and Van Staden M.C. (1986) Immunoproliferative small-intestinal disease with lymphoma: diagnostic difficulties and pitfalls. South African Medical Journal *69*:260–262.

Gilinsky N.H., Mee A.S., Beatty D.W., Novis B.H., Young G., Price S., Purves L.R. and Marks I.N. (1985) Plasma cell infiltration of the small bowel: lack of evidence for a non-secretory form of alpha-heavy chain disease. Gut *26*:928–934.

Gillberg R., Dotevall G. and Ahren C. (1982) Chronic inflammatory bowel disease in patients with coeliac disease. Scandinavian Journal of Gastroenterology *17*:491–496.

Gillon J., Thamery D.A. and Ferguson A. (1982) Features of small intestinal pathology (epithelial cell kinetics, intraepithelial lymphocytes, disaccharidases) in a primary Giardia muris infection. Gut *23*:498–506.

Gleason T.H. and Patterson S.D. (1982) The pathology of Yersinia enterocolitica ileocolitis. American Journal of Surgical Pathology 6:347–355.

Gleeson M.H., Bloom S.R., Polak J.M., Henry K. and Dowling R.H. (1970) An endocrine tumour in kidney affecting small bowel structure, motility, and function. (Abstract) Gut *11*:1066.

Glew R.H., Basu A., Prence E.M. and Remaley A.T. (1985) Lysosomal storage diseases. Laboratory Investigation *53*:250–269.

Goldgar C.M. and Vanderhoof J.A. (1986) Lack of correlation of small bowel biopsy and clinical course of patients with intractable diarrhea of infancy. Gastroenterology *90*:527–531.

Good R.A. Peterson R.D.A., Percy D.Y., Finstad J. and Cooper M.D. (1968) Immunological deficiency diseases in man. Birth defects: Original Article Series IV, 1, p. 17. Edited by D. Bergsma and R.A. Good. New York. The National Foundation–March of Dimes.

Goodwin C.S. (1988) Duodenal ulcer, campylobacter pylori, and the "leaking roof" concept. Lancet *ii*:1467–1469.

Gorbach S.L. and Tabaqchali S. (1969) Bacteria, bile and the small bowel. Gut *10*:963–972.

Gordon J. and Smith J.L. (1980) Immunoglobulin synthesis by neoplastic cells: models of a clonal transition from IgM to IgG synthesis. Journal of Clinical Pathology *33*:539–554.

Gouffier E., Phan A., Paraf A., Boddaert A. and Chevrel J-P. (1977) Recurrent ulcerative jejuno-ileitis. Report of a case with operative and endoscopic observations. Gastroenterologie Clinique et Biologique *1*:545–552.

Green F. and Heyworth B. (1980) Immunoglobulin-containing cells in jejunal mucosa of children with protein-energy malnutrition and gastroenteritis. Archives of Diseases in Childhood 55:380–383.

Green P.H.R., Lefkowitch J.H., Glickman R.M., Riley J.W., Quinet E. and Blum C.B. (1982) Apoprotein localization and quantitation in the human intestine. Gastroenterology *83*:1223–1230.

Greenwood N. (1976) The jejunal mucosa in two cases of A-beta-lipoproteinemia. The American Journal of Gastroenterology *65*:160–162.

Grefte J.M.M., Bouman J.G., Grond J., Jansen W. and Kleibeuker J.H. (1988) Slow and incomplete histological and functional recovery in adult gluten sensitive enteropathy. Journal of Clinical Pathology *41*:886–891.

Gregg J.A. and Garabedian M. (1974) Duodenitis. American Journal of Gastroenterology *61*:177–184.

Guerra R., Wheby M.S. and Bayless T.M. (1965) Long-term antibiotic therapy in tropical sprue. Annals of Internal Medicine *63*:619–634.

Guix M., Skinner J.M. and Whitehead R. (1979) Measuring intraepithelial lymphocytes, surface area, and volume of lamina propria in the jejunal mucosa of coeliac patients. Gut *20*:275–278.

Gupta S., Pinching A.J., Onwubalili J., Vince A., Evans D.J. and Hodgson H.J.F. (1986) Whipple's disease with unusual clinical, bacteriologic and immunologic findings. Gastroenterology *90*:1286–1289.

Gupta T.P. and Weinstock J.V. (1986) Duodenal pseudomelanosis associated with chronic renal failure. Gastrointestinal Endoscopy *32*:358–360.

Gushurst T.P. and Lesesne H.R. (1984) Isolated duodenal varix: an unusual cause of gastrointestinal hemorrhage. Southern Medical Journal 77:915–918.

Gustavsson S., Weiland L.H. and Kelly K.A. (1987) Relationship of backwash ileitis to ileal pouchitis after ileal pouch-anal anastomosis. Diseases of the Colon and Rectum *30*:25–28.

Haeney M.R., Goodwin B.J.F., Barratt M.E.J., Mike N. and Asquith P. (1982) Soya protein antibodies in man: their occurrence and possible relevance in coeliac disease. Journal of Clinical Pathology *35*:319–322.

Hall P.A., Jass J.R., Levison D.A., Morson B.C., Shepherd N.A., Sobin L.H. and Stansfeld A.G. (1988) Classification of primary gut lymphomas. Lancet *ii*:958.

Hallgren R., Colombel J.F., Dahl R., Fredens K., Kruse A., Jacobsen N.O., Venge P. and Rambaud J.C. (1989) Neutrophil and eosinophil involvement of the small bowel in patients with celiac disease and Crohn's disease: studies on the secretion rate and immunohistochemical localisation of granulocyte granule constituents. American Journal of Medicine *86*:56–64.

Halliday C.E.W. and Farthing M.J.G. (1986) Giardiasis. Gastroenterology *5*:3–7.

Halliday K., Edmeades R. and Shepherd R. (1982) Persistent post-enteritis diarrhoea in childhood. A prospective analysis of clinical features, predisposing factors and sequelae. Medical Journal of Australia *1*:18–20.

Halphen M., Galian A., Certin M., Ink F., Filali A. and Rambaud J-C. (1989) Clinicopathological study of a patient with idiopathic villous atrophy and small vessel alterations of the ileum. Digestive Diseases and Sciences *34*:111–117.

Halphen M., Najjar T., Jaafoura H., Cammoun M. and Tufrali G. (1986) Diagnostic value of upper intestinal fiber endoscopy in primary small intestinal lymphoma. Cancer *58*:2140–2145.

Halstead C.H., Sheir S. and Raasch F.O. (1969) The small intestine in human schistosomiasis. Gastroenterology *57*:622–623.

Hand N.M. (1987) Enzyme histochemistry on jejunal tissue embedded in resin. Journal of Clinical Pathology *40*:346–352.

Hara M., Harasawa S., Tani N., Miwa T. and Tsutsumi Y. (1988) Gastric metaplasia in duodenal ulcer. Acta Pathologica Japonica *38*:1011–1018.

Harris M., Burton I.E. and Scarffe J.H. (1983) Macroglobulinaemia and intestinal lymphangiectasia: a rare association. Journal of Clinical Pathology *36*:30–36.

Harris O.D., Cooke W.T., Thompson M. and Waterhouse J.A.H. (1967) Malignancy in adult celiac disease and idiopathic steatorrhea. American Journal of Medicine *42*:899–912.

Hasan M., Hay F., Sircus W. and Ferguson A. (1983) Nature of the inflammatory cell infiltrate in duodenitis. Journal of Clinical Pathology *36*:280–288.

Hauer-Jensen M., Poulakos L., Milani F.X. and Osborne J.W. (1988) Effects of exocrine pancreatic secretions on hyperthermic injury of rat small intestine. International Journal of Hyperthermia *4*:417–426.

Helmy I. (1980) Endoscopic diagnosis of immunoproliferative small intestinal disease (IPSID). Endoscopy *12*:114–116.

Hendrix T.R. and Yardley J.H. (1970) Modern trends in gastroenterology. Vol 4. p. 229. Edited by W.I. Card and B. Creamer. London: Butterworth.

Hennig A. (1956) Inhalt einer aus papilleu oder zotten gebildeten flache. Mikroscopie *11*:206–213.

Henry K., Bird R.G. and Doe W.F. (1974) Intestinal coccidiosis in a patient with alpha-chain disease. British Medical Journal *1*:542–543.

Henson D. (1972) Cytomegalovirus inclusion bodies in the gastrointestinal tract. Archives of Pathology *93*:477–482.

Herbert P.N., Assmann G., Gotto A.M. and Fredrickson D.S. (1982) Familial lipoprotein deficiency: abetalipoproteinemia, hypobetalipoproteinemia and Tangier disease. In: The Metabolic Basis of Inherited Disease. 4th Edition. Edited by J.B. Stanbury, J.B. Wyngaarden and D.S. Fredrickson. New York: McGraw-Hill, pp. 589–621.

Hermans P.E., Huizenga K.A., Hoffman H.N., Brown A.L. and Markowitz H. (1966) Dysgammaglobulinemia associated with nodular lymphoid hyperplasia of the small intestine. American Journal of Medicine *40*:78–79.

Hermos J.A., Cooper H.L., Kramer P. and Trier J.S. (1970) Histological diagnosis by peroral biopsy of Crohn's disease of the proximal intestine. Gastroenterology *59*:868–873.

Hibi T., Asakura H., Kobayashi K., Munakata Y., Kano S., Tsuchiya M., Teramoto T. and Uematsu Y. (1982) Alpha heavy chain disease lacking secretory alpha chain, with cobblestone appearance of the small intestine and duodenal ulcer demonstrated by endoscopy. Gut *23*:422–427.

Hoang C., Halphen M., Galian A., Brouet J-C., Marsan C., Leclerc J-P. and Rambaud J-C. (1985) Small bowel involvement and exudative enteropathy in Waldenstrom's macroglobulinemia. Gastroenterologie Clinique et Biologique *9*:444–448.

Hobbs J.R. and Hepner G.W. (1968) Deficiency of gamma-M-globulin in coeliac disease. Lancet *i*:217–220.

Hobbs J.R., Hepner G.W., Douglas A.P., Crabbe P.A. and Johansson S.G.O. (1969) Immunological mystery of coeliac disease. Lancet *ii*:649–650.

Hockenstrom T., Kock N.G., Norlen L.J., Ahren C. and Philipson B.M. (1986) Morphologic changes in ileal reservoir mucosa after long-term exposure to urine. Scandinavian Journal of Gastroenterology *21*:1224–1234.

Holdstock G., Eade O.E., Isaacson P. and Smith C.L. (1979) Endoscopic duodenal biopsies in coeliac disease and duodenitis. Scandinavian Journal of Gastroenterology *14*:717–720.

Holmes G.K.T., Asquith P., Stokes P.L. and Cooke W.T. (1974) Cellular infiltrate of jejunal biopsies in adult coeliac disease in relation to gluten withdrawal. Gut *15*:278–283.

Holmes G.K.T., Prior P., Lane M.R., Pope D. and Allan R.N. (1989) Malignancy in coeliac disease: effect of a gluten free diet. Gut *30*:333–338.

Holmes G.K.T., Stokes P.L., Sorahan T.M., Prior P., Waterhouse J.A.H. and Cooke W.T. (1976) Coeliac disease, gluten-free diet and malignancy. Gut *17*:612–619.

Horn T., Svendsen L.B., Johansen A. and Backer O. (1985) Brown bowel syndrome. Ultrastructural Pathology *8*:357–361.

Horowitz A. and Shiner M. (1981) The recognition of premalignant change in jejunal mucosal biopsies of patients with malabsorption. Journal of Submicroscopic Cytology *13*:423–443.

Hosler J.P., Kimmel K.K. and Moeller D.D. (1982) The "Brown Bowel Syndrome": a case report. American Journal of Gastroenterology *77*:854–855.

Hourihane D.O'B. (1963) Diarrhoea of small bowel origin. The histology of small intestinal biopsies. Proceedings of the Royal Society of Medicine *56*:1073–1077.

Hourihane D.O'B. and Weir D.G. (1970) Malignant celiac syndrome. Report of two cases with malabsorption and microscopic foci of intestinal lymphoma. Gastroenterology *59*:130–139.

Howard F.M., Carter C.O., Candy D.C.A. and Harries J.T. (1981) A family study of protracted diarrhea in infancy. Journal of Medical Genetics *18*:81–86.

Ikeda K., Sannohe Y., Murayama H., Ikeda R. and Inutsuka S. (1982) Heterotopic gastric mucosa in the duodenum: reaction to congo red under fiberscopic observation. Endoscopy *14*:168–170.

Inge P.M.G., Edson C.M. and Farthing M.J.G. (1988) Attachment of Giardia lamblia to rat intestinal epithelial cells. Gut *29*:795–801.

Isaacson P. (1980) Malignant histiocytosis of the intestine: the early histological lesion. Gut *21*:381–386.

Isaacson P. (1981) Primary gastrointestinal lymphoma. Virchows Archiv (A) *391*:1–8.

Isaacson P.G. (1985) B-cell lymphomas of the gastrointestinal tract. American Journal of Surgical Pathology *9*(Suppl):117–128.

Isaacson P.G., Jones D.B., Sworn M.J. and Wright D.H. (1982) Malignant histiocytosis of the intestine: report of three cases with immunological and cytochemical analysis. Journal of Clinical Pathology 35:510–516.

Isaacson P.G., Maclennan K.A. and Subbuswamy S.G. (1984) Multiple lymphomatous polyposis of the gastrointestinal tract. Histopathology 8:641–656.

Isaacson P.G., O'Connor N.T., Spencer J., Bevan D.H., Connolly C.E., Kirkham N., Pollock D.J., Wainscoat J.S., Stein H. and Mason D.Y. (1985) Malignant histiocytosis of the intestine: A T-cell lymphoma. Lancet ii:688–691.

Isaacson P.G. and Spencer J. (1987) Malignant lymphoma of mucosa-associated lymphoid tissue. Histopathology 11:445–462.

Isaacson P.G. and Wright D.H. (1978) Malignant histiocytosis of the intestine: its relationship to malabsorption and ulcerative jejunitis. Human Pathology 9:661–677.

Isselbacher K.J., Scheig R., Plotkin G.R. and Caulfield J.B. (1964) Congenital b-lipoprotein deficiency; a hereditary disorder involving a defect in the absorption and transport of lipids. Medicine (Baltimore) 43:347–361.

Iyngkaran N., Yadav M., Boey C.G., Kamath K.R. and Lam K.L. (1989) Causative effect of cow's milk protein and soy protein on progressive small bowel mucosal damage. Journal of Gastroenterology and Hepatology 4:127–136.

Iyngkaran N., Yadav M., Boey C.G., Meng L.L., Puthucheary S.D. and Lam K.L. (1988a) Effect of diet on the clinical course and repair of the small bowel mucosa in infantile gastroenteritis. Journal of Gastroenterology and Hepatology 3:337–344.

Iyngkaran N., Yadav M., Looi L.M., Boey C.G., Lam K.L., Balabaskaran S., and Puthucheary S.D. (1988) Effect of soy protein on the small bowel mucosa of young infants recovering from acute gastroenteritis. Journal of Pediatric Gastroenterology and Nutrition 7:68–75.

Jackson P.G., Lessof M.H., Baker R.W.R., Ferrett J. and MacDonald D.M. (1981) Intestinal permeability in patients with eczema and food allergy. Lancet 1:1285–1286.

James A.H. (1964) Gastric epithelium in the duodenum. Gut 5:285–294.

Jeffries G.H., Steinberg H. and Sleisenger M.H. (1968) Chronic ulcerative (nongranulomatous) jejunitis. American Journal of Medicine 44:47–59.

Jenkins D., Goodall A., Gillet F.R. and Scott B.B. (1985) Defining duodenitis: quantitative histological study of mucosal responses and their correlations. Journal of Clinical Pathology 38:1119–1126.

Jewell D.P. (1983) Ulcerative enteritis. British Medical Journal 287:1740–1741.

Johansen A. (1974) Enzyme histochemical investigations of heterotopic gastric epithelium in the duodenum. Acta Pathologica et Microbiologica Scandinavica 82:613–617.

Johansen A. and Hansen O.H. (1973) Heterotopic gastric epithelium in the duodenum and its correlation to gastric disease and acid level. Acta Pathologica et Microbiologica Scandinavica 81:676–680.

Johnson C.D. and White H. (1988) Colonic metaplasia with colonic-type polyps on an ileostomy stoma in polyposis coli. Diseases of the Colon and Rectum 31:405–407.

Jones B., Fishman E.K., Bayless T.M. and Siegelman S.S. (1983) Villous hypertrophy of the small bowel in a patient with glucagonoma. Journal of Computer Assisted Tomography 7:334–337.

Jones M.A., Griffith L.M. and West A.B. (1989) Adenocarcinoid tumor of the periampullary region: a novel duodenal neoplasm presenting as biliary tract obstruction. Human Pathology 20:198–200.

Judd E.S. and Nagel W.G. (1927) Duodenitis. Annals of Surgery 85:380.

Kagnoff M.F., Paterson Y.J., Kumar P.J., Kasarda D.D., Carbone F.R., Unsworth D.J. and Austin R.K. (1987) Evidence for the role of a human intestinal adenovirus in the pathogenesis of coeliac disease. Gut 28:995–1001.

Kamath K.R. and Murugasu R. (1974) A comparative study of four methods for detecting Giardia lamblia in children with diarrheal disease and malabsorption. Gastroenterology 66:16–21.

Kang J.Y., Wu A.Y.T., Chia J.L.S., Wee A., Sutherland I.H. and Hori R. (1987) Clinical and ultrastructural studies in duodenal pseudomelanosis. Gut 28:1673–1681.

Kanof M.E., Rance N.E., Hamilton S.R., Luk G.D. and Lake A.M. (1987) Congenital diarrhea with intestinal inflammation and epithelial immaturity. Journal of Pediatric Gastroenterology and Nutrition 6:141–146.

Kavin H. (1981) Celiac disease complicated by chronic nongranulomatous ulcerative enterocolitis, nodular lymphoid hyperplasia, and disseminated intravascular coagulation. Digestive Diseases and Sciences 26:73–80.

Keeling J.W. and Harries J.T. (1973) Intestinal malabsorption in infants with histiocytosis X. Archives of Diseases in Childhood 48:350–354.

Kelly J., O'Farrelly C., O'Mahony C., Weir D.G. and Feighery C. (1987) Immunoperoxidase demonstration of the cellular composition of the normal and coeliac small bowel. Clinics of Experimental Immunology 68:177–188.

Kent T.H. (1964) Malabsorption syndrome with malignant lymphoma. Archives of Pathology 78:97–103.

Keren D.F., Weisburger W.R., Yardley J.H., Salyer W.R., Arthur R.R. and Charache P. (1976) Whipple's disease: demonstration by immunofluorescence of similar bacterial antigens in macrophages from three cases. Johns Hopkins Medical Journal 139:51–59.

Kerr C. (1984) Diagnosis of lysosomal storage disorders. Medical Journal of Australia 140:188–189.

Khojasteh A., Haghshenass M. and Haghighi P. (1983) Immunoproliferative small intestinal disease. A "Third-World Lesion." New England Journal of Medicine 308:1401–1405.

Kikindjanin V., Vukavic T., Opric M. and Novakov G. (1985) Local immunodeficiency of the intestinal mucosa: a contribution to etiopathogenesis of recurrent urticaria and diarrhoea. Allergie und Immunologie *31*:183–188.

King C.E. and Toskes P.P. (1979) Small intestinal bacterial overgrowth. Gastroenterology *76*:1035–1055.

Kingham J.G., Levison D.A. and Fairclough P.D. (1981) Diarrhoea and reversible enteropathy in Zollinger-Ellison syndrome. Lancet *ii*:610–612.

Klipstein F.A. and Schenk E.A. (1975) Enterotoxigenic intestinal bacteria in tropical sprue. II. Effect of the bacteria and their enterotoxins on intestinal structure. Gastroenterology *68*:642–655.

Kluge F., Koch H.K., Grosse-Wilde H., Lesch R. and Gerok W. (1982) Follow-up of treated adult celiac disease: Clinical and morphological studies. Hepato-gastroenterology *29*:17–23.

Knight R. and Wright S.G. (1978) Progress report intestinal protozoa. Gut *19*:940–953.

Kokkonen J., Simila S. and Herva R. (1980) Gastrointestinal findings in atopic children. European Journal of Pediatrics *134*:249–254.

Konjetzny G.E. (1924) Zur pathologie und chirurgischen Behandlung des Ulcus duodeni. Deutsche Zeitschrift der Chirurgie *184*:85.

Kosnai I. Karpati S., Savilahti E., Verkasalo M., Bucsky P. and Torok E. (1986) Gluten challenge in children with dermatitis herpetiformis: a clinical, morphological and immunohistological study. Gut *27*:1464–1470.

Kosnai I., Kuitunen P., Savilahti E. and Sipponen P. (1984). Mast cells and eosinophils in the jejunal mucosa of patients with intestinal cow's milk allergy and celiac disease of childhood. Journal of Pediatric Gastroenterology and Nutrition *3*:368–372.

Kosztolanyi G. and Pap M. (1986) Severe growth failure associated with atrophic intestinal mucosa and ring chromosome 15. Acta Paediatrica Scandinavica *75*:326–331.

Kreuning J., Bosman F.T., Kuiper G., v.d. Wal A.M. and Lindeman J. (1978) Gastritis and duodenal mucosa in "healthy" individuals: an endoscopic and histopathological study of 50 volunteers. Journal of Clinical Pathology *31*:69–77.

Kumar P.J., O'Donoghue D.P., Stenson K. and Dawson A.M. (1979) Reintroduction of gluten in adults and children with treated coeliac disease. Gut *20*:743–749.

Kundrotas L.W., Camara D.S., Meenaghan M.A., Montes M., Wosick W.F. and Weiser M.M. (1985) Heterotopic gastric mucosa. A case report. American Journal of Gastroenterology *80*:253–256.

Kuo Y-C. and Wu C-S. (1988) Duodenal melanosis. Journal of Clinical Gastroenterology *10*:160–164.

Kwitko A.O., Shearman D.J.C., McKenzie P.E., La Brooy J.T., Rowland R. and Woodroffe A.J. (1980) Whipple's disease: a case with circulating immune complexes. Gastroenterology *79*:1318–1323.

Lake B.D. (1988) Microvillus inclusion disease: specific diagnostic features shown by alkaline phosphatase histochemistry. Journal of Clinical Pathology *41*:880–882.

Lamers C.B.H.W., Wagener D.J.T., Assmann K.J.M. and Van Tongeren J.H.M. (1980) Jejunal lymphoma in a patient with primary adult-onset hypogammaglobulinemia and nodular lymphoid hyperplasia of the small intestine. Digestive Diseases and Sciences *25*:553–557.

Lamy M., Frezal J., Polonovski J., Druez G. and Rey J. (1962) Congenital absence of beta-lipoproteins. Paediatrics *31*:277–289.

Lancaster-Smith M., Packer S., Kumar P.J. and Harries J.T. (1976a) Cellular infiltrate of the jejunum after re-introduction of dietary gluten in children with treated coeliac disease. Journal of Clinical Pathology *29*:587–591.

Lancaster-Smith M., Packer S., Kumar P.J. and Harries J.T. (1976b) Immunological phenomena in the jejunum and serum after re-introduction of dietary gluten in children with treated coeliac disease. Journal of Clinical Pathology *29*:592–597.

Lancet (1970) A new line on age pigment? Lancet *ii*:451–452.

Lancet (1974) Epidemic giardiasis. Lancet *ii*:1493.

Lancet (1979) Food allergy. Lancet *i*:249–250.

Lancet (1984) Cryptosporidiosis. Lancet *i*:492–493.

Landboe-Christensen E. (1944) The duodenal glands of Brunner in man, their distribution and quantity. Acta Pathologica et Microbiologica Scandinavica. Supplement *52*:240.

Landing B.H. and Nadorra R. (1986) Infantile systemic hyalinosis. Pediatric Pathology *6*:55–79.

Langman J.M. and Rowland R. (1986) The number and distribution of lymphoid follicles in the human large intestine. Journal of Anatomy *194*:189–194.

Lasser K.H., Lewin K.J. and Ryning F.W. (1979) Cryptosporidial enteritis in a patient with congenital hypogammaglobulinemia. Human Pathology *10*:234–240.

Lawson H.H. (1987) Is duodenitis related to duodenal ulceration as gastritis is to gastric ulceration? South African Journal of Surgery *25*:85–86.

Lazaro R.P., Dentinger M.P., Rodichok L.D., Barron K.D. and Satya-Murti S. (1986) Muscle pathology in Bassen-Kornzweig syndrome and vitamin E deficiency. American Journal of Clinical Pathology *86*:378–387.

Lebenthal E. and Branski D. (1981) Childhood celiac disease: a reappraisal. The Journal of Pediatrics *98*:681–690.

Lee H.H., O'Donnell D.B. and Keren D.F. (1987) Characteristics of melanosis duodeni: incorporation of endoscopy, pathology and etiology. Endoscopy *19*:107–109.

Lee S.P. and Nicholson G.I. (1976) Ceroid enteropathy and vitamin E deficiency. New Zealand Medical Journal *83*:318–320.

Lev R., Thomas E., Parl F.F. and Pitchumoni C.S. (1980) Pathological and histomorphometric study of the effects of alcohol on the human duodenum. Digestion 20:207–213.

Lin H-J., Tsay S-H., Chiang H., Tsai Y-T., Lee S-D., Yeh Y-S. and Lo G-H. (1988) Pseudomelanosis duodeni. Journal of Clinical Gastroenterology 10:155–159.

Loehry C.A. and Grace R. (1974) The dynamic structure of a flat small intestinal mucosa studied on the explanted rat jejunum. Gut 15:289–293.

London N.J.M., Leese T., Bingham P., O'Reilly K. and Self J.B. (1988) Invasive Paneth cell-rich adenocarcinoma of the duodenum. British Journal of Hospital Medicine 40:222–223.

Loughran T.P., Kadin M.E. and Deeg H.J. (1986) T-cell intestinal lymphoma associated with celiac sprue. Annals of Internal Medicine 104:44–47.

MacCarty W.C. (1924) Excised duodenal ulcers: a report of four hundred and twenty-five specimens. Journal of the American Medical Association 83:1894.

Mackinnon M., Willing R.L. and Whitehead R. (1982) Cimetidine in the management of symptomatic patients with duodenitis. A double-blind controlled trial. Digestive Diseases and Sciences 27:217–219.

McClave S.A., Goldschmid S., Cunningham J.T. and Boyd W.P. (1988) Dieulafoy's cirsoid aneurysm of the duodenum. Digestive Diseases and Sciences 33:801–805.

McDonald G.B., Schuffler M.D., Kadin M.E. and Tytgat G.N.J. (1985) Intestinal pseudoobstruction caused by diffuse lymphoid infiltration of the small intestine. Gastroenterology 89:882–889.

McNeish A.S. (1980) Coeliac disease: duration of gluten-free diet. Archives of Disease in Childhood 55:110–111.

Macromichalis J., Brueton M.J., McNeish A.S. and Anderson C.M. (1976) Evaluation of the intraepithelial lymphocyte count in the jejunum in childhood enteropathies. Gut 17:600–603.

Madanagopolan N., Shiner M. and Rowe B. (1965) Measurements of small intestinal mucosa obtained by peroral biopsy. American Journal of Medicine 38:42–53.

Magalhaes A.F.N., Trevisan M.A.S. and Pereira A.S. (1975) Jejunal biopsies in protein-calorie malnutrition and intestinal parasitic infestation in Brazil. American Journal of Gastroenterology 64:472–477.

Mahant T.S., Kohli P.K., Mathur J.M., Bhushurmath S.R., Wig J.D. and Kaushik S.P. (1983) Actinomycosis caecum: a case report. Digestion 27:53–55.

Maizel H., Ruffin J.M. and Dobbins W.O. (1970) Whipple's disease: a review of 19 patients from one hospital and a review of the literature since 1950. Medicine 49:175–205.

Major D.A. and Brandt F. (1976) Brunner's gland adenoma associated with high-output congestive heart failure. American Journal of Gastroenterology 66:562–565.

Maluenda C., Phillips A.D., Briddon A. and Walker-Smith J.A. (1984) Quantitative analysis of small intestinal mucosa in cow's milk-sensitive enteropathy. Journal of Pediatric Gastroenterology and Nutrition 3:349–356.

Mangla J.C., Pereira M. and Bhargava A. (1985) Nodular duodenitis in chronic maintenance hemodialysis patients. Gastrointestinal Endoscopy 31:318–321.

Manousos O.N., Economidou J.C., Georgiadou D.E., Pratsika-Ougourloglou K.G., Hadziyannis S.J., Merikas G.E., Henry K. and Doe W.F. (1974) Alpha-chain disease with clinical, immunological and histological recovery. British Medical Journal 2:409–412.

Maratka Z., Kocianova J., Kudrmann J., Jirk P. and Pirk F. (1979) Hyperplasia of Brunner's glands. Radiology, endoscopy and biopsy. Acta Hepato-Gastroenterology 26:64–69.

Marcial M.A. and Madara J.L. (1986) Cryptosporidium: cellular localization, structural analysis of absorptive cell-parasite membrane-membrane interactions in guinea pigs, and suggestion of protozoan transport by M cells. Gastroenterology 90:83–94.

Marks J. and Shuster S. (1970) Small intestinal mucosal abnormalities in various skin diseases: fact or fancy? Gut 11:281–291.

Marks R., Whittle M.W., Beard R.J., Robertson W.B. and Gold S.C. (1968) Small bowel abnormalities in dermatitis herpetiformis. British Medical Journal 1:552–555.

Marsh M.N. (1980) Studies of intestinal lymphoid tissue: III. Quantitative analyses of epithelial lymphocytes in the small intestine of human control subjects and of patients with coeliac sprue. Gastroenterology 79:481–492.

Marsh M.N. (1982) Studies of intestinal lymphoid tissue: IV. The predictive value of raised mitotic indices among jejunal epithelial lymphocytes in the diagnosis of gluten-sensitive enteropathy. Journal of Clinical Pathology 35:517–525.

Marsh M.N. (1985) Functional and structural aspects of the epithelial lymphocyte, with implications for coeliac disease and tropical sprue. Scandinavian Journal of Gastroenterology 20(suppl 114):55–75.

Marsh M.N. and Haeney M.R. (1983) Studies of intestinal lymphoid tissue. VI. Proliferative response of small intestinal epithelial lymphocytes distinguishes gluten from non-gluten-induced enteropathy. Journal of Clinical Pathology 36:149–160.

Marsh M.N. and Hinde J. (1985) Inflammatory component of celiac sprue mucosa. I. Mast cells, basophils, and eosinophils. Gastroenterology 89:92–101.

Marsh M.N., Mathan M. and Mathan V.I. (1983) Studies of intestinal lymphoid tissue. VII. The secondary nature of lymphoid cell "activation" in the jejunal lesion of tropical sprue. American Journal of Pathology 112:302–312.

Marshall A.R., Al-Jumaili I.J., Fenwick G.A., Bint A.J. and Record C.O. (1987) Cryptosporidiosis in patients at a large teaching hospital. Journal of Clinical Microbiology 25:172–173.

Mathan M., Hughes J. and Whitehead R. (1987) The morphogenesis of the human Paneth cell. An immunocytochemical ultrastructural study. Histochemistry *87*:91–96.

Mathan M., Mathan V.I. and Baker S.J. (1975) An electron microscopic study of jejunal mucosal morphology in control subjects and in patients with tropical sprue in Southern India. Gastroenterology *68*:17–32.

Mathan M.M., Ponniah J. and Mathan V.I. (1986) Epithelial cell renewal and turnover and relationship to morphologic abnormalities in jejunal mucosa in tropical sprue. Digestive Diseases and Sciences *31*:586–592.

Matuchansky C., Colin R., Hemet J., Touchard G., Babin P., Eugene C., Bergue A., Zeitoun P. and Barboteau M.A. (1984) Cavitation of mesenteric lymph nodes, splenic atrophy, and a flat small intestinal mucosa. Gastroenterology *87*:606–614.

Matuchansky C., Morichau-Beauchant M., Touchard G., Lenormand Y., Bloch P., Tanzer J., Alcalay D. and Babin P. (1980) Nodular lymphoid hyperplasia of the small bowel associated with primary jejunal malignant lymphoma. Gastroenterology *78*:1587–1592.

Mazzanti R. and Jenkins W.J. (1987) Effect of chronic ethanol ingestion on enterocyte turnover in rat small intestine. Gut *28*:52–55.

Mead G.M., Whitehouse J.M., Thompson J., Sweetenham J.W., Williams C.J. and Wright D.H. (1987) Clinical features and management of malignant histiocytosis of the intestine. Cancer *60*:2791–2796.

Mee A.S., Burke M., Vallon A.G., Newman J. and Cotton P.B. (1985) Small bowel biopsy for malabsorption: comparison of the diagnostic adequacy of endoscopic forceps and capsule biopsy specimens. British Medical Journal *291*:769–772.

Meisel J.L., Perera D.R., Meligro C. and Rubin C.E. (1976) Overwhelming watery diarrhea associated with a cryptosporidium in an immunosuppressed patient. Gastroenterology *70*:1156–1160.

Meyers W.M., Neafie R.C. and Connor D.H. (1976) Ancylostomiasis. In: Pathology of Tropical and Extraordinary Diseases, Volume 2. Edited by C.H. Binford and D.H. Connor. Washington: Armed Forces Institute of Pathology, pp. 421–427.

Millan M.S., Morris G.P., Beck I.T. and Henson J.T. (1980) Villous damage induced by suction biopsy and by acute ethanol intake in normal human small intestine. Digestive Diseases and Sciences *25*:513–525.

Minford A.M.B., MacDonald A. and Littlewood J.M. (1982) Food intolerance and food allergy in children: a review of 68 cases. Archives of Disease in Childhood *57*:742–747.

Mirakian R., Richardson A., Milla P.J., Walker-Smith J.A., Unsworth J., Savage M.O. and Bottazzo G.F. (1986) Protracted diarrhea of infancy: evidence in support of an autoimmune variant. British Medical Journal *293*:1132–1136.

Mistilis S.P., Skyring A.P. and Stephen D.D. (1965) Intestinal lymphangiectasia. Mechanism of enteric loss of plasma protein and fat. Lancet *i*:77–79.

Monges H., Aubert L., Chamlian A., Remacle J-P., Mathieu B., Cougard A. and Arroyo H. (1975) Maladie des chaines alpha a forme intestinale. Archives Francaises des Maladie de l'Appareil Digestif *64*:223–231.

Monges H., Aubert L., Remacle J-P., Chamlian A., Mathieu B., Cougard A., Quilichini R. and Chaffanjon P. (1980) Survenue d'une maladie de Hodgkin quatre ans apres remission complete d'une maladie des chaines alpha. Gastroenterologie Clinique et Biologique *4*:181–187.

Montero C. and Erlandsen S.L. (1978) Immunocytochemical and histochemical studies on intestinal epithelial cells producing both lysozyme and mucosubstance. Anatomical Record *190*:127–141.

Montgomery R.D., Beale D.J., Sammons H.G. and Schneider R. (1973) Postinfective malabsorption: a sprue syndrome. British Medical Journal *2*:265–268.

Montgomery R.D. and Shearer A.C.I. (1974) The cell population of the upper jejunal mucosa in tropical sprue and postinfective malabsorption. Gut *15*:387–391.

Moore J.V. (1984) Death of intestinal crypts and of their constituent cells after treatment by chemotherapeutic drugs. British Journal of Cancer *49*:25–32.

Moorthy S., Nolley G. and Hermos J.A. (1977) Whipple's disease with minimal intestinal involvement. Gut *18*:152–155.

Morecki R. and Parker J.G. (1967) Ultrastructural studies of the human giardia lamblia and subadjacent jejunal mucosa in a subject with steatorrhea. Gastroenterology *52*:151–164.

Morecki R., Paunier L. and Hamilton J.R. (1968) Intestinal mucosa in cystinosis. Archives of Pathology *86*:297–307.

Morgensen A.M., Bulow S. and Hage E. (1989) Duodenal adenomas in familial adenomatous polyposis: their structure and cellular composition with particular reference to endocrine hyperplasia. Virchows Archiv (A) *414*:315–319.

Morgensen A.M., Hage E. and Bulow S. (1989) Electron microscopic studies of endocrine hyperplasia in duodenal adenomas in familial adenomatous polyposis. Virchows Archiv (A) *414*:321–324.

Moritz M., Moran J.M. and Patterson J.F. (1971) Chronic ulcerative jejunitis. Gastroenterology *60*:96–102.

Muigai R., Gatei D.G., Shaunak S., Wozniak A., and Bryceson A.D.M. (1983) Jejunal function and pathology in visceral leishmaniasis. Lancet *ii*:476–479.

Nabeyama A. and Leblond C.P. (1974) "Caveolated cells" characterized by deep surface invaginations and abundant filaments in mouse gastro-intestinal epithelia. American Journal of Anatomy *140*:147–166.

Nagura H., Kohler P.F. and Brown W.R. (1979) Immunocytochemical characterization of the lymphocytes in nodular lymphoid hyperplasia of the bowel. Laboratory Investigation *40*:66–73.

Nakanishi T., Takeuchi T., Hara K. and Sugimoto A. (1984) A great Brunner's gland adenoma of the duodenal bulb. Digestive Diseases and Sciences 29:81–85.

Nakayama M., Kamuro Y., Sagara K., Sato T., Togami K. and Tashiro S. (1983) A case of bleeding duodenal varices located in the third portion. Gastroenterologica Japonica 18:599–602.

Nash J.R.G., Gradwell E. and Day D.W. (1986) Large-cell intestinal lymphoma occurring in coeliac disease: morphological and immunohistochemical features. Histopathology 10:195–205.

Nasr K., Haghighi P., Bakhshandeh K., Abadi P. and Lahimgarzadeh A. (1976) Primary upper small intestinal lymphoma. A report of 40 cases from Iran. American Journal of Digestive Diseases 21:313–323.

Nime F.A., Burek J.D., Page D.L., Holscher M.A. and Yardley J.H. (1976) Acute enterocolitis in a human being infected with the protozoan cryptosporidium. Gastroenterology 70:592–598.

Norton A.J. and Isaacson P.G. (1989a) Lymphoma phenotyping in formalin-fixed and paraffin wax-embedded tissues. I. Range of antibodies and staining patterns. Histopathology 14:437–446.

Norton A.J. and Isaacson P.G. (1989b) Lymphoma phenotyping in formalin-fixed and paraffin wax-embedded tissues. II. Profiles of reactivity in the various tumour types. Histopathology 14:557–559.

Obertop H., Nundy S., Malamud D. and Malt R.A. (1977) Onset of cell proliferation in the shortened gut. Rapid hyperplasia after jejunal resection. Gastroenterology 72:267–270.

O'Brien B.D., Shnitka T.K., McDougall R., Walker K., Costopoulos L., Lentle B., Anholt L., Freeman H. and Thomson A.B.R. (1982) Pathophysiologic and ultrastructural basis for intestinal symptoms in Fabry's disease. Gastroenterology 82:957–962.

O'Donoghue D.P., Lancaster-Smith M., Laviniere P. and Kumar P.J. (1976) T cell depletion in untreated adult coeliac disease. Gut 17:328–331.

O'Farrelly C., Graeme-Cook F., Hourihane D.O'B., Feighery C. and Weir D.G. (1987) Histological changes associated with wheat protein antibodies in the absence of villous atrophy. Journal of Clinical Pathology 40:1228–1230.

O'Grady J.G., Stevens F.M. and McCarthy C.F. (1985) Celiac disease: Does hyposplenism predispose to the development of malignant disease? American Journal of Gastroenterology 80:27–29.

Oliva H., Gonzalez-Campos C., Navarro V. and Mogena H.H. (1972) Two cases of Whipple's disease showing clinical and morphological similarity. Gut 13:430–437.

Olsson R., Kagevi I. and Rydberg L. (1982) On the concurrence of primary biliary cirrhosis and intestinal villous atrophy. Scandinavian Journal of Gastroentrology 17:625–628.

Olubuyide I.O., Williamson R.C.N., Bristol J.B. and Read A.E. (1984) Goblet cell hyperplasia is a feature of the adaptive response to jejunoileal bypass in rats. Gut 25:62–68.

Orchard J.L., Luparello F. and Brunskill D. (1979) Malabsorption syndrome occurring in the course of disseminated histoplasmosis. American Journal of Medicine 60:331–335.

Orenstein S.R. (1986) The small bowel biopsy in intractable diarrhea of infancy. Gastroenterology 90:785–787.

Otto H.F., Bettman I., Weltzien J.V. and Gebbers J-O. (1981) Primary intestinal lymphomas. Virchows Archiv (A) 391:9–31.

Owen R.L. (1977) Sequential uptake of horseradish peroxidase by lymphoid follicle epithelium of Peyer's patches in the normal unobstructed mouse intestine: an ultrastructural study. Gastroenterology 72:440–451.

Owen R.L., Allen C.L. and Stevens D.P. (1981) Phagocytosis of Giardia muris by macrophages in Peyer's patch epithelium in mice. Infection and Immunity 33:591–601.

Owen R.L. and Nemanic P. (1978) Antigen processing structures of the mammalian intestinal tract: an SEM study of lymphoepithelial organs. Scanning Electron Microscopy 2:367–378.

Owen R.L., Nemanic P.C. and Stevens D.P. (1979) Ultrastructural observations on giardiasis in a murine model. I. Intestinal distribution, attachment, and relationship to the immune system of Giardia muris. Gastroenterology 76:757–769.

Paerregaard A., Vilien M., Krasilnikoff P.A. and Gudmand-Hoyer E. (1988) Supposed coeliac disease during childhood and its presentation 14–38 years later. Scandinavian Journal of Gastroenterology 23:65–70.

Paimela H., Tallgren L.G., Stenman S., Numers H.V. and Scheinin T.M. (1984) Multiple duodenal polyps in uraemia: a little known clinical entity. Gut 25:259–263.

Paoluzi P., Pallone F., Palazzesi P., Marcheggiano A. and Iannoni C. (1982) Frequency and extent of bulbar duodenitis in duodenal ulcer, endoscopic and histological study. Endoscopy 14:193–195.

Partin J.C. and Schubert W.K. (1969) Small intestinal mucosa in cholesterol ester storage disease. Gastroenterology 57:542–558.

Patrick W.J.A., Denham D. and Forrest A.P.M. (1974) Mucous change in the human duodenum: a light and electron microscopic study and correlation with disease and gastric acid secretion. Gut 15:767–776.

Pena A.S., Callender S.T., Truelove S.C. and Whitehead R. (1972) Small intestinal mucosal abnormalities and disaccharidase activity in pernicious anemia. British Journal of Haematology 23:313–321.

Pena A.S., Truelove S.C. and Whitehead R. (1972) Disaccharidase activity and jejunal morphology in coeliac disease. Quarterly Journal of Medicine 41:457–476.

Pena A.S., Truelove S.C. and Whitehead R. (1973) Morphology and disaccharidase levels of jejunal biopsy specimens from healthy British subjects. Digestion 8:317–323.

Penna F.J., Hill I.D., Kingston D., Robertson K., Slavin G. and Shiner M. (1981) Jejunal mucosal morphometry in children with and without gut symptoms and in normal adults. Journal of Clinical Pathology *34*:386–392.

Perlmutter D.H., Leichtner A.M., Goldman H. and Winter H.S. (1985) Chronic diarrhea associated with hypogammaglobulinemia and enteropathy in infants and children. Digestive Diseases and Sciences *30*:1149–1155.

Petersen H. (1972) Giardiasis (lambliasis). Scandinavian Journal of Gastroenterology 7(Suppl. 14):4–44.

Phillips A.D., Avigad S., Sacks J., Rice S.J., France N.E. and Walker-Smith J.A. (1980) Microvillous surface area in secondary disaccharidase deficiency. Gut *21*:44–48.

Phillips A.D., Jenkins P., Raafat F. and Walker-Smith J.A. (1985) Congenital microvillous atrophy: specific diagnostic features. Archives of Diseases in Childhood *60*:135–140.

Pietroletti R., Bishop A.E., Carlei F., Bonamico M., Lloyd R.V., Wilson B.S., Ceccamea A., Lezoche E., Speranza V. and Polak J.M. (1986) Gut endocrine cell population in coeliac disease estimated by immunocytochemistry using a monoclonal antibody to chromogranin. Gut *27*:838–843.

Pink I.J. and Creamer B. (1967) Response to gluten-free diet of patients with coeliac syndrome. Lancet *i*:300–304.

Pink I.J., Croft D.N. and Creamer B. (1970) Cell loss from small intestinal mucosa: a morphological study. Gut *11*:217–222.

Pinkerton C.R., Cameron C.H.S., Sloan J.M., Glasgow J.F.T. and Gwevava N.J.T. (1982) Jejunal crypt cell abnormalities associated with methotrexate treatment in children with acute lymphoblastic leukaemia. Journal of Clinical Pathology *35*:1272–1277.

Polak J.M., Pearse A.G.E., van Noorden S., Bloom S.R. and Rossiter M.A. (1973) Secretin cells in coeliac disease. Gut *14*:870–874.

Pollack D.J., Nagle R.E., Jeejeebhoy K.N. and Coghill N.F. (1970) The effect of jejunal mucosa of withdrawing and adding dietary gluten in cases of idiopathic steatorrhoea. Gut *11*:567–575.

Polanko I., Mearin M.L., Larrauri J., Biemond I., Wipkink-Bakker A. and Pena A.S. (1987) Effect of gluten supplementation in healthy siblings of children with celiac disease. Gastroenterology *92*:678–681.

Pomerantz M. and Waldmann T. (1963) Systemic lymphatic abnormalities associated with gastrointestinal protein loss secondary to intestinal lymphangiectasia. Gastroenterology *45*:703–711.

Pounder D.J., Ghadially F.N., Mukherjee T.M., Hecker R., Rowland R., Dixon B. and Lalonde J.M.A. (1982) Ultrastructure and electron-probe x-ray analysis of the pigment in melanosis duodeni. Journal of Submicroscopic Cytology *14*:389–400.

Pruzanski W., Warren R., Goldie J. and Katz A. (1973) Malabsorption syndrome with infiltration of the intestinal wall by extracellular monoclonal macroglobulin. American Journal of Medicine *54*:811–818.

Raizman R.E. (1976) Giardiasis: an overview for the clinician. American Journal of Digestive Diseases *21*:1070–1074.

Rambaud J-C., Bognel C., Prost A., Burnier J.J., Le Quintrec Y., Lambling A., Danon F., Hurez D. and Seligmann M. (1968) Clinico-pathological study of a patient with "Mediterranean" type of abdominal lymphoma and a new type of IgA abnormality ("alpha-chain disease"). Digestion *1*:321–336.

Rambaud J-C., Galian A., Danon F.G., Preudhomme J-L., Brandtzaeg P., Wassef M., Carrer M.L., Mehaut M.A., Voinchet O.L., Perol R.G. and Chapman A. (1983) Alpha-chain disease without qualitative serum IgA abnormality. Report of two cases, including a "nonsecretory" form. Cancer *51*:686–693.

Rao S.S.C., Dundas S. and Holdsworth C.D. (1987) Intestinal lymphangiectasia secondary to radiotherapy and chemotherapy. Digestive Diseases and Sciences *32*:939–942.

Rayford P.L., Miller T.A. and Thompson J.C. (1976a) Secretin, cholecystokinin and newer gastrointestinal hormones. Part 1. New England Journal of Medicine *294*:1093–1101.

Rayford P.L., Miller T.A. and Thompson J.C. (1976b) Secretin, cholecystokinin and newer gastrointestinal hormones. Part 2. New England Journal of Medicine *294*:1157–1164.

Reisberg I.R. and Oyakawa S. (1987) Mastocytosis with malabsorption, myelofibrosis, and massive ascites. American Journal of Gastroenterology *82*:54–60.

Reunala T., Kosnai I., Karpati S., Kuitunen P., Torok E. and Savilahti E. (1984) Dermatitis herpetiformis: jejunal findings and skin response to gluten-free diet. Archives of Disease in Childhood *59*:517–522.

Rex D.K. and Jersild R.A. (1988) Further characterization of the pigment in pseudomelanosis duodeni in three patients. Gastroenterology *95*:177–182.

Rhee J.W., Gryboski J.D., Sheahan D.G., Dolan T.F. Jr. and Dwyer J.M. (1975) Reversible enteritis and lymphopenia in infantile x-linked agammaglobulinemia. American Journal of Digestive Diseases *20*:1071–1075.

Rhodes J. (1964) Experimental production of gastric epithelium in the duodenum. Gut *5*:454–458.

Rhodes J., Evans K.T., Lawrie J.H. and Forest A.P.M. (1968) Coarse mucosal folds in the duodenum. Quarterly Journal of Medicine *37*:151–169.

Richards W.C.D. (1959) Pigmentation of gastrointestinal muscle. Lancet *i*:683.

Ridley M.J. and Ridley D.S. (1976) Serum antibodies and jejunal histology in giardiasis associated with malabsorption. Journal of Clinical Pathology *29*:30–34.

Riecken E.O. (1970) In Modern Trends in Gastroenterology. Volume 4. Edited by W.I. Card and B. Creamer. London: Butterworth, p. 20.

Riemann J.F. and Schmidt H. (1981) Synopsis of endoscopic and other morphological findings in intestinal lymphangiectasia. Endoscopy 13:60–63.

Rijke R.P.C., Hanson W.R., Plaisier H.M. and Osborne J.W. (1976) The effect of ischemic villus cell damage on crypt cell proliferation in the small intestine. Evidence for a feedback control mechanism. Gastroenterology 71:786–792.

Robertson D.A.F., Dixon M.F., Scott B.B., Simpson F.G. and Losowsky M.S. (1983) Small intestinal ulceration: diagnostic difficulties in relation to coeliac disease. Gut 24:565–574.

Robinson J.E., Brown N., Andiman W., Halliday K., Francke U., Robert M.F., Andersson-Anvret M., Horstman D. and Miller G. (1980) Diffuse polyclonal B-cell lymphoma during primary infection with Epstein-Barr virus. New England Journal of Medicine 302:1293–1297.

Robinson J.W.L. (1972) Intestinal malabsorption in the experimental animal. Gut 13:938–945.

Roca M., Truelove S.C. and Whitehead R. (1975) The histological state of the gastric and duodenal mucosa in healthy volunteers. Gut 16:404.

Roehrkasse R.L., Roberts I.M., Wald A., Talamo T.S. and Mendelow H. (1986) Celiac sprue complicated by lymphoma presenting with multiple gastric ulcers. Gastroenterology 91:740–745.

Rosch W. and Hoer P.W. (1983) Hyperplasiogenic polyp in the duodenum. Endoscopy 15:117–118.

Rosekrans P.C.M., Lindeman J. and Meijer C.J.L.M. (1981) Quantitative histological and immunohistochemical findings in jejunal biopsy specimens in giardiasis. Virchows Archiv (A) 393:145–151.

Rosekrans P.C.M., Meijer C.J.L.M., Cornelisse C.J., Wal A.M. and Lindeman J. (1980) Use of morphometry and immunohistochemistry of small intestinal biopsy specimens in the diagnosis of food allergy. Journal of Clinical Pathology 33:125–130.

Rossi T.M., Lebenthal E., Nord K.S. and Fazili R.R. (1980) Extent and duration of small intestinal mucosal injury in intractable diarrhea of infancy. Pediatrics 66:730–735.

Roy C.C., Levy E., Green P.H.R., Sniderman A., Letarte J., Buts J-P., Orquin J., Brochu P., Weber A.M., Morin C.L., Marcel Y. and Deckelbaum R.J. (1987) Malabsorption, hypocholesterolemia and fat-filled enterocytes with increased intestinal apoprotein B. Gastroenterology 92:390–399.

Rubin C.E., Brandborg L.L., Phelps P.D., Taylor H.C., Murray C.V., Steinler R., Howry C. and Volwiler W. (1960) Studies of celiac disease. II. Gastroenterology 38:517–535.

Rubin C.E. and Dobbins W.O. (1965) Peroral biopsy of the small intestine. Gastroenterology 49:676–697.

Rufenacht H., Kasper M., Heitz Ph. U., Streule K. and Harder F. (1986) "Brunneroma": Hamartoma or tumor? Pathology, Research and Practice 181:107–109.

Ryan D.P., Schapiro R.H. and Warshaw A.L. (1986) Villous tumors of the duodenum. Annals of Surgery 203:301–306.

Sadek A. (1965) In Proceedings of the 1st National Symposium on Bilharziasis 1964, Volume 2. Cairo, Ministry of Scientific Research, p. 270.

Saha T.K. and Ghosh T.K. (1977) Invasion of small intestinal mucosa by giardia lamblia in man. Gastroenterology 72:402–405.

Salata H.H., Mercader J., Navarro A., Cortes J.M. and Gonzales-Campos C. (1984) Lymphangioma of the duodenum. Endoscopy 16:30–32.

Salem P., El-Hashimi L., Anaissie E., Geha S., Habboubi N., Ibrahim N., Khalyl M. and Allam C. (1987) Primary small intestinal lymphoma in adults. Cancer 59:1670–1676.

Sallon S., Deckelbaum R.J., Schmid I.I., Harlap S., Baras M. and Spira D.T. (1988) Cryptosporidium, malnutrition, and chronic diarrhea in children. AJDC 142:312–315.

Salt H.B., Wolff O.H., Lloyd J.K., Fosbrooke A.S., Cameron A.H. and Hubble D.V. (1960) On having no beta-lipoprotein. A syndrome comprising a-beta-lipoproteinaemia, acanthocytosis and steatorrhoea. Lancet ii:325–329.

Sandow M.J. and Whitehead R. (1979) The Paneth cell. Gut 20:420–431.

Sanfilippo G., Pantane R., Fusto A., Passanisi G., Valenti R. and Russo A. (1986) Endoscopic approach to childhood coeliac disease. Acta Gastroenterologica (Bel.) 49:401–408.

Savage M.O., Mirakian R., Wozniak E.R., Jenkins H.R., Malone M., Phillips A.D., Milla P.J., Bottazzo G.F. and Harrie J.T. (1985) Specific autoantibodies to gut epithelium in two infants with severe protracted diarrhea. Journal of Pediatric Gastroenterology and Nutrition 4:187–195.

Schenk E.A., Samloff I.M. and Klipstein F.A. (1965) Morphologic characteristics of jejunal biopsy in celiac disease and tropical sprue. Americal Journal of Pathology 47:765–781.

Schlossberg D., Rudy F.R., Jackson F.W. and Dumalag L.B. (1984) Syphilitic enteritis. Archives of Internal Medicine 144:811–812.

Schmitz-Moormann P., Pittner P.M., Reichmann L. and Massarat S. (1984) Quantitative histological study of duodenitis in biopsies. Pathology, Research and Practice 178:499–507.

Schreibman D., Brenner B., Jacobs R., Ben-Arieh Y., Tatarsky I. and Alroy G. (1988) Small intestinal myeloid metaplasia. Journal of the American Medical Association 259:2580–2582.

Schuffler M.D. and Chaffee R.G. (1979) Small intestinal biopsy in a patient with Crohn's disease of the duodenum: The spectrum of abnormal findings in the absence of granulomas. Gastroenterology 76:1009–1014.

Schuger L., Peretz T., Goldin E., Durst A.L. and Okon E. (1988) Duodenal epithelial atypia. Cancer 61:663–666.

Scott B.B., Goodall A., Stephenson P. and Jenkins D. (1985) Duodenal bulb plasma cells in duodenitis and duodenal ulceration. Gut 26:1032–1037.

Scott B.B., Hardy G.J. and Losowsky M.S. (1975) Involvement of the small intestine in systemic mast cell disease. Gut 16:918–924.

Scott B.B. and Losowsky M.S. (1976) Patchiness and duodenal-jejunal variation of the mucosal abnormality in coeliac disease and dermatitis herpetiformis. Gut *17*:984–992.

Scott B.B., Miller J.P. and Losowsky M.S. (1979). Hypobetalipoproteinaemia: a variant of the Bassen-Kornzweig syndrome. Gut *20*:163–168.

Selby W.S. and Gallagher N.D. (1979) Malignancy in a 19-year experience of adult celiac disease. Digestive Diseases and Sciences *24*:684–688.

Selby W.S., Janossy G. and Jewell D.P. (1981) Immunohistological characterisation of intraepithelial lymphocytes of the human gastrointestinal tract. Gut *22*:169–176.

Seligmann M., Mihaesco E. and Frangione B. (1971) Alpha chain disease. Annals of the New York Academy of Science *190*:487–500.

Shaw E.B. Jr. and Hennigar G.R. (1974) Intestinal lymphoid polyposis. American Journal of Clinical Pathology *61*:417–422.

Sheehy T.W., Artenstein M.S. and Green R.W. (1964) Small intestinal mucosa in certain viral diseases. Journal of the American Medical Association *190*:1023–1028.

Sheehy T.W., Meroney W.H., Cox R.S. and Soler J.E. (1962) Hookworm disease and malabsorption. Gastroenterology *42*:148–156.

Shepherd N.A., Blackshaw A.J., Hall P.A., Bostad L., Coates P.J., Lowe D.G., Levison D.A., Morson B.C. and Stansfeld A.G. (1987a) Malignant lymphoma with eosinophilia of the gastrointestinal tract. Histopathology *11*:115–130.

Shepherd N.A., Jass J.R., Duval I., Moskowitz R.L., Nicholls R.J. and Morson B.C. (1987b) Restorative proctocolectomy with ileal reservoir: pathological and histochemical study of mucosal biopsy specimens. Journal of Clinical Pathology *40*:601–607.

Sherif S.M. (1970) Malabsorption and schistosomal involvement of jejunum. British Medical Journal *1*:671–672.

Sheth K.J., Werlin S.L., Freeman M.E. and Hodach A.E. (1981) Gastrointestinal structure and function in Fabry's disease. American Journal of Gastroenterology *76*:246–251.

Shilken K.B., Zerman B.J. and Blackwell J.B. (1968) Lymphangiectatic cysts of the small bowel. Journal of Pathology and Bacteriology *96*:353–358.

Shiner M. (1973) Ultrastructural changes suggestive of immune reaction in the jejunal mucosa of coeliac children following gluten challenge. Gut *14*:1–12.

Shiner M., Ballard J., Brook C.G.D. and Herman S. (1975) Intestinal biopsy in the diagnosis of cow's milk protein intolerance without acute symptoms. Lancet *ii*:1060–1063.

Shiner M., Ballard J. and Smith M.E. (1975) The small intestinal mucosa in cow's milk allergy. Lancet *i*:136–140.

Shiner M. and Pearson J.R. (1981) Abnormalities in the jejunal mucosa in Arab children. Gastroenterologie Clinique et Biologique *5*:663–673.

Shiner M., Redmond A.O.B. and Hansen J.D.L. (1973) The jejunal mucosa in protein-energy malnutrition. A clinical, histological, and ultrastructural study. Experimental and Molecular Pathology *19*:61–78.

Shiner M. and Shmerling D.H. (1970) The pathogenesis of coeliac disease (Abstract) Gut *11*:1058–1059.

Short R.H.D. (1950) Alveolar epithelium in relation to growth of the lung. Philosophical Transactions B *235*:35–86.

Shousha S., Spiller R.C. and Parkins R.A. (1983) The endoscopically abnormal duodenum in patients with dyspepsia: biopsy findings in 60 cases. Histopathology *7*:23–34.

Shwachman H., Lloyd-Still J.D., Khaw K-T. and Antonowicz I. (1973) Protracted diarrhea of infancy treated by intravenous alimentation. American Journal of Diseases in Children *125*:365–368.

Silva M.T., Macedo P.M. and Nunes J.F.M. (1985) Ultrastructure of bacilli and the bacillary origin of the macrophagic inclusions in Whipple's disease. Journal of General Microbiology *131*:1001–1013.

Simmonds J.P. and Rosenthal F.D. (1981) Lymphadenopathy in coeliac disease. Gut *22*:756–758.

Singleton J., Kern F. and Waddell W. (1965) Diarrhea and pancreatic islet cell tumor. Report of a case with a severe jejunal mucosal lesion. Gastroenterology *49*:197–208.

Sircus W. (1985) Duodenitis: a clinical, endoscopic and histopathological study. Quarterly Journal of Medicine *56*:593–600.

Sjolund K., Alumets J., Berg N-O., Hakanson R. and Sundler F. (1979) Duodenal endocrine cells in adult coeliac disease. Gut *20*:547–552.

Sjolund K., Sanden G., Hakanson R. and Sundler F. (1983) Endocrine cells in human intestine: an immunocytochemical study. Gastroenterology *85*:1120–1130.

Skellenger M.E., Kinner B.M. and Jordan P.H. (1983) Brunner's gland hamartomas can mimic carcinoma of the head of the pancreas. Surgery, Gynecology and Obstetrics *156*:774–776.

Skinner J.M. and Whitehead R. (1976) Morphological methods in the study of the gut immune system in man. Journal of Clinical Pathology *29*:564–567.

Slavin G., Sowter C., Robertson K., McDermott S. and Paton K. (1980) Measurement in jejunal biopsies by computer-aided microscopy. Journal of Clinical Pathology *33*:254–261.

Sleisenger M.H., Almy T.P. and Barr D.P. (1953) The sprue syndrome secondary to lymphoma of the small bowel. American Journal of Medicine *15*:666–674.

Smallman L.A., Young J.A., Shortland-Webb W.R., Carey M.P. and Michael J. (1986) Strongyloides stercoralis hyperinfestation syndrome with Escherichia coli meningitis: report of two cases. Journal of Clinical Pathology *39*:366–370.

Socinski M.A., Frankel J-P., Morrow P.L. and Krawitt E.L. (1984) Painless diarrhea secondary to intestinal ischemia. Diagnosis of atheromatous emboli by jejunal biopsy. Digestive Diseases and Sciences *29*:674–677.

Solcia E., Capella C., Buffa R., Fiocca R., Frigerio B. and Usellini L. (1980) Identification, ultrastructure and classification of gut endocrine cells and related growths. Investigative and Cell Pathology *3*:37–49.

Solhaug J.H. (1976) Morphometric studies of the small intestine following jejuno-ileal shunt operation. Scandinavian Journal of Gastroenterology *11*:155–160.

Solthoft J. and Soeberg B. (1972a) Immunoglobulin-containing cells in the small intestine in viral hepatitis. Acta Pathologica et Microbiologica Scandinavica *80*:379–387.

Solthoft J. and Soeberg B. (1972b) Immunoglobulin-containing cells in the small intestine during acute enteritis. Gut *13*:535–538.

Sorensen R.U., Halpin T.C., Abramowsky C.R., Hornick D.L., Miller K.M., Naylor P. and Incefy G.S. (1985) Intestinal lymphangiectasia and thymic hypoplasia. Clinical and Experimental Immunology *59*:217–226.

Spencer J., Cerf-Bensussan N., Jarry A., Brousse N., Guy-Grand D., Krajewski A.S. and Isaacson P.G. (1988) Enteropathy-associated T cell lymphoma (malignant histiocytosis of the intestine) is recognized by a monoclonal antibody (HML–1) that defines a membrane molecule on human mucosal lymphocytes. American Journal of Pathology *132*:1–5.

Spencer J., MacDonald T.T., Diss T.C., Walker-Smith J.A., Ciclitira P.J. and Isaacson P.G. (1989) Changes in intraepithelial lymphocyte subpopulations in coeliac disease and enteropathy associated T cell lymphoma (malignant histiocytosis of the intestine). Gut *30*:339–346.

Sprinz H., Sribhibhadh E.J., Gangarosa E.J., Benyajata C., Kundel D. and Halstead S. (1962) Biopsy of small bowel of Thai people. American Journal of Clinical Pathology *38*:43–51.

Stamp G.W.H. and Evans D.J. (1987) Accumulation of ceroid in smooth muscle indicates severe malabsorption and vitamin E deficiency. Journal of Clinical Pathology *40*:798–802.

Stern M., Gruttner R. and Krumbach J. (1980) Protracted diarrhoea: secondary monosaccharide malabsorption and zinc deficiency with cutaneous manifestations during total parenteral nutrition. European Journal of Pediatrics *135*:175–180.

Stessens L., Van Den Oord J.J., Geboes K., De Wolf-Peeters C. and Desmet V.J. (1986) GI lymphomatous polyposis. Gastroenterology *90*:2041–2042.

Stevens F.M., Flanagan R.W., O'Gorman D. and Buchanan K.D. (1984) Glucagonoma syndrome demonstrating giant duodenal villi. Gut *25*:784–791.

Stewart J.S., Pollock D.J., Hoffbrand A.V., Mollin D.L. and Booth C.C. (1967) A study of proximal and distal intestinal structure and absorptive function in idiopathic steatorrhoea. Quarterly Journal of Medicine *36*:425–444.

Stolte M., Schwabe H. and Prestele H. (1981) Relationship between diseases of the pancreas and hyperplasia of Brunner's glands. Virchows Archiv (A) *394*:75–87.

Strobel S., Busuttil A. and Ferguson A. (1983) Human intestinal mucosal mast cells: expanded population in untreated coeliac disease. Gut *24*:222–227.

Sukigara M., Koyama I., Komazaki T., Matsuda T., Ishii T. and Omoto R. (1987) Bleeding varices located in the second portion of the duodenum. Japanese Journal of Surgery *17*:130–135.

Swanson V.L. and Thomassen R.W. (1965) Pathology of the jejunal mucosa in tropical sprue. American Journal of Pathology *46*:511–551.

Swanson V.L., Wheby M.S. and Bayless T.M. (1966) Morphological effects of folic acid and vitamin B12 on the jejunal lesion of tropical sprue. American Journal of Pathology *49*:167–191

Swinson C.M., Slavin G., Coles E.C. and Boothe C.C. (1983) Coeliac disease and malignancy. Lancet *i*:111–115.

Tabaqchali S. and Booth C.C. (1970) In Modern Trends in Gastroenterology. Volume 4. Edited by W.I. Card and B. Creamer. London: Butterworth, p. 143.

Talbot I.C., Neoptolemos J.P., Shaw D.E. and Carr-Locke D. (1988) The histopathology and staging of carcinoma of the ampulla of Vater. Histopathology *12*:156–165.

Tandon B.N., Tandon R.K., Satpathy B.K. and Shriniwas (1977) Mechanism of malabsorption in giardiasis: a study of bacterial flora and bile salt deconjugation in upper jejunum. Gut *18*:176–181.

Tankel H.I., Clark D.H. and Lee F.D. (1965) Radiation enteritis with malabsorption. Gut *6*:560–569.

Taylor C.R. (1976) An immunohistological study of follicular lymphoma, reticulum cell sarcoma and Hodgkin's disease. European Journal of Cancer *12*:61–75.

Thompson H. (1976) Pathology of coeliac disease. Current Topics in Pathology *63*:49–75.

Thomson W.O., Joffe S.N., Robertson A.G., Lee F.D., Imrie C.W. and Blumgart L.H. (1977) Is duodenitis a dyspeptic myth? Lancet *i*:1197–1198.

Thurlbeck W.M., Benson J.A. and Dudley H.R. (1960) The histopathologic changes of sprue and their significance. American Journal of Clinical Pathology *34*:108–117.

Tofler A.H., Hukill P.B. and Spiro H.M. (1963) Brown bowel syndrome. Annals of Internal Medicine *58*:872–877.

Tomkins A. (1981) Tropical malabsorption: recent concepts in pathogenesis and nutritional significance. Clinical Science *60*:131–137.

Tomkins A.M., Drasar B.S. and James W.P.T. (1975) Bacterial colonisation of jejunal mucosa in acute tropical sprue. Lancet *i*:59–62.

Townley R.R.W., Cass M.H. and Anderson C.M. (1964) Small intestinal mucosal patterns of coeliac disease and idiopathic steatorrhoea seen in other situations. Gut *5*:51–55.

Trier J.S. (1962) Morphologic alterations induced by methotrexate in the mucosa of the human proximal intestine. Gastroenterology 42:295–305.

Trier J.S. and Browning T.H. (1966) Morphologic response of the mucosa of human small intestine to x-ray exposure. Journal of Clinical Investigation 45:194–204.

Trier J.S. and Madara J.L. (1981) Functional morphology of the mucosa of the small intestine. In: Physiology of the Gastrointestinal Tract. Edited by L.R. Johnson. New York: Raven Press, pp. 925–961.

Tsadilas T. (1984) Duodenal polyp composed of ectopic gastric mucosa. Digestive Diseases and Sciences 29:475–477.

Tsubone M., Kozura S., Taki T., Hoshino M., Yasui A. and Hachisuka K. (1984) Heterotopic gastric mucosa in the small intestine. Acta Pathologica Japonica 34:1425–1431.

Tylki-Szymanska A., Maciejko D., Wozniewicz B. and Muszynska B. (1987) Two cases of cholesteryl ester storage disease (CESD) acid lipase deficiency. Hepato-gastroenterology 34:98–99.

Tytgat G.N., Hoogendijk J.L., Agenant D. and Schellekens P.T. (1977) Etiopathogenetic studies in a patient with Whipple's disease. Digestion 15:309–321.

Tzipori S., Angus K.W., Campbell I. and Gray E.W. (1982) Experimental infection of lambs with cryptosporidium isolated from a human patient with diarrhoea. Gut 23:71–74.

Ulshen M.H. and Rollo J.L. (1980) Pathogenesis of escherichia coli gastroenteritis in man: another mechanism. New England Journal of Medicine 302:99–101.

Vanderhoof J.A., Rich K.C., Stiehm E.R. and Ament M.E. (1977) Esophageal ulcers in immunodeficiency with elevated levels of IgM and neutropenia. American Journal of Children 131:551–552.

Van Der Valk P., Lindeman J. and Meijer C.J.L.M. (1988) Non-Hodgkin's lymphomas of the gastrointestinal tract: a review with special reference to the gut-associated lymphoid tissue. In: Digestive Disease Pathology. Volume 1. Edited by S. Watanabe, M. Wolff and S.C. Sommers. Philadelphia: Field and Wood Inc, pp. 105–119.

Van Spreeuwel J.P., Lindeman J., Van Maanen J. and Meyer C.J.L.M. (1984) Increased numbers of IgE containing cells in gastric and duodenal biopsies. An expression of food allergy secondary to chronic inflammation? Journal of Clinical Pathology 37:601–606.

Variend S., Phillips A.D. and Walker-Smith J.A. (1984) The small intestinal mucosal biopsy in childhood. Perspectives in Pediatric Pathology 1:57–78.

Variend S., Placzek M., Raafat F. and Walker-Smith J.A. (1984) Small intestinal mucosal fat in childhood enteropathies. Journal of Clinical Pathology 37:373–377.

Veloso F.T. and Saleiro J.V. (1982) Mast cells in Whipple's disease. Journal of Submicroscopic Cytology 14:515–520.

Veloso F.T. and Saleiro J.V. (1987) Small bowel changes in recurrent ulceration of the mouth. Hepato-gastroenterology 34:36–37.

Veloso F.T., Saleiro J.V., Baptista F. and Ribeiro E. (1981). Whipple's disease. Report of a case with clinical immunological studies. American Journal of Gastroenterology 75:419–425.

Venables C.W. (1985) Duodenitis. Scandinavian Journal of Gastroenterology 20(suppl. 109):91–97.

Vitoria J.C., Camarero C., and Solaguren R. (1979) Cow's milk protein-sensitive enteropathy. Clinical and histological results of the cows' milk provocation test. Helvetica Paediatrica Acta 34:309–318.

Vitoria J.C. Camerero C., Sojo A., Ruiz A. and Rodriguez-Soriano J. (1982) Enteropathy related to fish, rice and chicken. Archives of Disease in Childhood 57:44–48.

Walan A. (1981) Non-ulcer dyspepsia. Proceedings of a symposium held in the Swedish Society of Medical Sciences, Stockholm, November 6/7/81. Smith, Kline and French A.B., Stockholm.

Waldmann T.A. (1970) In Modern Trends in Gastroenterology. Volume 4. Edited by W.I. Card and B. Creamer. London: Butterworth, p. 136.

Waldmann T.A., Wochner R.D., Laster L. and Gordon R.S. (1967) Allergic gastroenteropathy. New England Journal of Medicine 276:761–769.

Walker-Smith J.A. (1970) Transient gluten intolerance. Archives of Disease in Childhood 45:523–526.

Walker-Smith J.A. (1972) Variation of small intestinal morphology with age. Archives of Disease in Childhood 47:80–83.

Walker-Smith J.A. (1978) Gastrointestinal allergy. The Practitioner 220:562–573.

Walker-Smith J.A., Unsworth D.J., Hutchins J., Phillips A.D. and Holborow E.G. (1982) Autoantibodies against gut epithelium in child with small intestinal enteropathy. Lancet i:566–567.

Wall A.J., Douglas A.J., Booth C.C. and Pearse A.G.E. (1970) Response of the jejunal mucosa in adult coeliac disease to oral prednisolone. Gut 11:7–14.

Ward H., Jalan K.N., Maitra T.K., Agarwal S.K. and Mahalanabis D. (1983) Small intestinal nodular lymphoid hyperplasia in patients with giardiasis and normal serum immunoglobulins. Gut 24:120–126.

Warnke R., Miller R., Grogan T., Pederson M., Dilley J. and Levy R. (1980) Immunologic phenotype in 30 patients with diffuse large-cell lymphoma. New England Journal of Medicine 303:293–300.

Watson A.J., Appleton D.R. and Wright N.A. (1982) Adaptive cell-proliferative changes in the small intestinal mucosa in coeliac disease. In: Basic Science in Gastroenterology: Structure of the Gut. Edited by J.M. Polak, S.R. Bloom, N.A. Wright and M.J. Daly. Ware (U.K.) Glaxo Group Research Ltd, pp. 431–443.

Watson A.J. and Parkin J.M. (1970) Jejunal biopsy findings during prodromal stage of measles in a child with coeliac disease. Lancet ii:1134–1135.

Watson J.H.L. and Haubrich W.S. (1969) Bacilli bodies in the lumen and epithelium of the jejunum in Whipple's disease. Laboratory Investigation 21:347–357.

Watt J., Pincott J.R. and Harries J.T. (1983) Combined cow's milk protein and gluten-induced enteropathy: common or rare? Gut *24*:165–170.

Webster A.D.B. (1980) Giardiasis and immunodeficiency diseases. Transactions of the Royal Society of Tropical Medicine and Hygiene *74*:440–443.

Webster A.D.B., Kenwright S., Ballard J., Shiner M., Slavin G., Levi A.J., Loewi G. and Asherson G.L. (1977) Nodular lymphoid hyperplasia of the bowel in primary hypogammaglobulinaemia: study of in vivo and in vitro lymphocyte function. Gut *18*:364–372.

Webster A.D.B., Slavin G., Shiner M., Platts-Mills T.A.E. and Asherson G.L. (1981) Coeliac disease with severe hypogammaglobulinaemia. Gut *22*:153–157.

Weibel E.R. (1963) Principles and methods for the morphometric study of the lung and other organs. Laboratory Investigation *12*:131–155.

Weinstein L., Edelstein S.M., Madara J.L., Falchuk K.R., McManus B.M. and Trier J.S. (1981) Intestinal cryptosporidiosis complicated by disseminated cytomegalovirus infection. Gastroenterology *81*:584–591.

Weinstein W.M., Saunders D.R., Tytgat G.N. and Rubin C.E. (1970) Collagenous sprue: an unrecognized type of malabsorption. New England Journal of Medicine *283*:1297–1301.

Weir D.G. and Hourihane D.O'B. (1974) Coeliac disease during the teenage period: the value of serial serum folate estimations. Gut *15*:450–457.

West B. (1988) Pseudomelanosis duodeni. Journal of Clinical Gastroenterology *10*:127–129.

Whalen G.E., Rosenberg E.B., Strickland G.T., Gutman R.A., Cross J.H., Watten R.H., Uylangeo C. and Dizou J.J. (1969) Intestinal capillariasis. A new disease in man. Lancet *i*:13–16.

Wheeler E.E. and Challacombe D.N. (1984) Quantification of enterochromaffin cells with serotonin immunoreactivity in the duodenal mucosa in coeliac disease. Archives of Disease in Childhood *59*:523–527.

Whipple G.H. (1907) A hitherto undescribed disease characterised anatomically by deposits of fat and fatty acids in the intestinal and mesenteric lymphatic tissues (intestinal lipodystrophy). Johns Hopkins Hospital Bulletin *18*:382–391.

Whitehead R. (1968a) Primary lymphadenopathy complicating idiopathic steatorrhoea. Gut *9*:569–575.

Whitehead R. (1968b) Recent Advances in Clinical Pathology. Series V. Edited by S.C. Dyke. London: Churchill, P. 385.

Whitehead R. (1973) Mucosal biopsy of the gastrointestinal tract. In Major Problems in Pathology. Volume 3. London: W.B. Saunders Co.

Whitehead R., Roca M., Meikle D.D., Skinner J. and Truelove S.C. (1975) The histological classification of duodenitis in fibreoptic biopsy specimens. Digestion *13*:129–136.

Whitehead R., Roca M. and Truelove S.C. (1972) Antroduodenitis in duodenal ulcers and non-ulcer dyspepsia. In Chronic Duodenal Ulcer. Edited by C. Wastell. London: Butterworth, pp. 17–23.

Wiernik G. (1966) In vivo cell kinetics of a normal human tissue. British Medical Journal *2*:385–387.

Wiernik G., Shorter R.G. and Creamer B. (1962) The arrest of intestinal epithelial "turnover" by the use of x-irradiation. Gut *3*:26–31.

Wilcox G.M., Tronic B.S., Schecter D.J., Arron M.J., Righi D.F. and Weiner N.J. (1987) Periodic acid-Schiff-Negative granulomatous lymphadenopathy in patient with Whipple's disease. American Journal of Medicine *83*:165–170.

Williamson R.C.N. (1982) Intestinal adaption: factors that influence morphology. In: Basic Science in Gastroenterology: Structure of the Gut. Edited by J.M. Polak, S.R. Bloom, N.A. Wright and M.J. Daly. Ware (U.K.), Glaxo Group Research Limited, pp. 337–345.

Witham R.R. and Mosser R.S. (1979) An unusual presentation of schistosomiasis duodenitis. Gastroenterology *77*:1316–1318.

World Health Organisation (1976) Alpha-chain disease and related small intestinal lymphoma. A Memorandum Bulletin *54*:615–624

Wright N., Watson A., Morley A., Appleton D., Marks J. and Douglas A. (1973a) The cell cycle time in the flat (avillous) mucosa of the human small intestine. Gut *14*:603–606.

Wright N., Watson A., Morley A., Appleton D., Marks J. and Douglas A. (1973b) Cell kinetics in flat (avillous) mucosa of the human small intestine. Gut *14*:701–710.

Wright S.G. and Tomkins A.M. (1978) Quantitative histology in giardiasis. Journal of Clinical Pathology *31*:712–716.

Yamase H., Norris M. and Gillies C. (1985) Pseudomelanosis duodeni: a clinicopathologic entity. Gastrointestinal Endoscopy *31*:83–86.

Zuckerman M.J., Pittman D.L., Boman D. and Farley P.C. (1986) Multiple lymphomatous polyposis of the gastrointestinal tract with immunologic marker studies. Journal of Clinical Gastroenterology *8*:295–300.

Zukerman G.R., Mills B.A., Koehler R.E., Siegel A., Harter H.R. and DeSchryver-Kecskemeti K. (1983) Nodular duodenitis. Pathologic and clinical characteristics in patients with end-stage renal disease. Digestive Diseases and Sciences *28*:1018–1024.

Colonic Biopsy

IV

15

NORMAL APPEARANCES IN COLONIC BIOPSY SPECIMENS

The mucous membrane of the colon (Fig. 15–1) has a comparatively smooth surface, since there are no villi. Straight tubular glands extend from the surface down through the entire thickness of the lamina propria to abut the muscularis mucosa. A detailed examination of the human large-intestinal epithelium is reported by Shamsuddin, Phelps and Trump (1982). They have shown that significant differences occur in the different regions of the large bowel although the basic structure is the same. Undifferentiated stem cells occupy the base of the crypts. They are the only ones capable of mitotic division and clearly give rise to the goblet cell population that is the predominant cell type lining the crypts. They have large supranuclear mucous vacuoles and small apical vesicles. The apical vesicles show variable electron density, maximum in the ascending colon and progressively less dense distally to become lucent in the rectum.

Histochemically the mucins are predominantly sulphomucins in the lower two thirds of the crypt and sialomucin in the upper crypt and surface epithelium. There are also said to be changes in mucin composition in different parts of the colon. Utilising a panel of monoclonal antibodies against purified colonic mucins, Podolsky, Fournier and Lynch (1986) have shown that in humans the colonic mucosa contains several subpopulations of goblet cells. It is claimed that they produce distinctive combinations of mucin glycoprotein subtypes, but their functional roles have not been elucidated. Interspersed among the goblet or mucous cells, at the surface between the crypt openings, are the occasional columnar cells that in the past have been equated to the absorptive cells of the small intestine because by light microscopy they have an eosinophilic cytoplasm and on electron microscopy a well-defined microvillous border. Shamsuddin, Phelps and Trump (1982) prefer to call them columnar cells and believe them to be a variant of goblet cells that have discharged their large mucous vacuoles. They have all the ultrastructural apparatus for potential mucus secretion.

Endocrine cells can also be recognised in the lower half of the glands, especially in the rectum, where they occur with greater frequency than in the rest of the colon. The increasingly important enterochromaffin system has already been mentioned in the sections on the gastric and small-intestinal mucosa. In the superficial and crypt epithelium there is an occasional intraepithelial lymphocyte. Paneth cells may be seen in tissue from the very proximal colon, especially in children, but in rectal or distal colonic biopsy tissues the presence of these cells is invariably abnormal.

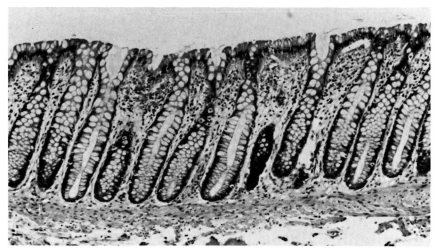

Figure 15–1. Rectal biopsy. Normal colonic mucosa; gland tubules cut longitudinally (H & E × 70).

Surrounding the crypts there is a sheath of cells that in the past have been thought of as fibroblasts. A role in maintaining the crypt form and function has been postulated. More recently these cells are being regarded as myofibroblasts (see also Collagenous Colitis, Chap. 17) on the basis of electron microscopic observations and on their reaction with specific monoclonal antibodies (Richman et al 1987).

The lamina propria, which consists of a delicate connective tissue and is richly vascular, contains a few plasma cells and lymphocytes, an occasional mast cell and eosinophil together with a histiocyte, and sometimes a solitary lymphoid follicle (Fig. 15–2). Histiocytes predominate in the more superficial aspects of the lamina propria as do plasma cells, and Leonard and MacLennan (1982) have stressed the need to bear this in mind when enumerating plasma cells, in order to arrive at

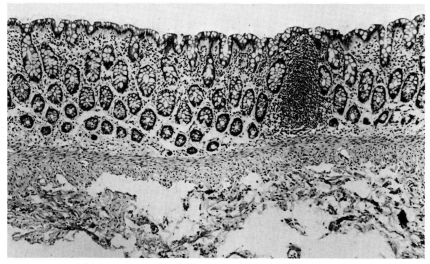

Figure 15–2. Rectal biopsy. Normal colonic mucosa with a lymphoid follicle; gland tubules cut transversely (H & E × 38).

accurate estimations. There is little information concerning the changes in cellularity of the lamina propria along the length of the colon, but a personal subjective observation is that there is a definite increase in lymphocytes and plasma cells in the caecum and neighbouring ascending colon as compared with the distal bowel and rectum. The density, on occasion, prompts the observer to question the possibility of a colitis, but lack of polymorphs and degenerative epithelial features or architectural distortion allows this to be ruled out. Neutrophil polymorphs are very uncommon in the entirely normal biopsy, except inside capillaries, but, particularly in the submucosa, occasional mast cells occur. Lymphoid follicles are often encountered in rectal biopsies and, like the Peyer's patches of the small intestine, are most numerous at the time of puberty (Cornes 1965). With increasing age they become less frequent and are rare in senility. They characteristically split the muscularis mucosa, partially extending into the submucosa. Sometimes they are accompanied by a few tubular glands, which may actually extend into the submucosa (Fig. 15–3).

It has been claimed that the lymphoid glandular complexes (microbursae) constitute weak points in the colonic wall, and they have been implicated in the pathogenesis of diverticular disease (Kealy 1976a). This appears highly unlikely, for too frequently diverticulae exist in the absence of mural lymphoid tissue. O'Leary and Sweeney (1986) studied these complexes by both immunohistochemistry and electron microscopy and have concluded that they are the sites of antigen processing. Indeed, cells that are the equivalent of M cells of the small intestine are found in the epithelium related to these follicles. Jacob, Baker and Swaminathan (1987) believe that these cells have an antigen-sampling function and that their presence may explain the localisation of the early aphthous lesions of Crohn's disease to the lymphoid glandular complexes.

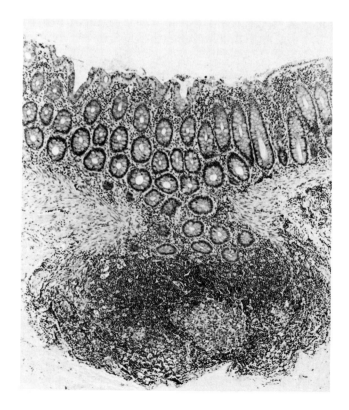

Figure 15–3. Lymphoglandular complex (microbursa) in normal rectal mucosa. The superficial epithelium shows a traumatic artefact (H & E × 130).

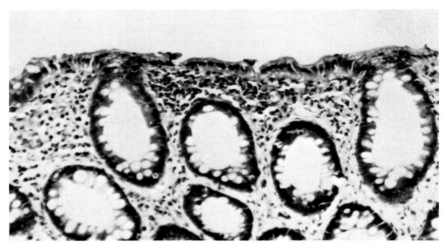

Figure 15–4. Rectal biopsy. Flattening of the superficial epithelium and a localised increase in round cells in the lamina propria (H & E × 188).

Minor changes of the superficial epithelium, consisting of a decrease in goblet cells and reversion to a flatter and more simple type of epithelium, are seen fairly often (Fig. 15–4). It is usual for there to be an accompanying increase, slight but perceptible, in inflammatory cells in the lamina propria, although invasion of the surface epithelium and that lining the crypts is unusual. Rarely, however, in circumstances such as constipation or more frequently in chronic obstruction, e.g., Hirschsprung's disease, an occasional, rather poorly formed crypt abscess may be seen. These minor changes, however, are not usually related to the clinical picture. Nevertheless, whenever colonic biopsy appearances are being assessed, it is always advisable to consider the possibility that factors such as the preparation of the colon for instrumentation, the instrumentation itself or some other form of trauma or injury may be contributing to the overall picture. The energetic use of enemas can result in an appreciable although non-specific acute inflammatory reaction. Acute degenerative epithelial changes are well described following the use of a variety of enemas (Meisel et al 1977, Leriche et al 1978) (see also Chapter 17). Indeed, in certain societies where the use of repeated enemas is part of the culture, as in the South African black races, severe inflammation and bowel perforation not uncommonly result (Segal et al 1979). It clearly is extremely helpful if the pathologist is made aware of any circumstance that could possibly influence the interpretation of a particular biopsy specimen.

Although much has been written about the racial variation in jejunal morphology, there is little in the literature concerning the colon and rectum in this respect. Changes in cellularity of the lamina propria of the colon, however, may even be attributable to differences in the luminal environment of the gut as a whole. Thus in assessing rectal biopsy appearances, a possible racial variation should be borne in mind. Increased cellularity of the lamina propria with more than the usual complement of lymphocytes and plasma cells may have a more specific connotation, for it could possibly reflect a generalised reaction of the gut-associated lymphoid system to a more localised stimulus. When such changes are seen in rectal biopsy specimens, for example, it could be that there is an inflammatory lesion in another part of the gastrointestinal tract. Indeed, Crucioli (1972) has shown that a sigmoidoscopically normal rectum may show an increased lymphoid component in rectal biopsy specimens if there is Crohn's disease in the more proximal parts of the colon. Moreover, Soltoft (1969) found that there were increased numbers of IgM and IgG cells in the lamina propria of jejunal biopsies in patients who have ulcerative colitis. Except when rectal biopsy is being used for a specific diagnostic purpose, e.g., in amyloidosis, clinicians have a tendency to biopsy the colonic mucosa only when it appears abnormal to them. There are several instances in which endoscopically normal mucosa will reveal histological abnormalities. It cannot be stressed too strongly that if there is an indication for diagnostic endoscopy, there is also invariably an indication for mucosal biopsy.

This allows pathologists to build an experience of rectal biopsy appearances. They will then be aware of normal variations, age changes and artefactual appearances and thus be better equipped to diagnose significant abnormalities.

16

ULCERATIVE COLITIS, CROHN'S COLITIS, ISCHAEMIC COLITIS, PSEUDOMEMBRANOUS AND ANTIBIOTIC-ASSOCIATED COLITIS

Rectal and low colonic biopsies have long been employed in the diagnosis and management of neoplasia. However, because of increasing interest in the diagnosis and treatment of inflammatory disease of the large bowel, colonic biopsy has attained a new importance. The clinician faced with the differential diagnosis between ulcerative colitis and other inflammatory conditions of the colon, in particular Crohn's disease, ischaemic colitis, pseudomembranous colitis, amoebic colitis and the more recently recognised forms of colitis, will increasingly rely on the expert interpretation of colonic biopsy material. With fibreoptic colonoscopes it is possible to obtain tissue as far proximally as the terminal ileum, and although the pieces of mucosa are small and somewhat superficial, when the same principles of interpretation are applied to them as to the larger more conventional sigmoido-scopic biopsies, useful if sometimes limited information will be revealed. This was particularly well illustrated in the study by Myeren, Serck-Hanssen and Solberg (1976), who not only confirmed the value of fibreoptic colonoscope biopsy examination in ulcerative colitis but also proved the importance of experience in pathological interpretation and the value of biopsy even when endoscopic appearances are normal. The importance of stepwise colonic biopsy in patients being investigated for diarrhoea cannot be stressed too strongly. Microscopic colitis, collagenous colitis and other less frequent causes of diarrhoea are usually associated with unremarkable endoscopic appearances, which invariably are non-diagnostic (Stolte 1988). Even Crohn's disease may be diagnosed histologically when endoscopic appearances are normal (Sanderson et al 1986).

ULCERATIVE COLITIS

Classical ulcerative colitis is an inflammatory process of the mucosa involving the rectum and a variable length of colon in continuity with the rectum, not infrequently extending as far as the last few inches of the terminal ileum. There is ample evidence (Farmer and Brown 1972, Myers, Humphries and Cox 1976, Das et al 1977, Ritchie, Powel-Tuck and Lennard-Jones 1978) that so-called ulcerative idiopathic or haemorrhagic proctitis is the same disease but in a milder form. Sometimes rectal involvement appears minimal or absent sigmoidoscopically when there is evidence of severe disease in the proximal large bowel. Previous local treatment with steroid retention enemas, for example, may account for such a distribution in some cases, but not all. Even in such circumstances, however, the rectal biopsy generally will reveal abnormality. It is not sufficiently widely recognised that rectal mucosa judged to be normal sigmoidoscopically may reveal marked histological changes in ulcerative colitis. The abnormalities brought to light may be minimal, and in some circumstances the mucosa may not differ greatly from normal, but if there have been sequential biopsies, typical changes will almost always be seen in previous tissues. In ulcerative colitis, therefore, colonic biopsy is of paramount importance, not only in diagnosis but also in the assessment of therapy.

The course of ulcerative colitis is typically one of remission and exacerbation, and this is reflected in the range of histological appearances in biopsy material.

In the acute stage during the first attack (Fig. 16–1) the mucosa shows oedema and prominent vascular congestion of the lamina propria. There is an obvious increase in inflammatory cells, lymphocytes and plasma cells predominating with conspicuous eosinophils. Polymorphs are most obvious where they show margination on the capillary endothelium, or as they migrate through the glandular epithelium to fill the lumen and so constitute so-called crypt abscesses. The pus discharges and can often be seen on the surface of the mucosa. The superficial and crypt epithelium loses its goblet cell component as an early feature, sometimes preceding marked inflammatory cell infiltration (Fig. 16–2). It is replaced by a simple basophilic epithelium, and the gland tubular pattern later becomes distorted by the inflammatory exudate and crypt abscess formation (Fig. 16–3). This process is usually limited to the mucosa proper and generally does not extend beyond the

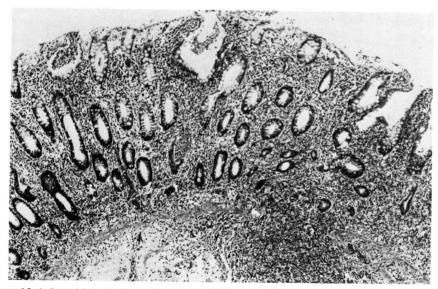

Figure 16–1. Rectal biopsy. Acute ulcerative colitis in an early stage. Marked inflammatory infiltrate, some crypt abscesses but gland pattern only slightly distorted (H & E × 84).

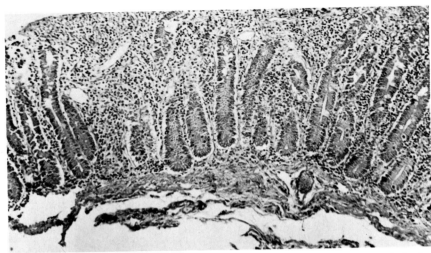

Figure 16–2. Rectal biopsy. Acute ulcerative colitis showing early severe goblet cell depletion and replacement by simple columnar epithelium (H & E × 100).

muscularis mucosa to any significant degree unless there is ulceration, although in the very acute phase the submucosa may show oedema and vascular dilatation (Fig. 16–4). If there is more severe epithelial destruction, ulceration occurs. This varies from superficial erosions to huge areas of total mucosal loss, and in biopsy material this is often manifested by the luminal surface being represented simply by granulation tissue.

Resolution of the inflammatory process with diminution of the infiltration and epithelial regeneration and repair can produce a variety of appearances. A mild first attack may be followed by a complete restoration of the mucosa. More usually,

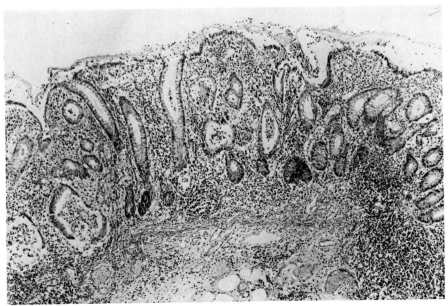

Figure 16–3. Rectal biopsy. Acute ulcerative colitis showing distortion of the gland tubular pattern by the inflammatory process (H & E × 72).

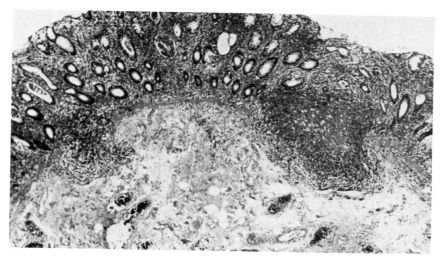

Figure 16–4. Rectal biopsy. Acute ulcerative colitis showing oedema and vascular congestion of the submucosa but no significant inflammatory cell infiltration (H & E × 350).

however, there will be residual abnormality even if this is slight, and it is common to find that the bases of the regenerating tubules have fallen short of the muscularis mucosa (Fig. 16–5) despite having regained a relatively normal appearance. Recurrent attacks and their subsequent resolution result in a variety of abnormalities characterised by a relative loss of tubules, and by branching and irregularity of size and orientation of those that remain (Figs. 16–6 to 16–8). As the attack subsides the simple type of regenerating epithelium is gradually replaced by increasing numbers of goblet cells. Between attacks, therefore, the mucosa may show a variety of appearances that range from normal to one which is distorted, atrophic and sometimes without significant inflammatory infiltrate. It is of some

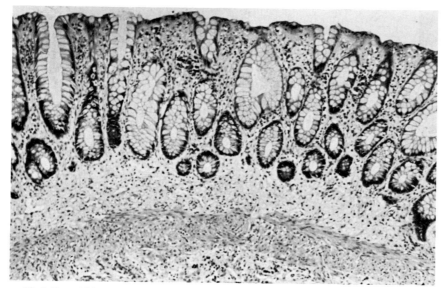

Figure 16–5. Rectal biopsy. Resolution after an acute attack of ulcerative colitis. The gland tubules are irregular although the goblet cell population is restored, but they fall short of the muscularis mucosa (H & E × 140).

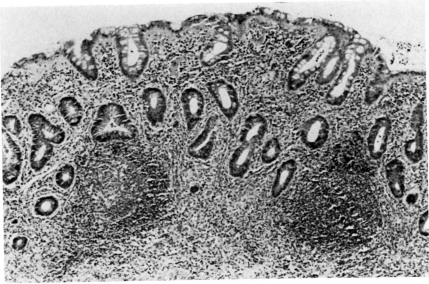

Figure 16–6. Chronic resolving ulcerative colitis revealing progressively more marked tubular loss with abnormalities of shape and size (H & E × 70).

interest that in a quantitative study of ulcerative colitis patients who were in remission the most important feature that differentiated colitic from non-colitic patients was the diameter of the lumen of the glands of the rectal mucosa (Rubio, Johansson and Kock 1982). A further characteristic appearance in the inactive chronic remitting form is a more or less dense collagenosis of that zone of the lamina propria where successive generations of regenerated tubules have fallen short of the muscularis mucosa (Fig. 16–9).

Instead of the chronic remitting form, some patients have chronic persistent disease, and the mucosa never loses the features of active inflammation. The

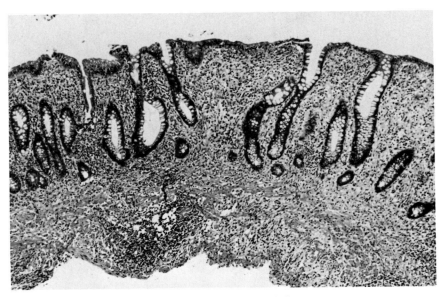

Figure 16–7. Same as Figure 16–6.

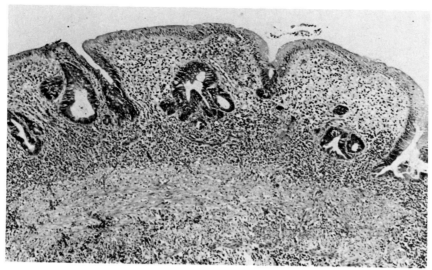

Figure 16–8. Same as Figure 16–6.

features predictably are a mixture of those seen in the acute stage superimposed on an incompletely restored mucosa showing chronic inflammation. Persistent ulceration and attempted healing proceed hand in hand, and it is by this interplay that inflammatory pseudopolyps are produced. They evolve as areas of granulation tissue and an overexuberant regenerative reaction of the mucosal elements. Sometimes these inflammatory polyps are so large that they become symptomatic in their own right due to partial obstruction or blood loss (Kelly et al 1986). When biopsied these lesions not infrequently cause a problem because of pseudomalignant appearances. Beneath the ulcer surface, in a zonal distribution, one may see a layer of quite bizarre pleomorphic or spindle-shaped cells with large ganglion cell-like nuclei. Immunohistochemistry and electron microscopy prove that they are not epithelial, and although their true nature is not established, they are

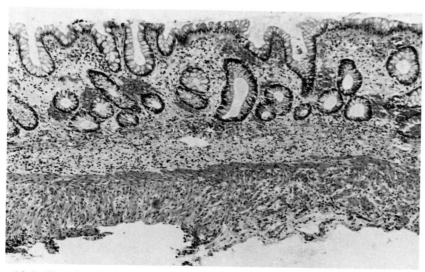

Figure 16–9. Chronic quiescent ulcerative colitis. Goblet cell population normal but tubular pattern abnormal. There is a zone of collagen between the tubules and muscularis mucosa (H & E × 70).

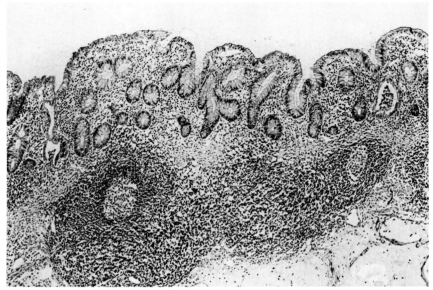

Figure 16–10. Chronic active ulcerative colitis. Note some tubules have a normal goblet cell component; others show crypt abscesses and there is lymphoid hyperplasia (H & E × 70).

probably mesenchymal (Jessurun et al 1986). A marked reactive hyperplasia of the mucosal lymphoid tissue may also occur (Fig. 16–10), and on occasion this may progress and become so marked that a macroscopically polypoidal state is produced. Flejou et al (1988) have made the claim that when lymphoid follicular hyperplasia is associated with disease limited to the rectum, an absence of ulceration and acute inflammation, and failure to respond to steroid therapy, it constitutes the separate disease entity of chronic follicular proctitis. However, it seems curious that rectal bleeding is said to characterise this disease when it is claimed that ulceration of the mucosa is absent. One must presume that what the authors mean by absence of ulceration is full thickness loss of the mucosa. If bleeding occurs there obviously must be some breach in the epithelial surface.

There appears to be a somewhat different clinical picture of ulcerative colitis in the elderly. The onset is usually abrupt and severe, but if the acute phase is overcome, the further course is milder with a lower relapse rate. Brandt et al (1981) have recommended caution in making a diagnosis of ulcerative colitis over the age of 50 years, for in a review of 81 patients, in 75 per cent a retrospective diagnosis of ischaemic colitis was made.

In longstanding ulcerative colitis Watson and Roy (1960) describe Paneth cell metaplasia, and although this occurs more often in the right side of the colon it can also be seen not infrequently in rectal biopsy tissues. The same authors gained the impression that argentaffin cells were also increased in number, but Skinner, Whitehead and Piris (1971) made a quantitative study in rectal biopsy material and found argentaffin cells to be decreased in number. They also showed that argentaffin cells could be found in all parts of the distorted mucous membrane and not only in the crypts, as in a normal mucosa. This has been confirmed using a glyoxylic-acid–induced fluorescence method by Kyosola, Penttila and Salaspuro (1977). Using the Grimelius silver technique, however, Gledhill, Enticott and Howe (1986) claimed that there was an increase in argyrophil cells in ulcerative colitis, but that there was a marked variation from case to case. This apparent discrepancy might well be related to the different techniques used, since the Grimelius method would demonstrate both argyrophil and argentaffin cells. An increase in eosinophils occurs in the mucosa in ulcerative colitis (Anthonisen and Riis 1971), and it is claimed that tissue eosinophilia could be used to distinguish between ulcerative colitis and Crohn's colitis. Further work, however, showed that this was only true of longstanding disease, for the eosinophil count was not raised above normal in a first attack, even if severe (Willoughby, Piris and Truelove 1979). Heatley and James (1978), moreover, claimed that a raised eosinophil count occurred only in relatively benign disease, and that those with aggressive disease not responsive to treatment had significantly smaller numbers.

There is a controversy as to whether or not IgE plasma cells are also increased in number in ulcerative colitis. This may be partly explained by the fact that some cases of ulcerative proctitis referred to earlier may be quite different from ulcerative colitis. Rosekrans et al (1980), for example, showed that whereas in ulcerative colitis IgE cell numbers were normal, in some cases described as allergic proctitis, IgE containing lamina propria plasma cells were increased in number. The patients with this disease responded to the drug disodium chromoglycate, which is known to be beneficial in IgE-mediated immune reactions. Further evidence that IgE plasma cells play no role in ulcerative colitis is provided by Murdoch and Piris (1982). By using a monoclonal antibody, in a peroxidase study, they were able to show that IgE plasma cells were rare in the lamina propria in both normal and diseased mucosa. Furthermore, Scott et al (1983) claim that in a comparison of ulcerative colitis, Crohn's disease and infective colitis, changes in plasma cell counts of the lamina propria are a non-specific response to mucosal damage and do not differentiate the type of inflammatory bowel disease. In a more comprehensive investigation of the lymphoid cells in inflammatory bowel disease, using immunohistochemistry, Hirata et al (1986) failed to show specific changes in a variety of lymphoid cell subgroups in ulcerative colitis. Dendritic cells and scavenger macrophages, however, tend to aggregate around ulcers in both ulcerative colitis and Crohn's disease (Seldenrijk et al 1989).

The muscularis mucosa not infrequently shows involvement by the inflammatory infiltrate, and it is common to see it split and disrupted by hyperplastic lymphoid aggregates. Extension of inflammation into the submucosa is unusual, however, except in the region of deep ulceration and in the very acute form of the disease known as toxic dilatation. Unless the patient has survived such an attack with the aid of intensive medical treatment, fibrosis of the submucosa is not a usual feature of ulcerative colitis. It is associated with clear evidence of deep ulceration that has effaced the muscularis mucosa, the latter having no capacity for regeneration. In longstanding disease the muscularis mucosa may also show fibromuscular hyper-plasia (Fig. 16–11), which, if severe, may result in stricture formation (Goulston and McGovern 1969).

It is widely accepted that patients with ulcerative colitis are liable to develop carcinoma of the large intestine (Morson 1966). Those who seem particularly prone are patients with total colitis and a history of more than ten years duration. It is a traditional concept that patients with an onset of disease in childhood have a higher incidence than patients whose colitis begins in later life, but this has been challenged (Sachar and Greenstein 1981). Patients with mild disease of long standing seem especially vulnerable, but there is disagreement whether those with continuous symptoms (Edwards and Truelove 1964) or quiescent disease (Svartz and Ernberg 1949, Kornman 1971, Sachar and Greenstein 1981) account for the majority. In a recent critical review Collins, Feldman and Fordtran (1987) have cast serious doubt on the value of colonoscopic surveillance of colitic patients

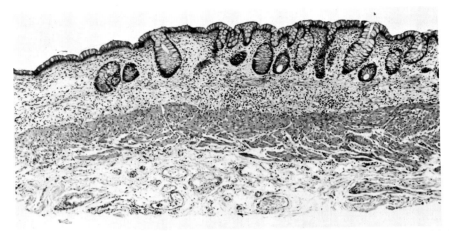

Figure 16–11. Chronic quiescent ulcerative colitis. The muscularis mucosa is hypertrophied and appears as thick as the atrophic gland layer (H & E × 35).

seemingly at risk of developing colonic cancer. Furthermore, Gyde et al (1988) provide evidence in a large cohort study from three centres that patients with extensive colitis have a genetic predisposition to colorectal cancer and that longstanding inflammation is not of primary importance. Nevertheless, others (Jones, Grogono and Hoare 1988) still advocate surveillance even in those patients with distal disease. It is probably true that earlier diagnosis and treatment is obtained by those under continuous medical care, and in centres that see their colitic patients regularly a low incidence is often recorded. The explanation for this probably lies in the fact that, on the whole, more patients in the high-risk group will have a colectomy before any malignant change can occur. Early work in this field by Morson and Pang (1967) provided evidence suggesting that sequential rectal biopsy had value in such cases as an aid to cancer control. This was disputed by Evans and Pollock (1972) and Cook and Goligher (1975), who described cancer cases in which the rectum was normal, precancer in cases without cancer, and no precancer in the presence of cancer. In common with other epithelial surfaces that undergo precancerous changes, the colonic mucosa may exhibit a wide range of dysplastic features before the stage of frank carcinoma in situ or cancer proper is reached. The difficulty for the pathologist lies in deciding at which stage a firm diagnosis of precancer can be made.

The situation was seemingly clarified by Riddell (1976), who reassessed the available material from St. Mark's Hospital, London, from whence Morson and Pang's original article was published. The importance of clear diagnostic criteria is obvious when one considers that a total colectomy is the only operative procedure that theoretically can offer hope of a cure. However, it seems there is still much work to be done in this interesting and important field. Riddell has highlighted the need for a set of working definitions to enable pathologists faced with the problem of diagnosis of precancer in ulcerative colitis to assess each patient. Cases such as those recorded by McGovern (1972) show that precancerous changes may precede the development of invasive cancer by as much as six years, and it is in this interim period that diagnosis and subsequent treatment will effect a certain cure.

The problem is the recognition of the specific pathological criteria upon which a decision to advocate colectomy can be based (Riddell et al 1983). Riddell (1984) and Ransohoff, Riddell and Lewin (1985) have addressed the problem time and again, and despite formulated detailed classifications upon which clinical decisions can be based, the problem is still current. Dundas et al (1987) have shown, for example, that for some aspects of the assessment for dysplasia that concern columnar mucous cells and dystrophic goblet cells, there is very poor interobserver agreement. Clearly the distribution of dysplasia in the colon is also important (Vatn, Elgjo and Bergan 1984) and that it may not be recognisable endoscopically. Thus biopsy of dysplastic areas may be a hit-and-miss affair, and patients, although under surveillance, may develop a carcinoma. Allen and Biggart (1986) have even drawn attention to the event of invading carcinomas probably arising from dysplastic misplaced epithelium deep in the colonic wall being covered by non-dysplastic mucosa. Despite claims that other markers of dysplasia may be useful, such as those demonstrated by monoclonal antibodies (Olding et al 1985), mucin stains (Ehsanullah et al 1985, Filipe, Edwards and Ehsanullah 1985, Habib et al 1986), lectins (Pihl et al 1985, Ahnen et al 1987, Fozard et al 1987), morphometric analysis (Allen et al 1987, Cuvelier, Morson and Roels 1987), and ploidy studies (Fozard et al 1986, Svendsen et al 1987), none have overcome the central problem that despite the acceptance of a dysplasia cancer sequence in ulcerative colitis, cases of cancer still develop undetected. Furthermore, there is still no single criterion upon which to base a decision to advocate colectomy for the prevention of cancer in patients with ulcerative colitis. The problem is accentuated by the fact that on investigation ostensibly normal, asymptomatic people may have active ulcerative colitis (Mayberry et al 1989).

However, there are certain macroscopic appearances that should lead the endoscopist to the likeliest diagnostic site for biopsy. One is mucosa of velvet-like appearance due to an underlying villous microscopic structure, but this need not be dysplastic (Lee 1987). Polypoidal mucosa is another, despite the fact that this will usually be of inflammatory type. In ulcerative colitis true adenomatous polyps also occur, and Dawson and Pryse-Davies (1959) have shown that polyps in ulcerative colitis may show a spectrum of features from truly inflammatory through mixed types to those that are truly neoplastic (Figs. 16–12, 16–13). This was confirmed in a later study (Blackstone et al 1981) that stressed the point that patients with a polyp or plaque showing epithelial dysplasia were more likely to harbour a separate carcinoma than those patients with dysplasia in a flat mucosa. It is probable that when a mass lesion is found it is chronologically an older one and more likely to be associated with actual carcinoma in another part of the bowel (Butt and Morson 1981). This notion is at variance, however, with the report by Rubio et al (1982) of relatively non-dysplastic villous adenomas in association with separate invasive carcinomas. The most frequent macroscopic appearance, unfortunately, is less easy to recognise. It is flat and not unlike the usual featureless mucosa of chronic ulcerative colitis. If the underlying vessels are difficult to see, however, biopsy may be rewarding, since the overlying mucosa, although flat, is thickened.

Microscopically, Riddell (1976) described two common changes, adenomatous and basal cell. Three others may be seen rarely: in situ anaplasia, clear cell change, and pancellular change. The adenomatous change is cytologically the same as that seen in ordinary adenomatous polyps of the colon. It occurs, however, in macroscopically flat, villous and polypoidal lesions. Increasing nuclear atypia in the form of enlargement, pleomorphism, hyperchromasia, mitotic rate and loss or modification of goblet cell appearance can be seen (Figs. 16–14 to 16–16). The basal cell change is commonest in flat mucosae and is characterised by tubules formed by intensely hyperchromatic cells arranged in a linear fashion parallel to the basement membrane at the basal pole of the cell. The cell size and shape vary

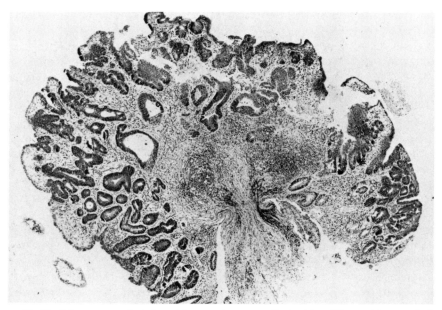

Figure 16–12. Polyp removed at sigmoidoscopy from a patient with a 12 year history of ulcerative colitis. The lesion has many of the features of a true adenomatous polyp (H & E × 20).

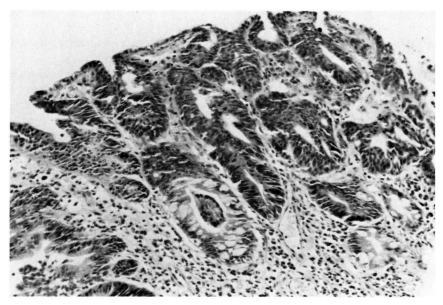

Figure 16–13. Detail of Figure 16–12 showing branched and irregular tubules composed of dysplastic epithelium (H & E × 150).

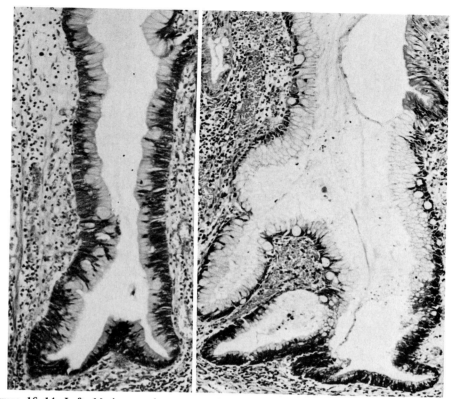

Figure 16–14. Left, Moderate adenomatous dysplasia with retained mucin production (H & E × 120). **Right,** Mild dysplasia, but some goblet cells have an in situ signet ring appearance (H & E × 120).

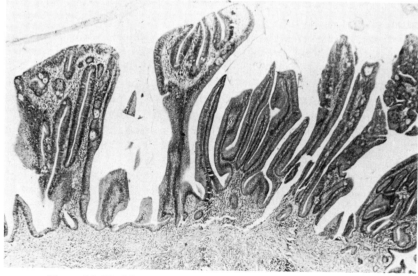

Figure 16–15. Adenomatous dysplasia of villous type (H & E × 48).

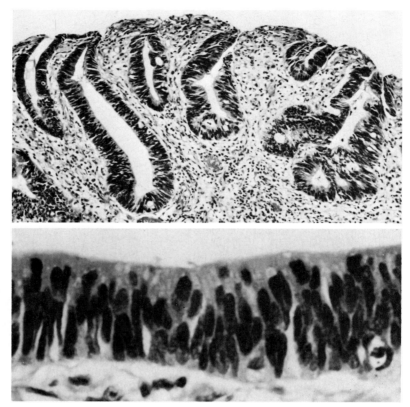

Figure 16–16. Upper, Adenomatous dysplasia in a flat area of mucosa. Irregular budding of tubules has produced a back-to-back arrangement of crypts on the right and all show severe cellular dysplasia (H & E × 190). **Lower,** Detail of dysplastic epithelium. Note the absence of goblet cells (H & E × 750).

little, and the absence of pleomorphism and changes in cell polarity is typical, but mitotic figures are increased in number. The cytoplasm is characteristically eosinophilic, and the cells occupy most of the tubules, so that goblet cells are often scanty and may be poorly formed (Figs. 16–17 to 16–19).

In situ anaplasia occurs only in flat mucosa, often in the company of basal cell change. It is composed of single malignant cells in sheets, with or without signet ring forms, that are confined by the muscularis mucosa. The appearance is likened to superficial spreading carcinoma of the stomach (see Fig. 8–15). Clear cell change at first glance often appears innocuous. It forms a slightly raised lesion macroscopically and basically has a tubular configuration. The cytoplasm of the cells is clear or has a ground-glass appearance. The tubules nearer the surface have a saw-toothed outline similar to that seen in metaplastic polyps of the colon (Fig. 16–20). In pancellular dysplasia the mucosa is flat and shows enlarged and atypical cells arising from all the normal cell types, i.e., goblet cells, so-called absorptive cells, Paneth cells and even argentaffin cells. One or other cell type may predominate, and Riddell even describes an appearance resembling an in situ argentaffinoma. Argyrophil cell hyperplasia, an atypical carcinoid tumour (Miller and Sumner 1982) and frankly malignant carcinoid complicating chronic ulcerative colitis have also been described (Owen et al 1981, Gledhill et al 1986). Rarely, squamous metaplasia of the colonic mucosa occurs in chronic ulcerative colitis, and Adamsen, Ostberg and Norryd (1988) describe such a phenomenon, but with superimposed severe squamous dysplasia.

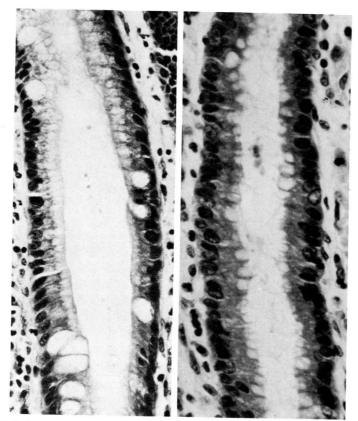

Figure 16–17. Left, Earliest recognisable basal cell dysplasia. Nuclear hyperchromasia and pleomorphism are apparent. Mucin secretion is still present, but some goblet cells are atypical (H & E × 300). **Right,** More severe nuclear changes and atypical mucin production (H & E × 480).

By and large the histological diagnosis of precancer as described should only be made in the absence of significant active inflammation because of the difficulties, even for experienced observers, of evaluating purely reactive epithelial changes, which can appear remarkably bizarre, especially in childhood. Although, as illustrated, it is possible to subdivide dysplasia according to the predominant cytological appearance, mixtures are not infrequent. From a practical point of view, until objective methods of increasing dysplasia can be devised, the pathologist needs to make a subjective decision. If the dysplasia is severe, i.e., architecturally and cytologically approaching an appearance of carcinoma, a confident diagnosis should make a colectomy the first choice of management. However, this is a clinical decision that is often complex. Even greater difficulty arises in the situation when the dysplasia is definite, but mild in severity. As many arguments can be raised for follow-up of such patients with regular rebiopsy as can for the recommendation of colectomy.

It is now clear that routine rectal biopsy in the search of precancer will miss a group of cases, not only of precancer elsewhere but also of established cancer in the more proximal colon. With increasing practice of colonoscopy and multiple sampling of the mucosa of the whole colon, some but not all of the problems related to colitis cancer have been solved. In the at-risk patient, Lennard-Jones et al (1983) follow the practice of stepwise biopsy of the whole colonic mucosa every 10 cm when it appears flat and also biopsy any macroscopically abnormal area.

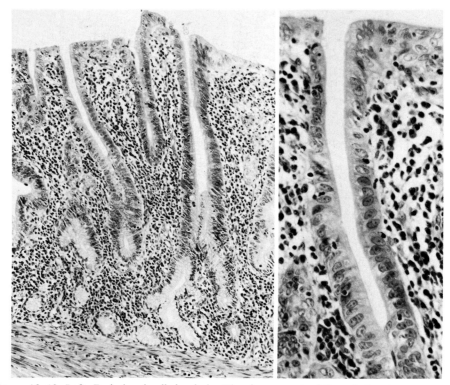

Figure 16–18. Left, Early basal cell dysplasia. The deep aspect of the tubules shows non-specific pseudopyloric metaplasia, but the upper parts exhibit loss of goblet cells and obvious nuclear enlargement (H & E × 120). **Right,** High-power of left photomicrograph showing abnormal but basally situated nuclei (H & E × 480).

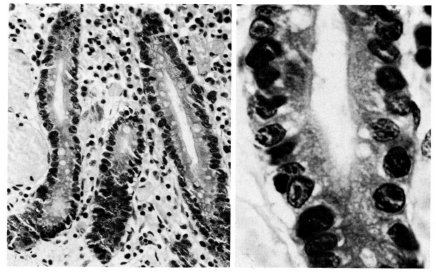

Figure 16–19. Left, Basal cell dysplasia is obvious with more or less loss of mucin production and severe nuclear dysplasia, but no significant loss of polarity (H & E × 300). **Right,** Detail of left. Retention of polarity by cells with markedly dysplastic nuclei (H & E × 1000).

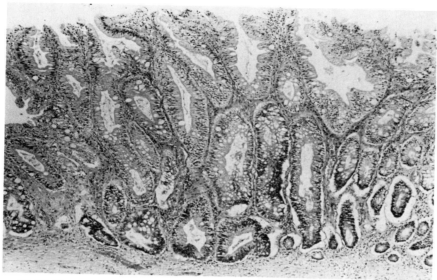

Figure 16–20. Clear cell dysplasia. There is a resemblance to a hyperplastic polyp of the colon. The upper parts of the tubules have a saw-toothed appearance. Most cells have a ground glass cytoplasmic appearance which contrasts with the retained goblet cells (H & E × 75).

Some recommend that this be performed annually (Yardley et al 1983), but this depends on resources and, as already pointed out, some (Collins, Feldman and Fordtran 1987) feel that annual biopsy is not justified. It is possible with increasing experience in the recognition of earlier and earlier stages of precancer, perhaps by objective methodologies, that the recommendation that total colectomy be performed will be made with confidence. This decision may, however, not be palatable for patients without symptoms or with only minor symptoms. Nevertheless, it is hoped that eventually no colitic patient in the cancer-prone group will ever come to operation when carcinoma is already present. It may be that for the reasons outlined colonoscopic biopsy surveillance will prove not to be the optimum method. Certainly it is less cost effective than when used in cancer detection in those with positive occult blood tests. Fozard and Dixon (1989) have recently reviewed the problem and concluded that perhaps the answer lies in the newer molecular biology techniques. Theoretically these could be used with good effect in detecting genetic abnormalities in early malignant cells derived from total colonic samples.

CROHN'S COLITIS

Although Crohn's colitis was originally described as a disease of the terminal ileum (Crohn, Ginzburg and Oppenheimer 1932), it was soon realised that any part of the small intestine could be involved. Two years after Crohn's original paper, Colp (1934) stressed that the disease could also involve the colon, and other papers citing colonic involvement followed. There was, however, a general reluctance to accept colonic Crohn's disease as an entity until almost 30 years later, when the criteria for differentiating Crohn's disease of the colon from the more common condition of ulcerative colitis were published (Lockhart-Mummery and Morson 1960). It is now plain that Crohn's disease can involve the mouth, larynx, pharynx, oesophagus, stomach, small and large intestines, anus, musculoskeletal system and the skin (Whitehead 1987). Crohn's disease limited to the colon accounts for between 15 and 20 per cent of all cases and is only slightly less common than cases showing involvement of both small and large intestine. In the elderly, distal colonic involvement is common (Fabricius et al 1985). However, the very presence of small-bowel lesions renders the diagnosis of Crohn's disease of the colon easier to make. In a similar way, the diagnosis of Crohn's disease of the skin or mouth can be made with confidence only when there is typical intestinal disease. Crohn's disease confined to the large intestine, therefore, poses a diagnostic challenge to the clinician and pathologist alike.

The importance of colonic biopsy in the diagnosis of this disease cannot be overemphasised (Dyer, Stansfeld and Dawson 1970). When rectal tissue is obtained, whether a suction instrument or forceps are used, every effort should be made to ensure that submucosal tissues are included. If there is obvious sigmoidoscopic inflammation and ulceration, several biopsies should be obtained. Ideally, ulcerative lesions, inflamed but intact mucosa and mucosa that seems more normal should be sampled when possible. It is claimed that biopsies from ulcers are diagnostically superior (Potzi et al 1989). Rectal biopsies should also be taken when the sigmoidoscopic appearances are apparently normal, as should multiple colonic biopsies during colonoscopic procedures. One of the fields of greatest difficulty for both clinician and pathologist is the differential diagnosis between Crohn's colitis and ulcerative colitis: if the rectal biopsy is histologically normal, an inflammatory lesion in a more proximal part of the colon is most unlikely to be due to ulcerative colitis and more likely to be due to Crohn's disease or some other segmental lesion.

The histological features of Crohn's disease as seen in colonic biopsies reflect the pathology of the disease as a whole. It is basically an inflammatory disorder, usually included in the chronic granulomatous group. However, as in tuberculosis, one may rarely observe more acute inflammatory reaction at one end of the scale and the more common and very chronic hyperplastic fibrous reaction at the other. It is the fulminating, acute-onset cases of Crohn's colitis that pose extremely difficult problems in differential diagnosis. Early in the course of the disease, tissue reactions may be non-specific, and some of these cases are no doubt similar to the so-called indeterminate colitis (to be referred to). Others with a similar history finally evolve into more histologically typical disease (Linssen and Tytgat 1982). The problem of the relationship of these more acute cases to the more classical cases of colonic disease is in many ways comparable to the relationship of acute terminal ileitis to chronic regional ileitis of the older literature. The evidence seems to point to the fact that when acute terminal ileitis due to other causes such as *Yersinia enterocolitica* infection is excluded, a small proportion of cases of acute disease does go on to develop into classical Crohn's (Jess 1981).

In typical disease rectal or colonic biopsies of non-ulcerated areas situated near ulcers may appear relatively normal but will usually show a plasma cell and lymphocytic infiltration of the lamina propria (Fig. 16–21). Polymorphs, either within capillaries or around the basement membranes of tubules, also are not infrequently present, and an occasional collection of polymorphs within the lumen of a gland tubule is not unusual. Rarely the inflammatory exudate within the crypt is granulomatous (Fig. 16–22). Gross crypt abscess formation and marked epithelial invasion by polymorphs is not seen, however, in non-ulcerated mucosa. It is a relatively important diagnostic feature that these inflammatory changes are not usually associated with any significant distortion of gland tubular pattern or goblet cell depletion, and within the biopsy itself they are less evenly distributed than in ulcerative colitis. The inflammation, moreover, is frequently more marked

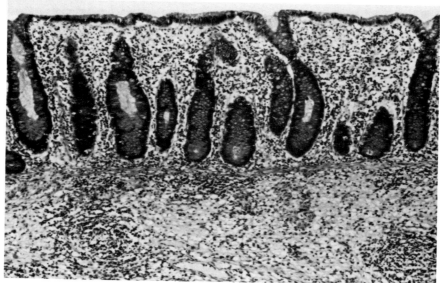

Figure 16–21. Rectal biopsy in Crohn's colitis. The tubules retain a good goblet cell component and their pattern is relatively normal, although they are more widely separated than normal by the inflammatory infiltrate (H & E × 75).

in the submucosa than in the lamina propria and also has a tendency to be perilymphatic. This disproportionate inflammation is another useful feature, especially when attended by denser and more clearly demarcated lymphoid aggregates (Fig. 16–23). The submucosal infiltrate may be associated with lymphatic and vascular dilation or, when the reaction is more chronic, by a fibroplasia. These features are less likely to be evaluable in the more superficial colonoscopic biopsies.

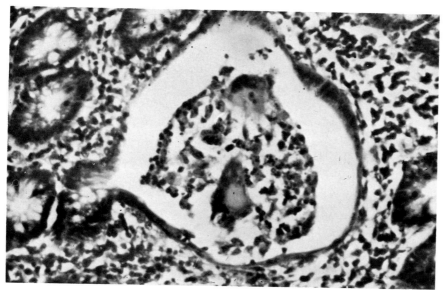

Figure 16–22. Dilated crypt in Crohn's colitis. The exudate contains multinucleate giant cells (H & E × 450).

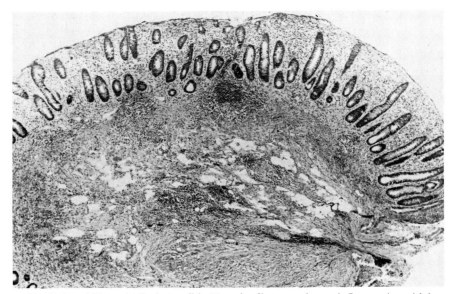

Figure 16–23. Rectal biopsy in Crohn's colitis. Note the disproportionate inflammation with lymphoid aggregates in the submucosa. Mucosal distortion and goblet cell depletion is minimal (H & E × 38).

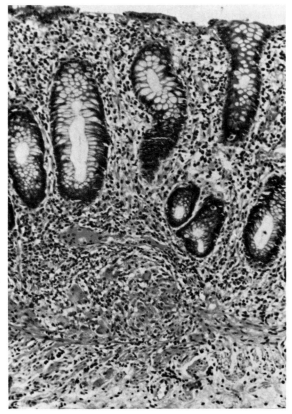

Figure 16–24. Rectal biopsy in Crohn's colitis. There is an epithelioid and multinucleate giant cell granuloma splitting the muscularis mucosa (H & E × 180).

Diagnostically the most significant of the more chronic tissue reactions is the presence of epithelioid cell granulomata (Fig. 16–24), which usually contain one or more multinucleate giant cells. They may be seen in the lamina propria but are most common in the submucosa (McGovern and Goulston 1968). With a tendency to form near lymphatics, they sometimes bulge into the lumen. These granulomata are more variable in size, and the component cells are less tightly packed together than the usual sarcoid granulomata, although the loose cellular arrangement may simply reflect a generalised tissue oedema. The giant cells (which are not always present) may contain Schaumann bodies, and the overall appearance of the granulomata is similar to that of sarcoidosis. They are particularly diagnostically significant if seen in the submucosa and in areas distant from ulceration. It is important to remember that a giant cell and histiocyte reaction may be of foreign body type (Figs. 16–25, 16–26) or appear as a reaction to mucin (Fig. 16–27), and they may be seen occasionally in ulcerative colitis (Figs. 16–28, 16–29). However, giant cells and small granulomata also appear to form in relation to degenerating tubules and are associated with a few polymorphs (Figs. 16–30 to 16–33). The importance of these microgranulomata is referred to later.

In relation to the significance of granulomata in rectal biopsies it is necessary to address the question as to whether systemic sarcoidosis can involve the gastrointestinal tract. It has been stated in the past that while gastric sarcoidosis occurs occasionally, involvement of the intestine is very rare and it may be that something about the gut-associated lymphoid tissue makes it resistant to involvement. There are, however, a few cases of both small and large bowel sarcoidosis that have been described (Macfarlane 1955, Aaronson, Meir and Ulin 1957,

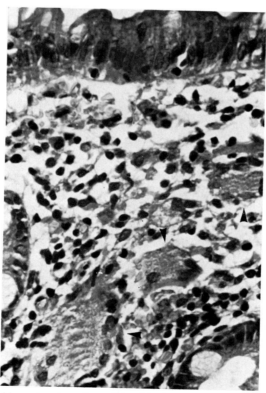

Figure 16–25. Rectal biopsy in ulcerative colitis with subepithelial multinucleate giant cells (arrowheads) (H & E × 360).

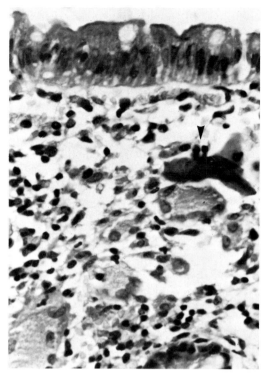

Figure 16–26. Same biopsy as Figure 16–25, but serially sectioned to locate foreign body (arrowhead) (H & E × 360).

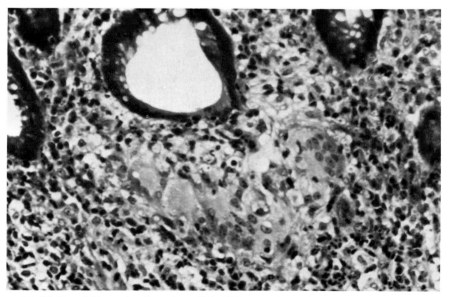

Figure 16–27. Rectal biopsy in ulcerative colitis. This granuloma situated just above the muscularis gave a strong positive reaction with mucin stains (H & E × 360).

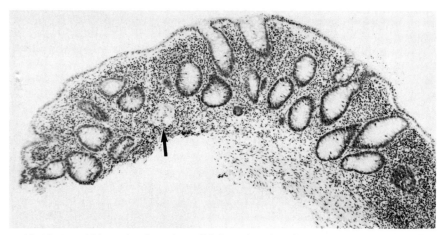

Figure 16–28. Rectal biopsy in ulcerative colitis in a chronic quiescent stage. A single multinucleate giant cell (arrow) is apparent (H & E × 70).

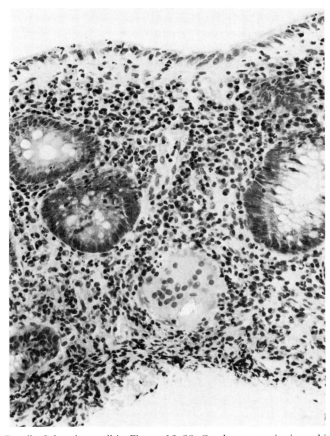

Figure 16–29. Detail of the giant cell in Figure 16–28. On deeper sectioning a birefringent foreign body inclusion was seen in the cytoplasm (H & E × 350).

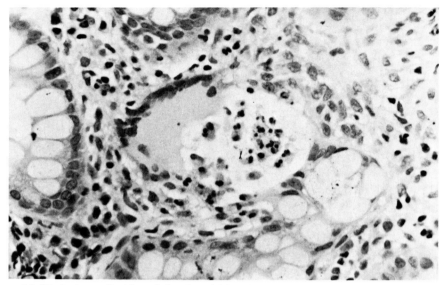

Figure 16–30. A giant cell with peripheral nuclei in relation to degenerating polymorphs and to the right a few epithelioid cells (H & E × 500).

Gourevitch and Cunningham 1959, Gould, Handley and Barnardo 1973, Kondo et al 1980, Tobi, Kobrin and Ariel 1982, Bulger et al 1988).

Biopsy specimens from ulcer margins in Crohn's colitis will show distortion of gland tubular patterns, crypt abscesses and epithelial cell degenerative and regenerative changes. As a consequence, the goblet cell population will be reduced, but this is rarely as marked a feature as in ulcerative colitis. Many of the ulcers in Crohn's colitis have no special features, but biopsy tissues may reveal evidence of two types of ulceration that deserve special mention. The first is the histological

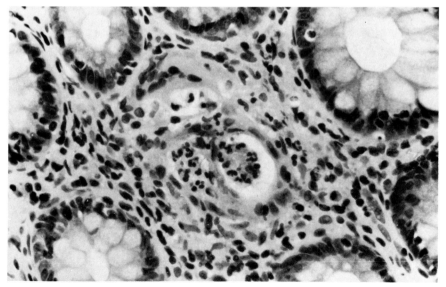

Figure 16–31. Step serial section of a degenerating tubule surrounded by epithelioid histiocytes and containing polymorphs (H & E × 500).

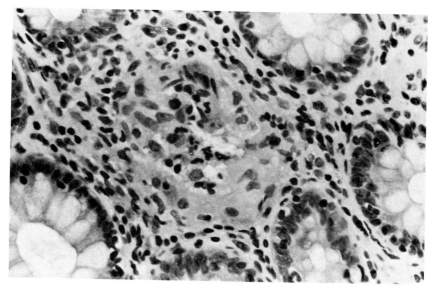

Figure 16–32. Same as Figure 16–31.

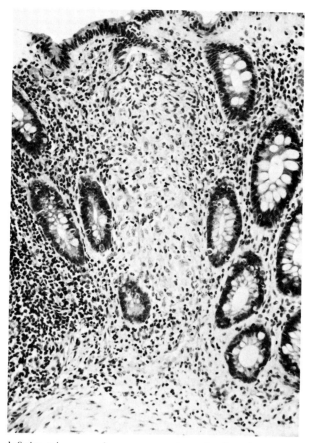

Figure 16–33. A definite microgranuloma composed predominantly of epithelioid histiocytes in relation to an effaced tubule (H & E × 350).

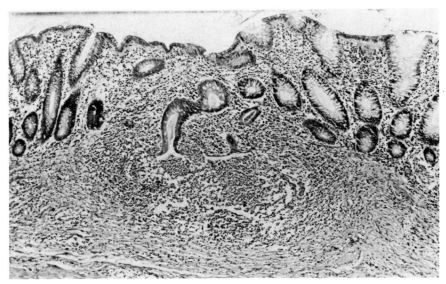

Figure 16–34. Early aphthoid lesion. Central microabscess within a lymphoid aggregate involving the base of a gland. The other glands are relatively normal and have a good goblet cell population (H & E × 75).

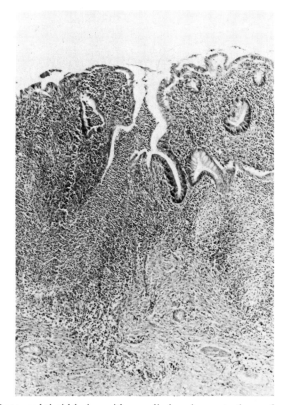

Figure 16–35. Later aphthoid lesion with pus discharging onto the surface (H & E × 75).

equivalent of the aphthoid ulcer seen macroscopically. The early lesion (Fig. 16–34) is composed of a central microabscess, sometimes appearing to occur actually within a lymphoid aggregate at the mucosal-submucosal junction. The abscess nearly always seems to involve the base of a dilated tubular gland that shows necrosis of its walls and pus streaming up into the lumen (Fig. 16–35). Focal superficial ulceration is seen in older lesions (Fig. 16–36), and suppuration may thus obliterate any original lymphoid follicle. Biopsy evidence of the fissuring type of ulceration may also be present. These ulcers, which occur at right angles to the long axis of the bowel, often contain pus and are lined by a granulation tissue that has a conspicuous histiocytic element. The pale, plump cells are very similar to and probably identical with the epithelioid histiocytes that occur in the granulomata. The cells occasionally form multinucleate giant cells of the Langhans type with peripheral nuclei, but in the region of ulcers obvious foreign body giant cells may also be seen. These tend to have more numerous and centrally placed nuclei. It is not always possible to be absolutely certain of the significance of isolated giant cells (Figs. 16–37, 16–38).

In the absence of endoscopic abnormality Goodman, Skinner and Truelove (1976) have shown that although conventional light microscopic examination may reveal no significant abnormality, a quantitative assessment of the volume of lamina propria and the plasma cell per unit length of muscularis mucosa is greater than normal. The mucosal level of glucosamine synthetase is also significantly higher than normal, and these authors conclude that apparently normal rectal mucosa in Crohn's colitis is always abnormal. These subtle abnormalities apparently also exist outside the gastrointestinal tract. Crama-Bohbouth et al (1983) have shown an increase in IgA plasma cells in biopsies from the apparently normal lip of patients with Crohn's disease elsewhere. In a much larger series, using ordinary light microscopy and subjective assessments of inflammatory cells and features such as granulomas, disproportionate inflammation and lymphoid aggregates, Korelitz and Sommers (1977) found evidence of inflammatory involvement of the rectal mucosa when it was sigmoidoscopically normal in 45 per cent of 99 patients with Crohn's disease in another part of the bowel. In 18 per cent of the cases granulomas were recognised.

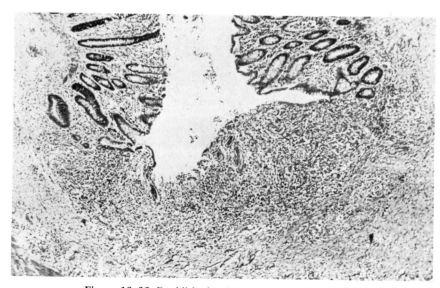

Figure 16–36. Established aphthoid ulcer (H & E × 75).

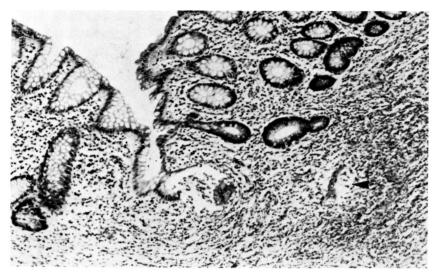

Figure 16–37. Rectal biopsy in Crohn's colitis. A giant cell with centrally placed and abundant nuclei apparently within a gland. A further giant cell is seen to the right (arrowhead) (H & E × 75).

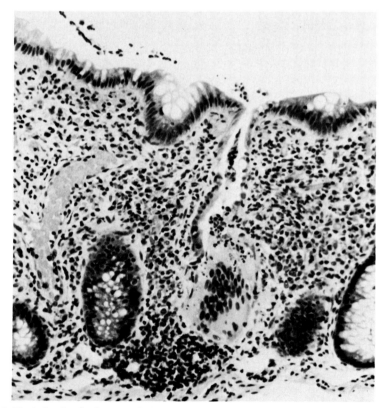

Figure 16–38. A foreign body type of giant cell at the base of a degenerating tubule containing pus (H & E × 200).

In another paper concerning the same cases, Rotterdam, Korelitz and Sommers (1977) drew attention to the importance of superficial, small and poorly defined collections of histiocytes and lymphocytes with or without giant cells, which they termed microgranulomata. If foreign body or mucin granulomata can be excluded, it is now becoming clear that if associated in the same biopsy with patchy chronic inflammation they can nearly always be regarded as positively indicative of Crohn's diease. They are usually seen in association with other chronic inflammatory cells or a few polymorphs invading a neighbouring tubule and are of greater significance if neighbouring tubules are entirely normal. When present along with other pathological and clinical features they are clearly of greater diagnostic significance. Microgranulomas will not infrequently be found if endoscopists biopsy areas of aphthous ulceration or microerosions (Poulsen, Pedersen and Jarnum 1984). The importance of microgranulomas in colon biopsies is obvious from the serial sectioning study performed on colectomy specimens by Kuramoto et al (1987). These workers found microgranulomas were common in the surface layers of the mucosa, whereas more mature epithelioid and giant cell lesions occurred in deeper tissues. These microgranulomas, which range in size from 80 to 160 μm and contain between 10 and 30 immature macrophages thus assume great diagnostic importance in superficial colonoscopic biopsy tissues (Fig. 16–39). Because of this,

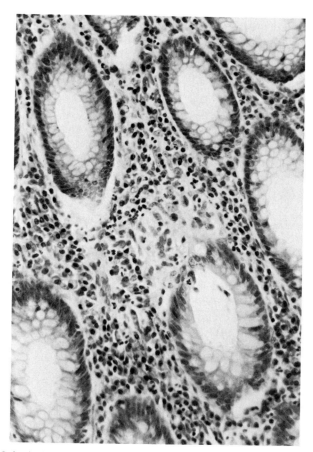

Figure 16–39. Colonic biopsy with a focally distributed chronic colitis and a microgranuloma centrally, adjacent to a segmental degeneration of a mucosal gland tubule. Note also occasional polymorphs in the infiltrate (H & E × 500).

a growing practice is to subject rectal or colonic biopsies in patients suspected of Crohn's disease to serial section. Petri et al (1982) have shown that in a single rectal biopsy in patients with colonic Crohn's disease, 30 per cent will show granulomas if serial sections are examined. This is certainly a better yield than when a few sections of a rectal biopsy are examined when the figure for detecting granulomas is only 15 per cent (Iliffe and Owen 1981). Schmitz-Moormann et al (1984) have even shown that if several biopsies are examined by serial section in Crohn's colitis, granulomas can be found in 40–50 per cent of patients. In a transmission electron microscope study Dvorak et al (1980) describe an increase in mast cells in the submucosa in Crohn's disease. The claim was entirely subjective and based on relatively minute samples of tissue. Whether or not it is substantiated, it has not been found to have diagnostic significance and may be regarded simply as a non-specific manifestation of the inflammatory response. The lack of diagnostic significance also probably applies to the finding of an increase in chromogranin-positive cells in Crohn's disease (Bishop et al 1987).

In a prospective study of rectal biopsies in Crohn's colitis patients, Ward and Webb (1977) produced evidence that the severity of histological involvement as revealed by a semiquantitative method is related to the severity and final outcome of the disease. The presence of either fissuring or ulceration suggests a poor prognosis; whereas granulomas in the large bowel and anus are of good prognostic significance, this does not hold true for the small bowel (Chambers and Morson 1979).

Differential Diagnosis Between Ulcerative Colitis and Crohn's Colitis

The differential diagnosis between ulcerative colitis and Crohn's colitis is a difficult problem frequently posed. Although there are claims that they may be different manifestations of a basically similar disease (Lewin and Swales 1966, Lewkonia and McConnell 1976), there are well-documented cases of coexistent disease (McDermott et al 1982, White et al 1983). That there is an overlap of features, however, cannot be denied, and this is observed particularly in specimens from patients with a short history of severe disease who undergo surgery for toxic megacolon. This type of disease corresponds to the "colitis indeterminate" of Price (1978), who used the term because the pathological features of deep ulceration and transmural inflammation can occur in fulminant ulcerative colitis as well as Crohn's disease. However, if previous surgical or biopsy material from such patients is reviewed, it is often possible to place them in one or other category. Nevertheless, there are cases of idiopathic inflammatory bowel disease that are difficult to classify. Bonfils et al (1977), for example, described what they claimed as a distinct form of colitis, often in younger patients, characterised by a discrepancy between the moderate clinical severity and the evidence of total severe colitis on radiological and histological examination. The colitis recovered spontaneously and did not recur. Except for the course of the disease the presentation had more the features of Crohn's colitis. The author also has experience of such cases in which there was dramatic recovery, and of others treated surgically because of the evidence of total colitis and the severity of the radiological changes. Histologically the striking features are deep ulceration of mucosa, which characteristically shows intense vascular dilatation and an inflammatory reaction with a relative absence of polymorphonuclear neutrophils and only a slight round cell and histiocyte component. The mucosa bordering the ulcers retains its goblet cell component and features oedema, vascular congestion and haemorrhage, rather than acute purulent inflammation as in the more typical ulcerative colitis case. There are thus arguable grounds for retaining the term "colitis indeterminate" for this type of case.

The presence of deeply situated granulomata in rectal biopsy tissues makes the diagnosis of Crohn's disease a simple matter, but even in their absence differentiation from ulcerative colitis is often possible. A relative sparing of the mucosa by an inflammatory process that is more obvious in the submucosa is an important sign. The uneven distribution of the inflammation in the same site or biopsies from different sites is another. A normal mucosa or one showing goblet cell preservation and a normal gland pattern despite inflammatory infiltration of the lamina propria would favour a diagnosis of Crohn's disease. Lymphoid aggregates may be seen in both Crohn's disease and ulcerative colitis; when they lie in the submucosa and are well separated from the muscularis mucosa, and when there is also submucosal oedema or fibrosis in the presence of an intact mucosa and muscularis mucosa, the diagnosis indicated is that of Crohn's disease.

Perhaps of greatest practical importance in the differentiation of ulcerative colitis from Crohn's colitis and other forms of colitis is that the pathologist should receive multiple biopsies. Pieces of mucosa should be taken from areas that appear both normal and abnormal by endoscopy. This provides valuable information concerning the focal, as opposed to a more diffuse, inflammatory involvement of the mucosa in Crohn's colitis and ulcerative colitis respectively. In view of the fact that granulomata may be found in as many as 30 per cent of rectal biopsies in known Crohn's disease of the colon if serial sections are examined, at least three biopsies should be taken from different sites. Anthonisen and Riis (1971) have reported that eosinophilia in biopsy smear preparations is indicative of ulcerative colitis rather than Crohn's disease. This author has no personal experience of this method, but in view of the more obvious overall polymorphonuclear nature of the cellular infiltrate in ulcerative colitis this phenomenon might be expected. Nevertheless, in an individual case in the absence of more specific features, an eosinophil count of the lamina propria by itself can not be used as a reliable diagnostic criterion. Eosinophils are also probably just as frequently seen in other forms of colitis, particularly those of infective origin. In a morphometric analysis of 16 variables Schmitz-Moormann and Himmelmann (1988) claimed an improved rate of discrimination between Crohn's disease and ulcerative colitis. However, it was conceded that the method had no application in daily routine pathology practice.

In addition to rectal biopsy, tissues for histological examination should also be removed from other easily accessible sites (perianal, skin, mouth, oesophagus, stomach) if these show evidence of disease. They may contain granulomata, and if so a diagnosis of Crohn's disease can be made. This assumes great importance, particularly when a histological diagnosis of a coincident bowel lesion has not been obtained.

There is evidence that patients with Crohn's colitis of long standing are more prone to develop adenocarcinoma than the normal population (Weedon et al 1973, Gyde et al 1980). In some cases the cancer has occurred in an unaffected area, but precancerous changes similar to those that occur in ulcerative colitis have also been described in both colon and small intestine (Craft et al 1981, Simpson, Traube and Riddell 1981, Perzin et al 1984). There is some evidence that colorectal cancer is now as common in Crohn's disease and ulcerative colitis patients (Softley et al 1988). However, although dysplastic changes have been described in resection specimens in the region of or separate from the carcinoma, there has been no systematic study to determine the frequency of dysplasia in patients with longstanding Crohn's colitis who do not have adenocarcinoma. This is because patients with widespread disease of long standing are much more likely because of stenosis, fistulae, etc., to be subjected to surgery, and thus the identification and characterisation of a precancer to cancer sequence in Crohn's disease is made much less likely than in ulcerative colitis.

ISCHAEMIC COLITIS

If the viability of the tissues of the bowel is in any way endangered, the result will be invasion of the wall by the many pathogenic organisms that normally pass through or reside in the lumen. The mechanisms of intestinal ischaemia are complex, and secondary factors modify or accentuate the ordinary ischaemic lesion; as a consequence the range of pathological and clinical entities is extremely wide, resulting in a confusing terminology. As far as the colon is concerned, some of these entities have been given better definitions (Marston et al 1966, Whitehead 1971, 1972, 1976, Marston 1977).

Ischaemic colitis can be considered in two broad categories. The first is characterised clinically by abdominal pain of sudden onset and the passage of blood and clots per rectum. It is frequently associated with narrowing or occlusion of the mesenteric vessels, although accurate information concerning this is difficult to acquire during life even by advanced radiological techniques. Recovery either with or without surgical intervention is usual, and resolution with or without scarring and stricture is the end result. Thromboatheromatous disease of the mesenteric vessels is the usual predisposing cause, and thus it is commonest in the older age group. It is, however, seen occasionally in young adults when it usually occurs as a single episode with complete resolution. Clarke, Lloyd-Mostyn and Sadler (1972) described four such cases and reviewed the previous literature, which contained ten others. They commented on the prevalence of right-sided lesions and the low incidence of stricture formation. The precise aetiology in these is not known, although in young females it has been ascribed to the use of oral contraceptive agents (Cotton and Lea Thomas 1971), but this is purely speculative and largely unsupported by the available evidence. Lamy et al (1988), however, describe a marked intimal hyperplasia and thrombosis of the visceral arteries in a young woman with extensive bowel ischaemia and ascribe it to a combination of oral contraception and smoking. Acute reversible ischaemic colitis in a young, female, long-distance runner is also recorded (Heer et al 1987). Nevertheless, the reported incidence of the less severe form of this disease in young men is rising (Neto and Ribeiro 1974), and the author has personal experience with three typical cases of males who obtained spontaneous and complete recovery. Archibald et al (1980) were able to demonstrate inferior mesenteric vein thrombosis in their male patient with ischaemic colitis, and further cases are described by Duffy (1981) and by Heron et al (1981), who refer to the condition as evanescent colitis. Despite the prevalence of right-sided lesions in this group, the part of the colon at maximum risk from an ischaemic insult is the watershed area between the superior and inferior mesenteric vessels, and thus the commonest site for ischaemic lesions of this type is the splenic flexure. Surgical interference with the inferior mesenteric vessels, abdominal aorta and iliac arteries or aortic aneurysms may be associated with colonic (Kim et al 1983) and rectosigmoid lesions (Stenberg and Risberg 1984, Welling et al 1985), but these also occur spontaneously (Kilpatrick et al 1968). Devroede et al (1982) have shown that faecal incontinence and rectal angina are also part of the spectrum of ischaemic bowel disease, and Archibald, Jirsch and Bear (1978) have described an association with renal transplantation. An unusual case of ischaemic proctitis was apparently the result of fibromuscular dysplasia of the superior rectal artery (Quirke, Campbell and Talbot 1984) or of all the mesenteric vessels, a condition that may be familial (Meacham and Brantley 1987).

Apart from thromboatheromatous lesions such as may be seen in quite young patients if, say, they are diabetic (Spotnitz et al 1984), other forms of vascular pathology, in particular the necrotising arteritis group, on occasion may be associated with colonic ischaemia, e.g., polyarteritis nodosa (Wood et al 1979, Lee et al 1984, Roikjaer 1987), rheumatoid vasculitis (Burt et al 1983) and systemic lupus erythematosus (Gore et al 1983, Helliwell et al 1985, Papa, Shiloni and McDonald 1986, Ho, Teh and Goh 1987). It is the subject of rare case reports in association with Kawasaki disease (Fan, Lau and Wong 1986), Buerger's disease (Soo et al 1983, Rosen, Sommer and Knobel 1985), blunt abdominal trauma (Davidson and Everson 1987) and malignant atrophic papulosis or Degos' disease (Barlow et al 1988). Low intestinal flow states also play their part, and colonic obstruction with the attendant decrease in mucosal circulation is a frequent association. Hunt and Mildenhall (1975) claim a connection between ischaemic colonic strictures and pancreatitis, but the aetiology of ischaemia in these cases is obscure. It has been described in association with chronic intermittent peritoneal dialysis (Koren et al 1984, Jablonski, Putzki and Heymann 1987) and in renal transplant recipients (Komorowski et al 1986). Occasionally, ischaemic colitis is complicated by significant dilatation of the bowel (Carr et al 1986). For a full discussion on the pathology of intestinal ischaemia the reader is referred to Whitehead (1976).

In biopsy tissues, appearances are characteristic. The mild cases (Fig. 16–40 A, B, C) will show an ischaemic necrosis of the superficial epithelium and a variable extent of the luminal two thirds or so of the mucosa. The surface epithelium and upper parts of the tubules show ischaemic degeneration and sloughing, and the lamina exhibits an oedema, ballooning of capillaries and sludging of red cells. Rarely does a capillary show a tiny plug of thrombus (Fig. 16–41). Lesions of this severity resolve completely as long as the bases of the crypts are not damaged, and a completely normal mucosa may be seen five to seven days later (Fig. 16–42). More severe lesions (Fig. 16–43) will show ischaemic necrosis of the full thickness of the mucosa and extension into the deeper layers (Fig. 16–44). In these, secondary infection, ulceration (Fig. 16–45) and scarring are usual, and in the healing and healed stages mucosal biopsy tissues reveal a variety of abnormalities. Regenerating gland tubules tend to be irregular in shape, size and orientation (Fig. 16–46), and the component cells of simple type are often a little bizarre and show numerous mitoses (Fig. 16–47). In areas of regenerated mucosa, glandular distortion persists (Fig. 16–48) and there is frequently a fibrosis of the lamina propria that often extends into the submucosa through the breaches of the muscularis mucosa (Fig. 16–49), which has no capacity for regeneration. The fibrosis is attended by a progressive devascularisation, becoming typically dense and hyaline (Fig. 16–50), and is often associated with collections of haemosiderin-filled histiocytes. Levine et al (1986) describe inflammatory polyposis of the colon following ischaemic colitis. An occasional observation in biopsies that also show features of ischaemic colitis, especially in the elderly, is not only severe hyaline sclerosis of small vessels but also atheromatous embolisation (Figs. 16–51, 16–52).

The second type of ischaemic lesion is described variously as "ischaemic enterocolitis" (McGovern and Goulston 1965), "haemorrhagic enterocolitis" (Wilson and Qualheim 1954), "necrotising enterocolitis" (Killingback and Williams

Text continued on page 329

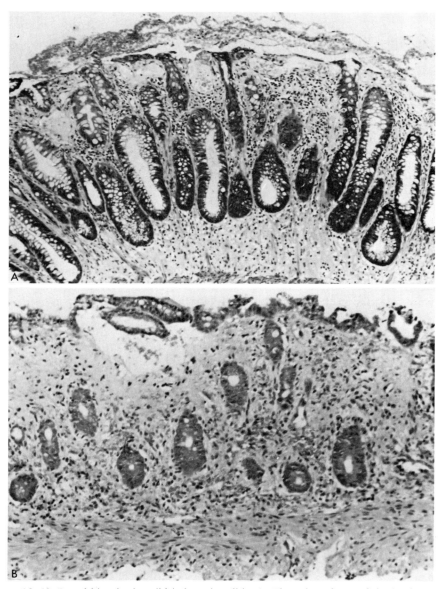

Figure 16–40. Rectal biopsies in mild ischaemic colitis. **A,** There is oedema of the lamina propria, capillary dilatation and superficial mucosal necrosis with haemorrhage (H & E × 20). **B,** There is more extensive ischaemic change, but the bases of the crypts are still intact (H & E × 180).

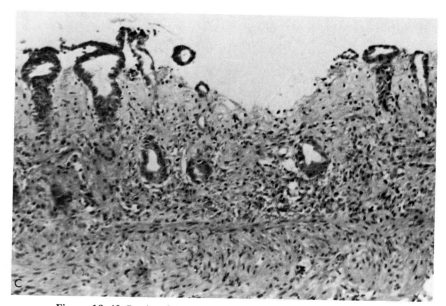

Figure 16–40 *Continued* **C,** Early sloughing and ulceration (H & E × 180).

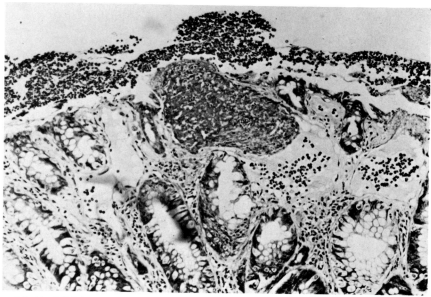

Figure 16–41. Mild ischaemic colitis. There is a tiny fibrin plug in a dilated capillary (H & E × 280).

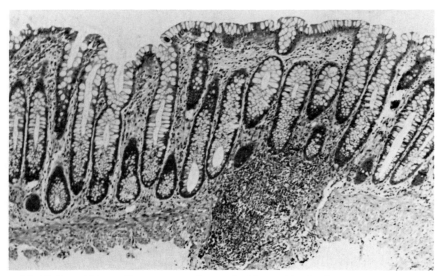

Figure 16–42. Rectal biopsy from same patient as in Figure 16–40 taken one week later, showing almost perfect resolution of mucosa (H & E × 70).

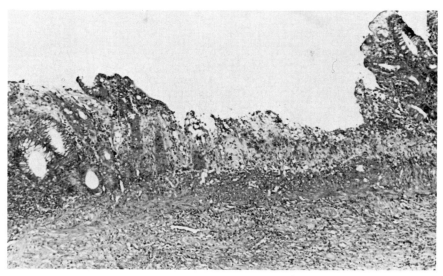

Figure 16–43. Rectal biopsy in ischaemic colitis with full thickness mucosal necrosis and sloughing ulceration (H & E × 70).

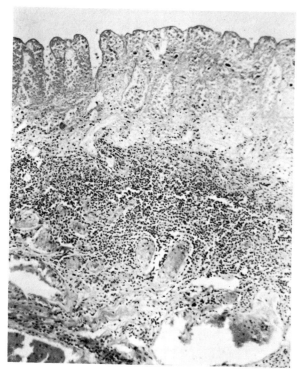

Figure 16–44. Complete ischaemic necrosis of mucosa and part of the submucosa with secondary inflammatory infiltration. Note the vascular dilation in the submucosa (H & E × 70).

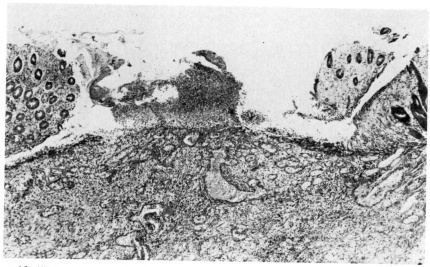

Figure 16–45. Rectal biopsy showing ischaemic ulceration with typical vascular granulation tissue at base and attempted regeneration by marginal epithelium (H & E × 70).

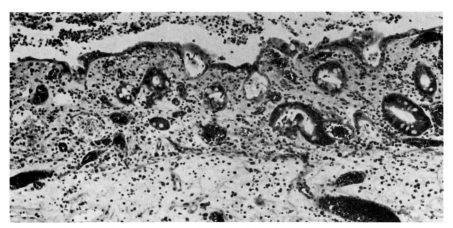

Figure 16–46. Regenerating mucosa in ischaemic colitis. The tubular pattern is abnormal. There is still oedema and vascular congestion (H & E × 75).

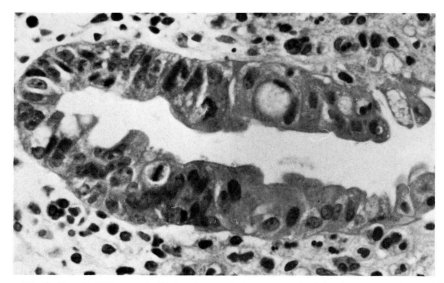

Figure 16–47. Detail of Figure 16–46 showing a tubule composed of simple regenerating epithelium and cells in mitoses (H & E × 450).

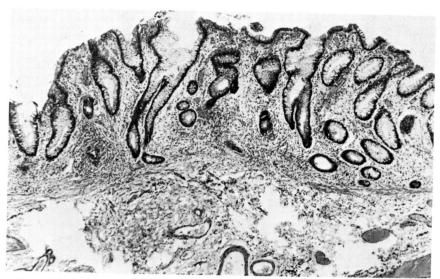

Figure 16–48. Healed ischaemic colitis. Note the glandular distortion (H & E × 75).

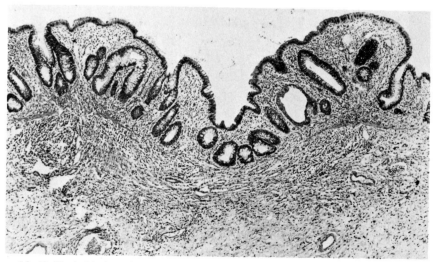

Figure 16–49. Healed ischaemic colitis. Fibrosis of the lamina propria extends through the breaches in the muscularis mucosa into the submucosa (H & E × 75).

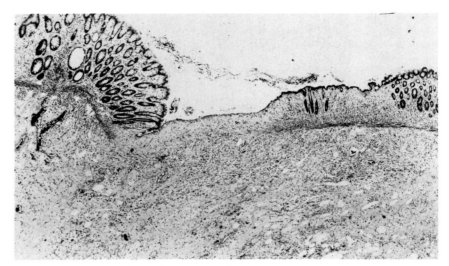

Figure 16–50. Ischaemic colitis with persistent ulcer. The fibrosis of the submucosa is characteristically hyaline and dense (H & E × 38).

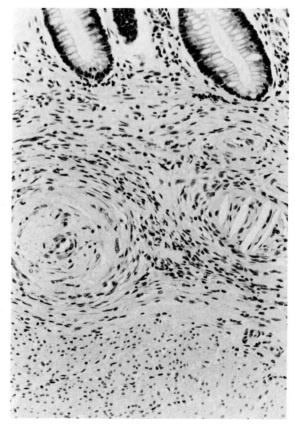

Figure 16–51. Colonic biopsy with mild ischaemic fibrosis of the lamina propria and submucosa. Note the hyalinised, thickened submucosal vessel **(left)** and atheromatous cholesterol crystal embolism **(right).** (H & E × 350).

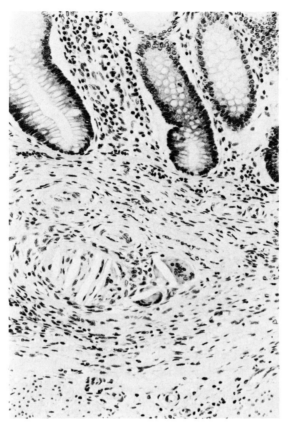

Figure 16–52. Atheromatous embolism with foreign body giant cell reaction to the crystals of cholesterol (H & E × 350).

1961), "postoperative enterocolitis," "uraemic enterocolitis," "non-occlusive intestinal infarction" (Renton 1972, Byrd, Cunningham and Goldman 1987) and "acute intestinal failure" (Marston 1977). It is often a terminal condition, presenting with bloody diarrhoea, usually but not always in patients seriously ill owing to some other disease, frequently being associated with the postoperative period or an episode of shock. There is no special localisation of lesions in or near the splenic flexure, and sometimes the whole of the large bowel and part of the small bowel are involved. No age group is exempt but it is commoner in old age.

In adults the diagnosis is only made at autopsy; in the usual circumstances of its occurrence it does not pose a diagnostic problem. Rarely, however, it arises without obvious predisposing cause and then must be distinguished from acute-onset ulcerative colitis and Crohn's disease. Rectal biopsy is rarely performed but typically shows mucosal necrosis, submucosal haemorrhage and oedema, and a variable, secondary inflammatory infiltrate, depending on the duration of the lesion. The obvious feature is the ballooning of capillaries and venules, which are stuffed with red cells and are invariably occluded by numerous recent fibrin plugs (Fig. 16–53). Gas formation, probably due to secondary invasion by bacteria, is not evident in biopsies. The aetiology of this lesion is complex and includes many factors, one or other of which may appear to assume greater importance in any individual case. They include partial or complete blocks in the blood supply and

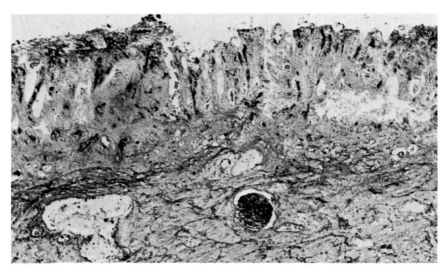

Figure 16–53. Ischaemic enterocolitis. The mucosa is infarcted, and the mucosal and submucosal vessels are occluded by thrombus (fibrin stain × 75).

variations in the blood flow controlled by various shunting mechanisms, the nature of the intestinal contents including the bacterial flora and various intestinal enzymes, the effectiveness of the mucosal barrier to entry of endotoxin or similar agents, and the priming of the mucosal immune mechanism to agents such as endotoxin. The vascular thrombosis already referred to was previously thought to be secondary, but Whitehead (1971) has produced evidence that it may well be primary, the ischaemic necrosis being the local manifestation of disseminated intravascular coagulation. It is therefore of some interest that Craner and Burdick (1976) and Dillard (1983) describe a colitis in the haemolytic-uraemic syndrome with which disseminated intravascular coagulation is intimately associated. Many cases of so-called clostridial and staphylococcal enterocolitis probably also belong to this group, and simply represent primary ischaemia with superimposed massive overgrowth of organisms already within the bowel.

Pseudomembranous lesions that are typical of pseudomembranous enterocolitis (Goulston and McGovern 1965) may also be seen in this condition. A range of appearances are noted between predominantly haemorrhagic and predominantly pseudomembranous, and it was postulated by Whitehead (1971) that in the latter cases the process of intravascular coagulation is less severe and evolves much more slowly. Margaretten and McKay (1971), in a paper concerned with thrombotic ulcerations of the gastrointestinal tract, made particular comment on the association of microthrombosis with pseudomembranous enterocolitis. These authors were also able to show evidence not only of widespread microthrombosis at autopsy but also of alteration in clotting factors, indicating an episode of intravascular coagulation occurring during life. The relationship to pseudomembranous enterocolitis is as puzzling as the overall aetiology of ischaemic enterocolitis in its normal form, and this is discussed in greater depth by Whitehead (1976), who examines the role of the Shwartzman phenomenon in these disorders.

More recently further evidence for this is provided by Behan and Mills (1982), who demonstrated complement consumption in four patients with pseudomembranous colitis. Nevertheless, the way in which these final pathogenetic mechanisms are triggered is far from being understood. That an element of mesenteric vasoconstriction is involved is provided by Bailey et al (1986), who in an experimental study on pigs concluded that non-occlusive ischaemic colitis is mediated by a sensitivity of the colonic vasculature to the renin-angiotensin axis. The association of pseudomembranous colitis and ischaemic enterocolitis is also highlighted by the occurrence of both types of lesions in association with Hirschsprung's disease, either before or immediately following operation. The toxin of *Clostridium difficile*, which is so frequently demonstrated in association with pseudomembranous colitis, has been recovered from patients with neonatal necrotising colitis (Cashore et al 1981) and in Hirschsprung's disease complicated by enterocolitis (Thomas et al 1982). The condition of neonatal necrotising enterocolitis also falls into this category of disease and has been studied more intensely than ischaemic enterocolitis in adults. Not only does the disease affect neonates, usually in the setting of an intensive care unit, but it is described in older infants and children up to the age of 17 years. (Takayanagi and Kapila 1981, Moss and Adler 1982). Its aetiology is also obscure, and although clostridrial organisms have been implicated in its aetiology (Sturm et al 1980, Arseculeratne, Panabokke and Navaratnam 1980), their precise role is unclear. The fact that it occurs in unfed premature infants (Marchildon, Buck and Abdenour 1982) makes it likely that ischaemia, rather than gut flora, is the most important aetiological factor. Based upon the examination of so-called intestinal atresia, when meconium can be found in the distal part of the intestine, showing that it was once patent, and in the absence of evidence for vascular occlusion, it is believed that non-occlusive ischaemia can occur in utero. Vasoconstrictive agents such as Cafergot ingested by a pregnant woman have been cited as a cause of intestinal atresia in a prematurely born infant (Graham, Marin-Padilla and Hoefnagel 1983). The intestine of infants in utero is, of course, sterile, which makes it likely that gut organisms cannot be wholly implicated in this disease, and they may indeed be only secondary invaders.

PSEUDOMEMBRANOUS COLITIS AND ANTIBIOTIC-ASSOCIATED COLITIS

Two facts are clear: first, pseudomembranous enterocolitis was an entity before the antibiotic era; and second, the condition has become much more common with increasing antibiotic usage. Its occurrence in patients who have not received antibiotics has been noted in association with colonoscopy (Patterson, Johnson and Schmulen 1984), leukaemia (Panachi et al 1985), paraquat poisoning (Imamura et al 1986), and Hirschsprung's disease (Brearly et al 1987). The list of antibiotics associated with pseudomembranous colitis is now extremely long, and it is perhaps salutary that the very antibiotic that is commonly used to treat the condition, i.e., metronidazole, has also been cited as a cause (Thomson et al 1981, Daly and Chowdary 1983). Bingley and Harding (1987) even describe a case following combined therapy with metronidazole and vancomycin that resolved after treatment with vancomycin alone.

An important consequence of the recent connection with antibiotics has been a greater awareness of the fact that pseudomembranous enterocolitis can present in many clinical settings. It may arise spontaneously in the previously healthy or more commonly after major surgery, during or after therapy with broad-spectrum antibiotics, as a complication of colonic obstruction, and in patients with debilitating diseases such as uraemia or leukaemia. The clinical picture varies from a mild diarrhoeal illness to fulminant colitis with fever, dehydration and shock. Small intestine, colon or both may be involved, and the characteristic plaques seen endoscopically are strongly suggestive of the disease. It is usually a self-limited disease in its mildest form, and non-debilitated patients improve within a few days. Treatment, therefore, should be medical in the first instance and recourse to surgery avoided if feasible. When it is not possible to differentiate between pseudomembranous and ulcerative colitis the fulminating form usually requires surgery. The mortality in all published series is high, but mild forms are being recognised increasingly. These are probably part of the spectrum of antibiotic-associated diarrhoeas. The aetiology is unknown, but as already stated it also has a relationship with ischaemic enterocolitis, which may represent the other end of the spectrum.

It was postulated that a Shwartzman-like reaction may be the basic pathological process, and absorption of a toxin of bacterial origin with or without a change in intestinal flora, with or without a fall in splanchnic perfusion, could be the triggering mechanism (Whitehead 1971, 1976, Lancet 1977). It was of considerable interest, therefore, when Larson and Price (1977) described a faecal toxin that closely resembled that produced by *Clostridium sordellii* in nine patients with pseudomembranous colitis. Subsequently the toxin was shown by Bartlett et al (1978) and Larson, Price and Honour (1978) to be produced by *Clostridium difficile*. In fact a number of different toxins are now known to be produced by *C. difficile*. Toxin A is an enterotoxin; toxin B is a cytotoxin, which is usually assayed in diagnosis; and toxin C is a motility altering factor (Taylor, Thorne and Bartlett 1981, Justus et al 1982, Mitchell et al 1986). *Clostridium difficile* also produces a factor that inhibits neutrophil migration and phagocytosis (Bolton et al 1985). The exact relationship of colonisation of the bowel by this anaerobe and production of toxins is not, however, entirely clear in relation to the mechanisms of the colitis. Lishman, Al-Jumaili and Record (1981) and George, Rolfe and Finegold (1982) have found that some patients remain clinically well despite high concentrations of faecal toxin. Faecal toxin can be demonstrated in a normal population, particularly in infants (George 1984), even in titres as high as in patients with colitis, and some patients with typical pseudomembranous colitis do not have the toxin or *Clostridium difficile* in their faeces (Dickinson, Rampling and Wight 1985). Moreover, sometimes pseudomembranous colitis is described in association with clostridial infection not of the difficile subtype (Chiu and Abraham 1982), and pseudomembranous colitis has progressed and proved fatal even when the organism and toxin have successfully been cleared from the bowel (Hawker et al 1981).

Clostridium difficile has also been implicated in exacerbation of inflammatory bowel disease (British Medical Journal 1981), but this was not substantiated in the study by Hyams and McLaughlin (1985), at least in children. It is becoming clear that *Clostridium difficile*-associated colitis is a disorder with a wide clinicopathological spectrum. It can vary from a mild, short-lived disease associated with diarrhoea to a severe illness associated with toxic dilatation (Burke, Wilson and Mehrez 1988). It can present as a localised lesion and mimic carcinoma (Arber et al 1987). *Clostridium difficile* can be responsible for endemic disease in institutions (Bender et al 1986) or epidemic disease with spread within several hospitals (Nolan et al 1987). In essence it seems that the presence of *Clostridium difficile* and its toxin merely reflects the extent to which the ecosystem of the intestine is disturbed by a variety of factors, e.g., the effect of antibiotics or intestinal blood flow. The importance of rectal biopsy in the recognition of pseudomembranous colitis is made plain by Tedesco, Corless and Brownstein (1982), who showed that membranes will be noted by flexible sigmoidoscopy in 91 per cent of patients. The fully developed dome-shaped plaque lesion is characteristic, but earlier and later phases also need consideration. Price and Davies (1977) describe three lesions. This is rather artificial since there is a continuum of appearances, but it serves to characterise the histological features. Type 1, the earliest, consists of focal epithelial necrosis of surface epithelium in the interglandular space (Fig. 16–54). The subjacent lamina propria contains an eosinophilic exudate of polymorphs and nuclear debris. Showers of polymorphs and fibrin erupt into the lumen. Type 2 lesions consist of the typical dome-shaped plaque where a well-defined group of glands are distended by mucin and polymorphs at their bases, and are covered by a plaque of fibrin, mucin, cellular debris and polymorphs (Fig. 16–55). The intervening mucosa between plaques is normal, but in several cases large areas of "membrane" may be present (Fig. 16–56). Type 3 lesions show complete structured necrosis of the mucosa with few surviving glands and a covering of cellular inflammatory debris, mucin and fibrin (Fig. 16–57).

There is also a series of changes seen in the resolving or healing phase. These consist of regenerative changes and reconstitution of the damaged mucosa from residual crypts in the original lesion or from neighbouring healthy mucosa (Figs. 16–58 to 16–61). Residual glandular irregularity may be seen, but complete restitution of the mucosa also occurs. This may well be accounted for by the fact that only the less severe cases survive, death being the rule for the more serious cases, especially if associated with another severe systemic disease. However, occasional cases are seen that are characterised by localised recurrent lesions often without significant systemic illness. The mucosa then may show a marked regen-

Text continued on page 339

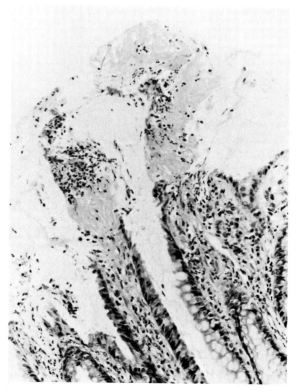

Figure 16–54. Early lesion (Type 1) which consists of necrosis of interglandular superficial epithelium and an exudate of fibrin and polymorphs into the gut lumen (H & E × 300).

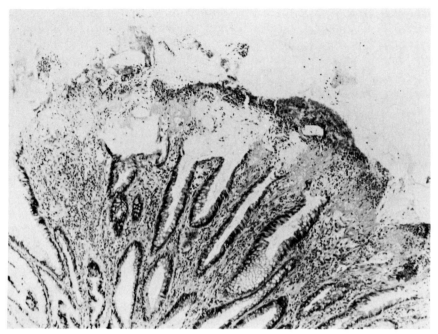

Figure 16–55. A later lesion (Type 2) with fusion of exudate covering the necrosed upper part of neighbouring glands (H & E × 150).

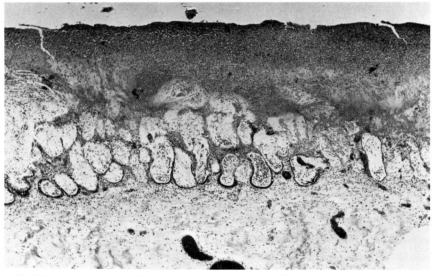

Figure 16–56. Extensive Type 2 lesion with distended mucin-filled gland bases and a covering layer of fibrin, mucin and cellular debris. This constitutes the typical membrane (trichrome × 70).

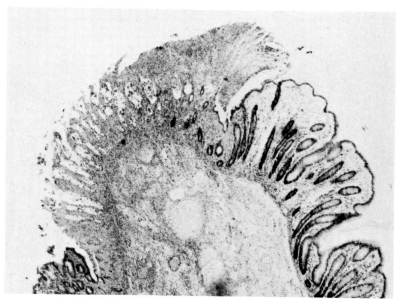

Figure 16–57. Type 3 lesion showing complete structured necrosis of the mucosa with a covering of inflammatory debris, mucin and fibrin (H & E × 25).

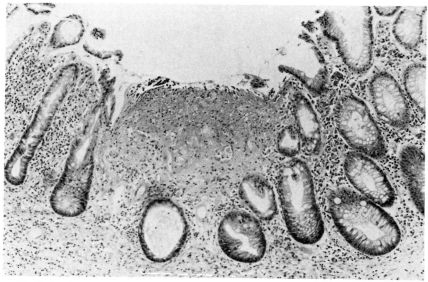

Figure 16–58. Early healing changes in a focal lesion. The residual crypt bases show regenerative changes (H & E × 180).

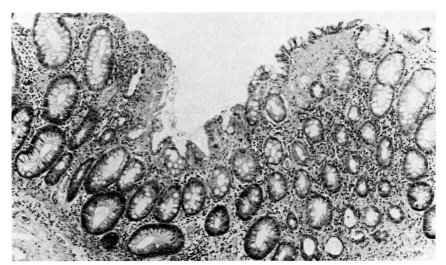

Figure 16–59. Nearly healed focal lesion with residual architectural abnormality (H & E × 180).

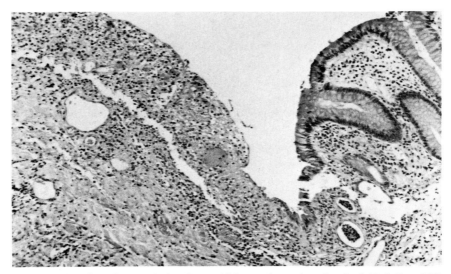

Figure 16–60. Edge of severe lesion from which membrane has sloughed (H & E × 180).

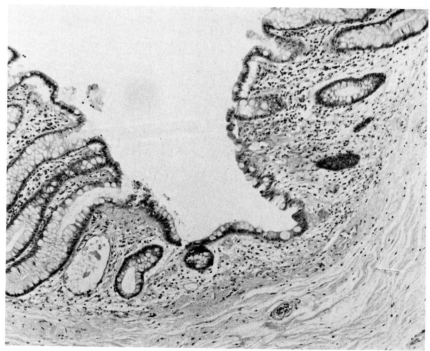

Figure 16–61. Healed deep lesion with a single layer of simple regenerated epithelium (H & E × 180).

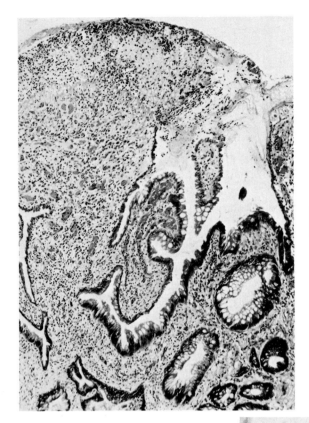

Figure 16–62. Marked irregular hyperplastic crypts in relation to persistent lesion in antibiotic-associated colitis (H & E × 250).

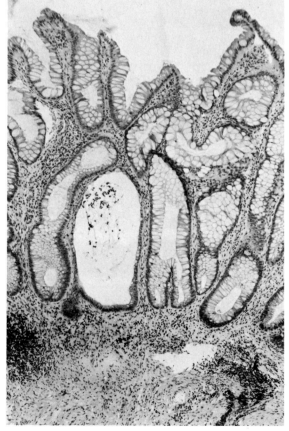

Figure 16–63. Irregular hyperplastic regenerative reaction in persistent antibiotic-associated colitis (H & E × 200).

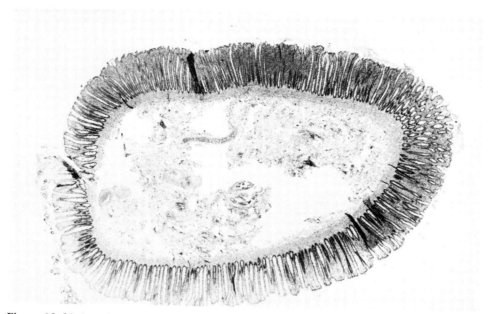

Figure 16–64. Rectal biopsy in antibiotic-associated colitis. Note the distinctive patchy distribution of the inflammation (H & E × 40).

erative reaction with thickening and a gross polypoidal appearance (Figs. 16–62, 16–63). It is usual for there to be accompanying pseudomembranous lesions at the apex of these excrescences, and it is pertinent that significant hyperplastic reactions of a similar nature occur in the experimental hamster model in which the caecum is affected (Price, Larson and Crow 1979).

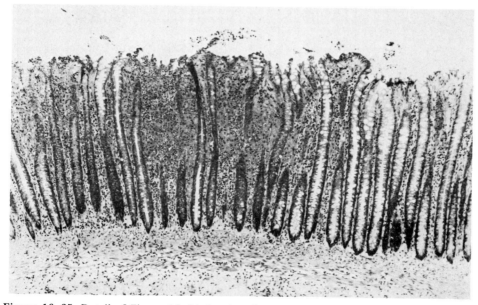

Figure 16–65. Detail of Figure 16–64 showing the variation in intensity of the inflammation (H & E × 180).

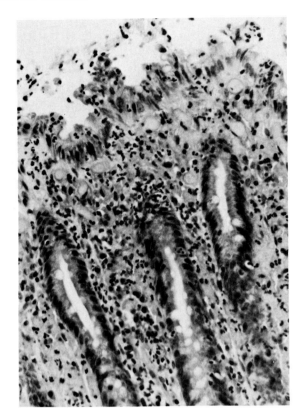

Figure 16–66. Antibiotic-associated colitis with superficial vascular dilatation and polymorph infiltration of rather degenerative superficial epithelium and upper crypts (H & E × 450).

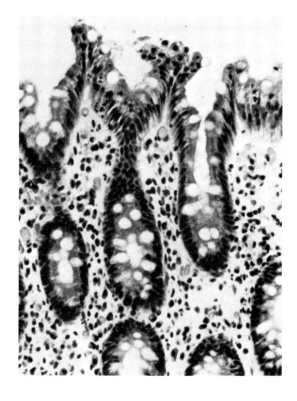

Figure 16–67. Antibiotic-associated colitis with pronounced syncytial appearance of degenerative epithelial cells between crypt mouths (H & E × 450).

A further and not infrequent appearance is seen in the clinical situation of mild but significant diarrhoea, usually without blood, in patients who have recently received antibiotics. It is characterised by a non-specific mild inflammation of the rectal mucosa. The inflammation often tends to be patchy even within the lamina propria of a single biopsy (Figs. 16–64, 16–65). The changes tend to involve the superficial epithelium and the upper quarter or half of the crypts. The lamina shows an increase in inflammatory cells, particularly of acute type, and this is associated with some vascular dilatation. There are always changes in the superficial epithelium, which appears flattened, and occasionally desquamated cells are trapped in adherent mucin. A common appearance is the presence of polymorphs in degenerating and damaged surface and upper crypt epithelium which often forms syncytial knot-like projections between the crypt mouths (Figs. 16–66, 16–67).

The polymorphs themselves often show degenerative changes but are not usually present in large numbers, so that classical dilated crypt abscesses are not found, although a few polymorphs may appear in the lumen. Pus overlying a normal mucosa is occasionally seen, but this is a completely non-specific appearance that may be due to focal sepsis elsewhere in the large bowel, in association with diverticular disease or neoplasm. There is evidence based upon the finding of *Clostridium difficile* toxin in the stool that these changes are related to or constitute the earliest lesions of pseudomembranous colitis. Their association was reviewed by Gibson, Rowland and Heckler (1975) and Rocca et al (1984).

OTHER FORMS OF COLITIS

17

INFECTIVE COLITIS

Bacillary dysentery occurs in most countries either as an epidemic or endemic infection. Epidemics of major proportions tend to occur in tropical countries that have low standards of hygiene, but in temperate zones bacillary dysentery occurs as an endemic disease. Sporadic cases or small outbreaks in these circumstances thus constitute a possible source of diagnostic error. Although bacillary dysentery is commonly equated with *Shigella* infection, of late it has been increasingly recognised that in some infections with *Salmonella*, traditionally regarded as primarily a small bowel pathogen, the colon is also involved and may bear the brunt of the disease (Boyd 1985). The same applies to *Campylobacter jejuni*, to certain strains of *Escherichia coli* (Skirrow 1977, Lambert et al 1979, Longfield et al 1979, Blaser, Parsons and Wang 1980, Colgan 1980, Sack 1981, Levine 1987) and to rarities like enterocolitis due to *Edwardsiella tarda* (Marsh and Gorbach 1982), a gram-negative rod normally found in snakes, toads and turtles. It is possible that there are a good many organisms that affect the colon still to be discovered. There is evidence, for example, that *Aeromonas* species may have a role in a cause of infectious diarrhoea not only in children but also in adults (George et al 1985, Doman et al 1989), and even group A streptococci have been shown to cause a proctitis in prepubertal females (Figueroa-Colon et al 1984, Guss and Larsen 1984). Infectious colitis can certainly simulate inflammatory bowel disease clinically and endoscopically (Tedesco et al 1983).

Apart from enteroinvasive forms of *E. coli* there is a recent vast literature concerning the verotoxin-producing enterohaemorrhagic *E. coli* serotype 0157, which is now a well-established cause of colitis characterised by bleeding (Remis et al 1984, Pai et al 1984, Smith et al 1987, Levine 1987). This can be a severe illness associated with the haemolytic uraemic syndrome (Symonds 1988). The association of an acute colitis with the haemolytic uraemic syndrome had in fact been noted well before verotoxin-induced *E. coli*-associated colitis was described (Gore 1982, Dillard 1983). Rectal biopsy appearances can be remarkably similar to a first attack of mild ulcerative colitis (Figs. 17–1, 17–2). The lamina propria shows oedema and there is a mixed inflammatory infiltration of the lamina propria with focal aggregates of polymorphs around gland tubules, and there is polymorph margination of the capillaries, which also show dilatation. The inflammatory cells can be seen invading the epithelium, and an occasional rather poorly developed crypt abscess may be seen (Fig. 17–3). These tend not to be the cystic enlarged crypts filled with polymorphs as in ulcerative colitis, but are often small atrophic and thin-walled. A useful differentiating feature is that there tends to be less goblet cell depletion than would be the case with an equally inflamed mucosa in

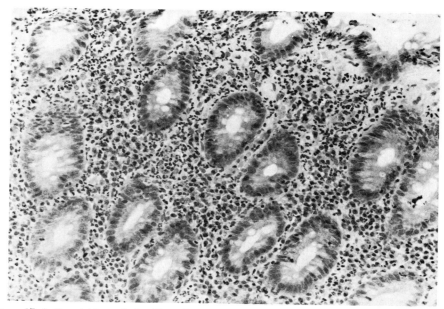

Figure 17–1. Rectal biopsy in bacillary dysentery. There is a diffuse inflammatory infiltration and slight goblet cell depletion (H & E × 70).

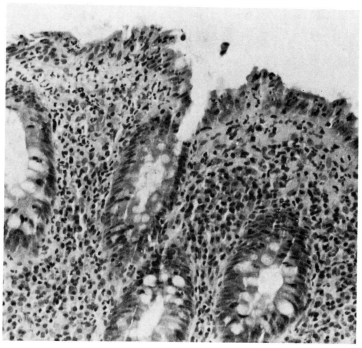

Figure 17–2. Detail of Figure 17–1 showing non-specific invasion of epithelium by inflammatory cells (H & E × 210).

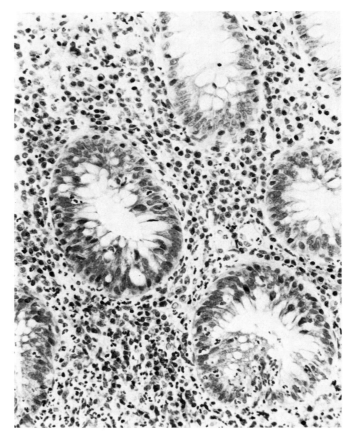

Figure 17–3. Colonic mucosa in infective colitis. The infiltrate is mixed with a noticeable neutrophil polymorph component and poorly developed crypt abscess (H & E × 400).

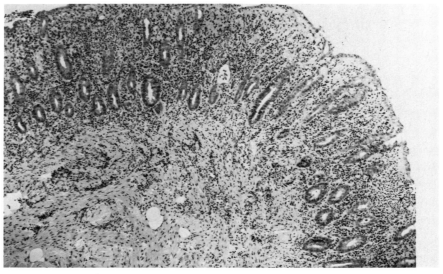

Figure 17–4. Colonic mucosa in infective colitis (H & E × 250).

ulcerative colitis, although when seen in the healing phase the glands do tend to be composed of immature, poorly developed goblet cells. Another histological feature is the shrinkage and beaded appearance of the mucosal gland profiles, which sometimes appear to melt away; this is unusual in other forms of colitis (Figs. 17–4 to 17–6). Kumar, Nostrant and Appelman (1982) stress that the absence of basal lamina propria plasmacytosis is a feature helpful in differentiating the lesion from ulcerative colitis. Some cases of *Shigella* colitis and more characteristically *Campylobacter* colitis and verotoxin-associated *E. coli* colitis have a distinctive haemorrhagic appearance, and bloody diarrhoea characterises the clinical picture (Chowdhury 1984, Van Spreeuwel et al 1985, Kelly et al 1987). The biopsy appearances reflect this in that the lesion is severe with superficial haemorrhagic necrosis of the mucosa, which is superimposed on a diffuse acute colitis. The paucity of crypt abscesses is also a feature (Figs. 17–7, 17–8).

It must be stressed that despite assertions that on the whole infective colitis and ulcerative colitis have a different histopathological appearance, individual cases can pose diagnostic problems (Price, Jewkes and Sanderson 1979, McKendrick, Geddes and Gearty 1982). Loss, Mangla and Pereira (1980) describe a case of *Campylobacter* colitis presenting as inflammatory bowel disease with segmental colonic ulceration and colonoscopic appearances suggesting Crohn's disease. A similar case with mucosal giant cells was described by Green et al (1984). Kalkay et al (1983) have reported the association of *Campylobacter* colitis and toxic megacolon. The enteroinvasive character of *Campylobacter* infection was confirmed by Van Spreeuwel et al (1985), who demonstrated intramucosal organisms, using specific antiserum in an immunohistochemical study. The increasingly common

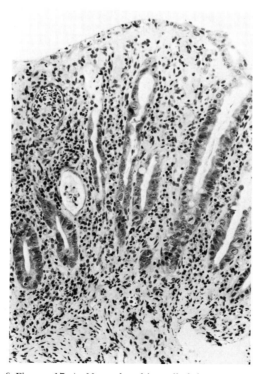

Figure 17–5. Detail of Figure 17–4. Note the thin-walled but not excessively enlarged crypts containing neutrophil polymorphs and the shrinkage and beaded appearance of the glands in longitudinal section (H & E × 350).

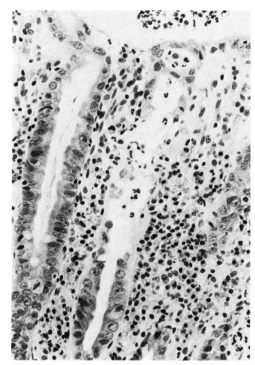

Figure 17–6. The glands in infective colitis sometimes appear to "melt away" (H & E × 450).

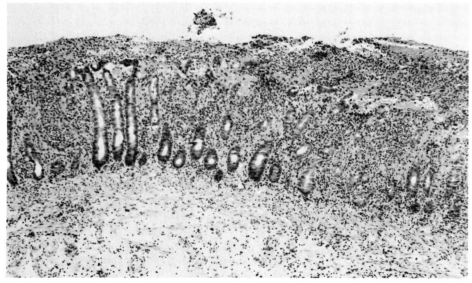

Figure 17–7. Rectal biopsy in *Campylobacter* colitis. It has a distinctive haemorrhagic quality and the mucosa is superficially necrosed (H & E × 50).

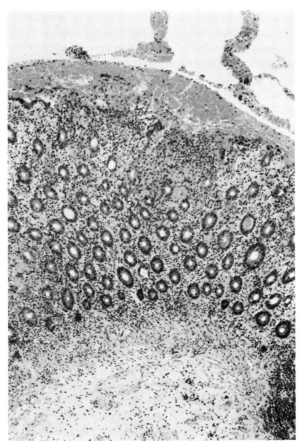

Figure 17–8. Detail of Figure 7–7. The surface exudate is largely composed of blood elements. Note the absence of crypt abscesses (H & E × 250).

practice of rectal biopsy in the investigation of patients with diarrhoea has resulted in recognition of surprisingly large numbers of cases with these histological features, which resolve completely but only some of which are proven to be due to a recognised pathogen.

The terminology of transient colitis syndrome (Mandal, Schofield and Morson 1982) has been applied to such cases in order to highlight the clinicopathological entity. Transient colitis equates to what has also been described as acute, self-limited colitis (Holdsworth 1984). Surawicz and Belic (1984) in a retrospective blind study of rectal biopsies claim the seven histological features are highly discriminative in favour of idiopathic inflammatory bowel disease and when present can virtually rule out acute, self-limited colitis as a diagnosis. The seven features are distorted crypt architecture, increase in both round cells and neutrophils in the lamina propria, a villous surface, epithelial granulomata, crypt atrophy, basal lymphoid aggregates and basally situated isolated giant cells. Similar results were found by Allison et al (1987), who also noted, however, a considerable degree of interobserver error. Thus basically the diagnosis of acute, self-limited colitis depends on the absence of the criteria usual for ulcerative colitis or Crohn's disease. However, although this schema may well be helpful in established idiopathic inflammatory bowel disease, in both first attack ulcerative colitis and

Crohn's disease, especially in ulcerative colitis, it is less useful. Anand et al (1986), for example, have shown that in *Shigella* dysentery it is extremely difficult to identify changes recognisably different from inflammatory bowel disease. It is pertinent, for example, that Nostrant, Kumar and Appelman (1987), in a study similar to but more detailed than that of Surawicz and Belic, found that in first attack ulcerative colitis the features most helpful in differentiating this from acute, self-limited colitis were crypt distortion and plasmacytosis of the lamina propria. Should any doubt remain as to a firm diagnosis, and there are undoubtedly cases in this category, follow-up studies are indicated (Lancet 1988). It is well to remember, however, that idiopathic inflammatory bowel disease can seemingly be triggered by an infective episode (Dronfield, Fletcher and Langman 1974, Taylor-Robinson et al 1989).

Yersinia enterocolitica also causes an ileocolitis with a characteristic histopathology in resection specimens (Gleason and Patterson 1982), but there are only occasional reports of the appearance of *Yersinia* colitis in endoscopic biopsies (Vantrappen et al 1977). Basically these were reported as non-specific microulcerations. Brown et al (1986), however, describe a case originally believed to be antibiotic associated on the basis of a patchy, mainly superficial, acute colitis. Rarely it seems *Yersinia enterocolitica* colitis can cause toxic dilatation (Stuart et al 1986).

Tuberculous Colitis

Tuberculosis of the colon is uncommon and likely to be mistaken for Crohn's disease or carcinoma (Knutson and Arosenius 1984) except in certain countries such as India where the disease is still prevalent. The primary form is not likely to be diagnosed in biopsy material, and the secondary form usually involves the terminal ileum, appendix and caecum. Colonoscopy and biopsy have been used to make the diagnosis of ileocaecal disease. Hiatt (1978) and Breiter and Hajjar (1981) also describe the biopsy diagnosis of the segmental colitic form, which radiologically and clinically closely mimics Crohn's disease. Indeed, in areas where tuberculosis is common, diagnosis of colonic tuberculosis in colonic biopsy is possible when the organisms are demonstrated, but differentiation from Crohn's disease is extremely difficult in their absence and in the absence of caseation (Figs. 17–9, 17–10). Fujisawa et al (1989) report three cases in which colonic tuberculosis was due to atypical mycobacteria.

Intestinal Spirochaetosis

Harland and Lee (1967) first described intestinal spirochaetosis as a non-treponemal infestation of the microvilli of rectal mucosal epithelial cells. The organism has been categorised as *Brachyspira aalborgi* by Hovind-Hougen et al (1982) but as a treponeme species by others (Cooper et al 1986). The spirochaetes are embedded at right angles to the microvilli, and in ordinary preparations the condition is suspected if a blue haze is recognised at the surface of the epithelial cells (Fig. 17–11). Electron microscopy (Fig. 17–12) will show the spirochaetes measuring 3 μm in length and 0.15 μm in diameter adherent to the epithelium lying parallel to and between the microvilli. There have been other similar observations (Toner, Carr and Wyburn 1971), and in the past it was generally agreed that the condition was without significance. However, this has been challenged (Gad et al 1977, Kaplan and Takeuchi 1979, Douglas and Crucioli

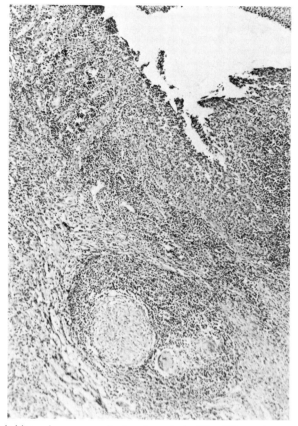

Figure 17–9. Colonic biopsy in proven colonic tuberculosis. The differentiation from Crohn's disease in ordinary H & E preparations may not be possible (H & E × 350).

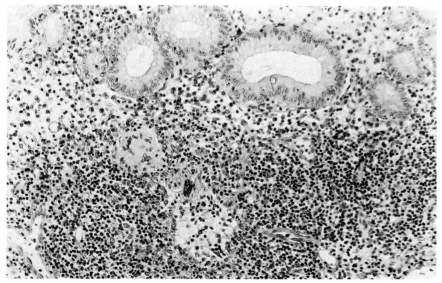

Figure 17–10. Colonic biopsy in proven tuberculosis. There is nothing diagnostic in the absence of caseation about these appearances (H & E × 450).

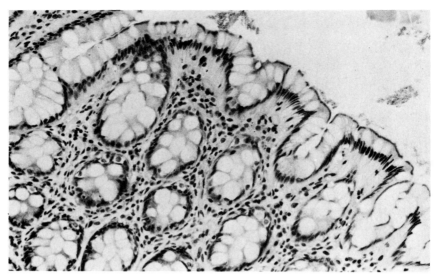

Figure 17–11. Rectal biopsy in intestinal spirochaetosis. The condition is evident as a haematoxophilic border to the surface epithelial cells. Note how it is interrupted by the goblet cells (H & E × 250).

1981, Crucioli and Bussuttil 1981, Gad 1983), and Rodgers et al (1986) describe blunting and destruction of the microvilli seen at electron microscopy. Apparently an association of heavy infestation and symptoms such as mucus discharge, diarrhoea and rectal bleeding may occur in the absence of any other pathology. The organism has also been reputedly transmitted by homosexual practices (Tompkins, Waugh and Cooke 1981). Antonakopoulos, Newman and Wilkinson (1982) and Gebbers et al (1987) describe cases in which the organism apparently invaded the epithelium. They may be seen in epithelial cells, macrophages and Schwann cells, but there was no colitis histologically. Nevertheless, eradication of

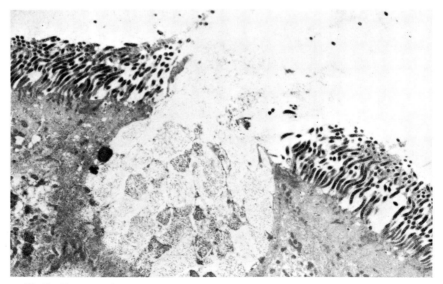

Figure 17–12. Electron micrograph of formalin-fixed tissue showing spirochaetes intimately woven with the surface microvilli. Note again their absence in relation to a discharging goblet cell (× 66,000).

the organism can result in alleviation of concomitant diarrhoea (Cooper et al 1986). It seems that the pathogenicity of the organism is still in doubt. However, in view of the increased reports of opportunistic infections in the acquired immunodeficiency syndrome associated with homosexuals, it is possible that in some circumstances the organism may prove to be pathogenic. In most instances, however (Nielsen et al 1983), the elimination of spirochaetes by antibiotic therapy does not affect symptoms, and when they are found in rectal biopsy of patients attending gastroenterology clinics, spirochaetes are of little significance.

VIRAL COLITIS

Although herpesvirus infection is a well-recognised complication in immune-depressed patients, it usually affects the upper gastrointestinal tract. Boulton, Slater and Hancock (1982), however, describe a case of extensive colonic ulceration in a patient with Hodgkin's disease treated with chemotherapy. Occasionally a painful proctitis occurs in otherwise normal people (White, Hanna and Stewart 1984). Colonic ulceration due to cytomegalovirus infection may also occur in renal transplant recipients (Foucar et al 1981) who are immunosuppressed, but it is also occasionally seen when the immune system is ostensibly normal (Bennett, Fine and Hanlon 1985). Berk et al (1985) have also drawn attention to the possible role of cytomegalovirus infection in the exacerbation of inflammatory bowel disease.

FUNGAL COLITIS

Histoplasmosis is endemic in many parts of North America, and the clinical features of involvement of the gastrointestinal tract are well documented (Boone and Allison 1969, Smith 1969). Primary infection is probably rare in the gut, and most gastrointestinal lesions result from haematogenous dissemination from the lungs. The pulmonary lesion, however, may be small, asymptomatic and difficult to identify even at autopsy. Sometimes colonic involvement is the presenting clinical feature (Kinder and Jourdan 1985, Lee et al 1985), and it sometimes mimics Crohn's disease (Alberti-Flor and Granda 1986). Rectal biopsy thus has a role to play in diagnosis in these cases and will show ulceration, inflammation and characteristic histiocytes in which the intracytoplasmic organisms can be identified. They can best be demonstrated in preparations especially designed to simplify the identification of fungi, but are usually obvious in a PAS stain, the capsule of the organism being strongly positive. Kirk, Lough and Warner (1971) have used rectal biopsy specimens in order to study the light and electron microscopic changes that occur in the organism during the course of treatment with amphotericin B. Other fungal infections rarely present as a colitis. Penna (1979) described a case due to *Paracoccidioides brasiliensis* that was confined to the colon and clinically resembled ulcerative colitis.

PARASITIC COLITIS

Amoebiasia

In countries where amoebiasis is non-endemic it is extremely important that pathogenic amoebae be considered as an aetiological agent in all cases of colitis. The histological diagnosis of amoebic colitis in biopsy specimens from ulcerated lesions usually causes little difficulty once the possibility is entertained, but unfortunately it is still far from a rare occurrence for the diagnosis to be made in surgical specimens. Pittman, El-Hashimi and Pittman (1973) describe eight cases that were "indistinguishable clinically and sigmoidoscopically from ulcerative or Crohn's colitis." This is further stressed by Pittman and Hennigar (1974), who studied nine cases and comment particularly on the histological similarities to ulcerative and Crohn's colitis in rectal biopsy specimens independent of whether or not amoebae were also seen. Inflammatory pseudopolyposis reverting to normal following specific therapy has also been reported in amoebic colitis (Berkowitz and Bernstein 1975).

The earliest mucosal lesion of amoebic colitis (Fig. 17–13) has been described in detail by Prathap and Gilman (1970). Before there is ulceration the thickness of the mucosa may appear irregular so that the surface outline is wavy. The irregularity is due to focal areas of goblet cell depletion with reversion to a cubical or simple epithelium, and these areas adjoin others showing increased thickness. This latter is due to a combination of hyperaemia, oedema and cellular infiltration. The infiltrate consists of plasma cells, lymphocytes and a few eosinophils, with polymorphs tending to marginate the capillary endothelium and the basement membrane of the gland tubules. Prathap and Gilman did not see crypt abscesses, but this author has seen some polymorphs not only invading the epithelium of glands and surface but also passing into the gland lumen in small numbers so that rather poorly developed crypt abscesses were indeed formed (Fig. 17–14).

When superficial ulceration appears it tends to occur on the surface between the gland in areas of mucus depletion. A superficial zone of necrosis and an overlying exudate of fibrin, red cells and mixed inflammatory cells are the first characteristic components. It is in the mucus overlying these zones that amoebae will frequently be identified (Figs. 17–15, 17–16). This fact should be impressed upon the person taking the biopsy so that in early cases overlying mucin is included in the biopsy, and in the laboratory every effort should be made to ensure that any such mucin or mucinous debris is processed and subsequently examined. Deeper ulcers giving rise to the typical flask-shaped lesions (Fig. 17–17) are always characterised by a zone of tissue necrosis at their base that is

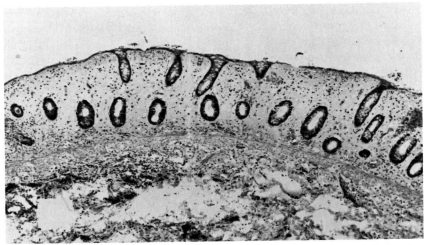

Figure 17–13. Amoebic colitis in the preulcerative stage. There is oedema of the lamina propria, dilatation of capillaries and a slight inflammatory infiltrate (H & E × 42).

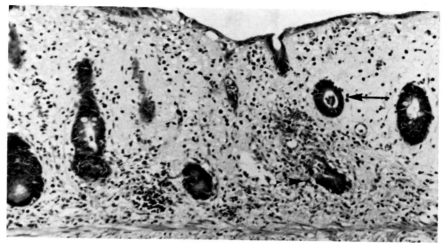

Figure 17–14. Detail of Figure 17–13 to show goblet cell depletion, degenerating crypt invaded by inflammatory cells (arrowhead) and poorly developed crypt abscess (arrow) (H & E × 105).

covered by exudate. The inflammatory exudate by this stage is marked, and the tissue reaction is complicated by secondary infection from faecal organisms. In the submucosa some of the blood vessels will show dilatation, others endothelial swelling, and sometimes there is occlusive thrombosis. At this stage amoebae will always be seen if searched for (Fig. 17–18), particularly in the zone of inflammatory infiltrate, and if found deeper in the tissues they will always appear within a halo of necrosis, sometimes surrounded by an artefactual retraction space.

The amoebae vary in size from 15 to 25 μm, have a single, small, spherical nucleus and in ordinary H & E-stained sections the cytoplasm is faintly granular in appearance and greyish-blue in colour. The vegetative forms of *Entamoeba histolytica* are difficult to differentiate from non-pathogenic amoebae in tissue sections and may be present coincidentally in other ulcerative bowel disorders. Important features in the diagnosis of amoebic colitis are the existence of engulfed red cells within the cytoplasm of the organisms and the presence of organisms actually within the tissues where they may rarely be seen within lymphatics or small vessels. They are more easily detected in iron haematoxylin and PAS preparations, the latter being widely advocated as the method of choice. However, macrophages that may have phagocytosed mucin are also positive, and as they are frequently found in ulcerative conditions they can cause some difficulty, especially since they may also contain engulfed red cells. The microscopist is helped to differentiate macrophages from amoebae by their smaller size, a nucleus that is oval or indented with a peripheral condensation of chromatin, and a nucleus that is relatively larger in relation to the overall size of the cell than is the case with a vegetative amoeba. Other PAS-positive cells, e.g., mast cells, the histiocytes of melanosis coli, cause no diagnostic difficulty.

A personal preference for a method that facilitates the easiest recognition of amoebae in tissues is the Goldner modification of Masson's trichrome. However, claims for easier detection by more specific methods such as the indirect immunofluorescent technique described by Parelkar, Stamm and Hill (1971) have been made, and in a comparison of six staining methods, including both direct and indirect fluorescent antibody procedures, Gilman et al (1980) showed that ethanol-fixed tissue stained by a fluorescent antibody or by PAS gave the best results.

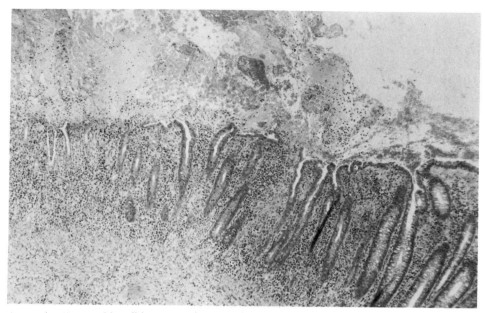

Figure 17–15. Amoebic colitis at an early stage of ulceration with surface exudate (H & E × 900).

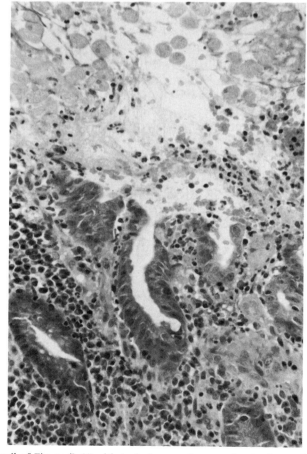

Figure 17–16. Detail of Figure 7–15 with typical vegetative amoebae in the surface exudate (H & E × 500).

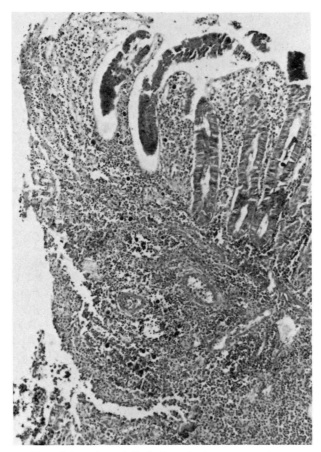

Figure 17–17. Amoebic colitis. Edge of flask-shaped ulcer. Vegetative amoebae visible as dark rounded bodies (PAS × 105).

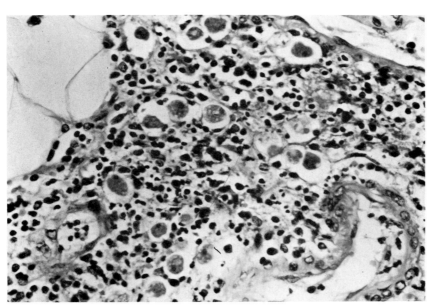

Figure 17–18. Detail of vegetative amoebae within the tissues. Note the small single round nucleus and vacuolated cytoplasm (H & E × 280).

It is only when amoebae are recognised with certainty in the biopsy specimen that a definite histological diagnosis can be made, but the additional morphological features already outlined are sufficiently characteristic to warrant suspicion of amoebiasis, even if the organisms are not seen. If, therefore, amoebiasis is suspected clinically or on biopsy appearances, a thorough stool examination for both vegetative and encysted organisms should follow; this sometimes proves positive in biopsy negative cases. It is only vegetative forms containing phagocytosed erythrocytes that indicate active disease as opposed to a carrier state.

Information from stool examination, biopsy and the results of serological tests (Sodeman and Dowda 1973) enable a diagnosis to be made in virtually all cases even when amoebiasis is complicating inflammatory bowel disease (Blumencranz et al 1983). The importance of early diagnosis and treatment cannot be overstressed, for not only is the likelihood of a liver abscess lessened but a particularly lethal complication is averted. It is not widely enough appreciated that amoebic colitis is a cause of fulminant toxic dilatation and bowel perforation (Kapur and Chopra 1978, Vajrabukka et al 1979, Wig, Talwar and Bushnurmath 1981). Furthermore amoebic colitis can seemingly precede the onset of otherwise typical idiopathic ulcerative colitis (Rampton, Salmon and Clark 1983). Sometimes amoebiasis takes on a protracted local form characterised by marked fibrosis and secondary infection. It is usually localised and commonly affects caecum or rectum (Ruiz-Moreno 1963). The lesion is often referred to as an amoebic granuloma or amoeboma and clinically behaves more like a mass lesion or neoplasm.

Balantidiasis

Balantidium coli is a ciliate and an intestinal commensal of the pig, monkey and rat that may infest man when the encysted form is ingested. In a small number of people harbouring the organism it gives rise to severe diarrhoea, haemorrhage and sometimes perforation. The common site of involvement is the right half of the colon and caecum, but the rectum and sigmoid are also frequently involved. Histological features are ulceration, with coagulative necrosis of ulcer base and margin. Adjacent tissues are oedematous and infiltrated by a mainly chronic inflammatory infiltrate. The characteristic vegetative parasites are oval in shape (Fig. 17–19), 50 to 100 μm long and 40 to 70 μm wide, with a large, kidney-shaped macronucleus and a smaller, round micronucleus situated at the hilum. The surface is covered with cilia and the cytoplasm usually contains vacuoles and granules. They are easily identified because of their size and, although they may be seen within venules and lymph nodes, liver involvement does not occur. The largest series described is probably that reported by Arean and Koppisch (1956), who describe the pathology in detail. Although in most descriptions the organism is in surgical or autopsy tissue, its characteristic morphology would obviously lend itself to diagnosis in biopsy material. This is beautifully illustrated in the report of two cases by Castro, Vazquez-Iglesias and Arnal-Monreal (1983) (Figs. 17–20 to 17–22).

Schistosomiasis

In the intestinal form of the disease it is the *Schistosoma mansoni* and *Schistosoma japonicum* that are responsible, and only heavy infestation produces the classic picture. The distal part of the intestine, the colon and rectum are the sites of

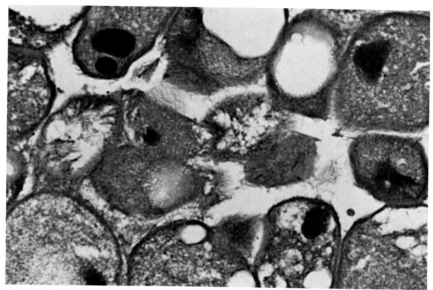

Figure 17–19. *Balantidium coli.* Peripheral cilia can just be discerned (H & E × 420).

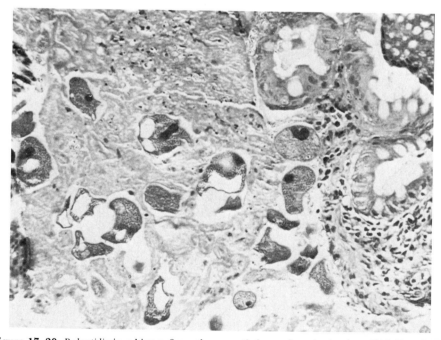

Figure 17–20. *Balantidia* in a biopsy from the necrotic base of a colonic ulcer (H & E × 250).

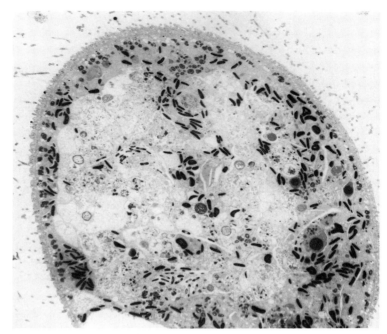

Figure 17–21. Electron micrograph of *Balantidium coli* showing engulfed colonic bacteria (× 1600).

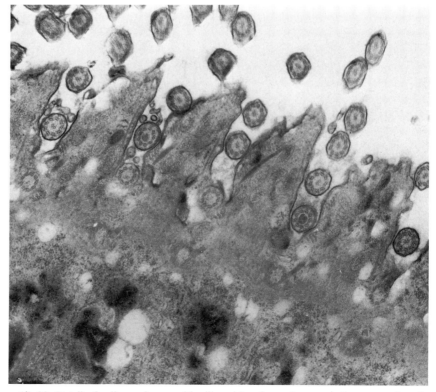

Figure 17–22. Detail of cell membrane with cilia arising from the grooved outer surface (× 6000). (Figures 17–20, 17–21 and 17–22 by courtesy of Dr. Francisco Arnal.)

severest involvement. The earliest tissue reaction (Fig. 17–23 A,B) around the newly laid eggs consists of plasma cells, lymphocytes and eosinophils, but later the characteristic inflammatory response involves histiocytes. Most ova produce a histiocytic granulomatous reaction (Fig. 17–24), which subsequently undergoes a concentric fibrosis. Outside the histiocytic granuloma, which may also form giant cells, the zone of mixed inflammatory cells occurs and later this has a conspicuous eosinophil component. Sometimes, especially in the oriental form of the disease, the eosinophil reaction is very pronounced and may delay the histiocytic response. Frequently in this form of reaction a zone of fibrinoid material is also deposited about the eggs. As the tissue reactions are developing, the shell dissolves slowly or becomes calcified and the embryo dies. The eggs of *Schistosoma mansoni* are oval and about 150 μm long and 50 μm wide, and they have a well-developed lateral

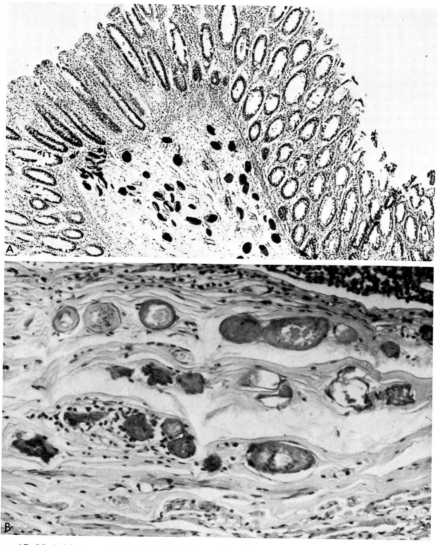

Figure 17–23. Schistosomiasis. **A,** Newly laid eggs in submucosa (H & E × 64). **B,** The earliest signs of tissue reaction to them (H & E × 375).

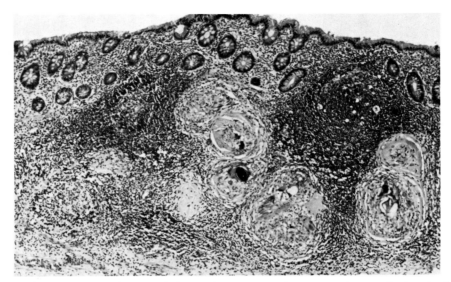

Figure 17–24. Schistosomiasis. Typical granulomatous reaction to eggs that are dead and calcified (H & E × 35).

spine. The eggs of *Schistosoma japonicum* are smaller and less oval, about 85 μm long and 60 μm wide with a subterminal hooklet, but this is often inconspicuous.

In the later stages of the disease, the granulomatous inflammatory fibrosis results in cicatrisation of the bowel wall, which is reflected in the biopsy tissues. Inflammatory pseudopolyps also occur, especially in *Schistosoma mansoni* infestations. Epithelial and glandular deformity, due to mucosal ulceration and subsequent healing, may also be seen. Gambescia et al (1976) review the colonic manifestations in schistosomiasis in greater detail. According to Nebel et al (1974) there is no hard evidence for an association between schistosomal polyposis and carcinoma of the colon. However, Ming-Chi et al (1965) describe 90 cases of large intestinal adenocarcinoma as a complication of schistosomiasis caused by *S. japonicum*. From the description of the lesions the pathogenesis may well be similar to that responsible for the malignancy occurring in ulcerative colitis in that it arises through a process of progressive dysplasia.

Other helminthic infestation is rarely a cause of mucosal pathology in colon and rectum. Leoutsakos, Agnadi and Kolisiatis (1977) describe a case and review the literature of colonic involvement in infestation with *Oesophagastomium brumpti*. The veins of the submucosa may contain adult worms, and mucosa and deeper tissues reveal an inflammatory and giant cell granulomatous reaction that would be revealed in rectal biopsy. No reports of a diagnosis being reached in biopsy tissues, however, are currently available. The same is true of the occasional case of strongyloidiasis hyperinfection, which causes a chronic colitis (Berry et al 1983). The subject of *Cryptosporidium* colitis in patients with acquired immunodeficiency syndrome is referred to in detail later. The question of whether cryptosporidiosis is a cause of chronic diarrhoea in normal children or adults, especially in undeveloped countries, is disputed. Some believe it is an important pathogen accounting for a significant proportion of cases of infective diarrhoea (Sallon et al 1988), but others find no firm evidence for this either in developed (Biggs et al 1987, Marshall et al 1987) or undeveloped countries (Mathan et al 1985). It seems highly probable that in common with many other opportunistic infective agents, on occasion it can cause a colitis even in normal people.

IRRADIATION COLITIS

Irradiation-induced lesions of the intestine are becoming less frequently encountered as the techniques of radiotherapy become increasingly sophisticated. The mucosa of the gastrointestinal tract has a susceptibility to irradiation injury comparable to that of lymphoid tissue and the bone marrow. The colon is less susceptible than the stomach and much less so than the small intestine, but it is the one area of the whole gastrointestinal tract that has been most frequently exposed. This is because of the widespread use of radiotherapy in the treatment of malignant disease of the female genital tract.

The early changes are now rarely seen; they come on within a few hours of exposure. There is prompt cessation of mitotic activity, and there may be an initial stage of hypersecretion of mucin, but soon the epithelial cells begin to show signs of degeneration, become swollen with bizarre, irregular nuclei and slough into the lumen with the formation of thin-walled crypt abscesses due to a secondary, sparse, acute inflammatory response (Figs. 17–25, 17–26). There is oedema and hyperaemia of the mucosa and submucosa and, in more severe exposure, hyaline degeneration and necrosis of the collagen. In severe cases ulcers may form, but gradually the normal crypt regenerative capacity is regained and after an interval of weeks or months recovery will occur. Its completeness depends on the initial

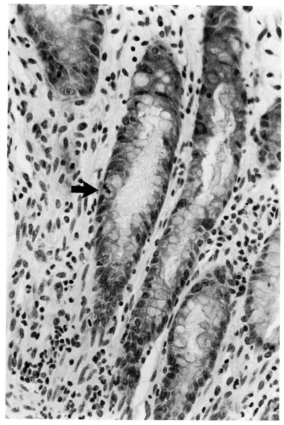

Figure 17–25. Earliest stage of irradiation damage to the colonic mucosa. There is swelling and atypia of epithelial cell nuclei and early cytoplasmic degeneration and sloughing, but a mitotic figure is evident (arrow) (H & E × 500).

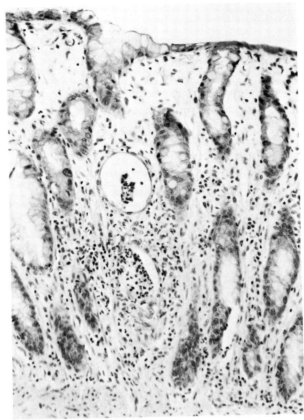

Figure 17–26. Early stage of irradiation injury of the colon. There is degeneration of some crypts that contain degenerate epithelial cells and a few polymorphs. Note the bizarre nuclear profiles and paucity of mitoses (H & E × 350).

injury, but a residuum of distortion or irregularity of the gland pattern is usual (Figs. 17–27, 17–28). Residual hyaline fibrosis of the mucosa and submucosa, and hyaline thickening of blood vessels will also persist.

Chronic irradiation injuries characterised macroscopically by ulceration and fibrosis may occur from six months to several years after the original exposure. The ulcer bed, like radiation ulcers elsewhere, is formed of poorly vascularised connective tissue that has a peculiar hyalinised appearance. Depending on the depth of ulceration it involves the mucosa, submucosa muscularis and even the serosa, so that stricture, either actual or functional, results. There is a superimposed non-specific inflammatory infiltrate and the ulcers tend not to heal. A characteristic of the granulation tissue is the bizarre nature of the fibroblast nuclei, which are large and often appear foamy with marginal polypoidal excrescences. New thin-walled and ectatic blood vessels are a feature, but the arterioles and small arteries also exhibit thickening and hyalinisation of their walls and a decrease in lumen size. Fibrin thrombi and fibrinoid necrosis of the walls of vessels are also seen, and some believe they are the main cause of the more chronic pathological changes (Hasleton, Carr and Schofield 1985, Haboubi, Schofield and Rowland 1988) and could account for the progressive nature of the disease (Galland and Spencer 1985, Yeoh and Horowitz 1987). Changes such as those described in the connective tissue and blood vessels of the submucosa may occur in areas where the mucosa is intact, but it will usually show some residual deformity of pattern.

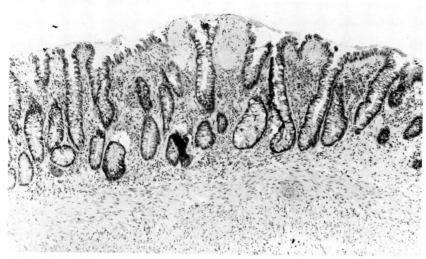

Figure 17–27. Rectal biopsy for bleeding one year after irradiation to carcinoma of the cervix. The mucosa shows some architectural distortion and there is a hyalinisation of the lamina propria. Centrally there is a defect in the epithelium (H & E × 80).

The pathology of irradiation damage to the intestine has been detailed in great depth by Friedman (1942) and Berthrong and Fajardo (1981). The latter authors also describe an unusual late hyperplastic response of the mucosa together with an appearance simulating colitis cystica profunda. There is some evidence that radiation-induced colonic mucosal damage may predispose to the development of adenocarcinoma (Castro, Rosen and Quan 1973), and Shamsuddin and Elias (1981) have described the appearance of dysplasia and carcinoma in situ in rectal biopsy tissue of flat non-polypoidal mucosa similar to that seen in ulcerative colitis. This observation clearly will require confirmation.

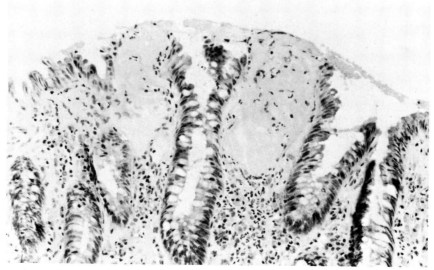

Figure 17–28. Detail of Figure 17–27. Polymorphs are included in the cellular infiltrate, but the principal feature is ectatic change in the superficial capillaries. The epithelium of the tubules shows variation in nuclear size and staining (H & E × 450).

COLLAGENOUS COLITIS

Lindstrom (1976) describes the first case of this condition in a patient with chronic watery diarrhoea and a thick collagenous deposit under the surface epithelium of the colorectal mucosa. It was proposed that the collagen layer prevented normal reabsorption of water and electrolytes, thus giving rise to the symptoms. A diagnosis of collagenous colitis can be made when the collagen layer measures more than 15 μm and it may reach as much as 60–70 μm. When this is seen in association with an increase in mixed inflammatory cell infiltration of the lamina propria and minor degenerative changes and flattening of the superficial epithelium, there can be no doubt that it is a distinct histological entity (Figs. 17–29A,B, 17–30A,B, 17–31, 17–32). Occasionally one sees Paneth cell metaplasia in the base of the colonic tubules. Flejou et al (1984) have noted an increase in lamina propria mast cells in their cases, but this was a subjective observation. In some cases intraepithelial lymphocytes are conspicuous. Not only is the collagen table abnormally thick, but it contains an increased number of fibroblasts, which sometimes are plump and active and sometimes rather more spindle shaped. It is possible that the activity of the fibroblasts and collagen production is phasic, which would account for the clinical picture of variation in the severity of symptoms (Palmer et al 1986).

Electron microscope observations (Figs. 17–33 to 17–35) have confirmed that basal lamina of the epithelium is in fact normal and the lesion is due to a collagen deposition under the epithelium. The collagen consists of a mixture of types I and III. The author's experience of more than 30 personal cases and observations on stepwise colonoscopic biopsies of the whole colon has revealed in addition to the features described in other reports (Bogomoletz et al 1980, Nielsen, Vetner and Harslof 1980, Teglbjaerg and Thaysen 1982, Grouls, Vogle and Sorger 1982, Bamford et al 1982, Galian et al 1982, Pieterse, Hecker and Rowland 1982, Farah et al 1985, Foerster and Fausa 1985, Coverlizza et al 1986, Danzi, McDonald and King 1988) that the lesion was not uniform throughout the colon. It was more marked in some areas than in others, the rectum often being less severely affected, and in places collagen occupied a position deeper in the lamina propria (Fig. 17–36). The variability in the collagen band with site has been confirmed in a study of 17 patients by Wang et al (1987). A further observation corroborated by Teglbjaerg, Thaysen and Jensen (1984) and Kingham et al (1986) is the development of the collagen band in sequential biopsies being preceded by an inflammatory phase (see microscopic colitis). The uneven distribution of collagen in some cases could cause problems in the interpretation of reversibility of the lesion in sequential biopsies. Evidence for this has been claimed by Bamford et al (1982), Pieterse, Hecker and Rowland (1982), Eaves et al (1983), Debongnie et al (1984), Morgensen, Olsen and Gudmand-Hoyer (1984), Fausa, Foerster and Hovig (1985). Most authors, however, believe the condition to be progressive and permanent (Kingham et al 1986). The collagen layer may be responsible for interference with function of the surface cells and thus impede absorption.

However, there is evidence that the diarrhoea is mediated by prostaglandins and is secretory in nature (Rask-Madsen et al 1983, Giardiello et al 1987). The normal colonic crypt of Lieberkühn is surrounded by a mesenchymal sheath that is a specialised part of the lamina propria. It consists of fibroblasts applied to the epithelium and collagen fibres oriented circumferentially to the crypt. Pascal, Kaye and Lane (1968) have demonstrated a steady-state renewal of the pericryptal fibroblasts and migration to the upper parts of the crypt in synchronisation with the epithelial migration. The fibroblast stem cells, like the epithelial cells, occupy

Text continued on page 370

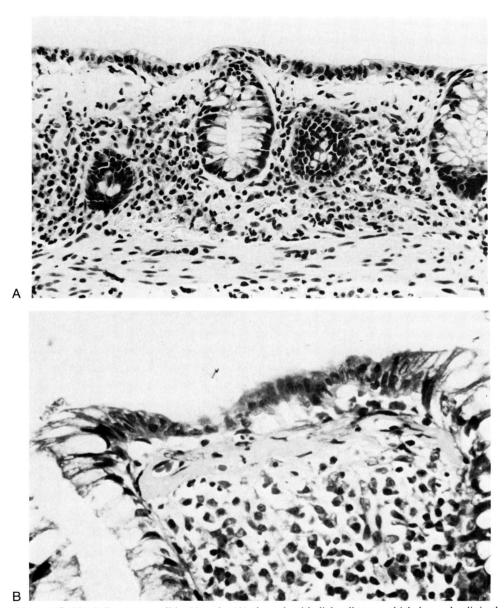

Figure 17–29. Collagenous colitis. Note in **(A)** the subepithelial collagen, which has a hyalinised appearance. In **(B)** fibroblast nuclei are thin and elongated. Note the density of inflammatory cells and the degenerative changes in the intercryptal superficial epithelial cells (trichrome, A × 250, B × 500).

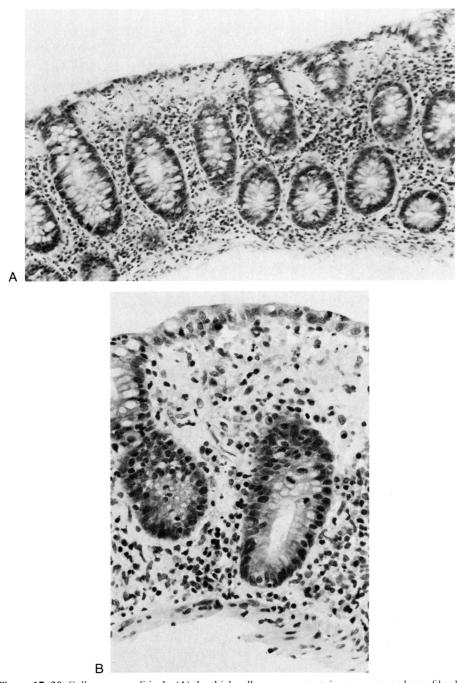

Figure 17–30. Collagenous colitis. In **(A)** the thick collagen zone contains numerous plump fibroblasts as well as inflammatory cells and nuclear debris detailed in **(B)** (H & E, A × 250, B × 500).

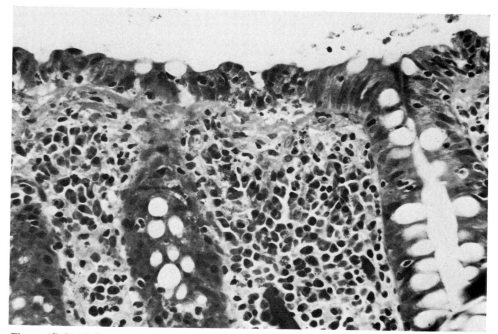

Figure 17–31. Collagenous colitis. In this case the inflammatory infiltration of tubules and epithelium is more marked and there are more severe degenerative changes of both crypt and surface epithelium (H & E × 500).

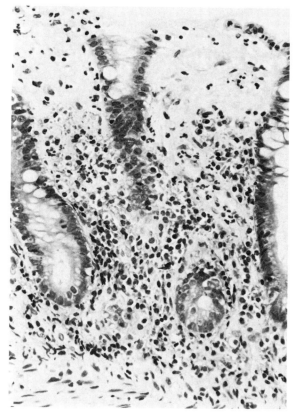

Figure 17–32. Collagenous colitis with a more pronounced neutrophil polymorph component in the lamina propria and in the collagen layer (H & E × 400).

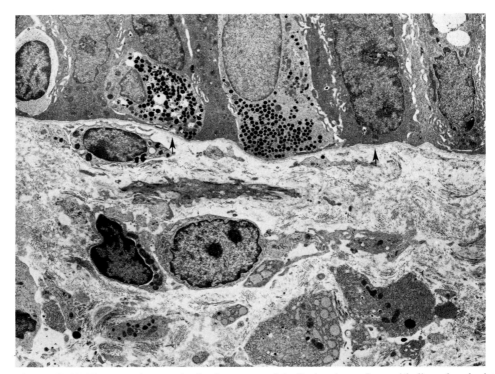

Figure 17–33. Electron micrograph of collagenous colitis. Under the surface epithelium that depicts two endocrine cells, the basal lamina (arrow) is normal. The subepithelial zone is occupied by typical collagen surrounding portions of neutrophils, plasma cells and a central active fibroblast (× 6637).

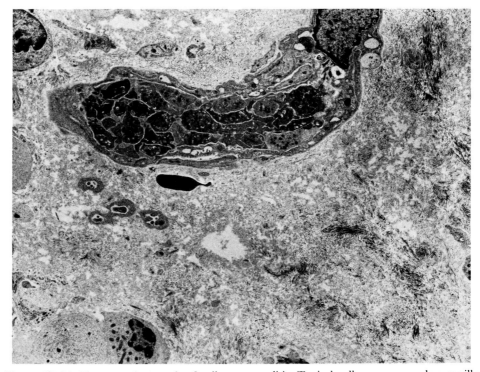

Figure 17–34. Electron micrograph of collagenous colitis. Typical collagen surrounds a capillary that is occluded by platelet thrombus and is indicative of an inflammatory reaction (× 6637).

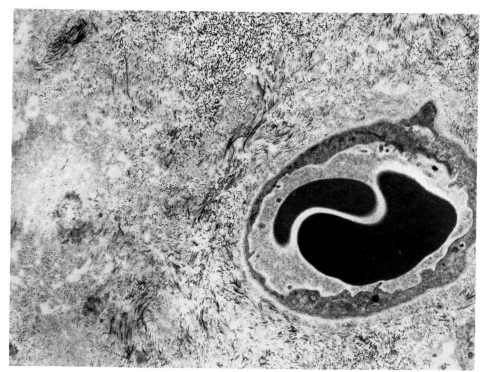

Figure 17–35. Collagenous colitis. A higher magnification of the dense collagen zone which in this field surrounds a capillary (× 15,525).

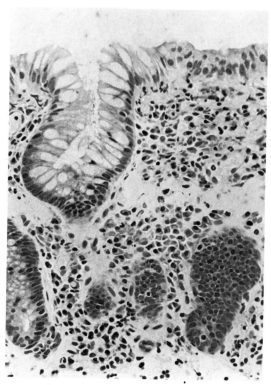

Figure 17–36. Collagenous colitis. In this biopsy the collagen layer occurs in the mid-zone of the lamina propria, but this is unusual (H & E × 400).

the lower one third of the crypt. The collagen table immediately under the surface epithelium is relatively thicker than elsewhere, and overall the evidence suggests a functional maturation of the pericryptal fibroblast layer as it ascends the crypt. The pericryptal fibroblasts and the epithelium thus act as a unit that maintains the structure and presumably also the function of the crypt. Minor changes in the kinetics involved might easily result in a thicker than normal collagen plate, and we have seen that this can occur in the small intestine in gluten-sensitive enteropathy. Why it should occur in either condition is not clear. It does not seem to be a result of longstanding inflammation, since it does not seem to occur in this site in chronic ulcerative colitis. However, Balazs et al (1988) did find similarities between collagenous and ulcerative colitis and in both describe an enhanced fibre-forming activity and proliferation of myofibroblasts.

In recent large series (Steadman et al 1987, Jessurun et al 1987), it has become apparent that not only is this condition much more common in middle aged to elderly females but it has a predilection to occur in association with thyroid and rheumatoid joint disease and autoimmune disease of other types. Thus it has been postulated that collagenous colitis itself may be an autoimmune disease. It has been reported, probably coincidentally, in association with colonic adenocarcinoma (Gardiner et al 1984) and Crohn's disease (Chandratre et al 1987). Collagenous colitis has also been reported in association with crypt hyperplastic villous atrophy in two patients, one of whom responded by a return to normal on a gluten-free diet (Hamilton et al 1986). These cases appear to be different from that described by Eckstein, Dowsett and Riley (1988) in which in addition to partial villous atrophy the small bowel also showed a thick subepithelial collagen band, but was thought not to be gluten related.

MICROSCOPIC COLITIS

Read et al (1980) reported minor histological changes in the colonic biopsies of 8 patients out of 27 investigated for intractable watery diarrhoea. The full significance of this was not at that time apparent, but Kingham et al (1982) coined the term microscopic colitis for the same condition, which is characterised by a mild total colitis, large-volume watery diarrhoea and with normal endoscopic and radiological appearances. Four of their six patients were female and all were middle aged. The condition was thought to be quite distinct from ulcerative colitis and Crohn's disease and in particular distinct from the so-called minimal change colitis described by Elliott et al (1982) in which normal sigmoidoscopy and barium enema are associated with histological evidence of overt Crohn's disease in the proximal large bowel, which less commonly proves to be due to ulcerative colitis. Bo-Linn et al (1985) put the existence of microscopic colitis on a firmer basis, and later the same group (Jessurun et al 1986) examined the evidence that microscopic colitis was the forerunner of collagenous colitis. Microscopic colitis affects the whole colon. It is, however, always characterised by a diffuse increase in lymphocytes and plasma cells in the lamina propria (Fig. 17–37). Eosinophils are usually prominent and neutrophils variable in number but are not uncommonly seen invading the epithelium of tubules, usually in their upper parts. The surface epithelium tends to be flatter than normal and shows degenerative changes accompanied by an increase in apoptotic bodies. There may also be an impressive increase in intraepithelial lymphocytes throughout the tubules, but this tends to occur later in the disease process (Figs. 17–38, 17–39). There is no architectural

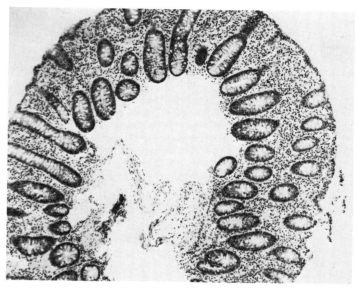

Figure 17–37. Microscopic colitis. A generalised increase in inflammatory cells of the lamina propria is obvious. Note the preservation of the overall mucosal architecture (H & E × 75).

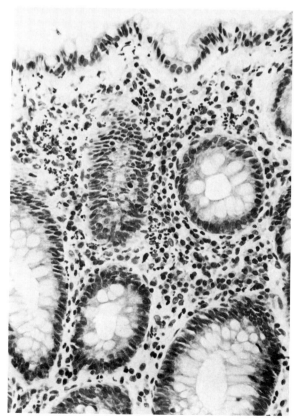

Figure 17–38. Microscopic colitis. In this case the infiltrate has a very prominent neutrophil polymorph infiltrate (H & E × 450).

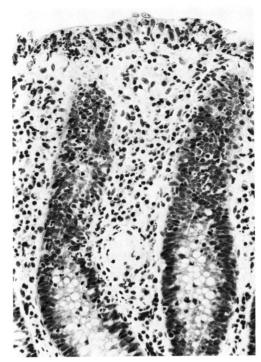

Figure 17–39. Microscopic colitis. In this case intraepithelial lymphocytes are unusually prominent (H & E × 450).

deformity or gross glandular inflammatory destruction such as is seen in ulcerative colitis, Crohn's or the various forms of infective or ischaemic colitis. In some cases a thin collagen band develops under the epithelium (Fig. 17–40), and there is a tendency for the inflammatory infiltrate to decrease in density, although an increased plasma cell and lymphocyte infiltrate persists. The picture is thus arguably identical with some cases of collagenous colitis. Lazenby et al (1989), however, feel that despite the striking similarities between microscopic colitis and collagenous colitis each has distinctive biopsy appearances. These authors were particularly struck with the intraepithelial lymphocyte component in microscopic colitis and have proposed that it be referred to as "lymphocytic colitis." The advantages of this new designation at a time when the relationship between microscopic colitis and collagenous colitis is far from clear are doubtful. As in coeliac disease and other lesions of the mucosa in other parts of the gastrointestinal tract, the intraepithelial lymphocytes are probably no more than a manifestation of an underlying pathogenetic mechanism.

The cause of microscopic/collagenous colitis is not known, but it is of interest that a similar collagenisation is also seen under the bronchial epithelium in asthma. Contrary to what has long been held, as in collagenous colitis, there is no abnormal thickening of the basement membrane (Roche et al 1989). One might thus postulate that the disease has an allergic basis, which would be in keeping with the prominent eosinophil component seen in the lamina propria. Rampton and Baithun (1987) describe a case of microscopic colitis that responded to cholestyramine therapy and postulated that at least some of these cases are due to bile salt malabsorption.

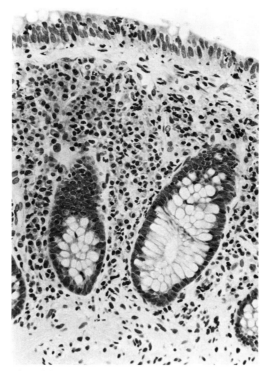

Figure 17–40. Microscopic colitis. A case in which a thin collagen band is present under the surface epithelium (H & E × 450).

COLITIS DUE TO FAECAL DIVERSION

Glotzer, Glick and Goldman (1981) drew attention to the mild focal epithelial degenerative changes and acute and chronic inflammatory infiltration, including crypt abscesses, that may follow diversion of the faecal stream by ileostomy or colostomy. It disappears when continuity is restored and is normally important only because it may be misinterpreted. On occasion, however, it can be severe enough to cause symptoms such as rectal bleeding (Bosshardt and Abel 1984, Ona and Boger 1985) when the inflammation is more severe and associated with ulceration. The ulceration may be aphthoid and mimic Crohn's disease (Lusk, Reichen and Levine 1984), which, of course, has significant implications when diversion of the faecal stream is performed in patients with this disease (Korelitz et al 1984). Diversion colitis is easily mistaken for further manifestations of Crohn's disease in these circumstances. Thorough evaluation of the bypassed colonic mucosa is thus essential. Murray et al (1987) have described not only inflammation and erosions but also occasional crypt abscesses, mucin granulomas and lymphoid hyperplasia in this condition. It has been proposed that faeces contain an essential trophic factor in the form of short chain fatty acids produced by the anaerobic faecal flora (Korelitz et al 1984, Lancet 1989). Thus it is of interest that Harig et al (1989) showed that local administration of these fatty acids to the diverted segment caused the inflammation to disappear.

COLITIS IN DIVERTICULAR DISEASE

Mucosal biopsy is usually unrewarding in the diagnosis of diverticular disease even if diverticulitis is present, although occasionally a pattern seen is normal mucosa with luminal pus cells. Cawthorn, Gibbs and Marks (1983) describe a segmental inflammation with histological features similar to the changes in solitary rectal ulcer in three patients with diverticular disease. This is probably due to recurrent prolapse of the mucosa lying between diverticulae as a result of the abnormal colonic muscular dynamics. It seems, however, that the more usual form of segmental colitis seen in association with diverticular disease is rather non-specific and to see fibromuscular obliteration of the lamina propria is unusual (Figs. 17–41 to 17–43). Generally biopsies show moderate acute and chronic inflammation with occasional crypt abscesses and some goblet cell depletion (Sladen and Filipe 1984).

COLITIS IN INFANTS

Gastrointestinal intolerance to cow's milk protein and soy protein is a well-established cause of enterocolitis in infants under the age of two or three years (Gryboski 1967). In this classic study sigmoidoscopic evidence of colitis disappeared when cow's milk was removed from the diet. There is more recent evidence for small-bowel injury, and the syndrome should properly be regarded as an enterocolitis. Lake, Whitington and Hamilton (1982) also describe an acute and chronic inflammation with an associated eosinophil infiltration in rectal biopsies from babies who developed rectal bleeding in the first month of life. A change from breast milk to soy protein or hydrolysed casein-based milk formula resulted in immediate remission. The problem of proctocolitis in babies and its relationship to milk or other protein intolerance was discussed in a leading article in the Lancet (1983), and since that time it has become plain that food allergy is a major cause of infantile colitis. Not only do colonic biopsies show a distinctive eosinophil infiltration and surface erosion, but there are numerous IgE-containing plasma cells in the lamina propria. Other allergic phenomena, increased serum IgE and blood eosinophilia are also commonly present (Jenkins et al 1984, Goldman and Proujansky 1986, Powell 1986). Proctocolitis and bloody stools in infants have many causes, and many can be excluded by colonic biopsy. Protein-induced colitis can be suspected by the colonoscopic aphthoid ulceration and biopsy appearances and then confirmed by manipulation of the diet. Food allergy would seem to be the commonest cause of colitis in this age group (Berezin et al 1989).

NEUTROPENIC COLITIS

Neutropenic colitis describes a distinctive caecal or right-sided colonic necrosis due to clostridial infection in association with agranulocytosis. It is also sometimes referred to as the ileocaecal syndrome or typhlitis, when only the caecum is involved. It is usually encountered in patients with acute leukaemia, lymphoma or myeloma, but also in association with neutropenia due to aplastic anaemia (Mulholland and Delaney 1983). The diagnosis is seldom made prior to death, and no case even in the largest series reported hitherto has been diagnosed on biopsy (Mower, Hawkins and Nelson 1986). Although *Clostridium septicum* is the usual organism implicated, other clostridial species are sometimes involved (Lancet 1987).

COLITIS DUE TO DRUGS OR CHEMICAL AGENTS

It is estimated that some 10 per cent of newly diagnosed colitis may be due to the ingestion of non-steroidal anti-inflammatory drugs (NSAID). Rectal biopsies

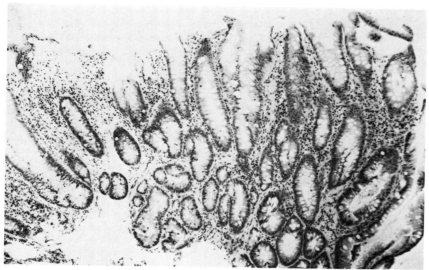

Figure 17–41. Colitis in diverticular disease. An uneven inflammation is associated with considerable architectural distortion of the glands (H & E × 150).

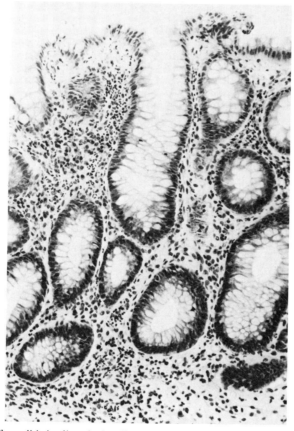

Figure 17–42. The colitis in diverticular disease has a patchy acute element (H & E × 450).

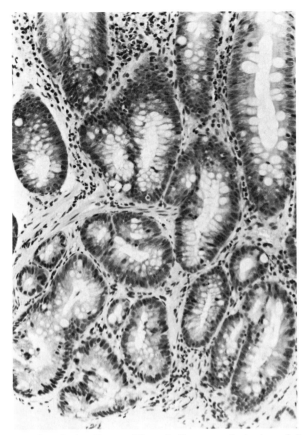

Figure 17–43. Colitis in diverticular disease. There is fibromuscularisation of the lamina propria as well as architectural distortion (H & E × 450).

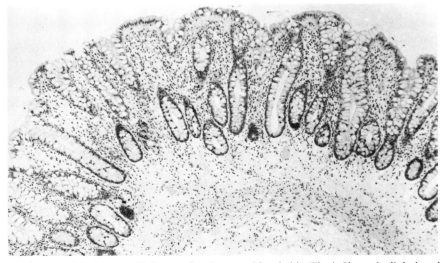

Figure 17–44. Colitis due to gold therapy for rheumatoid arthritis. The infiltrate is slight but definite and tends to involve the submucosa (H & E × 120).

in such patients generally show mild non-specific colitis with a neutrophil polymorph component in the inflammatory infiltrate; there may be occasional crypt
abscesses, but ulceration is unusual. The glandular pattern is usually preserved.
However, the precise relationship of ingestion of NSAID and colitis requires
further clarification because it is also recognised that these potent drugs may
activate quiescent inflammatory bowel disease. The subject is reviewed in two
recent publications (Kaufmann and Taubin 1987, Tanner and Raghunath 1988).

A colitis similar to Crohn's disease is described in patients taking oral contraceptives (Rhodes et al 1984), and a proctitis similar to ulcerative colitis is attributed
to salicylates (Pearson et al 1983). Innes et al (1988) report the onset of a total
severe colitis in a patient receiving cyclosporin, and toxic megacolon with severe
segmental colitis was attributed to methotrexate therapy by Atherton, Leib and
Kaye (1984). Drug-induced colitis has also been attributed to the therapeutic use
of methyldopa (Graham, Gallagher and Jones 1981) and gold (Martin et al 1981).
In the author's experience of the latter in patients treated for rheumatoid arthritis,
the colitis is mild, non-ulcerative and histologically non-specific except that eosinophilia of the lamina propria and submucosa is often a prominent feature (Figs.
17–44, 17–45).

Colitis varying from mild to severe with gangrenous change has been associated
with the use of various enemas, e.g., soap (Orchard and Lawson 1986), phosphate
(Sweeney et al 1986) and sorbitol (Lillemoe et al 1987), and has followed the

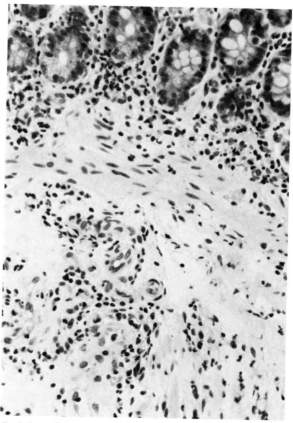

Figure 17–45. Detail of the colitis in Figure 17–44. The infiltrate is rich in eosinophils, which often
appear as bilobed polymorphonuclear cells (H & E × 500).

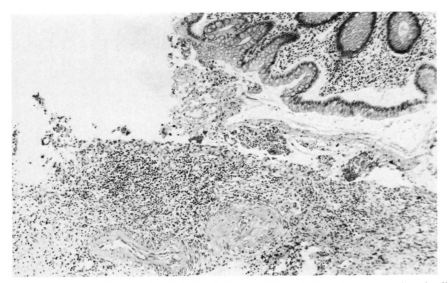

Figure 17–46. Biopsy of ulcer edge in Behçet's disease. The neighbouring mucosa is only slightly abnormal in that it is chronically inflamed (H & E × 400).

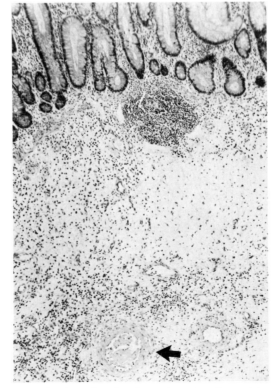

Figure 17–47. Behçet's colonic ulceration showing a thrombosed vessel (arrow) and oedema of the submucosa (H & E × 350).

inadvertent instillation of alcohol (Herrerias et al 1983) or cleaning solutions used for disinfective endoscopy (Jonas et al 1988). Strangely enough, sulfasalazine, the very drug used in the treatment of inflammatory bowel disease, has been incriminated as a cause of precipitating attacks of ulcerative colitis (Ruppin and Domschke 1984). Fishel et al (1985) report an unusual case of colitis associated with the use of cocaine. It had the pathological features of pseudomembranous colitis and was probably of ischaemic origin. An unusual and rare form of distal colitis was reported by Keefe and Girard (1985) in a patient thought to have a self-inflicted abrasive colonic injury secondary to daily consumption of quantities of peanuts while they were still in their indigestible shells.

THE COLITIS OF BEHÇET'S SYNDROME

This colitis is characterised by ulceration of the bowel wall, which may mimic Crohn's disease macroscopically. Usually the ulcers are more regular in outline and the surrounding mucosa is normal. The underlying pathology probably has an ischaemic basis, and a vasculitis is implicated. This takes the form in the bowel of a lymphoid venulitis or arteritis, occasionally with thrombosis (Figs. 17–46 to 17–48) (Katoh et al 1985, Lee 1986). In colonic or rectal mucosal biopsies the appearances are usually not diagnostic but confirm a localised inflammation in the mucosa next to the ulcers. However, the presence of entirely normal mucosa a short distance from the ulcers may give an indication of the diagnosis, especially if other manifestations of the disease such as oro-genital ulcers, iritis, arthritis, skin and nervous system involvement are present.

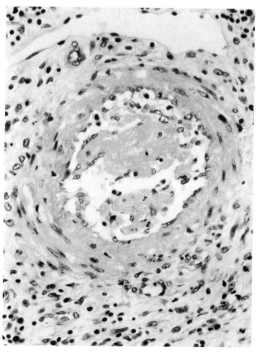

Figure 17–48. Detail of thrombosed vessel in Figure 17–47. The inflammatory infiltrate around this vessel is not striking (H & E × 500).

THE COLITIS OF CHRONIC GRANULOMATOUS DISEASE

This colitis may be virtually indistinguishable from Crohn's disease because similar granulomata are seen in association with patchy ulceration and inflammation. A histological clue to the diagnosis, however, is the additional feature of PAS-positive lipofuscin-filled histiocytes in both mucosa and submucosa (Werlin et al 1982, Isaacs et al 1985).

MISCELLANEOUS FORMS OF COLITIS

On rare occasions other conditions can present as and mimic inflammatory bowel disease. Such diseases as Wegener's granulomatosis (Sokol, Farrell and McAdams 1984, Haworth and Pusey 1984) and angioimmunoblastic lymphadenopathy (Rosenstein et al 1988) have been reported in this context.

18

MISCELLANEOUS LESIONS

PNEUMATOSIS CYSTOIDES INTESTINALIS

In this condition, air-filled gas cysts occur in the wall of the small or large intestine. At biopsy the clinician may hear a hissing pop as the gas, which is under some pressure, escapes. Histological examination reveals cystic spaces in the submucosa. The reaction at the margin of the spaces varies with the age of the lesion. Early cysts have no lining (Fig. 18–1) and at that stage can be clearly seen not to be dilated lymphatics, as was once thought. The first reaction is histiocytic and the spaces come to be lined by macrophages. Later there is a mild collagenisation outside this zone and the macrophages form multinucleate giant cells (Fig. 18–2). The reaction parallels that seen in subcutaneous tissues after air or its individual component gases are injected (Wright 1930).

The question arises as to how the air finds its way into the bowel wall. Koss (1952) noted a high incidence (58 per cent) in the reported cases of a coexistent organic lesion of the gut, e.g., ulceration, neoplasm, obstruction. It has been described in association with diverticular disease (Jorgensen and Wille-Jorgensen 1982). It seems to complicate the connective tissue diseases more frequently than by chance. Two cases occurring in association with mixed connective tissue disease are reported by Lynn et al (1984), who also review the previous literature. The condition has also been reported as a complication of enteral feeding via catheter jejunostomy (Zern and Clarke-Pearson 1985), after colonoscopy (Heer et al 1983) and of both bone marrow (Yeager et al 1987, Day, Ramsay and Letourneau 1988) and renal transplantation (Murphy and Weinfeld 1987). In such cases a mechanical theory of origin is usually postulated whereby gas is forced into the wall via a breach in the mucosa. Even when it seems reasonable to invoke this mechanism, as, for example, when the condition complicates jejunoileal bypass surgery for obesity (Doolas, Breyer and Franklin 1979), the anatomical site of anastomosis does not necessarily correspond to the location of the pneumatosis and sometimes the lesions appear many months after operation (Feinberg et al 1977). In many patients, however, no bowel lesion can be demonstrated, and both clinical (Doub and Shea 1960) and experimental (Keyting et al 1961) evidence have suggested another origin. Rupture of lung alveoli producing mediastinal emphysema is followed by the movement of gas downwards round the aorta. The path upwards is blocked by deep fascial attachments at the root of the neck. The gas moves along in the adventitia of branches of the aorta into the mesentery, subsequently entering and disrupting the bowel wall along the vascular planes. Namdaran, Dutz and Ovasepian (1979) were able to produce typical pneumatosis in two cadavers by using high-pressure oxygen insufflation of the lungs. The explanation is

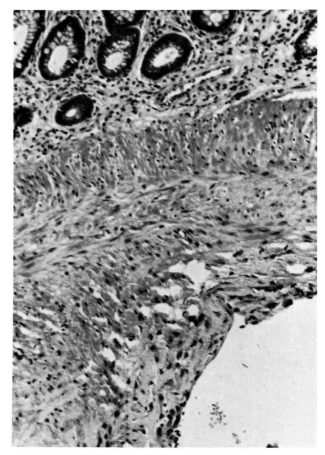

Figure 18–1. Pneumatosis cystoides intestinalis. Early cyst with no definitive lining (H & E × 210).

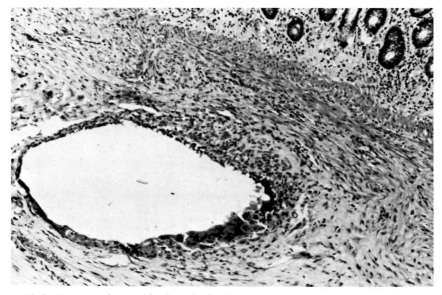

Figure 18–2. Pneumatosis cystoides intestinalis. Typical macrophage and giant cell lining of later lesion. There is early fibrosis outside the cyst (H & E × 105).

therefore tenable in patients with chronic lung diseases, but the claim that all cases can be explained in this way is unfounded. Certainly when pneumatosis is seen in the immediate vicinity of ulcerated lesions, and not elsewhere, a local origin is favoured.

In their analysis of 33 cases from the Armed Forces Institute of Pathology, Smith and Welter (1967) drew attention to the age distribution. All cases involved either children under one year or adults. There are cases in both children and adults that complicate severe ileocolitis, and in this author's experience these are the result of gas production by clostridial or other gas-forming organisms that are acting as secondary invaders in a primarily ischaemic lesion. It is of some interest in this respect that such cases have a fatal outcome, whereas the condition complicating lung disease or local bowel lesions is benign and self-limiting although it may be recurrent over several years. This conclusion was also reached in a study of 21 cases by Gruenberg, Grodsinsky and Ponka (1979), who also noted a bad prognosis when the disease process occurred in the setting of severe illness due to other causes. In an ultrastructural study Haboubi et al (1984) claimed that the cysts were dilated lymphatic channels. On the other hand, Pieterse, Leong and Rowland (1985) claimed that the gas enters from the bowel on the basis of an inflammatory process disrupting the crypts. This is certainly not the experience of most observers, and the small spaces Pieterse, Leong and Rowland observed are probably related to the lesion known as pseudolipomatosis referred to later.

COLITIS CYSTICA PROFUNDA AND SUPERFICIALIS

This is a benign condition characterised by the presence of mucin-filled epithelial cysts underneath the muscularis mucosa. Rectal biopsy includes part of these structures on occasion (Tedesco, Sumner and Kassens 1976), and awareness of the condition can help to prevent unnecessary surgical resections, not only because of histological misinterpretation, but because clinically it can present as a colonic mass lesion (Schein, Veller and Decker 1987) and it may be misdiagnosed as carcinoma. The wall of the cyst may be incomplete because of lack of depth in biopsy tissues, but the epithelial lining may also be absent because of rupture (Fig. 18–3). The presence of mucin can be verified by appropriate stains, and the condition can thus be easily differentiated from pneumatosis cystoides intestinalis and oil granuloma even if there is a foreign body reaction to the mucin. The condition may be present in localised form more commonly in the rectum, but occasionally elsewhere (Yashiro et al 1985) or as a more diffuse colonic lesion, and is usually associated with a local ulcerative disease process at least sometime in the course of its development (see solitary ulcer of rectum). There seems to be a further strong association with rectal prolapse in the distal form of the disease (Stuart 1984), but sometimes no antecedent bowel pathology can be established and it can be recurrent (Bentley et al 1985). It should be noted that the lesions of colitis cystica profunda are distinct from the colonic lymphoid glandular complexes (microbursa) as described by Kealy (1976a,b). These structures are a feature in about 10 per cent of normal colons (see Fig. 15–3). It is possible that a colon with numerous microbursae would be more likely to develop colitis cystica profunda lesions than a normal colon if it were subsequently the site of a mucosal inflammatory process associated with regenerative epithelial activity, such as occurs in chronic ulcerative or granulomatous colitis. An association with inflammatory bowel disease is well recognised (Wayte and Helwig 1967, Magidson and Lewin 1981, O'Donnell 1987), and it has complicated radiation-induced colonic structure

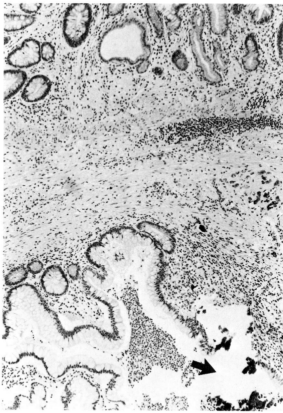

Figure 18–3. Colitis cystica profunda. This case was the result of an established chronic Crohn's disease. Note the incomplete lining of the submucosal glands, the pus in the lumen and the calcification (arrow) (H & E × 250).

(Gardiner, McAuliffe and Murray 1984). Morson and Dawson (1979) refer to a rare condition in children dying from leukaemia, pellagra and tropical sprue, called colitis cystica superficialis. The mucous membrane of the colon is atrophic and exhibits numerous small cysts due to ectasia of the glands. There is no record in the literature that the condition has been encountered in rectal biopsy specimens. However, it is not all that unusual to see on occasion thin-walled cystic glands in follow-up biopsies of patients with infective colitis, and this is probably a transient architectural abnormality, secondary to obstruction of the gland opening due to the healing process (Fig. 18–4).

AMYLOIDOSIS

Primary amyloidosis must be advanced before the Congo red test is positive and it is thus of little diagnostic value in early cases. Diagnosis by other means, especially by histological examination of biopsy tissues, has gradually become popular, therefore. Aspiration of tissues from internal organs carries a small but nevertheless real risk, and gingival biopsy (Calkins and Cohen 1960) or small-intestinal biopsy (Green et al 1961) gives a high false-negative rate. With rectal biopsy (Fig. 18–5) the diagnosis is achieved in 78 per cent of cases (Gafni and Sohar 1960), results which compare well with those obtained by renal biopsy and

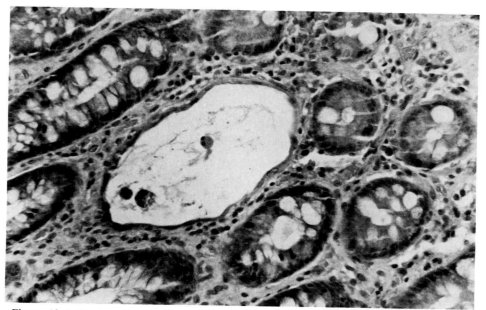

Figure 18–4. Cystic crypt in a follow-up biopsy from a case of infective colitis (H & E × 500).

are better than those for liver biopsy. The rectal biopsy must include the submucosa, since amyloid may be present at this site when absent from the lamina propria (Kyle, Spencer and Dahlin 1966). Amyloid deposits may be seen in the small arterioles of the lamina propria and submucosa, in the basement membrane of the surface epithelium and glands, and between fibres of the muscularis mucosa. Blood vessel involvement may be so marked that amyloid deposition may precipitate severe ischaemic lesions with quite gross secondary inflammatory

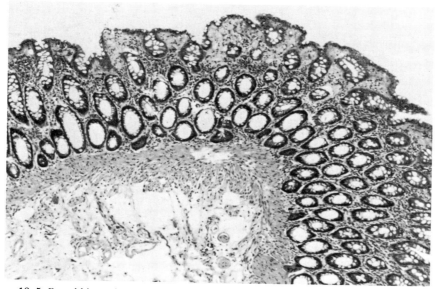

Figure 18–5. Rectal biopsy in severe amyloidosis. Even in H & E preparations the material is clearly visible under the superficial epithelium and in the upper one third of the lamina (H & E × 70).

disease (Vernon 1982, Perarnau et al 1982, Kumar et al 1983, Maher et al 1988). Although a great deal has been learned of the chemical composition of amyloid and its subtypes, for practical purposes, material that gives green birefringence in the polarising microscope when Congo red-stained sections are examined and an orange-red fluorescence in ultraviolet light can be regarded as amyloid (Zucker-Franklin, Pras and Franklin 1969). In such circumstances the more conventional methods will also be positive, but where there is serious doubt it may prove necessary to resort to more sophisticated methods that employ amyloid-specific fluorescein-conjugated antisera and electron microscopy (Zucker-Franklin and Franklin 1970).

MUCOVISCIDOSIS

There is a decrease in the diagnostic specificity of the sweat test with increasing age (Anderson and Freeman 1960, McKendrick 1962), and even in children it is sometimes falsely negative (Schwachman and Antonowicz 1962). All glandular epithelia may show abnormalities in this disorder, and this applies to the intestinal mucosa (Parkins et al 1963). A meconium ileus equivalent occurs in postneonatal children and young adults (Matseshe, Go and Dimagno 1977), and rectal biopsy therefore assumes increasing diagnostic importance. The goblet cells are conspicuous, the mouths of the colonic glands tend to gape and the crypts are widely dilated, being filled with lamellated mucin (Fig. 18–6). In some cases a mild inflammatory infiltrate is present in the lamina propria. Similar but less marked changes may occur normally in the region just above the mucocutaneous junction and occasionally also in healed inflammatory lesions of the colon, but they are then patchy; if marked changes are present in several biopsies, the diagnosis of mucoviscidosis is certain.

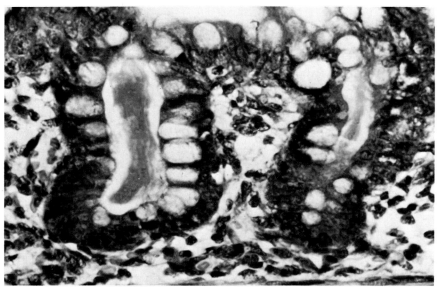

Figure 18–6. Mucoviscidosis in a rectal biopsy of a child. The glands contain thick inspissated secretion (H & E × 375).

SOLITARY ULCER OF THE RECTUM

This condition classically affects young adults of either sex who present with constipation and a combination of the following symptoms: difficulty in defaecation; sensations of incomplete evacuation; rectal prolapse; and rectal bleeding. Of late, however, it is being recognised more frequently in older age groups, and there are claims that it is underdiagnosed (Saul and Sollenberger 1985). Despite the title of the disease, in about one third of cases there is more than one ulcer and uncommonly there are several. Healing may occur, but reulceration is usual and the condition is chronic. A rectal biopsy from the healed area or the ulcer edge shows typical features (Madigan and Morson 1969). Apart from the expected changes due to ulceration and attempted healing, a characteristic feature is obliteration of the lamina propria by a fibromuscular proliferation (Figs. 18–7 and 18–8) continuous with the muscularis mucosa, which is hypertrophied and splayed. This can be shown to great effect in a connective tissue trichrome stain. In deep biopsies, a further feature sometimes seen is the presence of glandular epithelium and related lamina propria in the submucosa (Figs. 18–9, 18–10). These are prone to cystic dilation of the epithelial elements, which by virtue of their position are sometimes erroneously regarded as malignant. The lesion is a localised form of colitis cystica profunda and like the diffuse condition probably represents a regenerative reactive phenomenon. It is analogous to the lesions described in a previous chapter as gastritis cystica profunda. Its importance lies in the fact that it appears grossly as a mass lesion and may be misdiagnosed as carcinoma (Nagasako et al 1977).

Rectal biopsy carried out in the investigation of a variety of colorectal associated symptoms will occasionally reveal fibrous obliteration of the lamina propria and mild degenerate changes in the superficial epithelium (Fig. 18–11). It seems possible that these are the morphological consequences of repeated minimal mucosal trauma or ischaemia accompanying disorders of defaecation, either real

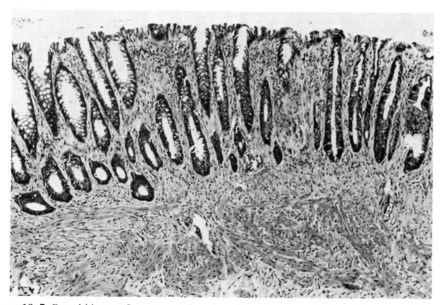

Figure 18–7. Rectal biopsy of mucosa at the edge of a solitary rectal ulcer. The muscularis mucosa is splayed, fibrotic and hypertrophied, and it merges with the lamina propria (H & E × 70).

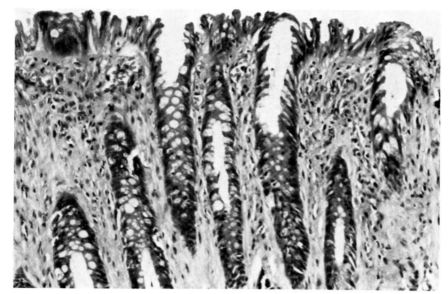

Figure 18–8. Detail of Figure 18–7 to show fibromuscular obliteration of the lamina propria (H & E × 210).

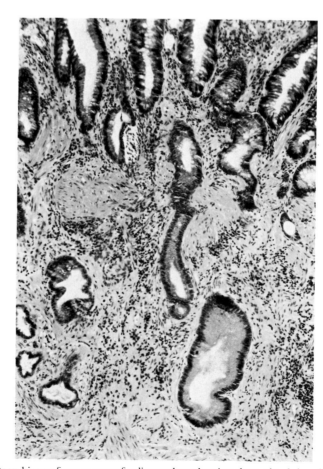

Figure 18–9. Deep biopsy from a case of solitary ulcer showing deep glandular elements embedded in hypertrophied muscularis (H & E × 350).

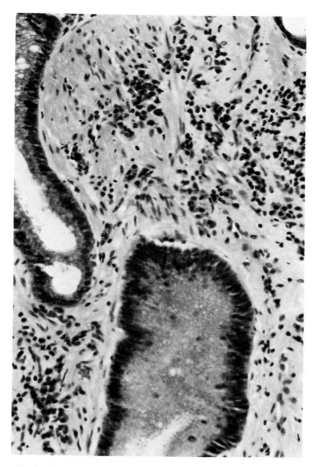

Figure 18–10. Detail of Figure 18–9 to show the intimate relationship between glandular elements and muscle (H & E × 500).

or otherwise, which result in straining at stool. Indeed, fibromuscular obliteration of the lamina propria is also seen in prolapsed rectal mucosa, prolapsed colostomy stomas and in the mucosa of chronically recurrent intussusception. Levine et al (1988) have drawn particular attention to this histological feature in differentiating the solitary ulcer syndrome from Crohn's disease and ulcerative colitis in biopsy tissues. If this is a manifestation of the low-grade mucosal trauma in these situations, similar but more severe trauma may be implicated in the mucosa, producing a solitary rectal ulcer. Parks, Porter and Hardcastle (1966) described the syndrome of the descending perineum in which chronic straining at stool results in a prolapse of the anterior rectal wall, further sensation of fullness and further straining. That a similar mechanism is involved in the aetiology of solitary ulcer seems likely. Martin, Parks and Biggart (1981) and Ford et al (1983) have shown that there is a spectrum of histological, gross and clinical abnormality culminating in frank ulceration in patients with abnormal rectal descent on straining. This has been further substantiated in the studies of Mackle and Parks (1986), Levine (1987) and Womack et al (1987). The regenerative and hyperplastic reactive changes that follow the repeated ischaemic trauma have been analysed histochemically (Ehsanullah, Filipe and Gazzard 1982, Franzin et al 1982), and it has been shown that a change from mainly sulphomucin to mainly sialomucin

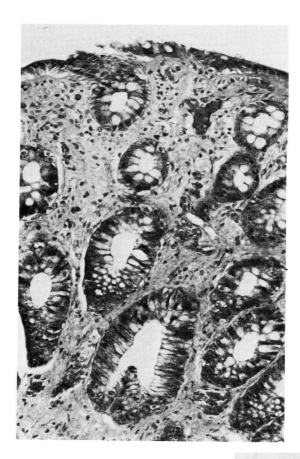

Figure 18–11. Slight architectural disturbance of glands and flattening of superficial epithelium in a mucosa from a patient with a long history of "difficulty" with defaecation (H & E × 175).

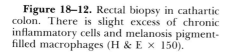

Figure 18–12. Rectal biopsy in cathartic colon. There is slight excess of chronic inflammatory cells and melanosis pigment-filled macrophages (H & E × 150).

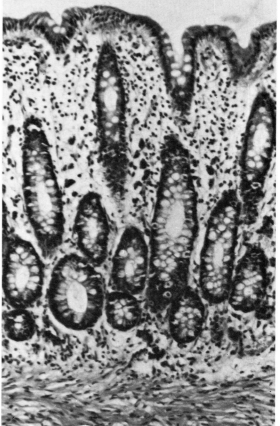

accompanies the histological abnormalities in the rectal mucosa. Similar changes in mucins and histological appearances are found in so-called cloacogenic polyps, and some if not all of these are due to mucosal prolapse (Saul 1987).

CATHARTIC COLON

The excessive and chronic use of purgatives may lead to either intractable diarrhoea with hypokalaemia (Houghton and Pears 1958) or protein-losing enteropathy (Heizer et al 1968). Reversible cachexia, hypogammaglobulinaemia and finger clubbing have also been described (Levine, Goode and Wingate 1981). It can also lead to increasing constipation, which in turn results in an increased drug dosage, so that a vicious circle is set up. The large bowel wall is thin and loses its haustra, its mobility is impaired, and there is melanosis coli if the anthracene group of drugs (aloe, senna, cascara, rhubarb) are being used. The lesion is most marked in the right side and it progresses distally. Rectal biopsy (Figs. 18–12, 18–13) is valuable in diagnosis, therefore, because it indicates a severe form due to long and significant exposure. Its presence also indicates recent exposure because the degree of pigmentation varies when the use of purgatives is periodic.

The exact nature of the pigment is the subject of doubt. It gives a positive PAS reaction and is autofluorescent. Lillee and Geer (1965) have shown that it has a protein component and a more or less closely bound glycolipid with free fatty acid residues. Rarely it is claimed that the pigment gives a reaction with Perls' stain for iron, but this author has not seen this phenomenon. The pigment is more or less similar to lipofuscin. The superficial cells of the mucosa may be flattened, but there are no destructive epithelial changes. The lamina propria may also contain an excess of chronic inflammatory cells, the muscularis mucosa is often markedly hypertrophied and the submucosa shows fatty infiltration (Fig. 18–14). There are also changes in the myenteric neurones (Smith 1972), which, of course, cannot be appreciated in mucosal biopsy tissues. The use of anthracene purgatives is so common that the finding of melanosis alone in colonic biopsies is not sufficient grounds to make a diagnosis of cathartic colon (Badiali et al 1985), and Balazs (1986) claims that in patients with melanosis, motility disorders are better correlated with electron microscopic evidence of ballooning and degeneration of autonomic neural elements in the mucosa. Indeed there is experimental evidence that the pigment itself is due to anthraquinone epithelial cell damage that results in increased apoptosis. The apoptotic bodies are then phagocytosed by intraepithelial macrophages that migrate into the lamina propria where the bodies are converted in heterolysosomes to lipofuscin (Walker, Bennett and Axelsen 1988). In early melanosis coli changes in humans, apoptotic bodies are a prominent feature in the overlying superficial epithelium (Fig. 18–15).

NEUROLOGICAL DISORDERS

In the past there was a great deal of controversy over the place of suction biopsy in the diagnosis of Hirschsprung's disease. Although the disease occurs in adolescents and adults (Parc, Douvin and Loygue 1979, Lefebvre et al 1984, Barnes et al 1986, Pescatori, Mattana and Castiglioni 1986, Starling, Croom and Thomas 1986), it is in the very young patient that precise diagnosis is a problem. This centres on the adequacy of examination of only the submucosal plexus instead of both the submucosal and myenteric plexuses as in full thickness biopsies.

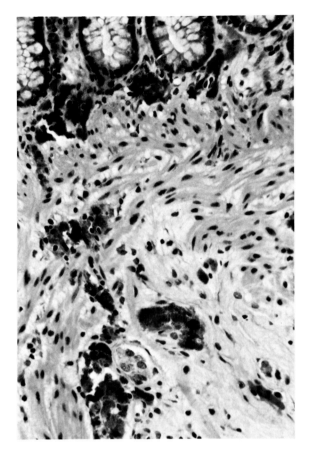

Figure 18–13. Melanosis coli pigmentation of a severe degree involving deeply situated macrophages in the submucosa and the submucosal neurones (H & E × 500).

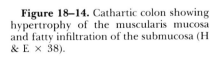

Figure 18–14. Cathartic colon showing hypertrophy of the muscularis mucosa and fatty infiltration of the submucosa (H & E × 38).

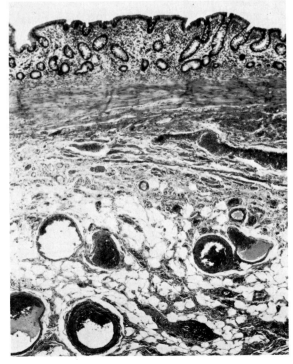

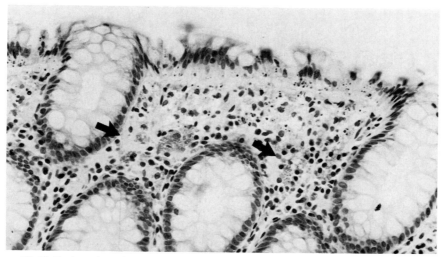

Figure 18–15. Early melanosis coli. Note occasional pigment macrophages (arrows) and the numerous apoptotic bodies in the epithelium and upper lamina propria (H & E × 500).

However, experienced observers became satisfied that histological examination of suction rectal and colonic biopsies has an established place in the diagnosis and treatment of this disease (Kurer, Lawson and Pambakian 1986). The tissue provided must include the submucosa where, in the normal biopsy, ganglion cells are easily recognised if sufficient sections are examined, and the biopsy must be taken at least 1 cm above the anorectal junction. Below this, ganglion cells are absent. As a rough guide any specimen that includes squamous epithelium and less submucosa than mucosa should be regarded as inadequate. In the usual case the involved segment of bowel exhibits not only an absence of ganglion cells but also non-myelinated nerve trunks (Figs. 18–16, 18–17), which are not present in the normal (Bodian 1960). A transitional zone often separates the aganglionic segment from the normal bowel, which may be considerably dilated and hypertrophied. In the transition zone ganglion cells are fewer and smaller than normal. Total colonic (Fekete et al 1986) and total intestinal aganglionosis occur but are less common (Caniano et al 1985, Fekete et al 1986, Rudin et al 1986).

The diagnosis of Hirschsprung's aganglionosis is very difficult in the neonate and in patients up to six months of age because of the immaturity of the submucosal neural elements (Smith 1968). With experience, however, these are easy to recognise, and Yunis, Dibbins and Sherman (1976) have described them in some detail. Rather than ganglion cells with obvious cytoplasm and prominent nucleoli the neural units appear as small, bare nuclei often set in a horseshoe pattern around central fibrillary neural tissue (Fig. 18–18). Their form, however, varies depending upon the plane of sectioning, and sometimes stages in mature neurone development among one or more of the primitive cells will be seen. When they are recognised the diagnosis of Hirschsprung's disease is excluded. As seems likely a group of clinically classic cases of this disease have only immature ganglia at a time when they would normally have matured. These and others with short distal segments showing an appearance characteristic of the transition zone, i.e., few ganglion cells but no abnormal nerve trunks, probably represent a less severe form of Hirschsprung's disease. Occasional cases with short incomplete distal aganglionosis and abnormal nerve trunks are also described (MacMahon, Moore and Cussen 1981), and there are instances of patients with Hirschsprung-

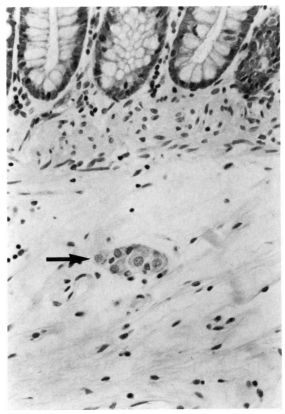

Figure 18–16. Rectal biopsy to show normal submucosal ganglion cells (arrow) (H & E × 225).

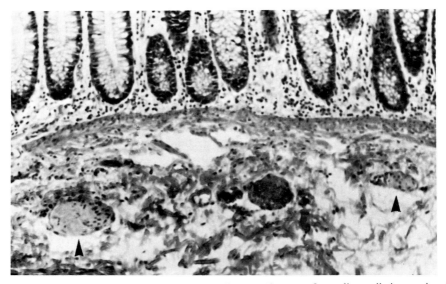

Figure 18–17. Rectal biopsy in Hirschsprung's disease. Absence of ganglion cells is associated with the presence of abnormal nerve trunks (arrowheads) (H & E × 113).

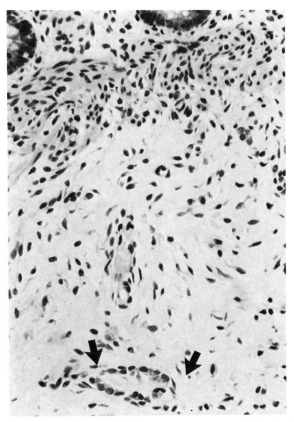

Figure 18–18. Neonatal rectal biopsy showing usual appearance of relatively immature ganglion cells (between arrows) that are not unlike the neighbouring inflammatory cells, but have a distinctive horseshoe-like configuration and sometimes central fibrils (H & E × 500).

like disease who have either quite localised or longer bowel segments in which submucosal ganglion cells are increased in number and show giant forms with ganglion cells as well as excessive nerve fibres in the lamina propria. These instances of so-called neuronal intestinal dysplasia may also occur in association with distal aganglionosis (Scharli and Meier-Ruge 1981, Ziegler et al 1984, Kessler and Campbell 1985, Munakata et al 1985). In the past, methods based on demonstration of acetyl cholinesterase, either by quantitative biochemical assay (Boston, Dale and Riley 1975, Dale et al 1979) or by a histochemical procedure, were used as adjuncts to the diagnosis of Hirschsprung's disease (Trigg et al 1974, Patrick, Besley and Smith 1980, Barr et al 1985). In expert hands they were useful, but it is pertinent that the value of these methods was always measured against the results of an examination by an expert observer of serial sections of the tissue under examination stained by ordinary haematoxylin and eosin (Challa et al 1987). If doubt persists a reappraisal of the clinical situation is undertaken. These histochemical methods proved useful in situations where biopsy material was limited to the mucosa by demonstrating an excessive permeation of nerve fibres throughout the lamina propria and muscularis mucosae in aganglionosis and positive ganglion cells in the lamina propria in neuronal dysplasia (Lake, Nixon and Claireaux 1978, Ziegler et al 1984).

Huntley et al (1982) described two types of acetyl cholinesterase nerve fibres. In type A the fibres are prominent in both the muscularis and the lamina, but in type B they are present mainly in the muscularis mucosa. Type B tends to be seen in infants aged one month or less, and the diagnosis of Hirschsprung's disease then needs to be substantiated by conventional routine histology. More recently still it has become apparent that the ganglion cells and nerve fibres in the rectal mucosa and submucosa can be much more easily visualised in immunohistochemical preparations using antibodies to neuron-specific enolase and S100 protein (Hall and Lampert 1985, Vinores and May 1985, Blisard and Kleinman 1986, Tam 1986) (Figs. 18–19, 18–20). Nevertheless, they need to be used in conjunction with routine serial sections stained by H & E, particularly because while the location of ganglion cells is facilitated, the delineation of mucosal nerve fibres is said not to be as good as with the acetyl cholinesterase method and both are liable to be misinterpreted and produce false-positive and false-negative results (Robey, Kuhajda and Yardley 1988). There are conflicting reports concerning changes in endocrine polypeptide cells in the excised bowel in Hirschsprung's disease. Cristina et al (1978) found no abnormalities in enteroglucagon and somatostatin cells, whereas Bishop et al (1981) found them increased, together with a vasoactive intestinal peptide content. There are no reports of the value of demonstrating changes in these cell types in rectal biopsies for the diagnosis of the disease.

McIver and Whitehead (1972) drew attention to a disease characterised by zonal aganglionosis in which a rectal biopsy may be normal. Rarely, therefore, in otherwise typical cases of Hirschsprung's disease is a normal low rectal biopsy seen, but this does not exclude the possibility of an aganglionic segment at a higher level. It is possible that this entity has a different aetiology, and zonal aganglionosis is described in the terminal ileum. Conceivably a different and temporary intrauterine insult could be involved. The neural elements migrate into the bowel in a cranio-caudal direction from the neural crest, and it could be postulated that whereas in Hirschsprung's disease the migration is terminated more or less abruptly and permanently, in zonal aganglionosis the interference is relatively short-lived. De Chadarevian, Slim and Akel (1982) and Seldenrijk et al (1986) report further cases of double zonal aganglionosis and provide a review of

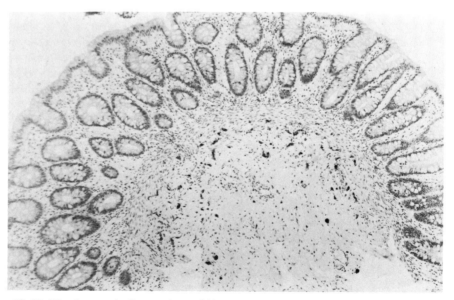

Figure 18–19. Hirschsprung's disease. A rectal biopsy showing abnormal nerve trunks (S100 × 150).

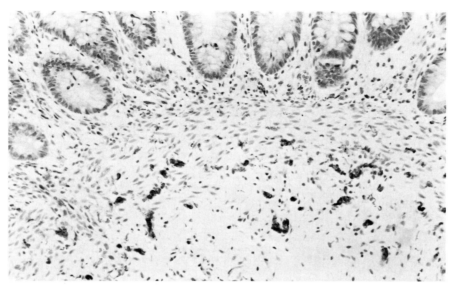

Figure 18–20. Detail of Figure 18–19 showing proliferation of nerve fibres in the submucosa and involving the muscularis mucosa (S100 × 500).

the literature on this curious variant. Another subtype or related disorder is segmental hypoganglionosis (Matsui et al 1987) and hypoganglionosis of the myenteric plexus with normal Meissner's plexus (Ariel et al 1985).

Early workers (Bodian and Lake 1963, Brett and Berry 1967) showed that rectal biopsy examination was helpful in the diagnosis of some central nervous system disorders. In neurolipidosis, metachromatic leukodystrophy and Hunter's syndrome, changes similar to those in the brain were found in the ganglion cells of the myenteric plexus. Jager, Den Hartog and Bethlem (1960) have also reported the Lewy body inclusions of Parkinson's disease, not only in the pigment-containing neurones within the brain but also in neurones of the autonomic ganglia. To be of maximum value, the biopsies should include the muscularis propria, and the technique for providing such biopsies via the rectum is not without risk.

With the refinement of biochemical procedures and advances in enzymology the need for biopsy procedures in the diagnosis of the storage disorders has decreased. Brett and Lake (1975) have reviewed the situation and concluded that although rectal neuronal involvement is present in many of these syndromes, easier, more reliable and safer methods are preferred. They suggest that with the exception of Batten's disease, which is really a group of diseases associated with the storage of ceroid-like pigment lipofuscin in which rectal biopsy is still used (Rapola, Santavuori and Savilahti 1984), it has been superseded as a diagnostic method. Nevertheless, rectal involvement has been described in the gangliosidoses, mucopolysaccharidoses and mucolipidoses, fucosidosis, monosidosis, Fabry's disease, Gaucher's disease, Niemann-Pick disease, Wolman's disease, Batten's disease, Tangier disease (Dechelotte et al 1985) and metachromatic leukodystrophy. An ultrastructural study of the rectal mucosa in a variety of storage diseases is reported by Yamano et al (1982). In addition to neuronal storage material, dense bodies and membrane bound vacuoles were seen in a variety of other cell types including plasma cells.

Colonic involvement is also described in systemic histiocytosis X and may cause ulceration (Moroz et al 1984, Hyams et al 1985).

In megacolon due to Chagas' disease the myenteric plexus shows a depletion of ganglion cells with an associated inflammatory cell infiltration of variable intensity that seems to be less marked the longer the history of the disease.

Smith (1972, 1982) has pointed out that many of the powerful drugs in everyday use are neurotoxic. Central neurones are usually protected by the blood-brain barrier, but the neurones of the autonomic nervous system are not. She describes in detail changes in myenteric neurones of the gut produced in experimental animals by a variety of therapeutic agents and in pseudo-obstruction of the intestine in the child and adult, but whether these results will have an application in detecting drug-induced or congenital neurone abnormality in human rectal biopsy material remains to be seen.

MALACOPLAKIA

Although more commonly found as a rare lesion of the bladder, malacoplakia can occur as a colonic lesion (Terner and Lattes 1963, Gonzalez-Angulo et al 1965). Even in the colon, it occurs most frequently in association with an obvious focus of suppuration, e.g., an abscess, carcinoma, diverticular disease and very rarely ulcerative colitis (MacKay 1978). Sometimes it mimics tumour and presents as lobulated masses in the mucosa, but occasionally it occurs as a diffuse lesion of the bowel. Lewin et al (1974) have reviewed the literature on intestinal malaco-plakia and stress the particularly aggressive nature of the disease when it involves this site. Histological examination of biopsy specimens reveals typical sheets of histiocytes (Fig. 18–21), some of which contain the rounded laminated and calcified Michaelis-Gutmann bodies. The histiocytes have been shown to contain alpha—1-antitrypsin (Callea, Van Damme and Desmet 1982).

Electron microscope studies (Lewin et al 1976, MacKay 1978, Chaudhry et al 1979, 1980) have revealed intact bacteria or bacteria showing various stages of destruction in macrophage lysosomes. The organisms show characteristics of

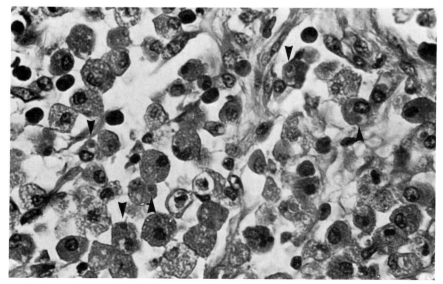

Figure 18–21. Malacoplakia of the colon. Typical histiocytes with their inclusions (arrowheads) (H & E × 460).

Escherichia coli, and the lysosomes are gradually filled with amorphous aggregates that become encrusted by calcium phosphate to form the typical Michaelis-Gutmann bodies. They also sometimes contain iron, and Stevens and McClure (1982) detail in depth a comprehensive histochemical study of these curious inclusions. The unusual reponse may represent the result of inadequate macrophage function. El-Mouzan et al (1988) report colonic disease in two children of the same family and propose that there may be a genetic predisposition.

HISTIOCYTOSIS AND OIL GRANULOMA

Macrophages containing mucoprotein (Azzopardi and Evans 1966) that stain positively with mucicarmine, Alcian blue and aldehyde fuchsin are not uncommonly seen in the lamina propria of the colon. They occur in otherwise normal biopsy specimens but also, and more commonly, in association with other mucosal abnormalities such as might be produced by previous inflammatory disruption (Fig. 18–22). They may be scattered throughout the lamina propria, but there is always a tendency for them to be more frequent on the mucosal aspect of the muscularis mucosa. This is invariably the site where muciphages will be found in otherwise normal mucosae (Fig. 18–23). The above staining reactions, which are probably due to the ingested mucin, serve to differentiate so-called muciphages from Whipple cells, which can occur in rectal mucosa, for both are PAS positive.

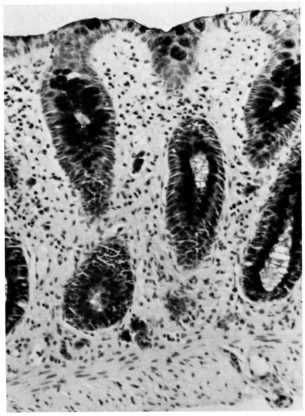

Figure 18–22. Rectal biopsy after resolution of a first mild attack of ulcerative colitis. Muciphages in the lamina propria stain in identical manner to goblet cells (Alcian blue × 140).

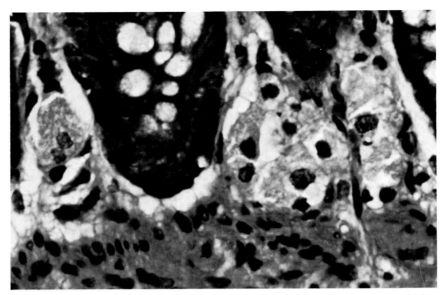

Figure 18–23. Normal rectal biopsy showing numerous muciphages next to muscularis mucosa below (H & E × 522).

There is some confusion in the literature surrounding the whole subject of colonic histiocytosis, and this is in part related to the fact that muciphages, macrophages containing lipofuscin, as seen par excellence in the brown-bowel syndrome, and melanosis coli macrophages all share one or more histochemical properties. In addition, these different types of macrophages may occur in the same biopsy material. What also is equally clear is that in some cases of systemic storage diseases, histiocytes of the lamina propria may be involved in addition to the neural elements. This happens, for example, in that rare disorder of congenital absence of high-density lipoproteins (Tangier disease) and the deposition in histiocytes throughout the reticuloendothelial system of cholesterol esters. The colon and rectum are also involved by the histiocytosis and this may be seen in the rectal biopsy tissues (Fig. 18–24). Cholesterol and other lipids are also involved in Wolman's disease, a much more severe type of histiocytosis that also affects the small intestine. It produces a malabsorption syndrome with diarrhoea and is usually fatal in the first six months of life. The histiocytes of the reticuloendothelial system in all areas outside the central nervous system are affected. In gangliosidosis the lamina propria histiocytes contain both a metachromatic water-soluble acid mucosubstance and some in an insoluble form (Fig. 18–25). Histiocytic involvement is also said to occur in Niemann-Pick disease and Gaucher's disease.

A local histiocytic and giant cell reaction also characterises the established lesion of oil granuloma that may follow the injection of oily sclerosants or the use of local ointments, lubricants or oral intake of paraffin oil associated with trauma or ulceration (Greaney and Jackson 1977, Mazier, Sun and Robertson 1978). It is sometimes an incidental finding, but it can present as a local rectal or anal canal tumefaction with or without ulceration. The severity of the histiocytic reaction probably varies with different oils and the time that the oil is in the tissues, but in some biopsy specimens it appears to be minimal and superficial and needs to be distinguished from so-called pseudolipomatosis (see later) (Figs. 18–26, 18–27). Histologically typical, the histiocytic and giant cell reaction surrounds circular

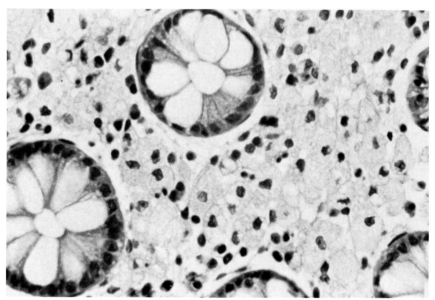

Figure 18–24. Rectal biopsy in Tangier disease. Pale histiocytes occupy the lamina propria (H & E × 510).

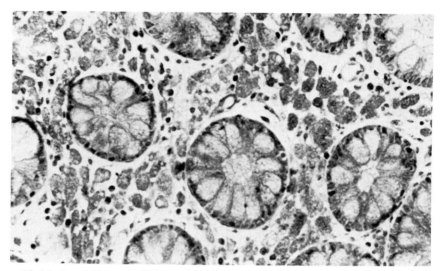

Figure 18–25. Rectal biopsy in GM_1 gangliosidosis. The histiocytes have been made more obvious by using the PAS method (PAS × 500).

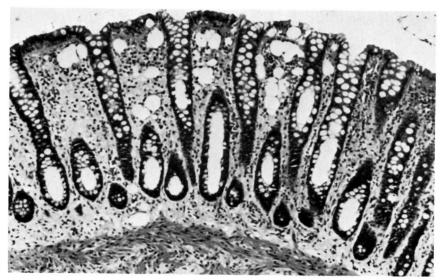

Figure 18–26. Incidental finding in rectal biopsy. The lamina propria shows numerous oil globule spaces (H & E × 70).

spaces, which before tissue processing contain the oil. Both mucosa and submucosa may be involved (Figs. 18–28, 18–29).

Another form of colonic histiocyte accumulation is so-called colonic xanthomatosis or lipid islands (Figs. 18–30, 18–31). They appear to be the colonic counterpart of gastric xanthomas or xanthelasmas. The light and electron microscopic appearances are similar (Remmele, Beck and Kaiserling 1988, Schaefer 1988). Scheiman et al (1988), however, in reporting two cases make a claim that xanthomatosis is associated with colonic dysmotility.

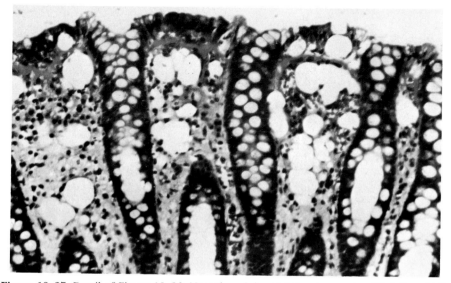

Figure 18–27. Detail of Figure 18–26. Note the minimal histiocytic reaction (H & E × 210).

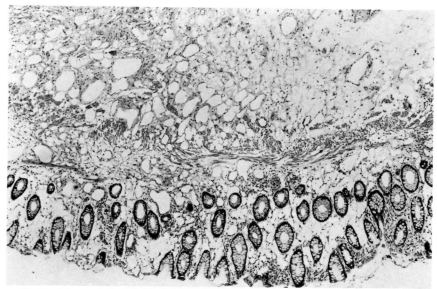

Figure 18–28. Oil granuloma in rectal biopsy. There is involvement of the mucosa and submucosa (H & E × 38).

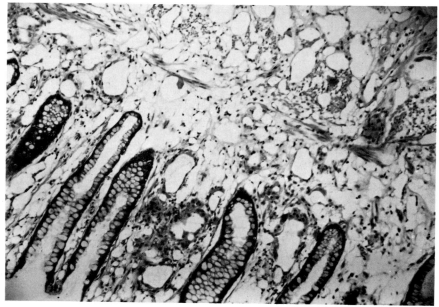

Figure 18–29. Detail of Figure 18–28. The histiocytic reaction is much more pronounced than in Figure 18–27 (H & E × 113).

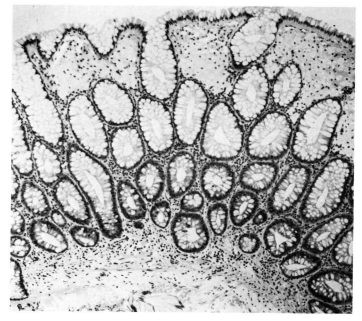

Figure 18–30. Colonic biopsy of a pale raised mucosal patch (H & E × 150).

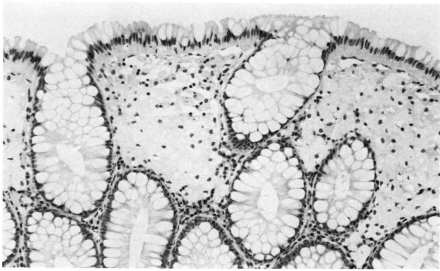

Figure 18–31. Detail of Figure 18–30. The collection of lipid-filled histiocytes is typical of colonic xanthoma or xanthelasma (H & E × 500).

DIABETIC ANGIOPATHY AND VASCULITIS

Biopsy has been used to detect microangiopathy in the capillaries of the rectal mucosa in patients with diabetes mellitus (Missmahl and Riemann 1968). Frank necrotising arteritis may also be seen in the biopsy tissues of patients with systemic autoimmune diseases (Fig. 18–32). A low posterior rectal biopsy, as a very safe procedure, has actually been used for the diagnosis of arteritis in patients with rheumatoid arthritis and related disorders (Schneider and Dobbins 1968). Tribe, Scott and Bacon (1981) found that an adequate biopsy is positive in 40 per cent of patients with a clinical vasculitis in rheumatoid arthritis patients. They advocated, however, the necessity to examine step serial sections. The problem of classifying necrotising vasculitis is exemplified by its occurrence in the gut. Kalla, Lee and Voss (1980) highlighted this in a case of necrotising and granulomatous arteritis with giant cells that was confined to the vessels of the right colon. It is not widely enough appreciated that the presence of arteritis in rectal biopsy tissues need not be associated with ischaemic lesions of the gut but is simply a reflection of its very good anastomotic blood supply. Many of the systemic autoimmune disorders, however, can be associated with a vasculitis so widespread and severe that it causes ischaemic colitis; this was referred to earlier.

BARIUM GRANULOMA

Rarely, following X-ray procedures and usually in association with inflammatory bowel disease, barium will be forced into or through the bowel wall. Small leaks

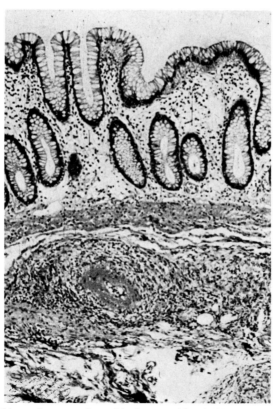

Figure 18–32. Rectal biopsy from a patient with rheumatoid arthritis. There is a necrotising vasculitis in the submucosa (H & E × 85).

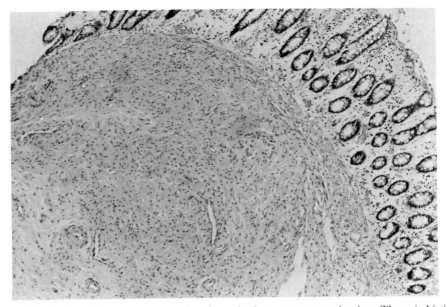

Figure 18–33. Rectal biopsy some months after a barium enema examination. There is histiocytic reaction involving the muscularis mucosa and submucosa (H & E × 75).

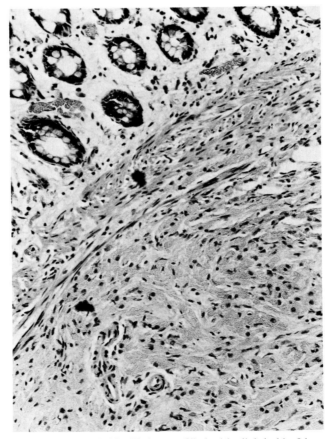

Figure 18–34. Detail of Figure 18–33. Histiocytes filled with slightly birefringent barium (H & E × 240).

are probably more common than is generally appreciated (Fielding and Lumsden, 1973). The medium excites a histiocytic reaction (Figs. 18–33, 18–34) that may subsequently be seen in rectal biopsy specimens. Barium can also be responsible for some unusual histological appearances and take the form of birefringent rhomboidal crystals (Womack 1984) or smaller birefringent particles within histiocytes (Levison et al 1984).

CRONKHITE-CANADA SYNDROME

This is referred to in Chapter 8. It is well to stress, however, that the whole intestine is involved to a greater or lesser extent. Nonetheless, even when there are no frankly polypoidal lesions, abnormality in size, shape and component goblet cells can be seen in biopsies from regions of the gastrointestinal tract other than the stomach (Fig. 18–35). Peart et al (1984), Freeman (1985) and Aanestad et al (1987) describe polypoid colonic lesions, and there are two reports (Katayama, Kimura and Konn 1985, Malhotra and Sheffield 1988) that describe adenomatous change in the polyps and coexistent adenocarcinoma.

PELVIC LIPOMATOSIS

This unusual condition comprises a non-tumoural, adipose infiltration of the pelvis that may cause visceral compression and interference with bladder and

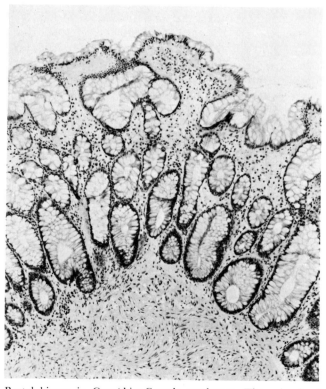

Figure 18–35. Rectal biopsy in Cronkhite-Canada syndrome. There is glandular enlargement, distortion, branching and variation in size. The individual goblet cells are also larger and more variable in shape than normal (H & E × 100).

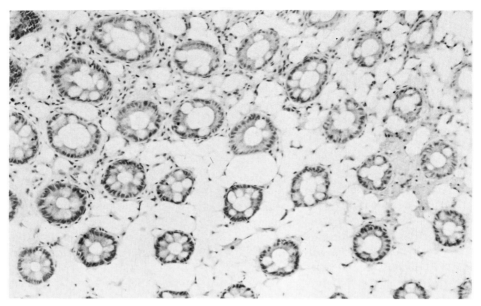

Figure 18–36. Rectal biopsy showing adipocyte infiltration (H & E × 500).

rectal function (Henriksson, Liljeholm and Lonnerholm 1984). Goldfain et al (1981) describe a case in which a rectal biopsy showed submucosal and mucosal adipocyte infiltration, which, taken in conjunction with the clinical features and radiology, allowed the diagnosis to be made, but this is unusual. It must be pointed out that rarely a few adipocytes may normally be seen in the rectal mucosa, especially in the aged and often at the site of atrophic lymphoid follicles, but it has no significance. It is usually an easy matter to differentiate this lesion from oil granuloma because there is no reactive histiocyte component (Figs. 18–36, 18–37). An appearance referred to as pseudolipomatosis (Snover, Sandstad and

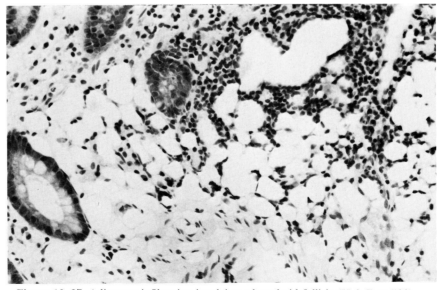

Figure 18–37. Adipocyte infiltration involving a lymphoid follicle (H & E × 500).

Hutton 1985) is similar, but apparently these authors found no evidence that fat was present in these small clear spaces. It is possible that this lesion is an artefact whereby luminal gas is introduced into the tissues during the biopsy procedure. Another biopsy artefact of interest is the appearance described by Dankwa and Davies (1988) of smooth muscle pseudotumours due to forceps pinching and rounding up a portion of muscularis propria so that it appears as a small tumour nodule arising in the submucosa.

GRAFT-VERSUS-HOST DISEASE

Sale et al (1979) and Epstein et al (1980) have utilised rectal biopsy in the evaluation of graft-versus-host disease (GVHD). Patients undergoing marrow transplantation were shown to have crypt epithelial degenerative changes and occasional crypt abscesses. The changes proved to be a good indication of graft-versus-host disease if the biopsy was performed after resolution of radiation or chemotherapeutic effects. Sviland et al (1988) have shown that rectal mucosa is a sensitive indicator of GVHD, with single cell necrosis, degeneration of crypts and crypt abscesses all being seen. In personal observations the most sensitive indicator is the appearance of apoptotic bodies in the crypt bases (Figs. 18–38, 18–39). Sometimes gross changes with epithelium denudation are described (Beschorner 1984, Thorning and Howard 1986) or widespread ulceration (Spencer et al 1986). Lampert et al (1985) describe a selective sparing of enterochromaffin cells so that small groups of these cells occupied crypt bases at the sites of destroyed crypt epithelium. Cytotoxic drug or irradiation may produce similar changes, however (Fig. 18–40).

SARCOIDOSIS

Rectal involvement in sarcoidosis has already been referred to, and although it is apparently a rare finding, it may be seen more frequently if rectal biopsy is performed routinely in known cases.

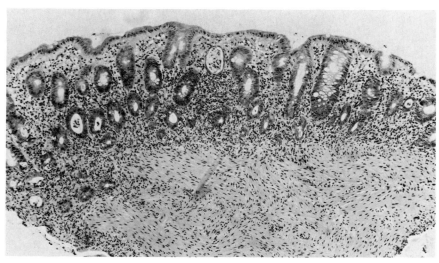

Figure 18–38. Rectal biopsy from a child with graft-versus-host disease following marrow transplantation. There is an obvious mild colitis and patchy tubular abnormalities with focal atrophy (H & E ×150).

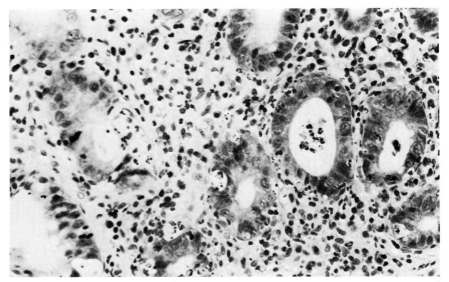

Figure 18–39. Detail of Figure 18–38. There is prominent apoptosis of crypt epithelial cells and cellular apoptotic debris in the dilated glands. A mild coincident colitis is present (H & E × 500).

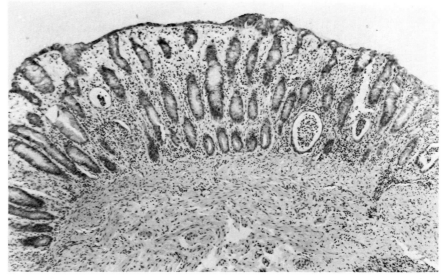

Figure 18–40. Colonic mucosa in cytotoxic drug therapy. The appearances are not unlike those of graft-versus-host disease, but the crypts contain more obvious collections of pus cells (H & E × 125).

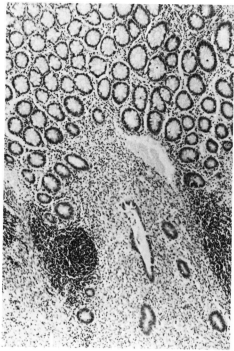

Figure 18–41. Colonic endometriosis. The abnormal tissue lies at the base of the mucosa (H & E × 250).

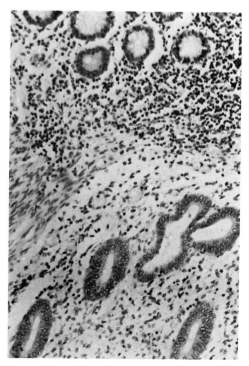

Figure 18–42. Detail of Figure 18–41. Note the subtle but distinct difference between colonic and endometrial glands, the surrounding lamina propria and the endometrial stroma (H & E × 500).

HETEROTOPIC GASTRIC MUCOSA AND SALIVARY GLAND OF THE RECTUM

Gastric heterotopia may be the cause of fresh rectal bleeding and usually presents in childhood. The abnormally located mucosa may be polypoidal or present as ulceration. Histologically, biopsies reveal a body type mucosa of usual histological appearance (Picard et al 1978, Edouard et al 1983, Pistoia et al 1987, Murray et al 1988). Sometimes gastric mucosa lines a rectal duplication (Schwarzenberg and Whitington 1983). Ectopic gastric mucosa sometimes presents in early adult life (Castellanos et al 1984). Weitzner (1983) described ectopic salivary gland tissue in the rectum. In previous cases on record it has usually been accompanied by gastric mucosa.

ALCOHOL-INDUCED CHANGES

Brozinsky et al (1978) studied 11 patients with a history of recent heavy drinking. A decrease in goblet cells, which returned to normal after two weeks abstinence, was seen in rectal biopsy specimens by light microscopy. These changes were accompanied by loss of microvilli, swollen mitochondria with distorted cristae, dilatation of the endoplasmic reticulum and Golgi and an increase in multivesicular bodies in an electron microscope evaluation.

COLONIC ENDOMETRIOSIS

The sigmoid colon is the commonest site of endometriosis, where it may give rise to obstruction and/or bleeding. It is not common for a diagnosis to be made in biopsy tissues, however (Croom, Donovan and Schwesinger 1984, Samper, Slagle and Hand 1984) (Figs. 18–41, 18–42).

REFERENCES—SECTION IV
COLONIC BIOPSY

Aanestad O., Raknerud N., Aase S.T. and Narverud G. (1987) The Cronkhite-Canada syndrome. Acta Chirurgia Scandinavica *153*:143–145.

Aaronson H.G., Meir J.H. and Ulin A.W. (1957) A case of sarcoidosis of the colon. Journal of the Albert Einstein Medical Center *6*:14–16.

Adamsen S., Ostberg G. and Norryd C. (1988) Squamous-cell metaplasia with severe dysplasia of the colonic mucosa in ulcerative colitis. Diseases of the Colon and Rectum *31*:558–562.

Ahnen D.J., Warren G.H., Greene L.J., Singleton J.W. and Brown W.R. (1987) Search for a specific marker of mucosal dysplasia in chronic ulcerative colitis. Gastroenterology *93*:1346–1355.

Alberti-Flor J.J. and Granda A. (1986) Ileocecal histoplasmosis mimicking Crohn's disease in a patient with Job's syndrome. Digestion *33*:176–180.

Allen D.C. and Biggart J.D. (1986) Misplaced epithelium in ulcerative colitis and Crohn's disease of the colon and its relationship to malignant mucosal changes. Histopathology *10*:37–52.

Allen D.C., Hamilton P.W., Watt P.C.H. and Biggart J.D. (1987) Morphological analysis in ulcerative colitis with dysplasia and carcinoma. Histopathology *11*:913–926.

Allison M.C., Hamilton-Dutoit S.J., Dhillon A.P. and Pounder R.E. (1987) The value of rectal biopsy in distinguishing self-limited colitis from early inflammatory bowel disease. Quarterly Journal of Medicine *65*:985–995.

Anand B.S., Malhotra V., Bhattacharya S.K., Datta P., Datta D., Sen D., Bhattacharya M.K., Mukherjee P.P. and Pal S.C. (1986) Rectal histology in acute bacillary dysentery. Gastroenterology *90*:654–660.

Anderson C.M. and Freeman M. (1960) "Sweat test" results in normal persons of different ages compared with families with fibrocystic disease of the pancreas. Archives of Disease in Childhood *35*:581–587.

Anthonisen P. and Riis P. (1971) Eosinophilic granulocytes in the rectal mucus of patients with ulcerative colitis and Crohn's disease of the ileum and colon. Scandinavian Journal of Gastroenterology *6*:731–734.

Antonakopoulos G., Newman J. and Wilkinson M. (1982) Intestinal spirochaetosis: an electron microscopic study of an unusual case. Histopathology *6*:477–488.

Arber N., Udassin R., Amir G., Zamir O. and Nissan S. (1987) Localized pseudomembranous colitis simulating carcinoma of the cecum. American Journal of Gastroenterology *82*:1193–1195.

Archibald R.B., Burnstein A.V., Knackstedt V.E., Tolman K.G. and Holbrook J.H. (1980) Ischemic colitis in a young adult due to inferior mesenteric vein thrombosis. Endoscopy *12*:140–143.

Archibald S.D., Jirsch D.W. and Bear R.A. (1978) Gastrointestinal complications of renal transplantation. 2. The colon. Canadian Medical Association Journal *119*:1301–1314.

Arean V.M. and Koppisch E. (1956) Balantidiasis. American Journal of Pathology *32*:1089–1115.

Ariel I., Hershlag A., Lernau O.Z., Nissan S. and Rosenmann E. (1985) Hypoganglionosis of the myenteric plexus with normal Meissner's plexus: a new variant of colonic ganglion cell disorders. Journal of Pediatric Surgery *20*:90–92.

Arseculeratne S.N., Panabokke R.G. and Navaratnam C. (1980) Pathogenesis of necrotising enteritis with special reference to intestinal hypersensitivity reactions. Gut *21*:265–278.

Atherton L.D., Leib E.S. and Kaye M.D. (1984) Toxic megacolon associated with methotrexate therapy. Gastroenterology *86*:1583–1588.

Azzopardi J.G. and Evans D.J. (1966) Mucoprotein-containing histiocytes (muciphages) in the rectum. Journal of Clinical Pathology *19*:368–374.

Badiali D., Marcheggiano A., Pallone F., Paoluzi P., Bausano G., Iannoni C., Materia E., Anzini F. and Corazziari E. (1985) Melanosis of the rectum in patients with chronic constipation. Diseases of the Colon and Rectum *28*:241–245.

Bailey R.W., Hamilton S.R., Morris J.B., Bulkley G.B. and Smith G.W. (1986) Pathogenesis of nonocclusive ischaemic colitis. Annals of Surgery *203*:590–599.

Bamford M.J., Matz L.R., Armstrong J.A. and Harris A.R.C. (1982) Collagenous colitis: a case report and review of the literature. Pathology *14*:481–484.

Balazs M. (1986) Melanosis coli. Ultrastructural study of 45 patients. Diseases of the Colon and Rectum *29*:839–844.

Balazs M., Egerszegi P., Vadasz G. and Kovacs A. (1988) Collagenous colitis: an electron microscopic study including comparison with the chronic fibrotic stage of ulcerative colitis. Histopathology *13*:319–328.

Barlow R.J., Heyl T., Simson I.W. and Schulz E.J. (1988) Malignant atrophic papulosis (Degos' disease); diffuse involvement of brain and bowel in an African patient. British Journal of Dermatology *118*:117–123.

Barnes P.R.H., Lennard-Jones J.E., Hawley P.R. and Todd I.P. (1986) Hirschsprung's disease and idiopathic megacolon in adults and adolescents. Gut *27*:534–541.

Barr L.C., Booth J., Filipe M.I. and Lawson J.O.N. (1985) Clinical evaluation of the histochemical diagnosis of Hirschsprung's disease. Gut *26*:393–399.

Bartlett J.G., Chang T.W., Curwith M., Gorbach S.L. and Onderdonk A.B. (1978) Antibiotic-associated pseudomembranous colitis due to toxin producing clostridia. New England Journal of Medicine *298*:531–534.

Behan W.M.H. and Mills P.R. (1982) Possible evidence for a Shwartzman reaction in pseudomembranous colitis. Digestion 23:141–150.

Bender B.S., Bennett R., Laughon B.E., Greenough W.B. III, Gaydos C., Sears S.D., Forman M.S. and Bartlett J.G. (1986) Is Clostridium difficile endemic in chronic-care facilities? Lancet ii:11–13.

Bennett M.R., Fine A.P. and Hanlon J.T. (1985) Cytomegalovirus hemorrhagic colitis in a nontransplant patient. Postgraduate Medicine 77:227–230.

Bentley E., Chandrasoma P., Cohen H., Radin R. and Ray M. (1985) Colitis cystica profunda: presenting with complete intestinal obstruction and recurrence. Gastroenterology 89:1157–1161.

Berezin S., Schwarz S.M., Glassman M., Davidian M. and Newman L.J. (1989) Gastrointestinal milk intolerance of infancy. American Journal of Disease in Children 143:361–362.

Berk T., Gordon S.J., Choi H.Y. and Cooper H.S. (1985) Cytomegalovirus infection of the colon: a possible role in exacerbations of inflammatory bowel disease. American Journal of Gastroenterology 80:355–360.

Berkowitz D. and Bernstein L.H. (1975) Colonic pseudopolyps in association with amoebic colitis. Gastroenterology 68:786–789.

Berry A.J., Long E.G., Smith J.H., Gourley W.K. and Fine D.P. (1983) Chronic relapsing colitis due to strongyloides stercoralis. American Journal of Tropical Medicine and Hygiene 32:1289–1293.

Berthrong M. and Fajardo L.F. (1981) Radiation injury in surgical pathology. Part II. Alimentary tract. American Journal of Surgical Pathology 5:153–178.

Beschorner W.E. (1984) Destruction of the intestinal mucosa after bone marrow transplantation and graft-versus-host disease. Surv. Synth. Path. Res. 3:264–274.

Biggs B-A., Megna R., Wickremesinghe S. and Dwyer B. (1987) Human infection with cryptosporidium spp.: results of a 24-month survey. Medical Journal of Australia 147:175–177.

Bingley P.J. and Harding G.M. (1987) Clostridium difficile colitis following treatment with metronidazole and vancomycin. Postgraduate Medical Journal 63:993–994.

Bishop A.E., Pietroletti R., Taat C.W., Brummelkamp W.H. and Polak J.M. (1987) Increased populations of endocrine cells in Crohn's ileitis. Virchows Archiv (A) 410:391–396.

Bishop A.E., Polak J.M., Lake B.D., Bryant M.G. and Bloom S.R. (1981) Abnormalities of the colonic regulatory peptides in Hirschsprung's disease. Histopathology 5:679–688.

Blackstone M.O., Riddell R.H., Rogers B.H.G. and Levin B. (1981) Dysplasia-associated lesion or mass (DALM) detected by colonoscopy in long-standing ulcerative colitis: an indication for colectomy. Gastroenterology 80:366–374.

Blaser M.J., Parsons R.B. and Wang W-L.L. (1980) Acute colitis caused by campylobacter fetus ss. jejuni. Gastroenterology 78:448–453.

Blisard K.S. and Kleinman R. (1986) Hirschsprung's disease: a clinical and pathologic overview. Human Pathology 17:1189–1191.

Blumencranz H., Kasen L., Romeu J., Waye J.D. and LeLeiko N.S. (1983). The role of endoscopy in suspected amebiasis. American Journal of Gastroenterology 78:15–18.

Bodian M. (1960) In: Recent Advances in Clinical Pathology. Series III. Edited by S.C. Dyke. London: Churchill, p. 384.

Bodian M. and Lake B.D. (1963) The rectal approach to neuropathology. British Journal of Surgery 50:702–714.

Bogomoletz W.V., Adnet J.J., Birembaut P., Feydy P. and Dupont P. (1980) Collagenous colitis: an unrecognised entity. Gut 21:164–168.

Bo-Linn G.W.. Vendrell D.D., Lee E. and Fordtran J.S. (1985) An evaluation of the significance of microscopic colitis in patients with chronic diarrhea. Journal of Clinical Investigation 75:1559–1569.

Bolton R.P., Cotter K.L. and Losowsky M.S. (1985) Inhibition of neutrophil chemotaxis and phagocytosis by Clostridium difficile. Clinical Science 68:53p.

Bonfils S., Hervoir P., Girodet J., le Quintrec Y., Bader J.P. and Gastard J. (1977) Acute spontaneously recovering ulcerating colitis. (ARUC). Report of 6 cases. American Journal of Digestive Diseases 22:429–436.

Boone W.T. and Allison F., Jr. (1969) Histoplasmosis. American Journal of Medicine 46:818–826.

Bosshardt R.T. and Abel M.E. (1984) Proctitis following fecal diversion. Diseases of the Colon and Rectum 27:605–607.

Boston V.E., Dale G. and Riley K.W.A. (1975) Diagnosis of Hirschsprung's disease by quantitative biochemical assay of acetylcholinesterase in rectal tissue. Lancet ii:951–953.

Boulton A.J.M., Slater D.N. and Hancock B.W. (1982) Herpesvirus colitis: a new cause of diarrhoea in a patient with Hodgkin's disease. Gut 23:247–249.

Boyd J.F. (1985) Pathology of the alimentary tract in salmonella typhimurium food poisoning. Gut 26:935–944.

Brandt L., Boley S., Goldberg L., Mitsudo S. and Berman A. (1981) Colitis in the elderly. A reappraisal. American Journal of Gastroenterology 76:239–245.

Brearly S., Armstrong G.R., Nairn R., Gornall P., Currie A.B.M., Buick R.G. and Corkery J.J. (1987) Pseudomembranous colitis: a lethal complication of Hirschsprung's disease unrelated to antibiotic usage. Journal of Pediatric Surgery 22:257–259.

Breiter J.R. and Hajjar J-J. (1981) Segmental tuberculosis of the colon diagnosed by colonoscopy. American Journal of Gastroenterology 76:369–373.

Brett E.M. and Berry C.L. (1967) Value of rectal biopsy in paediatric neurology: report of 165 biopsies. British Medical Journal iii:400–403.

Brett E.M. and Lake B.D. (1975) Reassessment of rectal approach to neuropathology in childhood. Review of 307 biopsies over 11 years. Archives of Disease in Childhood 50:753–762.

British Medical Journal (1981) Antibiotic-associated colitis: the continuing saga. British Medical Journal 282:1913–1914.

Brown R., Tedesco F.J., Assad R.T. and Rao R. (1986) Yersinia colitis masquerading as pseudomembranous colitis. Digestive Diseases and Sciences 31:548–551.

Brozinsky S., Fani K., Grosberg S.J. and Wapnick S. (1978) Alcohol ingestion-induced changes in the human rectal mucosa: light and electron microscopic studies. Diseases of the Colon and Rectum 21:329–335.

Bulger K., O'Riordan M., Purdy S., O'Brien M. and Lennon J. (1988) Gastrointestinal sarcoidosis resembling Crohn's disease. American Journal of Gastroenterology 83:1415–1417.

Burke G.W., Wilson M.E. and Mehrez I.O. (1988) Absence of diarrhea in toxic megacolon complicating Clostridium difficile pseudomembranous colitis. American Journal of Gastroenterology 83:304–307.

Burt R.W., Berenson M.M., Samuelson C.O. and Cathey W.J. (1983) Rheumatoid vasculitis of the colon presenting as pancolitis. Digestive Diseases and Sciences 28:183–188.

Butt J.H. and Morson B. (1981) Dysplasia and cancer in inflammatory bowel disease. Gastroenterology 80:865–868.

Byrd R.L., Cunningham M.W. and Goldman L.I. (1987) Nonocclusive ischemic colitis secondary to hemorrhagic shock. Diseases of the Colon and Rectum 30:116–118.

Calkins E. and Cohen A.S. (1960) Diagnosis of amyloidosis. Bulletin of Rheumatic Diseases 10:215–218.

Callea F., Van Damme B. and Desmet V.J. (1982) Alpha-1- antitrypsin in malakoplakia. Virchows Archiv A Pathology, Anatomy and Histology 395:1–9.

Caniano D.A., Ormsbee H.S., Polito W., Sun C-C., Barone F.C. and Hill J.L. (1985) Total intestinal aganglionosis. Journal of Pediatric Surgery 20:456–460.

Carr N.D., Wells S., Haboubi N.Y., Salem R.J. and Schofield P.F. (1986) Ischaemic dilatation of the colon. Annals of the Royal College of Surgeons of England 68:264–266.

Cashore W.J., Peter G., Lauermann M., Stonestreet B.S. and Oh W. (1981) Clostridia colonization and clostridial toxin in neonatal necrotizing enterocolitis. Journal of Pediatrics 98:308–311.

Castellanos D., Menchen P., López de la Riva M., Clemente G., Senen M., Rabago L., Garcia Andrade M. and Alcalá-Santaella R. (1984) Heterotopic gastric mucosa in the rectum. Endoscopy 16:197–199.

Castro E.B., Rosen P.P. and Quan S.H.Q. (1973) Carcinoma of large intestestine in patients irradiated for carcinoma of cervix and uterus. Cancer 31:45–52.

Castro J., Vazquez-Iglesias J.L. and Arnal-Monreal F. (1983) Dysentery caused by balantidium coli: report of two cases. Endoscopy 15:272–274.

Cawthorn S.J., Gibbs N.M. and Marks C.G. (1983) Segmental colitis: a new complication of diverticular disease. Gut 24:500.

Challa V.R., Moran J.R., Turner C.S. and Lyerly A.D. (1987) Histologic diagnosis of Hirschsprung's disease. The value of concurrent hematoxylin and eosin and cholinesterase staining in rectal biopsies. American Journal of Clinical Pathology 88:324–328.

Chambers T.J. and Morson B.C. (1979) The granuloma in Crohn's disease. Gut 20:269–274.

Chandratre S., Bramble M.G., Cooke W.M. and Jones R.A. (1987) Simultaneous occurrence of collagenous colitis and Crohn's disease. Digestion 36:55–60.

Chaudhry A.P., Saigal K.P., Intengan M. and Nickerson P.A. (1979) Malakoplakia of the large intestine found incidentally at necropsy: light and electron microscopic features. Diseases of the Colon and Rectum 22:73–81.

Chaudhry A.P., Satchidanand S.K., Anthone R., Baumler R.A. and Gaeta J.F. (1980) An unusual case of supraclavicular and colonic malakoplakia: a light and ultrastructural study. Pathology 131:193–208.

Chiu A.O. and Abraham A.A. (1982) Pseudomembranous colitis associated with an unidentified species of clostridium. American Journal of Clinical Pathology 78:398–402.

Chowdhury M.N.H. (1984) Campylobacter jejuni enteritis: a review. Tropical and Geographical Medicine 36:215–222.

Clarke A.W., Lloyd-Mostyn R.H. and Sadler M.R. de C. (1972) Ischaemic colitis in young adults. British Medical Journal iv:70–72.

Colgan T., Lambert J.R., Newman A. and Luk S.C. (1980) Campylobacter jejuni enterocolitis. A clinicopathologic study. Archives of Pathology and Laboratory Medicine 104:571–574.

Collins R.H., Feldman M. and Fordtran J.S. (1987) Colon cancer, dysplasia, and surveillance in patients with ulcerative colitis. New England Journal of Medicine 316:1654–1658.

Colp R. (1934) A case of non-specific granuloma of the terminal ileum and cecum. Surgical Clinics of North America 14:443–449.

Cook M.G. and Goligher J.C. (1975) Carcinoma and epithelial dysplasia complicating ulcerative colitis. Gastroenterology 68:1127–1136.

Cooper C., Cotton D.W.K., Hudson M.J., Kirkham N. and Wilmott F.E.W. (1986) Rectal spirochaetosis in homosexual men: characterisation of the organism and pathophysiology. Genitourinary Medicine 62:47–52.

Cornes J.S. (1965) Number, size and distribution of Peyer's patches in the human small intestine. Gut 6:225–233.

Cotton P.B. and Lea Thomas M. (1971) Ischaemic colitis and the contraceptive pill. British Medical Journal *iii*:27–28.

Coverlizza S., Ferrari A., Scevola F., Gemme C., Cavallero M., Spandre M., Risio M. and Rossini F.P. (1986) Clinico-pathological features of collagenous colitis: case report and literature review. American Journal of Gastroenterology *81*:1098–1103.

Craft C.F., Mendelsohn G., Cooper H.S. and Yardley J.H. (1981) Colonic "Precancer" in Crohn's disease. Gastroenterology *80*:578–584.

Crama-Bohbouth G., Bosman F.T., Vermeer B.J., van der Wal A.M., Biemond I., Weterman I.T. and Pena A.S. (1983) Immunohistological findings in lip biopsy specimens from patients with Crohn's disease and healthy subjects. Gut *24*:202–205.

Craner G.E. and Burdick G.E. (1976) Acute colitis resembling ulcerative colitis in the hemolytic-uremic syndrome. American Journal of Digestive Diseases *21*:74–76.

Cristina M.L., Lehy T., Voillemot N., Arhan P., Pellerin D. and Bonfils S. (1978) Endocrine cells of the colon in Hirschsprung's and control children. Virchows Archiv A. Pathology, Anatomy and Histology *377*:287–300.

Crohn B.B., Ginzburg L. and Oppenheimer G.D. (1932) Regional ileitis: a pathological and clinical entity. Journal of the American Medical Association *99*:1323–1328.

Croom R.D., Donovan M.L. and Schwesinger W.H. (1984) Intestinal endometriosis. American Journal of Surgery *148*:660–667.

Crucioli V. (1972) Rectal biopsy in Crohn's disease. Rendiconti di Gastroenterologia *4*:73–80.

Crucioli V. and Busuttil A. (1981) Human intestinal spirochaetosis. Scandinavian Journal of Gastroenterology *16*, Supplementary 70: 177–179.

Cuvelier C.A., Morson B.C. and Roels H.J. (1987) The DNA content in cancer and dysplasia in chronic ulcerative colitis. Histopathology *11*:927–939.

Dale G., Bonham J.R., Lowdon P., Wagget J., Rangecroft L. and Scott D.J. (1979) Diagnostic value of rectal mucosal acetylcholinesterase levels in Hirschsprung's disease. Lancet *i*:347–349.

Daly J.J. and Chowdary K.V.S. (1983) Pseudomembranous colitis secondary to Metronidazole. Digestive Diseases and Sciences *28*:573–574.

Dankwa E.K. and Davies J.D. (1988) Smooth muscle pseudotumours: a potentially confusing artefact of rectal biopsy. Journal of Clinical Pathology *41*:737–741.

Danzi J.T., McDonald T.J. and King J. (1988) Collagenous colitis. American Journal of Gastroenterology *83*:83–85.

Das K.M., Morecki R., Nair P. and Berkowitz J.M. (1977) Idiopathic proctitis. I. The morphology of proximal colonic mucosa and its clinical significance. American Journal of Digestive Diseases *22*:524–528.

Davidson B.R. and Everson N.W. (1987) Colonic stricture secondary to blunt abdominal trauma: report of a case and review of the aetiology. Postgraduate Medical Journal *63*:911–913.

Dawson I.M.P. and Pryse-Davies J. (1959) The development of carcinoma of the large intestine in ulcerative colitis. British Journal of Surgery *47*:113–128.

Day D.L., Ramsay N.K.C. and Letourneau J.G. (1988) Pneumatosis intestinalis after bone marrow transplantation. American Journal of Radiology *151*:85–87.

Debongnie J.C., De Galocsy C., Caholessur M.O. and Haot J. (1984) Collagenous colitis: a transient condition? Diseases of the Colon and Rectum *27*:672–676.

De Chadarevian J-P., Slim M. and Akel S. (1982) Double zonal aganglionosis in long segment Hirschsprung's disease with a "skip area" in transverse colon. Journal of Pediatric Surgery *17*:195–197.

Dechelotte P., Kantelip B., de Laguillaumie B.V., Labbe A. and Meyer M. (1985) Tangier disease. A histological and ultrastructural study. Pathology, Research and Practice *180*:424–430.

Devroede G., Vobecky S., Masse S., Arhan P., Leger C., Duguay C. and Hemond M. (1982) Ischemic fecal incontinence and rectal angina. Gastroenterology *83*:970–980.

Dickinson R.J., Rampling A. and Wight D.G.D. (1985) Spontaneous pseudomembranous colitis not associated with Clostridium difficile. Journal of Infection *10*:252–255.

Dillard R.P. (1983) Hemolytic-uremic syndrome mimicking ulcerative colitis. Lack of early diagnostic laboratory findings. Clinical Pediatrics *22*:66–67.

Doman D.B., Golding M.I., Goldberg H.J. and Doyle R.B. (1989) Aeromonas hydrophila colitis presenting as medically refractory inflammatory bowel disease. American Journal of Gastroenterology *84*:83–85.

Doolas A., Breyer R.H. and Franklin J.L. (1979) Pneumatosis cystoides intestinalis following jejunoileal by-pass. American Journal of Gastroenterology *72*:271–275.

Doub H.P. and Shea J.J. (1960) Pneumatosis cystoides intestinalis. Journal of American Medical Association *172*:1328–1242.

Douglas J.G. and Crucioli V. (1981) Spirochaetosis: a remediable cause of diarrhoea and rectal bleeding? British Medical Journal *283*:1362.

Dronfield M.W., Fletcher J. and Langman M.J.S. (1974) Coincident salmonella infections and ulcerative colitis: problems of recognition and management. British Medical Journal *19*:99–100.

Duffy T.J. (1981) Reversible ischaemic colitis in young adults. British Journal of Surgery *68*:34–37.

Dundas S.A.C., Kay R., Beck S., Cotton D.W.K., Coup A.J., Slater D.N. and Underwood J.C.E. (1987) Can histopathologists reliably assess dysplasia in chronic inflammatory bowel disease? Journal of Clinical Pathology *40*:1282–1286.

Dvorak A.M., Monahan R.A., Osage J.E. and Dickersin G.R. (1980) Crohn's disease: transmission electron microscopic studies. Human Pathology *11*:606–619.

Dyer N.H., Stansfeld A.G. and Dawson A.M. (1970) The value of rectal biopsy in the diagnosis of Crohn's disease. Scandinavian Journal of Gastroenterology *5*:491–496.

Eaves E.R., McIntyre R.L.E., Wallis P.L. and Korman M.G. (1983) Collagenous colitis: a recently recognised reversible clinico-pathological entity. Australian and New Zealand Journal of Medicine *13*:630–632.

Eckstein R.P., Dowsett J.F. and Riley J.W. (1988) Collagenous enterocolitis: a case of collagenous colitis with involvement of the small intestine. American Journal of Gastroenterology *83*:767–771.

Edouard A., Jouannelle A., Amar A., Doutone P., Maurice P. and Galand A. (1983) Heterotopie de muqueuse gastrique dans le rectum avec ulceration. Gastroenterology and Clinical Biology 7:39–42.

Edwards F.C. and Truelove S.C. (1964) The course and prognosis of ulcerative colitis. Gut *5*:15–22.

Ehsanullah M., Filipe M.I. and Gazzard B. (1982) Morphological and mucus secretion criteria for differential diagnosis of solitary ulcer syndrome and non-specific proctitis. Journal of Clinical Pathology *35*:26–30.

Ehsanullah M., Morgan M.N., Filipe M.I. and Gazzard B. (1985) Sialomucins in the assessment of dysplasia and cancer-risk patients with ulcerative colitis treated with colectomy and ileorectal anastomosis. Histopathology *9*:223–235.

Elliott P.R., Williams C.B., Lennard-Jones J.E., Dawson A.M., Bartram C.I., Thomas B.M., Swarbrick E.T. and Morson B.C. (1982) Colonoscopic diagnosis of minimal change colitis in patients with a normal sigmoidoscopy and normal air-contrast barium enema. Lancet *i*:650–651.

El-Mouzan M.I., Satti M.B., Al-Quorain A.A. and El-Ageb A. (1988) Colonic malacoplakia: occurrence in a family. Report of cases. Diseases of the Colon and Rectum *31*:390–393.

Epstein R.J., McDonald G.B., Sale G.E., Shulman H.M. and Thomas E.D. (1980) The diagnostic accuracy of the rectal biopsy in acute graft-versus-host disease: a prospective study of thirteen patients. Gastroenterology *78*:764–771.

Evans D.J. and Pollock D.J. (1972) In-situ and invasive carcinoma of the colon in patients with ulcerative colitis. Gut *13*:566–570.

Fabricius P.J., Gyde S.N., Shouler P., Keighley M.R.B., Alexander-Williams J. and Allan R.N. (1985) Crohn's disease in the elderly. Gut *26*:461–465.

Fan S.T., Lau W.Y. and Wong K.K. (1986) Ischemic colitis in Kawasaki disease. Journal of Pediatric Surgery *21*:964–965.

Farah D.A., Mills P.R., Lee F.D., McLay A. and Russell R.I. (1985) Collagenous colitis: possible response to sulfasalazine and local steroid therapy. Gastroenterology *88*:792–797.

Farmer R.G. and Brown C.H. (1972) Emerging concepts of proctosigmoiditis. Diseases of the Colon and Rectum *15*:142–146.

Fausa O., Foerster A. and Hovig T. (1985) Collagenous colitis. A clinical, histological and ultrastructural study. Scandinavian Journal of Gastroenterology *20*(suppl. 107):8–23.

Feinberg S.B., Schwartz M.Z., Clifford S., Buchwald H. and Varco R.L. (1977) Significance of pneumatosis cystoides intestinalis after jejunoileal bypass. American Journal of Surgery *133*:149–152.

Fekete C.N., Ricour C., Martelli H., Jacob S.L. and Pellerin D. (1986) Total colonic aganglionosis (with or without ileal involvement): a review of 27 cases. Journal of Pediatric Surgery *21*:251–254.

Fielding J.F. and Lumsden K. (1973) Large-bowel perforations in patients undergoing sigmoidoscopy and barium enema. British Medical Journal *1*:471–473.

Figueroa-Colon R., Grunow J.E., Torres-Pinedo R. and Rettig P.J. (1984) Group A streptococcal proctitis and vulvovaginitis in a prepubertal girl. Pediatric Infectious Disease *3*:439–441.

Filipe M.I., Edwards M.R. and Ehsanullah M. (1985) A prospective study of dysplasia and carcinoma in the rectal biopsies and rectal stump of eight patients following ileorectal anastomosis in ulcerative colitis. Histopathology *9*:1139–1153.

Fishel R., Hamamoto G., Barbul A., Jiji V. and Efron G. (1985) Cocaine colitis: is this a new syndrome? Diseases of the Colon and Rectum *28*:264–266.

Flejou J.F., Grimaud J.A., Molas G., Baviera E. and Potet F. (1984) Collagenous colitis. Ultrastructural study and collagen immunotyping of four cases. Archives of Pathology and Laboratory Medicine *108*:977–982.

Flejou J.F., Potet F., Bogomoletz W.V., Rigaud C., Fenzy A., Le Quintrec Y., Goldfain D. and Brousse N. (1988) Lymphoid follicular proctitis. A condition different from ulcerative proctitis? Digestive Diseases and Sciences *33*:314–320.

Foerster A. and Fausa O. (1985) Collagenous colitis. Pathology, Research and Practice *180*:99–104.

Ford M.J., Anderson J.R., Gilmour H.M., Holt S., Sircus W. and Heading R.C. (1983) Clinical spectrum of "Solitary Ulcer" of the rectum. Gastroenterology *84*:1533–1540.

Foucar E., Mukai K., Foucar K., Sutherland D.E.R. and Van Buren C.T. (1981) Colon ulceration in lethal cytomegalovirus infection. American Journal of Clinical Pathology *76*:788–801.

Fozard J.B.J. and Dixon M.F. (1989) Colonoscopic surveillance in ulcerative colitis: dysplasia through the looking glass. Gut *30*:285–292.

Fozard J.B.J., Dixon M.F., Axon A.T.R. and Giles G.R. (1987) Lectin and mucin histochemistry as an aid to cancer surveillance in ulcerative colitis. Histopathology *11*:385–394.

Fozard J.B.J., Quirke P., Dixon M.F., Giles G.R. and Bird C.C. (1986) DNA aneuploidy in ulcerative colitis. Gut *27*:1414–1418.

Franzin G., Dina R., Scarpa A. and Fratton A. (1982) "The evolution of the solitary ulcer of the rectum": an endoscopic and histopathological study. Endoscopy *14*:131–134.

Freeman K., Anthony P.P., Miller D.S. and Warin A.P. (1985) Cronkhite-Canada syndrome: a new hypothesis. Gut *26*:531–536.

Friedman N.B. (1942) Effects of radiation on the gastrointestinal tract including the salivary glands, the liver and the pancreas. Archives of Pathology *34*:748–787.

Fujisawa K., Watanabe H., Yamamoto K., Nasu T., Kitahara Y. and Nakano M. (1989) Primary atypical mycobacteriosis of the intestine: a report of three cases. Gut *30*:541–545.

Gad A. (1983) The pathogenicity of intestinal spirochaetosis. Histopathology *7*:140–141.

Gad A.A., Meyer P.R. and Taylor C.R. (1987) Papillomavirus antigens in anorectal condyloma and carcinoma in homosexual men. Journal of the American Medical Association *257*:337–340.

Gad A., Willen R., Furugard K., Forbes B. and Hradsky M. (1977). Intestinal spirochaetosis as a cause of longstanding diarrhoea. Upsala Journal of Medical Sciences *82*:49–54.

Gafni J. and Sohar E. (1960) Rectal biopsy for the diagnosis of amyloidosis. Americal Journal of Medical Science *240*:332–336.

Galian A., Le Charpentier Y., Goldfain D. and Chauveinc L. (1982) La colite collagene. A propos d'un nouveau cas avec etude ultrastructurale. Gastroenterology and Clinical Biology *6*:365–370.

Galland R.B. and Spencer J. (1985) The natural history of clinically established radiation enteritis. Lancet *i*:1257–1258.

Gambescia R.A., Kaufman B., Noy J., Young J. and Tedesco F.J. (1976) Schistosoma mansoni infection of the colon: a case report and review of the late colonic manifestations. American Journal of Digestive Diseases *21*:988–991.

Gardiner G.W., Goldberg R., Currie D. and Murray D. (1984) Colonic carcinoma associated with an abnormal collagen table. Cancer *54*:2973–2977.

Gardiner G.W., McAuliffe N., and Murray D. (1984) Colitis cystica profunda occurring in a radiation-induced colonic stricture. Human Pathology *15*:295–298.

Gebbers J-O., Ferguson D.J.P., Mason C., Kelly P. and Jewell D.P. (1987) Spirochaetosis of the human rectum associated with an intraepithelial mast cell and IgE plasma cell response. Gut *28*:588–593.

George W.L. (1984) Antimicrobial agent-associated colitis and diarrhea: historical background and clinical aspects. Reviews of Infectious Diseases *6*:S208-S213.

George W.L., Nakata M.M. Thompson J. and White M.L. (1985) Aeromonas-related diarrhea in adults. Archives of Internal Medicine *145*:2207–2211.

George W.L., Rolfe R.D. and Finegold S.M. (1982) Clostridium difficile and its cytotoxin in feces of patients with antimicrobial agent-associated diarrhea and miscellaneous conditions. Journal of Clinical Microbiology *15*:1049–1053.

Gerding D.N., Olson M.M., Peterson L.R., Teasley D.G., Gebhard R.L., Schwartz M.L. and Lee J.T. (1986) Clostridium difficile-associated diarrhea and colitis in adults. Archives of Internal Medicine *146*:95–100.

Giardiello F.M., Bayless T.M., Jessurun J., Hamilton S.R. and Yardley J.H. (1987) Collagenous colitis: physiologic and histopathologic studies in seven patients. Annals of Internal Medicine *106*:46–49.

Gibson G.E., Rowland R. and Heckler R. (1975) Diarrhoea and colitis associated with antibiotic treatment. A report of 16 cases. Australian and New Zealand Journal of Medicine *5*:340–347.

Gillin J.S., Shike M., Alcock N., Urmacher C., Krown S., Kurtz R.C., Lightdale C.J. and Winawer S.J. (1985) Malabsorption and mucosal abnormalities of the small intestine in the acquired immunodeficiency syndrome. Annals of Internal Medicine *102*:619–622.

Gilman R., Islam M., Paschi S., Goleburn J. and Ahmad F. (1980) Comparison of conventional and immunofluorescent techniques for the detection of entamoeba histolytica in rectal biopsies. Gastroenterology *78*:435–439.

Gleason T.H. and Patterson S.D. (1982) The pathology of Yersinia enterocolitica ileocolitis. American Journal of Surgical Pathology *6*:347–355.

Gledhill A., Enticott M.E. and Howe S. (1986) Variation in the argyrophil cell population of the rectum in ulcerative colitis and adenocarcinoma. Journal of Pathology *149*:287–291.

Gledhill A., Hall P.A., Cruse J.P. and Pollock D.J. (1986) Enteroendocrine cell hyperplasia, carcinoid tumours and adenocarcinoma in long-standing ulcerative colitis. Histopathology *10*:501–508.

Glotzer D.J., Glick M. E. and Goldman H. (1981) Proctitis and colitis following diversion of the fecal stream. Gastroenterology *80*:438–441.

Goldfain D., Potet F., Chauveinc L. and Rozenberg H. (1981) Lipomatose rectale. Association a une lipomatose pelvienne. Gastroenterology and Clinical Biology *5*:884–891.

Goldman H. and Proujansky R. (1986) Allergic proctitis and gastroenteritis in children. American Journal of Surgical Pathology *10*:75–86.

Gonzalez-Angulo A., Corral E., Garcia-Torres R. and Quijano M. (1965) Malakoplakia of the colon. Gastroenterology *48*:383–387.

Goodman M.J., Skinner J.M. and Truelove S.C. (1976) Abnormalities in the apparently normal bowel mucosa in Crohn's disease. Lancet *1*:275–278.

Gore R.M. (1982) Acute colitis and the hemolytic-uremic syndrome. Diseases of the Colon and Rectum *25*:589–591.

Gore R.M., Marn C.S., Ujiki G.T., Craig R.M., and Marquardt J. (1983) Ischemic colitis associated with systemic lupus erythematosus. Diseases of the Colon and Rectum *26*:449–451.

Gould S.R., Handley A.J. and Barnardo D.E. (1973) Rectal and gastric involvement in a case of sarcoidosis. Gut *14*:971–973.

Goulston S.J.M. and McGovern V.J. (1965) Pseudo-membranous colitis. Gut *6*:207–212.

Goulston S.J.M. and McGovern V.J. (1969) The nature of benign strictures in ulcerative colitis. New England Journal of Medicine *281*:290–295.

Gourevitch A. and Cunningham I.J. (1959) Sarcoidosis of the sigmoid colon. Postgraduate Medical Journal *35*:689–691.

Graham C.F., Gallagher K. and Jones J.K. (1981) Acute colitis with methyldopa. New England Journal of Medicine *304*:1044–1045.

Graham J.M., Marin-Padilla M. and Hoefnagel D. (1983) Jejunal atresia associated with Cafergot ingestion during pregnancy. Clinical Pediatrics *22*:226–228.

Greaney M.G. and Jackson P.R. (1977) Oleogranuloma of the rectum produced by Lasonil ointment. British Medical Journal *2*:997–998.

Green E.S., Parker N.E., Gellert A.R. and Beck E.R. (1984) Campylobacter infection mimicking Crohn's disease in an immunodeficient patient. British Journal of Medicine *289*:159–160.

Green P.A., Higgins J.A., Brown A.L., Jr., Hoffman H.N. and Sommerville R.L. (1961) Amyloidosis: appraisal of intubation biopsy of the small intestine in diagnosis. Gastroenterology *41*:452–456.

Grouls V., Vogel J. and Sorger M. (1982) Collagenous colitis. Endoscopy *14*:31–33.

Gruenberg J.C., Grodsinsky C. and Ponka J.L. (1979) Pneumatosis intestinalis: a clinical classification. Diseases of the Colon and Rectum *22*:5–9.

Gryboski J.D. (1967) Gastrointestinal mild allergy in infants. Pediatrics *40*:354–362.

Guss C. and Larsen J.G. (1984) Group A beta-hemolytic streptococcal proctocolitis. Pediatric Infectious Disease *3*:442–443.

Gyde S.N., Prior P., Allan R.N., Stevens A., Jewell D.P., Truelove S.C., Lofberg R., Brostrom O. and Hellers G. (1988) Colorectal cancer in ulcerative colitis: a cohort study of primary referrals from three centres. Gut *29*:206–217.

Gyde S.N., Prior P., Macartney J.C. and Thompson H. (1980) Malignancy in Crohn's disease. Gut *21*:1024–1029.

Habib N.A., Dawson P.M., Krausz T., Blount M.A., Kersten D. and Wood C.B. (1986) A study of histochemical changes in mucus from patients with ulcerative colitis, Crohn's disease, and diverticular disease of the colon. Diseases of the Colon and Rectum *29*:15–17.

Haboubi N.Y., Honan R.P., Hasleton P.S., Ali H.H., Anfield C., Hobbiss J. and Schofield P.F. (1984) Pneumatosis coli: a case report with ultrastructural study. Histopathology *8*:145–155.

Haboubi N.Y., Schofield P.F. and Rowland P.L. (1988) The light and electron microscopic features of early and late phase radiation-induced proctitis. American Journal of Gastroenterology *83*:1140–1144.

Hall C.L. and Lampert P.W. (1985) Immunohistochemistry as an aid in the diagnosis of Hirschsprung's disease. American Journal of Clinical Pathology *83*:177–181.

Hamilton I., Sanders S., Hopwood D. and Bouchier I.A.D. (1986) Collagenous colitis associated with small intestinal villous atrophy. Gut *27*:1394–1398.

Harig J.M., Soergel K.H., Komorowski R.A., and Wood C.M. (1989) Treatment of diversion colitis with short-chain fatty-acid irrigation. New England Journal of Medicine *320*:23–28.

Harland W.A. and Lee F.D. (1967) Intestinal spirochaetosis. British Medical Journal *iii*:718–719.

Hasleton P.S., Carr N. and Schofield P.F. (1985) Vascular changes in radiation bowel disease. Histopathology *9*:517–534.

Hawker P.C., Hine K.R., Burdon D.W., Thompson H. and Keighley M.R.B. (1981) Fatal pseudomembranous colitis despite eradication of Clostridium difficile. British Medical Journal *282*:109–110.

Haworth S.J. and Pusey C.D. (1984) Severe intestinal involvement in Wegener's granulomatosis. Gut *25*:1296–1300.

Heatley R.V. and James P.D. (1978) Eosinophils in the rectal mucosa. Gut *20*:787–791.

Heer M., Altorfer J., Pirovino M. and Schmid M. (1983) Pneumatosis cystoides coli: a rare complication of colonoscopy. Endoscopy *15*:119–120.

Heer M., Repond F., Hany A., Sulser H., Kehl O. and Jager K. (1987) Acute ischaemic colitis in a female long distance runner. Gut *28*:896–899.

Heizer W.D., Warshaw A.L., Waldmann T.A. and Laster L. (1968) Protein-losing gastroenteropathy and malabsorption associated with factitious diarrhoea. Annals of Internal Medicine *68*:839–852.

Helliwell T.R., Flook D., Whitworth J. and Day D.W. (1985) Arteritis and venulitis in systemic lupus erythematosus resulting in massive lower intestinal haemorrhage. Histopathology *9*:1103–1113.

Henriksson L., Liljeholm H. and Lonnerholm T. (1984) Pelvic lipomatosis causing constriction of the lower urinary tract and the rectum. Scandinavian Journal of Urology and Nephrology *18*:249–252.

Heron H.C., Khubchandani I.T., Trimpi H.D., Sheets J.A. and Stasik J.J. (1981) Evanescent colitis. Diseases of the Colon and Rectum *24*:555–561.

Herrerias J.M., Muniain M.A., Sanchez S. and Garrido M. (1983) Alcohol induced colitis. Endoscopy *15*:121–122.

Hiatt G.A. (1978) Miliary tuberculosis with ileocecal involvement diagnosed by colonoscopy. American Medical Association Journal *240*:561–563.

Hirata I., Berrebi G., Austin L.L., Keren D.F. and Dobbins W.O. (1986) Immunohistological characterization of intraepithelial and lamina propria lymphocytes in control ileum and colon and in inflammatory bowel disease. Digestive Diseases and Sciences *31*:593–603.

Ho M.S., Teh L.B. and Goh H.S. (1987) Ischaemic colitis in systemic lupus erythematosus: report of a case and review of the literature. Annals Academy of Medicine *16*:501–503.

Holdsworth C.D. (1984) Acute self limited colitis. British Medical Journal *289*:270–271.

Houghton B.J. and Pears M.A. (1958) Chronic potassium depletion due to purgation with cascara. British Medical Journal *i*:1328–1330.

Hovind-Hougen K., Birch-Andersen A., Henrik-Nielsen R., Orholm M., Pedersen J.O., Teglbjaerg P.S. and Thaysen E.H. (1982) Intestinal spirochetosis: morphological characterization and cultivation of the spirochete Brachyspira aalborgi gen. nov., sp. nov. Journal of Clinical Microbiology *16*:1127–1136.

Hunt D.R. and Mildenhall P. (1975) Etiology of strictures of the colon associated with pancreatitis. American Journal of Digestive Diseases *20*:941–946.

Huntley C.C., Shaffner L. de S., Challa V.R. and Lyerly A.D. (1982) Histochemical diagnosis of Hirschsprung disease. Pediatrics *69*:755–761.

Hyams J.S., Haswell J.E., Gerber M.A. and Berman M.M. (1985) Colonic ulceration in histiocytosis X. Journal of Pediatric Gastroenterology and Nutrition *4*:286–290.

Hyams J.S. and McLaughlin J.C. (1985) Lack of relationship between Clostridium difficile toxin and inflammatory bowel disease in children. Journal of Clinical Gastroenterology *7*:387–390.

Iliffe G.D. and Owen D.A. (1981) Rectal biopsy in Crohn's disease. Digestive Diseases and Sciences *26*:321–324.

Imamura T., Tsuruta J., Kambara T. and Maki S. (1986) Pseudomembranous colitis in a patient of Paraquat intoxication. Acta Pathologica Japonica *36*:309–316.

Innes A., Rowe P.A., Foster M.C., Steiger M.J. and Morgan A.G. (1988) Cyclosporin toxicity and colitis. Lancet *ii*:957.

Isaacs D., Wright V.M., Shaw D.G., Raafat F. and Walker-Smith J.A. (1985) Chronic granulomatous disease mimicking Crohn's disease. Journal of Pediatric Gastroenterology and Nutrition *4*:498–501.

Jablonski M., Putzki H. and Heymann H. (1987) Necrosis of the ascending colon in chronic hemodialysis patients. Diseases of the Colon and Rectum *30*:623–625.

Jacob E., Baker S.J. and Swaminathan S.P. (1987) "M" cells in the follicle-associated epithelium of the human colon. Histopathology *11*:941–952.

Jager W.A., Den Hartog and Bethlem J. (1960) The distribution of Lewy bodies in the central and autonomic nervous system in idiopathic paralysis agitans. Journal of Neurology, Neurosurgery and Psychiatry *23*:283–290.

Jenkins H.R., Pincott J.R., Soothill J.F., Milla P.J. and Harries J.T. (1984) Food allergy: the major cause of infantile colitis. Archives of Disease in Childhood *59*:326–329.

Jess P. (1981) Acute terminal ileitis. A review of recent literature on the relationship to Crohn's disease. Scandinavian Journal of Gastroenterology *16*:321–324.

Jessurun J., Paplanus S.H., Nagle R.B., Hamilton S.R., Yardley J.H. and Tripp M. (1986) Pseudosarcomatous changes in inflammatory pseudopolyps of the colon. Archives of Pathology and Laboratory Medicine *110*:833–836.

Jessurun J., Yardley J.H., Giardiello F.M., Hamilton S.R. and Bayless T.M. (1987) Chronic colitis with thickening of the subepithelial collagen layer (Collagenous Colitis). Human Pathology *18*:839–848.

Jessurun J., Yardley J.H., Lee E.L., Vendrell D.D., Schiller L.R. and Fordtran J.S. (1986) Microscopic and collagenous colitis: different names for the same condition? Gastroenterology *91*:1583–1584.

Jonas G., Mahoney A., Murray J. and Gertler S. (1988) Chemical colitis due to endoscope cleaning solutions: a mimic of pseudomembranous colitis. Gastroenterology *95*:1403–1408.

Jones H.W., Grogono J. and Hoare A.M. (1988) Surveillance in ulcerative colitis: burdens and benefit. Gut *29*:325–331.

Jorgensen A. and Wille-Jorgensen P. (1982) Pneumatosis intestinalis and pneumoperitoneum due to a solitary sigmoid diverticulum. Acta Chirurgica Scandinavica *148*:625–626.

Justus P.G., Martin J.L., Goldberg D.A., Taylor N.S., Bartlett J.G., Alexander R.W. and Mathias J.R. (1982) Myoelectric effects of Clostridium difficile: motility-altering factors distinct from its cytotoxin and enterotoxin in rabbits. Gastroenterology *83*:836–843.

Kalkay M.N., Ayanian Z.S., Lehaf E.A. and Baldi A. (1983) Campylobacter-induced toxic megacolon. American Journal of Gastroenterology *78*:557–559.

Kalla A.H., Lee K.U. and Voss E.C. Jr. (1980) The dilemma of colonic vasculitis: report of a unique case. Diseases of the Colon and Rectum *23*:590–596.

Kaplan L.R. and Takeuchi A. (1979) Purulent rectal discharge associated wih a nontreponemal spirochete. Journal of the American Medical Association *241*:52–53.

Kapur B.M.L. and Chopra P. (1978) Necrotizing amebic colitis: report of five cases. Diseases of the Colon and Rectum *21*:447–449.

Katayama Y., Kimura M. and Konn M. (1985) Cronkhite-Canada syndrome associated with a rectal cancer and adenomatous changes in colonic polyps. American Journal of Surgical Pathology *9*:65–71.

Katoh K., Matsunaga K., Ishigatsubo Y., Chiba J., Tani K., Kitamura H., Tani S. and Handwerger B.S. (1985) Pathologically defined neuro-, vasculo-, entero-Behçet's disease. Journal of Rheumatology *12*:1186–1190.

Kaufmann H.J. and Taubin H.L. (1987) Nonsteroidal anti-inflammatory drugs activate quiescent inflammatory bowel disease. Annals of Internal Medicine *107*:513–516.

Kealy W.F. (1976a) Colonic lymphoid-glandular complex (microbursa) nature and morphology. Journal of Clinical Pathology *29*:241–244.

Kealy W.F. (1976b) Lymphoid tissue and lymphoid-glandular complexes of the colon: relation to diverticulosis. Journal of Clinical Pathology 29:245–249.

Keefe E.B. and Girard D.E. (1985) Peanut shell colitis. Archives of Internal Medicine 145:1314–1315.

Kelly J.K., Langevin J.M., Price L.M., Hershfield N.B., Share S. and Blustein P. (1986) Giant and symptomatic inflammatory polyps of the colon in idiopathic inflammatory bowel disease. American Journal of Surgical Pathology 10:420–428.

Kelly J.K., Pai C.H., Jadusingh I.H., Macinnis M.L., Shaffer E.A. and Hershfield N.B. (1987) The histopathology of rectosigmoid biopsies from adults with bloody diarrhea due to verotoxin-producing escherichia coli. American Journal of Clinical Pathology 88:78–82.

Kessler S. and Campbell J.R. (1985) Neuronal colonic dysplasia associated with short-segment Hirschsprung's disease. Archives of Pathology and Laboratory Medicine 109:532–533.

Keyting W.S., McCarver R.R., Kovarik J.L. and Daywitt A.I. (1961) Pneumatosis intestinalis: a new concept. Radiology 76:733–741.

Killingback M.J. and Williams K.L. (1961) Necrotising colitis. British Journal of Surgery 49:175–185.

Kilpatrick Z.M., Farman J., Yesner R. and Spiro H.M. (1968) Ischemic proctitis. Journal of the American Medical Association 205:74–80.

Kim M.W., Hundahl S.A., Dang C.R., McNamara J.J., Straehley C.J. and Whelan T.J. (1983) Ischemic colitis after aortic aneurysmectomy. American Journal of Surgery 145:392–394.

Kinder R.B. and Jourdan M.H. (1985) Disseminated aspergillosis and bleeding colonic ulcers in renal transplant patient. Journal of the Royal Society of Medicine 78:338–339.

Kingham J.G.C., Levison D.A., Ball J.A. and Dawson A.M. (1982) Microscopic colitis: a cause of chronic watery diarrhoea. British Medical Journal 285:1601–1604.

Kingham J.G.C., Levison D.A., Morson B.C. and Dawson A.M. (1986) Collagenous colitis. Gut 27:570–577.

Kirk M.E., Lough J. and Warner H.A. (1971) Histoplasma colitis: an electron microscopic study. Gastroenterology 61:46–54.

Knutson L. and Arosenius K-E. (1984) Tuberculosis of the large bowel. Acta Chirurgica Scandinavica 150:345–348.

Komorowski R.A., Cohen E.B., Kauffman H.M. and Adams M.B. (1986) Gastrointestinal complications in renal transplant recipients. American Journal of Clinical Pathology 86:161–167.

Kondo J., Ruth M., Sassaris M. and Hunter F.M. (1980) Sarcoidosis of the stomach and rectum. American Journal of Gastroenterology 73:516–518.

Korelitz B.I. and Sommers S.C. (1977) Rectal biopsy in patients with Crohn's disease. Normal mucosa on sigmoidoscopic examination. Journal of the American Medical Association 237:2742–2744.

Korelitz B.I., Cheskin L.J., Sohn N. and Sommers S.C. (1984) Proctitis after fecal diversion in Crohn's disease and its elimination with reanastomosis: implications for surgical management. Report of four cases. Gastroenterology 87:710–713.

Koren G., Aladjem M., Militiano J., Seegal B., Jonash A. and Boichis H. (1984) Ischemic colitis in chronic intermittent peritoneal dialysis. Nephron 36:272–274.

Kornman B.S. (1971) Ulcerative colitis, autoimmune epiphenoma and colonic cancer. Cancer 28:82–88

Koss L.G. (1952) Abdominal gas cysts (pneumatosis cystoides intestinorum hominis):analysis with report of case and critical review of literature. Archives of Pathology 53:523–549.

Kumar S.S., Appavu S.S., Abcarian H. and Barreta T. (1983) Amyloidosis of the colon. Report of a case and review of the literature. Diseases of the Colon and Rectum 26:541–544.

Kumar N.B., Nostrant T.T. and Appelman H.D. (1982) The histopathologic spectrum of acute self-limited colitis (acute infectious-type colitis). American Journal of Surgical Pathology 6:523–529.

Kuramoto S., Oohara T., Ihara O., Shimazu R. and Kondo Y. (1987) Granulomas of the gut in Crohn's disease. Diseases of the Colon and Rectum 30:6–11.

Kurer M.H.J., Lawson J.O.N. and Pambakian H. (1986) Suction biopsy in Hirschsprung's disease. Archives of Disease in Childhood 61:83–84.

Kyle R.A., Spencer R.J. and Dahlin D.C. (1966) Value of rectal biopsy in the diagnosis of primary systemic amyloidosis. American Journal of Medical Science 251:501–506.

Kyösola K., Penttilä O. and Salaspuro M. (1977) Rectal mucosal adrenergic innervation and entero-chromaffin cells in ulcerative colitis and irritable colon. Scandinavian Journal of Gastroenterology 12:363–367.

Lake A.M., Whitington P.F. and Hamilton S.R. (1982) Dietary protein-induced colitis in breast-fed infants. Journal of Pediatrics 101:906–910.

Lake B.D., Nixon H.H. and Claireaux A.E. (1978) Hirschsprung's disease. An appraisal of histochemically demonstrated acetylcholinesterase activity in suction rectal biopsy specimens as an aid to diagnosis. Archives of Pathology and Laboratory Medicine 102:244–247.

Lambert M.E., Schofield P.F., Ironside A.G. and Mandal B.K. (1979) Campylobacter colitis. British Medical Journal 1:857–859.

Lampert I.A., Thorpe P., Van Noorden S., Marsh J., Goldman J.M., Gordon-Smith E.C. and Evans D.J. (1985) Selective sparing of enterochromaffin cells in graft versus host disease affecting the colonic mucosa. Histopathology 9:875–886.

Lamy A.L., Roy P.H., Morisette J-J. and Cantin R. (1988) Intimal hyperplasia and thrombosis of the visceral arteries in a young woman: possible relation with oral contraceptives and smoking. Surgery 103:706–710.

Lancet (1977) Pseudomembranous enterocolitis. Lancet *i*:839–840.

Lancet (1983) Colitis in term babies. Lancet *i*:1083–1084.

Lancet (1987) Clostridium septicum and neutropenic enterocolitis. Lancet *ii*:608.

Lancet (1988) Which type of colitis? Lancet *i*:336.

Lancet (1989) Diversion colitis. Lancet *i*:764.

Larson H.E. and Price A.B. (1977) Pseudomembranous colitis: presence of clostridial toxin. Lancet *ii*:1312–1314.

Larson H.E., Price A.B. and Honour P. (1978) Clostridium difficile and the aetiology of pseudomembranous colitis. The Lancet *i*:1063–1066.

Lazenby A.J., Yardley J.H., Giardiello F.M., Jessurun J. and Bayless T.M. (1989) Lymphocytic ("microscopic") colitis: a comparative histopathologic study with particular reference to collagenous colitis. Human Pathology *20*:18–28.

Lee E.L., Smith H.J., Miller G.L., Burns D.K. and Weiner H. (1984) Ischemic pseudomembranous colitis with perforation due to polyarteritis nodosa. American Journal of Gastroenterology *79*:35–38.

Lee R.G. (1986) The colitis of Behçet's syndrome. American Journal of Surgical Pathology *10*:888–893.

Lee R.G. (1987) Villous regeneration in ulcerative colitis. Archives of Pathology and Laboratory Medicine *111*:276–278.

Lee S.H., Barnes W.G., Hodges G.R. and Dixon A. (1985) Perforated granulomatous colitis caused by Histoplasma capsulatum. Diseases of the Colon and Rectum *28*:171–176.

Lefebvre M.P., Leape L.L., Pohl D.A., Safaii H. and Grand R.J. (1984) Total colonic aganglionosis initially diagnosed in an adolescent. Gastroenterology *87*:1364–1366.

Lennard-Jones J.E., Morson B.C., Ritchie J.K. and Williams C.B. (1983) Cancer surveillance in ulcerative colitis. Lancet *ii*:149–152.

Leonard R.C.F. and MacLennan I.C.M. (1982) Distribution of plasma cells in normal rectal mucosa. Journal of Clinical Pathology *35*:820–823.

Leoutsakos B., Agnadi N. and Kolisiatis S. (1977) Rectal bleeding due to oesophagostomum brumpti: Report of a case. Diseases of the Colon and Rectum *20*:632–634.

Leriche M., Devroede G., Sanchez G. and Rossano J. (1978) Changes in the rectal mucosa induced by hypertonic enemas. Diseases of the Colon and Rectum *21*:227–236.

Leung A.C.T., Orange G., McLay A. and Henderson I.S. (1985) Clostridium difficile-associated colitis in uremic patients. Clinical Nephrology *24*:242–248.

Levine D.S. (1987) "Solitary" rectal ulcer syndrome. Are "solitary" rectal ulcer syndrome and "localized" colitis cystica profunda analogous syndromes caused by rectal prolapse? Gastroenterology *92*:243–253.

Levine D., Goode A.W. and Wingate D.L. (1981) Purgative abuse associated with reversible cachexia, hypogammaglobulinaemia, and finger clubbing. Lancet *i*:919–920.

Levine D.S., Surawicz C.M., Ajer T.N., Dean P.J. and Rubin C.E. (1988) Diffuse excess mucosal collagen in rectal biopsies facilitates differential diagnosis of solitary rectal ulcer syndrome from other inflammatory bowel diseases. Digestive Diseases and Sciences *33*:1345–1352.

Levine D.S., Surawicz C.M., Spencer G.D., Rohrmann C.A. and Silverstein F.E. (1986) Inflammatory polyposis two years after ischemic colon injury. Digestive Diseases and Sciences *31*:1159–1167.

Levine M.M. (1987) Escherichia coli that cause diarrhea: enterotoxigenic, enteropathogenic, enteroinvasive, enterohemorrhagic, and enteroadherent. Journal of Infectious Diseases *155*:377–389.

Levison D.A., Crocker P.R., Smith A., Blackshaw A.J. and Bartram C.I. (1984) Varied light and scanning electron microscopic appearances of barium sulphate in smears and histological sections. Journal of Clinical Pathology *37*:481–487.

Lewin K.J., Fair W.R., Steigbigel R.T., Winberg C.D. and Droller M.J. (1976) Clinical and laboratory studies into the pathogenesis of malacoplakia. Journal of Clinical Pathology *29*:354–363.

Lewin K.J., Harell G.S., Lee A.S. and Crowley L.G. (1974) Malacoplakia. An electron-microscopic study: demonstration of bacilliform organisms in malacoplakic macrophages. Gastroenterology *66*:28–45.

Lewin K. and Swales J.D. (1966) Granulomatous colitis and atypical ulcerative colitis: histological features, behaviour, and prognosis. Gastroenterology *50*:211–223.

Lewkonia R.M. and McConnell R.B. (1976) Progress report: familial inflammatory bowel disease. Gut *17*:235–243.

Lillee R.D. and Geer J.C. (1965) On the relation of enterosiderosis pigments of man and guinea pig. Melanosis and pseudomelanosis of colon and villi and the intestinal iron uptake and storage mechanism. Histochemical and experimental studies. American Journal of Pathology *47*:965–1009.

Lillemoe K.D., Romolo J.L., Hamilton S.R., Pennington L.R., Burdick J.F. and Williams G.M. (1987) Intestinal necrosis due to sodium polystyrene (Kayexalate) in sorbitol enemas: clinical and experimental support for the hypothesis. Surgery *101*:267–272.

Lindstrom C.G. (1976) "Collagenous colitis" with watery diarrhoea: new entity? Pathologia Europaea *11*:87–89.

Linssen A. and Tytgat G.N. (1982) Fulminant onset of Crohn's disease of the colon (CDC). An observation of six cases. Digestive Diseases and Sciences *27*:731–736.

Lishman A.H., Al-Jumaili I.J. and Record C.O. (1981) Spectrum of antibiotic-associated diarrhoea. Gut *22*:34–37.

Lockhart-Mummery H.E. and Morson B.C. (1960) Crohn's disease (regional enteritis) of the large intestine and its distinction from ulcerative colitis. Gut *1*:87–105.

Longfield R., O'Donnell J., Yudt W., Lissner C. and Burns T. (1979) Acute colitis and bacteremia due to campylobacter fetus. Digestive Diseases and Sciences *24*:950–953.

Loss R.W. Jr., Mangla J.C. and Pereira M. (1980) Campylobacter colitis presenting as inflammatory bowel disease with segmental colonic ulcerations. Gastroenterology *79*:138–140.

Lusk L.B., Reichen J. and Levine J.S. (1984) Aphthous ulceration in diversion colitis. Clinical implications. Gastroenterology *87*:1171–1173.

Lynn J.T., Gossen G., Miller A. and Russell I.J. (1984) Pneumatosis intestinalis in mixed connective tissue disease: two case reports and literature review. Arthritis and Rheumatism *27*:1186–1189.

McDermott F.T., Pihl E.A., Kemp D.R. and Polglase A.L. (1982) Co-existing Crohn's disease and ulcerative colitis. Diseases of the Colon and Rectum *25*:600–602.

Macfarlane D.A. (1955) Intestinal sarcoidosis. British Journal of Surgery *42*:639–642.

McGovern V.J. (1972) Rectal biopsy in the differential diagnosis of colitis. Rendiconti di Gastroenterologia *4*:94–102

McGovern V.J. and Goulston S.J.M. (1965) Ischaemic enterocolitis. Gut *6*:213–220

McGovern V.J. and Goulston S.J.M. (1968) Crohn's disease of the colon. Gut *9*:164–176.

McIver A.G. and Whitehead R. (1972) Zonal colonic aganglionosis, a variant of Hirschsprung's disease. Archives of Disease in Childhood *47*:233–237.

MacKay E.H. (1978) Malakoplakia in ulcerative colitis. Archives of Pathology and Laboratory Medicine *102*:140–145.

McKendrick M.W., Geddes A.M. and Gearty J. (1982) Campylobacter enteritis: a study of clinical features and rectal mucosal changes. Scandinavian Journal of Infectious Diseases *14*:35–38.

McKendrick T. (1962) Sweat sodium levels in normal subjects, in fibrocystic patients and their relatives, and in chronic bronchitic patients. Lancet *i*:183–186.

MacMahon R.A., Moore C.C.M. and Cussen L.J. (1981) Hirschsprung-like syndromes in patients wih normal ganglion cells on suction rectal biopsy. Journal of Pediatric Surgery *16*:835–839.

Mackle E.J. and Parks T.G. (1986) The pathogenesis and pathophysiology of rectal prolapse and solitary rectal ulcer syndrome. Clinics in Gastroenterology *15*:985–1002.

Madigan M.R. and Morson B.C. (1969) Solitary ulcer of the rectum. Gut *10*:871–881.

Magidson J.G. and Lewin K.J. (1981) Diffuse colitis cystica profunda. Report of a case. American Journal of Surgical Pathology *5*:393–399.

Maher E.R., Dutoit S.H., Baillod R.A., Sweny P. and Moorhead J.F. (1988) Gastrointestinal complications of dialysis-related amyloidosis. British Medical Journal 297:265–266.

Malhotra R. and Sheffield A. (1988) Cronkhite-Canada syndrome associated with colon carcinoma and adenomatous changes in C-C polyps. American Journal of Gastroenterology *83*:772–776.

Mandal B.K., Schofield P.F. and Morson B.C. (1982) A clinicopathological study of acute colitis: the dilemma of transient colitis syndrome. Scandinavian Journal of Gastroenterology *17*:865–869.

Marchildon M.B., Buck B.E. and Abdenour G. (1982) Necrotizing enterocolitis in the unfed infant. Journal of Pediatric Surgery *17*:620–624.

Margaretten W. and McKay D.G. (1971) Thrombotic ulcerations of the gastrointestinal tract. Archives of Internal Medicine *127*:250–253.

Marsh P.K. and Gorbach S.L. (1982) Invasive enterocolitis caused by Edwardsiella tarda. Gastroenterology *82*:336–338.

Marshall A.R., AL-Jumaili I.J., Fenwick G.A., Bint A.J. and Record C.O. (1987) Cryptosporidiosis in patients at a large teaching hospital. Journal of Clinical Microbiology *25*:172–173.

Marston A. (1977) In Intestinal Ischaemia. London: Edward Arnold.

Marston A., Pheils M.T., Lea Thomas M. and Morson B.C. (1966) Ischaemic colitis. Gut *7*:1–15.

Martin C.J., Parks T.G. and Biggart J.D. (1981) Solitary rectal ulcer syndrome in Northern Ireland, 1971–1980. British Journal of Surgery *68*:744–747.

Martin D.M., Goldman J.A., Gilliam J. and Nasrallah S.M. (1981) Gold-induced eosinophilic enterocolitis: response to oral cromolyn sodium. Gastroenterology *80*:1567–1570.

Mathan M.M., Venkatesan S., George R., Mathew M. and Mathan V.I. (1985) Cryptosporidium and diarrhoea in Southern Indian children. Lancet *ii*:1172–1175.

Matseshe J.W., Go V.L.W. and Dimagno E.P. (1977) Meconium ileus equivalent complicating cystic fibrosis in postneonatal children and young adults. Report of 12 cases. Gastroenterology *72*:732–736.

Matsui T., Iwashita A., Iida M., Kume K. and Fujishima M. (1987) Acquired pseudoobstruction of the colon due to segmental hypoganglionosis. Gastrointestinal Radiology *12*:262–264.

Mayberry J.F., Ballantyne K.C., Hardcastle J.D., Mangham C. and Pye G. (1989) Epidemiological study of asymptomatic inflammatory bowel disease: the identification of cases during a screening programme for colorectal cancer. Gut *30*:481–483.

Mazier W.P., Sun K.M. and Robertson W.G. (1978) Oil-induced granuloma (eleoma) of the rectum: Report of four cases. Diseases of the Colon and Rectum *21*:292–294.

Meacham P.W. and Brantley B. (1987) Familial fibromuscular dysplasia of the mesenteric arteries. Southern Medical Journal *80*:1311–1316.

Meisel J.L., Bergman D., Graney D., Saunders D.R. and Rubin C.E. (1977) Human rectal mucosa: proctoscopic and morphological changes caused by laxatives. Gastroenterology *72*:1274–1279.

Miller R.R. and Sumner H.W. (1982) Argyrophilic cell hyperplasia and an atypical carcinoid tumor in chronic ulcerative colitis. Cancer *50*:2920–2925.

Ming-Chai C., Jen-Chun H., P'ei-Yu C., Ch'i-Yuan C., P'eng-Fei T., Shen-Hsing C., Fu-P'an W., Ts'u-Ling C. and Shun-Ch'uan C. (1965) Pathogenesis of carcinoma of the colon and rectum in Schistosomiasis Japonica: a study of 90 cases. Chinese Medical Journal *84*:513–525.

Missmahl H.P. and Riemann J. (1968) Einfacher nachweis der Mikroangiopathie an den Kapillaren der Rectumschleimhaut bei Diabetikern. Klinische Wochenschrift *46*:374–376.

Mitchell T.J., Ketley J.M., Haslam S.C., Stephen J., Burdon D.W., Candy D.C.A. and Daniel R. (1986) Effect of toxin A and B of Clostridium difficile on rabbit ileum and colon. Gut *27*:78–85.

Morgensen A.M., Olsen J.H. and Gudmand-Hoyer E. (1984) Collagenous colitis. Acta Medica Scandinavica *216*:535–540.

Moroz S.P., Schroeder M., Trevenen C.L. and Cross H. (1984) Systemic histiocytosis: an unusual cause of perianal disease in a child. Journal of Pediatric Gastroenterology and Nutrition *3*:309–311.

Morson B.C. (1966) Factors influencing the prognosis of early cancer of the rectum. Proceedings of the Royal Society of Medicine *59*:607–608.

Morson B.C. and Dawson I.M.P. (1979) Gastrointestinal Pathology. 2nd Edition. London: Blackwells, p. 514.

Morson B.C. and Pang L.S. (1967) Rectal biopsy as an aid to cancer control in ulcerative colitis. Gut *8*:423–434.

Moss T.J. and Adler R. (1982) Necrotizing enterocolitis in older infants, children, and adolescents. Journal of Pediatrics *100*:764–768.

Mower W.J., Hawkins J.A. and Nelson E.W. (1986) Neutropenic enterocolitis in adults with acute leukemia. Archives of Surgery *121*:571–574.

Mulholland M.W. and Delaney J.P. (1983) Neutropenic colitis and aplastic anemia. Annals of Surgery *197*:84–90.

Munakata K., Morita K., Okabe I. and Sueoka H. (1985) Clinical and histologic studies of neuronal intestinal dysplasia. Journal of Pediatric Surgery *20*:231–235.

Murdoch D.L. and Piris J. (1982) Immunoglobulin E in non-specific proctitis and ulcerative colitis: studies with a monoclonal antibody. Digestion *25*:201–204.

Murphy B.J. and Weinfeld A. (1987) Innocuous pneumatosis intestinalis of the right colon in renal transplant recipients. Diseases of the Colon and Rectum *30*:816–819.

Murray F.E., Lombard M., Dervan P., Fitzgerald R.J. and Crowe J. (1988) Bleeding from multifocal heterotopic gastric mucosa in the colon controlled by an H2 antagonist. Gut *29*:848–851.

Murray F.E., O'Brien M.J., Birkett D.H., Kennedy S.M. and LaMont J.T. (1987) Diversion colitis. Pathologic findings in a resected sigmoid colon and rectum. Gastroenterology *93*:1404–1408.

Myeren J., Serck-Hanssen A. and Solberg L. (1976) Routine and blind histological diagnoses on colonoscopic biopsies compared to clinical-colonoscopic observations in patients without and with colitis. Scandinavian Journal of Gastroenterology *11*:135–140.

Myers A., Humphries D.M. and Cox E.V. (1976) A ten year follow-up of haemorrhagic proctitis. Postgraduate Medical Journal *52*:224–228.

Nagasako K., Nakae Y., Kitao Y. and Aoki G. (1977) Colitis cystica profunda: report of a case in which differentiation from rectal cancer was difficult. Diseases of the Colon and Rectum *20*:618–624.

Namdaran F., Dutz W. and Ovasepian A. (1979) Pneumatosis cystoides intestinalis in Iran. Gut *20*:16–21.

Nebel O.T., El-Masry N.A., Castell D.O., Farid Z., Fornes M.F. and Sparks H.A. (1974) Schistosomal colonic polyposis. Gastrointestinal Endoscopy *20*:99–101.

Neto J.A.R. and Ribeiro A.P. (1974) Trombose mesenterica inferior. Revista da Associacao Medica Brasileira *20*:180–190

Nielsen R.H., Orholm M., Pedersen J.O., Hovind-Hougen K., Teglbjaerg P.S. and Thaysen E.H. (1983) Colorectal spirochetosis: clinical significance of the infestation. Gastroenterology *85*:62–67.

Nielsen V.T., Vetner M. and Harslof E. (1980) Collagenous colitis. Histopathology *4*:83–86.

Nolan N.P.M., Kelly C.P., Humphreys J.F.H., Cooney C., O'Connor R., Walsh T.N., Weir D.G. and O'Briain D.S. (1987) An epidemic of pseudomembranous colitis: importance of person to person spread. Gut *28*:1467–1473.

Nostrant T.T., Kumar N.B. and Appelman H.D. (1987) Histopathology differentiates acute self-limited colitis from ulcerative colitis. Gastroenterology *92*:318–328.

O'Donnell N. (1987) Enteritis cystica profunda - revisited. Human Pathology *18*:1300–1301.

Olding L.B., Ahren C., Thurin J., Karlsson K-A., Svalander C. and Koprowski H. (1985) Gastrointestinal carcinoma-associated antigen detected by a monoclonal antibody in dysplasia and adenocarcinoma associated with chronic ulcerative colitis. International Journal of Cancer *36*:131–136.

O'Leary A.D. and Sweeney E.C. (1986) Lymphoglandular complexes of the colon: structure and distribution. Histopathology *10*:267–283.

Ona F.V. and Boger J.N. (1985) Rectal bleeding due to diversion colitis. American Journal of Gastroenterology *80*:40–41.

Orchard J.L. and Lawson R. (1986) Severe colitis induced by soap enemas. Southern Medical Journal *79*:1459–1460.

Owen D.A., Hwang W.S., Thorlakson R.H. and Walli E. (1981) Malignant carcinoid tumor complicating chronic ulcerative colitis. American Journal of Clinical Pathology *76*:333–338.

Pai C.H., Gordon R., Sims H.V. and Bryan L.E. (1984) Sporadic cases of hemorrhagic colitis associated with escherichia coli 0157:H7. Annals of Internal Medicine *101*:738–742.

Palmer K.R., Berry H., Wheeler P.J., Williams C.B., Fairclough P., Morson B.C. and Silk D.B.A. (1986) Collagenous colitis: a relapsing and remitting disease. Gut *27*:578–580.

Panachi G., Pantosti A., Gentile G., Testore G.P., Venditti M., Martinos P. and Serra P. (1985) Clostridium difficile colitis in leukemia patients. European Journal of Cancer and Clinical Oncology *21*:1159–1163.

Papa M.Z., Shiloni E. and McDonald H.D. (1986) Total colonic necrosis. A catastrophic complication of systemic lupus erythematosus. Diseases of the Colon and Rectum *29*:576–578.

Parc R., Douvin D. and Loygue J. (1979) Le megacolon congenital de l'adulte. Etude de 15 cas. Gastroenterologie Clinique et Biologique *3*:321–328.

Parelkar S.N., Stamm W.P. and Hill K.R. (1971) Indirect immunofluorescent staining of entamoeba histolytica in tissues. Lancet *i*:212–213.

Parkins R.A., Eidelman S., Rubin C.E., Dobbins W.O. and Phelps P.C. (1963) The diagnosis of cystic fibrosis by rectal suction biopsy. Lancet *ii*:851–856.

Parks A.G., Porter N.H. and Hardcastle J. (1966) The syndrome of the descending perineum. Proceedings of the Royal Society of Medicine *59*:477–482.

Pascal R.R., Kaye G.I. and Lane N. (1968) Colonic pericryptal fibroblast sheath: replication, migration, and cytodifferentiation of a mesenchymal cell system in adult tissue. 1. Autoradiographic studies of normal rabbit colon. Gastroenterology *54*:835–851.

Patrick W.J.A., Besley G.T.N. and Smith I.I. (1980) Histochemical diagnosis of Hirschsprung's disease and a comparison of the histochemical and biochemical activity of acetylcholinesterase in rectal mucosal biopsies. Journal of Clinical Pathology *33*:336–343.

Patterson D.J., Johnson E.H. and Schmulen A.C. (1984) Fulminant pseudomembranous colitis occurring after colonoscopy. Gastrointestinal Endoscopy *30*:249–253.

Pearson D.J., Stones N.A., Bentley S.J. and Reid H. (1983) Proctocolitis induced by salicylate and associated with asthma and recurrent nasal polyps. British Medical Journal *287*:1675.

Peart A.G., Sivak M.V., Rankin G.B., Kish L.S. and Steck W.D. (1984) Spontaneous improvement of Cronkhite-Canada syndrome in a postpartum female. Digestive Diseases and Sciences *29*:470–474.

Penna F.J. (1979) Blastomycosis of the colon resembling clinically ulcerative colitis. Gut *20*:896–899.

Perarnau J.M., Raabe J.J., Courrier A., Peiffer G., Hennequin J.P., Bene M.C. and Arbogast J. (1982) A rare etiology of ischemic colitis: amyloid colitis. Endoscopy *14*:107–109.

Perzin K.H., Peterson M., Castiglione C.L., Fenoglio C.M. and Wolff M. (1984) Intramucosal carcinoma of the small intestine arising in regional enteritis (Crohn's disease). Cancer *54*:151–162.

Pescatori M., Mattana C. and Castiglioni G.C. (1986) Adult megacolon due to total hypoganglionosis. British Journal of Surgery *73*:765.

Petri M., Poulsen S.S., Christensen K. and Jarnum S. (1982) The incidence of granulomas in serial sections of rectal biopsies from patients with Crohn's disease. Acta Pathologica et Microbiologica Immunologica Scandinavica, Section A *90*:145–147.

Picard E.J., Picard J.J., Jorissen J. and Jardon M. (1978) Heterotopic gastric mucosa in the epiglottis and rectum. American Journal of Digestive Diseases *23*:217–221.

Pieterse A.S., Hecker R. and Rowland R. (1982) Collagenous colitis: a distinctive and potentially reversible disorder. Journal of Clinical Pathology *35*:338–340.

Pieterse A.S., Leong A.S.Y. and Rowland R. (1985) The mucosal changes and pathogenesis of pneumatosis cystoides intestinalis. Human Pathology *16*:683–688.

Pihl E., Peura A., Johnson W.R., McDermott F.T. and Hughes E.R.S. (1985) T-antigen expression by peanut agglutinin staining relates to mucosal dysplasia in ulcerative colitis. Diseases of the Colon and Rectum *28*:11–17.

Pistoia M.A., Guardagni S., Tuscano D., Negro P., Pistoia F. and Carboni M. (1987) Ulcerated ectopic gastric mucosa of the rectum. Gastrointestinal Endoscopy *33*:41–43.

Pittman F.E., El-Hashimi W.K. and Pittman J.C. (1973) Studies of human amebiasis. I. Clinical and laboratory findings in eight cases of acute amebic colitis. Gastroenterology *65*:581–587.

Pittman F.E. and Hennigar G.R. (1974) Sigmoidoscopic and colonic mucosal biopsy findings in amebic colitis. Archives of Pathology *97*:155–158.

Podolsky D.K., Fournier D.A. and Lynch K.E. (1986) Human colonic goblet cells. Journal of Clinical Investigation *77*:1263–1271.

Potzi R., Walgram M., Lochs H., Holzner H. and Gangl A. (1989) Diagnostic significance of endoscopic biopsy in Crohn's disease. Endoscopy *21*:60–62.

Poulsen S.S., Pedersen N.T. and Jarnum S. (1984) "Microerosions" in rectal biopsies in Crohn's disease. Scandinavian Journal of Gastroenterology *19*:607–612.

Powell G.K. (1986) Food protein-induced enterocolitis of infancy: differential diagnosis and management. Comprehensive Therapy *12*:28–37.

Prathap K. and Gilman R. (1970) The histopathology of acute intestinal amebiasis. A rectal biopsy study. American Journal of Pathology *60*:229–246.

Price A.B. (1978) Overlap in the spectrum of non-specific inflammatory bowel disease: "colitis indeterminate." Journal of Clinical Pathology *31*:567–577.

Price A.B. and Davies D.R. (1977) Pseudomembranous colitis. Journal of Clinical Pathology *30*:1–12.

Price A.B., Jewkes J. and Sanderson P.J. (1979) Acute diarrhoea: Campylobacter colitis and the role of rectal biopsy. Journal of Clinical Pathology *32*:990–997.

Price A.B., Larson H.E. and Crow J. (1979) Morphology of experimental antibiotic-associated enterocolitis in the hamster: a model for human pseudomembranous colitis and antibiotic-associated diarrhoea. Gut *20*:467–475.

Quirke P., Campbell I. and Talbot I.C. (1984) Ischaemic proctitis and adventitial fibromuscular dysplasia of the superior rectal artery. British Journal of Surgery *71*:33–38.

Rampton D.S. and Baithun S.I. (1987) Is microscopic colitis due to bile-salt malabsorption? Diseases of the Colon and Rectum *30*:950–952.

Rampton D.S., Salmon P.R. and Clark C.G. (1983) Nonspecific ulcerative colitis as a sequel to amebic dysentery. Journal of Clinical Gastroenterology *5*:217–219.

Ransohoff D.F., Riddell R.H. and Levin B. (1985) Ulcerative colitis and colonic cancer. Diseases of the Colon and Rectum *28*:383–388.

Rapola J., Santavuori P. and Savilahti E. (1984) Suction biopsy of rectal mucosa in the diagnosis of infantile and juvenile types of neuronal ceroid lipofuscinoses. Human Pathology *15*:352–360.

Rask-Madsen J., Grove O., Hansen M.G.J., Bukhave K., Scient C. and Henrik-Nielsen R. (1983) Colonic transport of water and electrolytes in a patient with secretory diarrhea due to collagenous colitis. Digestive Diseases and Sciences *28*:1141–1146.

Read N.W., Krejs G.J., Read M.G., Santa Ana C.A., Morawski S.G. and Fordtran J.S. (1980). Chronic diarrhoea of unknown origin. Gastroenterology *78*:264–271.

Remis R.S., MacDonald K.L., Riley L.W., Puhr N.D., Wells J.G., Davis B.R., Blake P.A. and Cohen M.L. (1984) Sporadic cases of hemorrhagic colitis associated with escherichia coli 0157.H7. Annals of Internal Medicine *101*:624–626.

Remmele W., Beck K. and Kaiserling E. (1988) Multiple lipid islands of the colonic mucosa. A light and electron microscopic study. Pathology, Research and Practice *183*:336–342.

Renton C.J.C. (1972) Non-occlusive intestinal infarction. Clinics in Gastroenterology *1*:655–671.

Rhodes J.M., Cockel R., Allan R.N., Hawker P.C., Dawson J. and Elias E. (1984) Colonic Crohn's disease and use of oral contraception. British Medical Journal *288*:595–596.

Richman P.I., Tilly R., Jass J.R. and Bodmer W.F. (1987) Colonic pericrypt sheath cells: characterisation of cell type with new monoclonal antibody. Journal of Clinical Pathology *40*:593–600.

Riddell R.H. (1976) The precarcinomatous phase of ulcerative colitis (1976). In Current Topics in Pathology: Pathology of the Gastrointestinal Tract. Edited by B.C. Morson. Berlin: Springer-Verlag, p. 179.

Riddell R.H. (1984) Dysplasia and cancer in ulcerative colitis: a soluble problem? Scandinavian Journal of Gastroenterology *19*(Suppl. 104):137–149.

Riddell R.H., Goldman H., Ransohoff D.F., Appelman H.D., Fenoglio C.M., Haggitt R.C., Ahren C., Correa P., Hamilton S.R., Morson B.C., Sommers S.C. and Yardley J.H. (1983) Dysplasia in inflammatory bowel disease: standardized classification with provisional clinical applications. Human Pathology *14*:931–968.

Ritchie J.K., Powell-Tuck J. and Lennard-Jones J.E. (1978) Clinical outcome of the first ten years of ulcerative colitis and proctitis. Lancet *i*:1140–1143.

Robey S.S., Kuhajda F.P. and Yardley J.H. (1988) Immunoperoxidase stains of ganglion cells and abnormal mucosal nerve proliferations in Hirschsprung's disease. Human Pathology *19*:432–437.

Rocca J.M., Hecker R., Pieterse A.S., Rich G.E. and Rowland R. (1984) Clostridium difficile colitis. Australian and New Zealand Journal of Medicine *14*:606–610.

Roche W.R., Beasley R., Williams J.H. and Holgate S.T. (1989) Subepithelial fibrosis in the bronchi of asthmatics. Lancet *i*:520–523.

Rodgers F.G., Rodgers C., Shelton A.P. and Hawkey C.J. (1986) Proposed pathogenic mechanism for the diarrhea associated with human intestinal spirochetes. American Journal of Clinical Pathology *86*:679–682.

Roikjaer O. (1987) Perforation and necrosis of the colon complicating polyarteritis nodosa. Acta Chirurgica Scandinavica *153*:385–386.

Rosekrans P.C.M., Meijer C.J.L.M., van der Wal A.M. and Lindeman J. (1980) Allergic proctitis, a clinical and immunopathological entity. Gut *21*:1017–1023.

Rosen N., Sommer I. and Knobel B. (1985) Intestinal Buerger's disease. Archives of Pathology and Laboratory Medicine *109*:962–963.

Rosenstein E.D., Rickert R.R., Gutkin M., Bacay A. and Kramer N. (1988) Colonic involvement in angioimmunoblastic lymphadenopathy resembling inflammatory bowel disease. Cancer *61*:2244–2250.

Rotterdam H., Korelitz B.I. and Sommers S.C. (1977) Microgranulomas in grossly normal rectal mucosa in Crohn's disease. American Journal of Clinical Pathology *67*:550–554.

Rubio C.A., Johansson C. and Kock Y. (1982) A quantitative method of estimating inflammation in the rectal mucosa. Scandinavian Journal of Gastroenterology *17*:1083–1087.

Rubio C.A., Nylander G., Johansson C. and Slezak P. (1982) Non-dysplastic villous changes in endoscopic biopsies in ulcerative colitis with carcinoma. Acta Pathologica Microbiologica Immuno-logica Scandinavica, Section A. *90*:277–282.

Rudin C., Jenny P., Ohnacker H. and Heitz P.U. (1986) Absence of the enteric nervous system in the newborn: presentation of three patients and review of the literature. Journal of Pediatric Surgery *21*:313–318.

Ruiz-Moreno F. (1963) Amoebic granuloma of the colon and rectum. Diseases of the Colon and Rectum *6*:201.

Ruppin H. and Domschke S. (1984) Acute ulcerative colitis: Rare complication of sulfasalazine therapy. Hepato-gastroenterology *31*:192–193.

Sachar D.B. and Greenstein A.J. (1981) Cancer in ulcerative colitis: good news and bad news. Annals of Internal Medicine *95*:642–644.

Sack R.B. (1981) Escherichia coli and acute diarrheal disease. Annals of Internal Medicine *94*:129–130.

Sale G.E., McDonald G.B., Shulman H.M. and Thomas E.D. (1979) Gastrointestinal graft-versus-host disease in man. American Journal of Surgical Pathology 3:291–299.

Sallon S., Deckelbaum R.J., Schmid I.I., Harlap S., Baras M. and Spira D.T. (1988) Cryptosporidium, malnutrition, and chronic diarrhea in children. American Journal of Diseases of Children 142:312–315.

Samper E.R., Slagle G.W. and Hand A.M. (1984) Colonic endometriosis: its clinical spectrum. Southern Medical Journal 77:912–914.

Sanderson I.R., Boyle S., Williams C.B. and Walker-Smith J.A. (1986) Histological abnormalities in biopsies from macroscopically normal colonoscopies. Archives of Disease in Childhood 61:274–277.

Saul S.H. (1987) Inflammatory cloacogenic polyp: relationship to solitary rectal ulcer syndrome, mucosal prolapse and other bowel disorders. Human Pathology 18:1120–1125.

Saul S.H. and Sollenberger L.C. (1985) Solitary rectal ulcer syndrome. American Journal of Surgical Pathology 9:411–421.

Schaefer H.E. (1988) Multiple lipid islands of the colonic mucosa: a light and electron microscopic study. Pathology, Research and Practice 183:343–346.

Scharli A.F. and Meier-Ruge W. (1981) Localized and disseminated forms of neuronal intestinal dysplasia mimicking Hirschsprung's disease. Journal of Pediatric Surgery 16:164–170.

Scheiman J., Elta G., Colturi T. and Nostrant T. (1988) Colonic xanthomatosis. Relationship to disorder motility and review of the literature. Digestive Diseases and Sciences 33:1491–1494.

Schein M., Veller M. and Decker G.A.G. (1987) Colitis cystica profunda simulating rectal carcinoma. South African Medical Journal 72:289–290.

Schmitz-Moormann P. and Himmelmann G.W. (1988) Does quantitative histology of rectal biopsy improve the differential diagnosis of Crohn's disease and ulcerative colitis in adults? Pathology, Research and Practice 183:481–488.

Schmitz-Moormann P., Pittner P.M., Malchow H. and Brandes J.W. (1984) The granuloma in Crohn's disease. Pathology, Research and Practice 178:467–476.

Schneider R.E. and Dobbins W.O. (1968) Suction biopsy of the rectal mucosa for diagnosis of arteritis in rheumatoid arthritis and related diseases. Annals of Internal Medicine 68:561–568.

Schwachman H. and Antonowicz I. (1962) The sweat test in cystic fibrosis. Annals of the New York Academy of Science 93:600–620

Schwarzenberg S.J. and Whitington P.F. (1983) Rectal gastric mucosa heterotopia as a cause of hematochezia in an infant. Digestive Diseases and Sciences 28:470–472.

Scott B.B., Goodall A., Stephenson P. and Jenkins D. (1983) Rectal mucosal plasma cells in inflammatory bowel disease. Gut 24:519–524.

Segal I., Tim L.O., Hamilton D.G., Lawson H.H., Solomon A., Kalk F. and Cooke S.A.R. (1979) Ritual-enema-induced colitis. Diseases of the Colon and Rectum 22:195–199.

Seldenrijk C.A., Drexhage H.A., Meuwissen S.G.M., Pals S.T. and Meijer C.J.L.M. (1989) Dendritic cells and scavenger macrophages in chronic inflammatory bowel disease. Gut 30:484–491.

Seldenrijk C.A., van der Harten H., Kluck P., Tibboel D., Moorman-Voestermans K. and Meijer C.J.L.M. (1986) Zonal aganglionosis. An enzyme and immuohistochemical study of two cases. Virchows Archiv (A) 410:75–81.

Shamsuddin A.K.M. and Elias E.G. (1981) Rectal mucosa. Malignant and premalignant changes after radiation therapy. Archives of Pathology and Laboratory Medicine 105:150–151.

Shamsuddin A.M., Phelps P.C. and Trump B.F. (1982) Human large intestinal epithelium: light microscopy, histochemistry and ultrastructure. Human Pathology 13:790–803.

Simpson S., Traube J. and Riddell R.H. (1981) The histologic appearance of dysplasia (precarcinomatous change) in Crohn's disease of the small and large intestine. Gastroenterology 81:492–501.

Skinner J.M., Whitehead R. and Piris J. (1971) Argentaffin cells in ulcerative colitis. Gut 12:636–638.

Skirrow M.B. (1977) Campylobacter enteritis: a "new" disease. British Medical Journal 2:9–11.

Sladen G.E. and Filipe M.I. (1984) Is segmental colitis a complication of diverticular disease? Diseases of the Colon and Rectum 27:513–514.

Smith B. (1968) Pre- and postnatal development of the ganglion cells of the rectum and its surgical implications. Journal of Pediatric Surgery 3:386–391.

Smith B. (1972) The Neuropathology of the Alimentary Tract. London, Edward Arnold, p. 80.

Smith B. (1982) The neuropathology of pseudo-obstruction of the intestine. Scandinavian Journal of Gastroenterology 17:103–109.

Smith B.H. and Welter L.H. (1967) Pneumatosis intestinalis. American Journal of Clinical Pathology 48:455–465.

Smith H.R., Rowe B., Gross R.J., Fry N.K. and Scotland S.M. (1987) Haemorrhagic colitis and verocytotoxin-producing escherichia coli in England and Wales. Lancet i:1062–1065.

Smith J.M.B. (1969) Mycoses of the alimentary tract. Gut 10:1035–1040.

Snover D.C., Sandstad J. and Hutton S. (1985) Mucosal pseudolipomatosis of the colon. American Journal of Clinical Pathology 84:575–580.

Sodeman W.A., Jr. and Dowda M.C. (1973) Rapid serological methods for the demonstration of entamoeba histolytica activity. Gastroenterology 65:604–607.

Softley A., Clamp S.E., Watkinson G., Bouchier I.A.D., Myren J. and De Dombal F.T. (1988) The natural history of inflammatory bowel disease: has there been a change in the last 20 years? Scandinavian Journal of Gastroenterology 23(Suppl. 144):20–23.

Sokol R.J., Farrell M.K. and McAdams A.J. (1984) An unusual presentation of Wegener's granulomatosis mimicking inflammatory bowel disease. Gastroenterology 87:426–432.

Soltoft J. (1969) Immunoglobulin-containing cells in normal jejunal mucosa and in ulcerative colitis and regional enteritis. Scandinavian Journal of Gastroenterology 4:353–360.

Soo K.C., Hollinger-Vernea S., Miller G., Pritchard G. and Frawley J. (1983) Buerger's disease of the sigmoid colon. Australian and New Zealand Journal of Surgery 53:111–112.

Spencer G.D., Shulman H.M., Myerson D., Thomas E.D. and McDonald G.B. (1986) Diffuse intestinal ulceration after marrow transplantation. A clinicopathologic study of 13 patients. Human Pathology 17:621–633.

Spotnitz W.D., Van Natta F.C., Bashist B., Wolff M., Green P. and Weber C.J. (1984) Localized ischemic colitis in a young woman with diabetes. Diseases of the Colon and Rectum 27:481–484.

Starling J.R., Croom R.D. and Thomas C.G. (1986) Hirschsprung's disease in young adults. American Journal of Surgery 151:104–109.

Steadman C., Teague C., Kerlin P., Harris O., Hourigan K. and Sampson J. (1987) Collagenous colitis: clinical and histological spectrum in ten patients. Journal of Gastroenterology and Hepatology 2:459–466.

Stenberg B. and Risberg B. (1984) Abdominal aortic aneurysm complicated by rectal necrosis. Acta Chirurgica Scandinavica 150:497–498.

Stevens S. and McClure J. (1982) The histochemical features of the Michaelis-Gutmann body and a consideration of the pathophysiological mechanisms of its formation. Journal of Pathology 137:119–127.

Stolte M. (1988) "Normal" endoscopic findings in the gastrointestinal tract—when should a biopsy be taken? Endoscopy 20:111–113.

Stuart M. (1984) Proctitis cystica profunda: incidence, etiology and treatment. Diseases of the Colon and Rectum 27:153–156.

Stuart R.C., Leahy A.L., Cafferkey M.T. and Stephens R.B. (1986) Yersinia enterocolitica infection and toxic megacolon. British Journal of Surgery 73:590.

Sturm R., Staneck J.L., Stauffer L.R. and Neblett W.W. III (1980) Neonatal necrotizing enterocolitis associated with penicillin-resistant, toxigenic clostridium butyricum. Pediatrics 66:928–931.

Surawicz C.M. and Belic L. (1984) Rectal biopsy helps to distinguish acute self-limited colitis from idiopathic inflammatory bowel disease. Gastroenterology 86:104–113.

Svartz N. and Ernberg T. (1949) Cancer coli in cases of colitis ulcerosa. Acta Medica Scandinavica 135:444.

Svendsen L.B., Sondergaard J.O., Hegnhoj J., Hojgard L., Lauritsen K.B., Bulow S., Horn T. and Danes B.S. (1987) In vitro tetraploidy in patients with ulcerative colitis. Scandinavian Journal of Gastroenterology 22:601–605.

Sviland L., Pearson A.D.J., Eastham E.J., Hamilton P.J., Proctor S.J., Malcolm A.J. and the Newcastle Upon Tyne Bone Marrow Transplant Group. (1988) Histological features of skin and rectal biopsy specimens after autologous and allogeneic bone marrow transplantation. Journal of Clinical Pathology 41:148–154.

Sweeney J.L., Hewett P., Riddell P. and Hoffmann D.C. (1986) Rectal gangrene: a complication of phosphate enema. Medical Journal of Australia 144:374–375.

Symonds J. (1988) Haemorrhagic colitis and Escherichia coli 0157: a pathogen unmasked. British Medical Journal 296:875–876.

Takayanagi K. and Kapila L. (1981) Necrotising enterocolitis in older infants. Archives of Disease in Childhood 56:468–471.

Tam P.K.H. (1986) An immunochemical study with neuron-specific-enolase and substance P of human enteric innervation: the normal developmental pattern and abnormal deviations in Hirschsprung's disease and pyloric stenosis. Journal of Pediatric Surgery 21:227–232.

Tanner A.R. and Raghunath A.S. (1988) Colonic inflammation and nonsteroidal anti-inflammatory drug administration. Digestion 41:116–120.

Taylor-Robinson S., Miles R., Whitehead A. and Dickinson R.J. (1989) Salmonella infection and ulcerative colitis. Lancet i:1145.

Taylor N.S., Thorne G. and Bartlett J.G. (1981) Comparison of two toxins produced by Clostridium difficile. Infection and Immunity 34:1036–1043.

Tedesco F.J., Corless J.K. and Brownstein R.E. (1982) Rectal sparing in antibiotic-associated pseudomembranous colitis: a prospective study. Gastroenterology 83:1259–1260.

Tedesco F.J., Hardin R.D., Harper R.N. and Edwards B.H. (1983) Infectious colitis endoscopically simulating inflammatory bowel disease: a prospective evaluation. Gastrointestinal Endoscopy 29:195–197.

Tedesco F.J., Sumner H.W. and Kassens W.D. Jr. (1976) Colitis cystica profunda. American Journal of Gastroenterology 65:339–343.

Teglbjaerg P.S. and Thaysen E.H. (1982) Collagenous colitis: an ultrastructural study of a case. Gastroenterology 82:561–563.

Teglbjaerg P.S., Thaysen E.H. and Jensen H.H. (1984) Development of collagenous colitis in sequential biopsy specimens. Gastroenterology 87:703–709.

Terner J. and Lattes R. (1963) Malacoplakia of the colon. Federation Proceedings 22, Abstract 2103:512.

Thomas D.F.M., Fernie D.S., Malone M., Bayston R. and Spitz L. (1982) Association between clostridium difficile and enterocolitis in Hirschsprung's disease. Lancet i:78–79

Thomson G., Clark A.H., Hare K. and Spilg W.G.S. (1981) Tea consumption: a cause of constipation. British Medical Journal 282:864–865.

Thorning D. and Howard J.D. (1986) Epithelial denudement in the gastrointestinal tracts of two bone marrow transplant recipients. Human Pathology *17*:560–566.

Tobi M., Kobrin I. and Ariel I. (1982) Rectal involvement in sarcoidosis. Diseases of the Colon and Rectum *25*:491–493.

Tompkins D.S., Waugh M.A. and Cooke E.M. (1981) Isolation of intestinal spirochaetes from homosexuals. Journal of Clinical Pathology *34*:1385–1387.

Toner P.G., Carr K.E. and Wyburn G.M. (1971) The Digestive System: An Ultrastructural Atlas and Review. London: Butterworths, p. 114.

Tribe C.R., Scott D.G.I. and Bacon P.A. (1981) Rectal biopsy in the diagnosis of systemic vasculitis. Journal of Clinical Pathology *34*:843–850.

Trigg P.H., Belin R., Haberkorn S., Long W.J., Nixon H.H., Plaschkes J., Spitz L. and Willital G.H. (1974) Experience with a cholinesterase histochemical technique for rectal suction biopsies in the diagnosis of Hirschsprung's disease. Journal of Clinical Pathology *27*:207–213.

Vajrabukka T., Dhitavat A., Kichananta B., Sukonthamand Y., Tanphiphat C. and Vongviriyatham S. (1979) Fulminating ameobic colitis: a clinical evaluation. British Journal of Surgery *66*:630–632.

Van Spreeuwel J.P., Duursma G.C., Meijer C.J.L.M., Bax R., Rosekrans P.C.M. and Lindeman J. (1985) Campylobacter colitis: histological, immunohistochemical and ultrastructural findings. Gut *26*:945–951.

Vantrappen G., Ponette E., Geboes K. and Bertrand P. (1977) Yersinia enteritis and enterocolitis. Gastroenterological aspects. Gastroenterology *72*:220–227.

Vatn M.H., Elgjo K., and Bergan A. (1984) Distribution of dysplasia in ulcerative colitis. Scandinavian Journal of Gastroenterology *19*:893–895.

Vernon S.E. (1982) Amyloid colitis. Diseases of the Colon and Rectum *25*:728–730.

Vinores S.A. and May E. (1985) Neuron-specific enolase as an immunohistochemical tool for the diagnosis of Hirschsprung's disease. American Journal of Surgical Pathology *9*:281–285.

Walker N.I., Bennett R.E. and Axelsen R.A. (1988) Melanosis coli. A consequence of anthraquinone-induced apoptosis of colonic epithelial cells. American Journal of Pathology *131*:465–476.

Wang K.K., Perrault J., Carpenter H.A., Schroeder K.W. and Tremaine W.J. (1987) Collagenous colitis: a clinicopathologic correlation. Mayo Clinic Proceedings *62*:665–671.

Ward M. and Webb J.N. (1977) Rectal biopsy as a prognostic guide in Crohn's colitis. Journal of Clinical Pathology *30*:126–131.

Watson A.J. and Roy A.D. (1960) Paneth cells in the large intestine in ulcerative colitis. Journal of Pathology and Bacteriology *80*:309–316.

Wayte D.M. and Helwig E.B. (1967) Colitis cystica profunda. American Journal of Clinical Pathology *48*:159–169.

Weedon D.D., Shorter R.G., Ilstrup D.M., Huizenga K.A. and Taylor W.F. (1973) Crohn's disease and cancer. New England Journal of Medicine *289*:1099–1103.

Weitzner S. (1983) Ectopic salivary gland tissue in submucosa of rectum. Diseases of the Colon and Rectum *26*:814–817.

Welling R.E., Roedersheimer L.R., Arbaugh J.J. and Cranley J.J. (1985) Ischemic colitis following repair of ruptured abdominal aortic aneurysm. Archives of Surgery *120*:1368–1370.

Werlin S.L., Chusid M.J., Caya J. and Oechler H.W. (1982) Colitis in chronic granulomatous disease. Gastroenterology *82*:328–331.

White C.L., Hamilton S.R., Diamond M.P. and Cameron J.L. (1983) Crohn's disease and ulcerative colitis in the same patient. Gut *24*:857–862.

White W.B., Hanna M., Stewart J.A. (1984) Systemic herpes simplex virus Type 2 infection. Proctitis, urinary retention, arthralgias, and meningitis in the absence of primary mucocutaneous lesions. Archives of Internal Medicine *144*:826–827.

Whitehead R. (1971) Ischaemic enterocolitis: an expression of the intravascular coagulation syndrome. Gut *12*:912–917.

Whitehead R. (1972) The pathology of intestinal ischaemia. Clinics in Gastroenterology *1*:613–637.

Whitehead R. (1976) The pathology of ischaemia of the intestines. In Pathology Annual. Edited by S.C. Sommers, pp. 1–52.

Whitehead R. (1987) Extra-intestinal Crohn's disease: Does it exist? In: Surgery of Inflammatory Bowel Disease. Clinical Surgery International, Volume 14. Edited by E.C.G. Lee and D.J. Nolan. London: Churchill Livingstone, pp 197–201.

Wig J.D., Talwar B.L. and Bushnurmath S.R. (1981) Toxic dilatation complicating fulminant amoebic colitis. British Journal of Surgery *68*:135–136.

Willoughby C.P., Piris J. and Truelove S.C. (1979) Tissue eosinophils in ulcerative colitis. Scandinavian Journal of Gastroenterology *14*:395–399.

Wilson R. and Qualheim R.E. (1954) A form of acute hemorrhagic colitis affecting chronically ill individuals. Gastroenterology *27*:431–444.

Womack C. (1984) Unusual histological appearances of barium sulphate: a case report with scanning electron microscopy and energy dispersive X ray analysis. Journal of Clinical Pathology *37*:488–493.

Womack N.R., Williams N.S., Holmfield J.H.M. and Morrison J.F.B. (1987) Pressure and prolapse: the cause of solitary rectal ulceration. Gut *28*:1228–1233.

Wood M.K., Read D.R., Kraft A.R. and Barreta T.M. (1979) A rare cause of ischemic colitis: polyarteritis nodosa. Diseases of the Colon and Rectum *22*:428–433.

Wright A.W. (1930) Local effect of injection of gases into the subcutaneous tissues. American Journal of Pathology *6*:87–124.

Yamano T., Shimada M., Okada S., Yutaka T., Kato T. and Yabuucki H. (1982) Ultrastructural study of biopsy specimens of rectal mucosa. Archives of Pathology and Laboratory Medicine 106:673–677.

Yardley J.H., Ransohoff D.F., Riddell R.H. and Goldman H. (1983) Cancer in inflammatory bowel disease: how serious is the problem and what should be done about it? (Editorial) Gastroenterology 85:197–200.

Yashiro K., Murakami Y., Iizuka B., Hasegawa K., Nagasako K. and Yamada A. (1985) Localized colitis cystica profunda of the sigmoid colon. Endoscopy 17:198–199.

Yeager A.M., Kanof M.E., Kramer S.S., Jones B., Saral R., Lake A.M. and Santos G.W. (1987) Pneumatosis intestinalis in children after allogeneic bone marrow transplantation. Pediatric Radiology 17:18–22.

Yeoh E.K. and Horowitz M. (1987) Radiation enteritis. Surgery, Gynaecology and Obstetrics 165:373–379.

Yunis E.J., Dibbins A.W. and Sherman F.E. (1976) Rectal suction biopsy in the diagnosis of Hirschsprung disease in infants. Archives of Pathology and Laboratory Medicine 100:329–333.

Zern R.T. and Clarke-Pearson D.L. (1985) Pneumatosis intestinalis associated with enteral feeding by catheter jejunostomy. Obstetrics and Gynecology 65:81S–83S.

Ziegler H.W., Heitz Ph.U., Kasper M., Spichtin H-P. and Ulrich J. (1984) Aganglionosis of the colon. Morphologic investigations in 524 patients. Pathology, Research and Practice 178:543–547.

Zucker-Franklin D. and Franklin E.C. (1970) Intracellular localization of human amyloid by fluorescence and electron microscopy. American Journal of Pathology 59:23–41.

Zucker-Franklin D., Pras M. and Franklin E.C. (1969) Studies on human amyloid. Journal of Clinical Investigation 48:93–94.

V

Human Immunodeficiency Virus Infection and Mucosal Biopsy

19

THE ACQUIRED IMMUNODEFICIENCY SYNDROME, OESOPHAGEAL AND GASTROINTESTINAL MANIFESTATIONS

In the late seventies and early eighties it was realised that an increasing range of gastroenterological conditions were being described in the homosexual population. Thus it was that these became collectively known as the "Gay Bowel Syndrome" (Kazal et al 1976), which was arguably bad terminology for a list of different disease states. Following the identification of the human immunodeficiency virus (HIV) and its association with the acquired immunodeficiency syndrome (AIDS), the pathological processes underlying these conditions are now better understood and it is now recognised that AIDS is not confined to the homosexual population. Some 50 per cent of AIDS victims will have gastroenterological clinical presentations, and virtually 100 per cent develop gut lesions during the course of their disease. For ease of description they are best considered on a regional basis but often more than one region of the gastrointestinal tract will be involved by the same pathological process. There are several review articles concerning the gastrointestinal tract and AIDS, several of which detail the various biopsy appearances (Weller 1985, Surawicz et al 1986, Boylston et al 1987, Stamm and Grant 1988, Gazzard 1988).

AIDS AND THE OESOPHAGUS

The commonest manifestation is oesophageal candidiasis, which may or may not be symptomatic. Candidiasis is the second most common infection in AIDS patients (Macher 1984). Cytomegaloviral (CMV) infection is the most common and can also cause oesophageal ulceration, as can herpes simplex virus (HSV) (Agha, Lee and Nostrant et al 1986). Rabeneck et al (1986) describe oesophageal ulceration, which by light microscopy was non-specific but at electron microscopy showed viral particles consistent with the morphology of a retrovirus and quite different from CMV or HSV. There is some evidence from studies in other immunocompromised patients (Walsh, Belitsos and Hamilton 1986) that bacterial oesophagitis is more common than has been recognised in the past in such patients. Involvement of the oesophagus by *Pneumocystis carinii* organisms (Grimes et al 1987) and by histoplasmosis (Cappell et al 1988) has also been described.

Other oesophageal lesions in AIDS patients include Kaposi's sarcoma (Friedman, Wright and Altman 1985) and malignant lymphoma (Bernal and del Junco 1986).

AIDS AND THE STOMACH

In addition to the conditions listed for the oesophagus, other unusual lesions described in the stomach include phlegmonous gastritis (Mittleman and Suarez 1985) and invasion of the mucosa by *Campylobacter pylori* (Meiselman et al 1988). The latter organism and its relationship to gastritis and peptic ulcer was discussed earlier when it was noted that normally it is seen in the superficial mucus layer and is non-invasive.

AIDS AND THE SMALL INTESTINE

Diarrhoea of small bowel origin is a frequent symptom in AIDS, and endoscopic biopsies often contribute to identifying the cause. Sometimes abnormalities at light microscopy are minimal, and a firm diagnosis can be reached only by electron microscopy. Such is the case with infection by some protozoa, of which *Cryptosporidia* is the commonest (Chiampi et al 1983, Current et al 1983, Guarda et al 1983, Ma and Soave 1983, Pitlik et al 1983, Cohen et al 1984, Gerstoft et al 1984). The identification of *Microsporidia* and *Isospora belli* as well as *Cryptosporidium* species is also described in AIDS patients with diarrhoea and malabsorption whose small-bowel mucosa was morphologically only minimally abnormal by light microscopy (Modigliani et al 1985, Forthal and Guest 1984, Dobbins and Weinstein 1985, Curry et al 1988). The biopsies showed only partial villous atrophy and a mild inflammation of the lamina propria. Developmental stages of *Microsporidia* and *Isospora* were visible in Giemsa-stained sections, actually within the enterocytes, while the *Cryptosporidia* were seen typically attached to the brush border. In a significant number of cases similar small-intestinal inflammation and villous abnormality are associated with diarrhoea without the recognition of an infective agent. It is possible that patients with AIDS are predisposed to as yet unidentified enteric pathogens (Gillin et al 1983). On the other hand, damage to the small-bowel mucosa has been ascribed to the HIV infection itself and compared to graft-versus-host disease (Batman et al 1989).

A Whipple-like small-bowel lesion due to infection with *Mycobacterium avium–intracellulare* is also described (Gillin et al 1983, Strom and Gruninger 1983, Kooijman and Poen 1984, Roth et al 1985). The histiocytes that occupy the bloated villi, in addition to being PAS positive, are seen to contain large numbers of Ziehl-Neelsen–positive tubercle bacilli.

Although *Pneumocystis carinii* infection usually involves the lungs in AIDS patients it is occasionally described in the small intestine (Carter et al 1988). Confluent lakes of eosinophilic foamy material in vessels and submucosa occur and in them cysts and trophozoites can be demonstrated.

AIDS AND THE COLORECTUM

Ano-rectal infections in homosexual males have been studied in depth both at sigmoidoscopy and by rectal biopsy (Quinn et al 1981, McMillan and Lee 1981, Goodell et al 1983), and there can be no doubt that they can mimic both ulcerative colitis and Crohn's disease grossly and microscopically. Although in the majority of cases the histological lesions will mimic ulcerative colitis, as does infective colitis acquired by usual routes, in chlamydial proctitis and in syphilis, the presence of granulomata or giant cells will introduce the possibility of Crohn's disease (Geller, Zimmerman and Cohen 1980, Quinn et al 1982).

The polymicrobial origin of colorectal infections in homosexual men is now well recognised (Quinn et al 1983). Acute proctitis due to gonococci and meningococci has been described in biopsy specimens (McMillan et al 1983a). Similar appearances are produced by *Campylobacter jejuni* and other *Campylobacter*-like organisms (Quinn et al 1984). Proctocolitis has also been ascribed to *Chlamydia, Salmonella, Shigella* species, *Treponema*, and *Aeromonas hydrophila*, in addition to amoebae (Quinn et al 1982, 1983, Klotz et al 1983, Mindel 1983, Owen 1986, Roberts, Parenti and Albert 1987, Antony et al 1988, Smith et al 1988, Connolly et al 1989). A colitis grossly resembling Crohn's disease due to tuberculosis may occur (Lax et al 1988), and rectal leishmaniasis is described (Rosenthal et al 1988). Herpes simplex virus (Guttman et al 1983, McMillan et al 1983b), and cytomegalovirus (Meiselman, Cello and Margaretten 1985) frequently cause a proctitis or a colitis, and in cytomegalovirus colitis it can be so severe as to cause toxic dilatation (Rene et al 1988). The inflamed mucosa may be ulcerated but has a non-specific appearance in herpes proctocolitis, although Guttman et al (1983) described ground-glass nuclei in endothelial and stromal cells. Likewise in cytomegalovirus colitis typical intranuclear inclusions are seen. As in the small intestine, *Mycobacterium avium–intracellulare* infection can occur and present as an ulcerating inflammation with typical histiocytes occupying the mucosa (Wolke et al 1984). Similarly, cryptosporidiosis occurs and occasionally causes toxic dilatation (Connolly and Gazzard 1987).

An interesting phenomenon is that described by James (1988), who reported a patient with an 18-year history of Crohn's disease of the colon, whose disease remitted completely on contracting AIDS. This suggests that CD4 T lymphocytes play a role in the pathogenesis of Crohn's disease. There are several studies describing an increase in the incidence of colorectal spirochaetosis in homosexuals (Surawicz et al 1987), but there is as yet no firm evidence that even in AIDS patients the organism is a confirmed pathogen.

Homosexuals are also known to show lymphoid hyperplasia of the rectal mucosa, and in AIDS patients follicular dendritic cell processes are shortened and fragmented (Bishop, McMillan and Gilmour 1987). In an electron microscopy biopsy study, intraepithelial lymphocytes in AIDS patients appear activated in that they possess more than the usual number of lysosomes and surface projections. It is postulated that it is these cells that play a role in the autoimmune injury of the intestinal mucosa that has been proposed in AIDS patients (Weber and Dobbins 1986). Kaposi's sarcoma can affect the whole of the gastrointestinal tract, including the colon in AIDS patients (Friedman, Wright and Altman 1985). There is also an increased incidence of other malignancy, including lymphoma (Ziegler et al 1984, Ioachim and Cooper 1986).

Finally, there is every possibility that even in the absence of a microbiological cause, a low-grade proctitis with or without superficial ulcers may result in passive homosexuals as the result of trauma or the use of enemas and lubricants.

AIDS AND THE ANAL CANAL

Homosexual men and AIDS patients are at high risk for anal condyloma, epithelial dysplasia and anal carcinoma (Sohn and Robilotti 1977, Gottlieb et al 1981, Nash, Allen and Nash 1986, Schofield, Lindley and Harcourt-Webster 1989). Using an immunohistochemical method Gal, Meyer and Taylor (1987) have shown a high incidence of human papilloma virus in the lesions.

REFERENCES—SECTION V
HUMAN IMMUNODEFICIENCY
VIRUS INFECTION AND
MUCOSAL BIOPSY

Agha F.P., Lee H.H. and Nostrant T.T. (1986) Herpetic esophagitis: a diagnostic challenge in immunocompromised patients. American Journal of Gastroenterology *81*:246–253.

Antony M.A., Brandt L.J., Klein R.S. and Bernstein L.H. (1988) Infectious diarrhea in patients with AIDS. Digestive Diseases and Sciences *33*:1141–1146.

Batman P.A., Miller A.R.O., Forster S.M., Harris J.R.W., Pinching A.J., and Griffin G.E. (1989) Jejunal enteropathy associated with human immunodeficiency virus infection: quantitative histology. Journal of Clinical Pathology *42*:275–281.

Bernal A. and del Junco G.W. (1986) Endoscopic and pathologic features of esophageal lymphoma: a report of four cases in patients with acquired immune deficiency syndrome. Gastrointestinal Endoscopy *32*:96–99.

Bishop P.E., McMillan A. and Gilmour H.M. (1987) A histological and immunocytochemical study of lymphoid tissue in rectal biopsies from homosexual men. Histopathology *11*:1133–1147.

Boylston A.W., Cook H.T., Francis N.D. and Goldin R.D. (1987) Biopsy pathology of acquired immune deficiency syndrome (AIDS). Journal of Clinical Pathology *40*:1–8.

Cappell M.S., Mandell W., Grimes M.M. and Neu H.C. (1988) Gastrointestinal histoplasmosis. Digestive Diseases and Sciences *33*:353–360.

Carter T.R., Cooper P.H., Petri W.A., Kim C.K., Walzer P.D. and Guerrant R.L. (1988) Pneumocystis carinii infection of the small intestine in a patient with acquired immune deficiency syndrome. American Journal of Clinical Pathology *89*:679–683.

Chiampi N.P., Sundberg R.D., Klompus J.P. and Wilson A.J. (1983) Cryptosporidial enteritis and pneumocystis pneumonia in a homosexual man. Human Pathology *14*:734–737.

Cohen J.D., Ruhlig L., Jayich S.A., Tong M.J., Lechago J. and Snape W.J. (1984) Cryptosporidium in acquired immunodeficiency syndrome. Digestive Diseases and Sciences *29*:773–777.

Connolly G.M. and Gazzard B.G. (1987) Toxic megacolon in cryptosporidiosis. Postgraduate Medical Journal *63*:1103–1104.

Connolly G.M., Shanson D., Hawkins D.A., Webster J.N.H. and Gazzard B.G. (1989) Non-cryptosporidial diarrhoea in human immunodeficiency virus (HIV) infected patients. Gut *30*:195–200.

Current W.L., Reese N.C., Ernst J.V., Bailey W.S., Heyman M.B. and Weinstein W.M. (1983) Human cryptosporidiosis in immunocompetent and immunodeficient persons. New England Journal of Medicine *308*:1252–1257.

Curry A., McWilliam L.J., Haboubi N.Y. and Mandal B.K. (1988) Microsporidiosis in a British patient with AIDS. Journal of Clinical Pathology *41*:477–478.

Dobbins W.O. and Weinstein W.M. (1985) Electron microscopy of the intestine and rectum in acquired immunodeficiency syndrome. Gastroenterology *88*:738–749.

Forthal D.N. and Guest S.S. (1984) Isospora belli enteritis in three homosexual men. American Journal of Tropical Medicine and Hygiene *33*:1060–1064.

Friedman S.L., Wright T.L. and Altman D.F. (1985) Gastrointestinal Kaposi's sarcoma in patients with acquired immunodeficiency syndrome. Gastroenterology *89*:102–108.

Gal A.A., Meyer P.R. and Taylor C.R. (1987) Papillomavirus antigens in anorectal condyloma and carcinoma in homosexual men. Journal of the American Medical Association *257*:337–340.

Gazzard B.G. (1988) HIV disease and the gastroenterologist. Gut *29*:1497–1505.

Geller S.A., Zimmerman M.J. and Cohen A. (1980) Rectal biopsy in early lymphogranuloma venereum proctitis. American Journal of Gastroenterology *74*:433–435.

Gerstoft J., Holten-Andersen W., Blom J., Nielsen J.O. (1984) Cryptosporidium enterocolitis in homosexual men with AIDS. Scandinavian Journal of Infectious Diseases *16*:385–388.

Gillin J.S., Urmacher C., West R. and Shike M. (1983) Disseminated Mycobacterium avium intracellulare infection in acquired immunodeficiency syndrome mimicking Whipple's disease. Gastroenterology *85*:1187–1191.

Goodell S.E., Quinn T.C., Mkrtichian E., Schuffler M.D., Holmes K.K. and Corey L. (1983) Herpes simplex virus proctitis in homosexual men. Clinical, sigmoidoscopic, and histopathological features. New England Journal of Medicine *308*:868–871.

Gottlieb M.S., Schroff R., Schanker H.M., Weisman J.D., Fan P.T., Wolf R.A. and Saxon A. (1981) Pneumocystis carinii pneumonia and mucosal candidiasis in previously healthy homosexual men: evidence of a new acquired cellular immunodeficiency. New England Journal of Medicine *305*:1425–1431.

Grimes M.M., LaPook J.D., Bar M.H., Wasserman H.S. and Dwork A. (1987) Disseminated pneumocystis carinii infection in a patient with acquired immunodeficiency syndrome. Human Pathology *18*:307–308.

Guarda L.A., Stein S.A., Cleary K.A. and Ordonez N.G. (1983) Human cryptosporidiosis in the acquired immune deficiency syndrome. Archives of Pathology and Laboratory Medicine *107*:562–566.

Guttman D., Raymond A., Gelb A., Ehya H., Mather U., Mildvan D. and Spigland I. (1983) Virus-associated colitis in homosexual men: two case reports. American Journal of Gastroenterology 78:167–169.

Ioachim H.L. and Cooper M.C. (1986) Lymphomas of AIDS. Lancet *i*:96–97.

James S.P. (1988) Remission of Crohn's disease after human immunodeficiency virus infection. Gastroenterology 95:1667–1669.

Kazal H.L., Sohn N., Carrasco J.I., Robilotti J.G. and Delaney W.E. (1976) The gay bowel syndrome: clinico-pathologic correlation in 260 cases. Annals of Clinical Laboratory Science 6:184–192.

Klotz S.A., Drutz D.J., Tam M.R. and Reed K.H. (1983) Hemorrhagic proctitis due to lymphogranu-loma venereum serogroup L2. New England Journal of Medicine 308:1563–1565.

Kooijman C.D. and Poen H. (1984) Whipple-like disease in AIDS. Histopathology 8:705–707.

Lax J.D., Haroutiounian G., Attia A., Rodriguez R., Thayaparan R. and Bashist B. (1988) Tuberculosis of the rectum in a patient with acquired immune deficiency syndrome. Diseases of the Colon and Rectum 31:394–397.

McMillan A. and Lee F.D. (1981) Sigmoidoscopic and microscopic appearance of the rectal mucosa in homosexual men. Gut 22:1035–1041.

McMillan A., Gilmour H.M., Slatford K. and McNeillage G.J.C. (1983a) Proctitis in homosexual men. British Journal of Venereal Diseases 59:260–264.

McMillan A., McNeillage G., Gilmour H.M. and Lee F.D. (1983b) Histology of rectal gonorrhoea in men, with a note on anorectal infection with Neisseria meningitidis. Journal of Clinical Pathology 36:511–514.

Ma P. and Soave R. (1983) Three-step stool examination for cryptosporidiosis in 10 homosexual men with protracted watery diarrhea. Journal of Infectious Diseases 147:824–828.

Macher A.M. (1984) Acquired immunodeficiency syndrome: epidemiologic, clinical, immunologic and therapeutic considerations. Annals of Internal Medicine 100:92–106.

Meiselman M.S., Cello J.P. and Margaretten W. (1985) Cytomegalovirus colitis. Report of the clinical, endoscopic and pathologic findings in two patients with the acquired immune deficiency syndrome. Gastroenterology 88:171–175.

Meiselman M.S., Miller-Catchpole R., Christ M. and Randall E. (1988) Campylobacter pylori gastritis in the acquired immunodeficiency syndrome. Gastroenterology 95:209–212.

Mindel A. (1983) Lymphogranuloma venereum of the rectum in a homosexual man. British Journal of Venereal Diseases 59:196–197.

Mittleman R.E. and Suarez R.V. (1985) Phlegmonous gastritis associated with the acquired immuno-deficiency syndrome/preacquired immunodeficiency syndrome. Archives of Pathology and Labora-tory Medicine 109:765–767.

Modigliani R., Bories C., Le Charpentier Y., Salmeron M., Messing B., Galian A., Ramboud J.C., Lavergne A., Cochand-Priollet B. and Desportes I. (1985) Diarrhoea and malabsorption in acquired immune deficiency syndrome: a study of four cases with special emphasis on opportunistic protozoan infestations. Gut 26:179–187.

Nash G., Allen W. and Nash S. (1986) Atypical lesions of the anal mucosa in homosexual men. Journal of the American Medical Association 256:873–876.

Owen R.L. (1986) Role of biopsy in diagnosis of rectal infections. Gastroenterology 91:770–772.

Pitlik S.D., Fainstein V., Garza D., Guarda L., Bolivar R., Rios A., Hopfer R.L. and Mansell P.A. (1983) Human cryptosporidiosis: spectrum of disease. Archives of Internal Medicine 143:2269–2275.

Quinn T.C., Corey L., Chaffee R.G., Schuffler M.D. Brancato F.P. and Holmes K.K. (1981) The etiology of anorectal infections in homosexual men. American Journal of Medicine 71:395–406.

Quinn T.C., Goodell S.E., Fennell C., Wang S-P., Schuffler M.D., Holmes K.K. and Stamm W.E. (1984) Infections with campylobacter jejuni and campylobacter-like organisms in homosexual men. Annals of Internal Medicine 101:187–192.

Quinn T.C., Goodell S.E., Mkrtichian E., Schuffler M.D., Wang S-P., Stamm W.E. and Holmes K.K. (1981) Chlamydia trachomatis proctitis. New England Journal of Medicine 305:195–200.

Quinn T.C., Lukehart S.A., Goodell S., Mkrtichian E., Schuffler M.D. and Holmes K.K. (1982) Rectal mass caused by treponema pallidum: confirmation by immunofluorescent staining. Gastroenterology 82:135–139.

Quinn T.C., Stamm W.E., Goodell S.E., Mkrtichian E., Benedetti J., Corey L., Schuffler M.D. and Holmes K.K. (1983) The polymicrobial origin of intestinal infections in homosexual men. New England Journal of Medicine 309:576–582.

Rabeneck L., Boyko W.J., McLean D.M., McLeod W.A. and Wong K.K. (1986) Unusual esophageal ulcers containing enveloped viruslike particles in homosexual men. Gastroenterology 90:1882–1889.

Rene E., Marche C., Chevalier T., Rouzioux C., Regnier B., Saimot A.G., Negesse Y., Matheron S., Leport C., Wolff B., Moriniere B., Katlama C., Godeberge B., Vittecoq B., Bricaire F., Brun-Vesinet C., Pangon B., Deluol A.M., Coulaud J.P., Modai J., Frottier J., Vilde J.L., Vachon F., Mignon M. and Bonfils S. (1988) Cytomegalovirus colitis in patients with acquired immunodeficiency syndrome. Digestive Diseases and Sciences 33:741–750.

Roberts I.M., Parenti D.M. and Albert M.B. (1987) Aeromonas hydrophilia: associated colitis in a male homosexual. Archives of Internal Medicine 147:1502–1503.

Rosenthal P.J., Chaisson R.E., Hadley W.K. and Leech J.H. (1988) Rectal leishmaniasis in a patient with acquired immunodeficiency syndrome. American Journal of Medicine 84:307–309.

Roth R.I., Owen R.L., Keren D.F. and Volberding P.A. (1985) Intestinal infection with mycobacterium avium in acquired immune deficiency syndrome (AIDS). Histological and clinical comparison with Whipple's disease. Digestive Diseases and Sciences *30*:497–504.

Schofield J.B., Lindley R.P. and Harcourt-Webster J.N. (1989) Biopsy pathology of HIV infection: experience at St Stephen's Hospital, London. Histopathology *14*:277–288.

Smith P.D., Lane H.C., Gill V.J., Manischewitz J.F., Quinnan G.V., Fauci A.S. and Masur H. (1988) Intestinal infections in patients with the acquired immunodeficiency syndrome (AIDS). Annals of Internal Medicine *108*:328–333.

Sohn N. and Robilotti J.G. (1977) The gay bowel syndrome. A review of colonic and rectal conditions in 200 male homosexuals. American Journal of Gastroenterology *67*:478–484.

Stamm B. and Grant J.W. (1988) Biopsy pathology of the gastrointestinal tract in human immunodeficiency virus-associated disease: a 5 year experience in Zurich. Histopathology *13*:531–540.

Strom R.L. and Gruninger R.P. (1983) AIDS with Mycobacterium avium intracellulare lesions resembling those of Whipple's disease. New England Journal of Medicine *309*:1323–1334.

Surawicz C.M., Goodell S.E., Quinn T.C., Roberts P.L., Corey L., Holmes K.K., Schuffler M.D. and Stamm W.E. (1986) Spectrum of rectal biopsy abnormalities in homosexual men with intestinal symptoms. Gastroenterology *91*:651–659.

Surawicz C.M., Roberts P.L., Rompalo A., Quinn T.C., Holmes K.K. and Stamm W.E. (1987) Intestinal spirochetosis in homosexual men. American Journal of Medicine *82*:587–592.

Walsh T.J., Belitsos N.J. and Hamilton S.R. (1986) Bacterial esophagitis in immunocompromised patients. Archives of Internal Medicine *146*:1345–1348.

Weber J.R. and Dobbins W.O. (1986) The intestinal and rectal epithelial lymphocyte in AIDS. American Journal of Surgical Pathology *10*:627–639.

Weller I.V.D. (1985) AIDS and the gut. Scandinavian Journal of Gastroenterology *20*(suppl. 114):77–89.

Wolke A., Meyers S., Adelsberg B.R., Bottone E.J., Damsker B., Schwartz I.S. and Janowitz H.D. (1984) Mycobacterium avium-intracellulare-associated colitis in a patient with the acquired immunodeficiency syndrome. Journal of Clinical Gastroenterology *6*:225–229.

Ziegler J.L., Beckstead J.A., Volberding P.A., Abrams D.I., Levine A.M. and Lukes R.J. et al (1984) Non-Hodgkin's lymphoma in 90 homosexual men: relationship to generalized lymphadenopathy and acquired immunodeficiency syndrome (AIDS). New England Journal of Medicine *311*:565–570.

Index

Note: Page numbers in *italics* refer to illustrations; page numbers followed by t refer to tables.